Scot

MW01528229

Differential Diagnosis for the Dermatologist

Second Edition

Springer

Scott M. Jackson, M.D.
Health Sciences Center
Dermatology
Louisiana State University
Baton Rouge, LA
USA

Lee T. Nesbitt Jr., M.D.
Health Sciences Center
Dermatology
Louisiana State University
New Orleans, LA
USA

ISBN 978-3-642-28005-4   ISBN 978-3-642-28006-1 (eBook)
DOI 10.1007/978-3-642-28006-1
Springer Heidelberg New York Dordrecht London

Library of Congress Control Number: 2012936977

Printed on acid-free paper

Springer is part of Springer Science+Business Media (www.springer.com)

Preface to the Second Edition

It is with great pleasure that I introduce the second edition of *Differential Diagnosis for the Dermatologist*. My goal with this book has been to create a quick and easily accessible source of information for practicing dermatologists. My dream is that this book will be placed in the work area and will be used "on the go" for a rapid source of information about the differential diagnosis of a given skin problem.

I had always wished for the text to have a section for treatment options but the task of compiling treatment options as well as compiling the differential diagnoses proved to be too daunting for me in the first edition. However, with this second edition, my efforts were focused in part to bring treatment options to the fingertips of the dermatologist. For all commonly treated skin diseases and skin lesions, the reader can find a list of the treatment options. While they are listed in no particular order, the first-line and most reliable treatments are underlined. Treatment options for genetic skin diseases and diseases that are treated by nondermatologists are not given.

The reader will also find several other changes in the second edition. There are 50 new photographs in the text, and there are 25 new diagnoses or entry headings. Many of the references have been updated to provide a more current supporting literature for the text. The last major change in the book involves the use of underlining to indicate to the reader the skin diseases that more closely simulate the heading diagnosis. In addition, the associations that are most commonly identified with a given diagnosis are underlined as well.

It is my sincere hope that dermatologists will find this information useful in their daily practice.

Scott M. Jackson, M.D.

Preface I to the First Edition

This book originated as a small reference manual that I created to serve as an educational supplement for the dermatology residents at Louisiana State University Health Sciences Center. Deeming the compiled information to be useful for all dermatologists, I decided to expand the text and publish it. Every major category of the patient evaluation, from the chief complaint to the diagnosis, is addressed with regard to the dermatological differential diagnosis.

The establishment of a precise differential diagnosis for a given cutaneous problem is the fundamental challenge that the dermatologist faces with every patient. This unique exercise is very intellectual; in a short period of time, the clinician must select from a list of perhaps several hundred diseases a few possibilities that match the clinical presentation. This is performed while also negotiating the patient interaction, examining the patient, and beginning to formulate a plan of action. Proficiency in the formulation of a differential diagnosis that is brief and simultaneously thorough allows for consideration of all possibilities, proper evaluation, and, hopefully, rapid diagnosis. We hope to provide the target readers (dermatologists and dermatologists in training) with some assistance in carrying out this frequently complicated task. For the confrontation with an atypical presentation of a common disease or the classic presentation of an uncommon disease, the reader will hopefully find this book very useful.

The dermatologist may move toward the diagnosis of a particular cutaneous presentation with a morphology-driven approach and/or a diagnosis-driven approach. Classically, the dermatologist is trained to first recognize the morphology of the disease and then ponder all of the causes of that type of lesion. For example, if a patient presents with a papulosquamous eruption, then several diagnoses are suggested on the basis of morphology alone. While morphology of lesions is essential, distribution, patient demographics, and associated features are left out in this approach. On the other hand, a diagnosis-driven approach is also advantageous and possibly more inclusive and yet still specific. With the exhaustive section organized by dermatologic diagnosis, we believe this text will help clinicians formulate a diagnosis-driven approach to the differential diagnosis. For example, if a patient presents with a rash that resembles a certain dermatosis (e.g., pityriasis rosea), the clinician now has quick access to the differential diagnosis of that dermatosis (and any subtypes or variants) so that all alternative diagnoses are considered, not just diagnoses that share morphology. While recognition and appreciation of morphology is still critical, a diagnosis-based approach to the differential diagnosis is sometimes also helpful when faced with a diagnostic dilemma. In addition, the book provides supporting information for each diagnosis, including recommended evaluative studies, diagnostic criteria, and a source article to reference.

Although inclusiveness was a primary goal of the project, we are aware of the limitations of this text. It was a difficult task to decide which of the many diagnoses in the dermatologic literature to include in the large chapter on diagnosis. There is a tremendous amount of controversy surrounding the existence of many diagnoses, and we were forced to take a position on the controversies when including or excluding certain diseases. An effort was made to exclude diseases that have not been described in over 20 years. We also wanted to include many of the more recently described diagnoses from the past 2 years. It was also difficult to generate the lists under each diagnosis with an acceptable level of sensitivity and specificity. We felt that erring on the side of too many diagnoses was more acceptable than missing a potential important diagnostic alternative. We welcome any criticisms or suggestions that would improve the sensitivity and specificity of the lists for future editions.

We sincerely hope that you find this text useful in your training or in your daily practice.

Scott M. Jackson, M.D.

Preface II to the First Edition

Ah, but a man's reach should exceed his grasp....

ROBERT BROWNING

Probably, the most satisfying aspect of being a chairman or residency program director in academic medicine is to be associated with, and help, bright young people who are anxious to learn and contribute to our body of medical knowledge. In my 35 years in academic dermatology, Scott Jackson is one of the brightest people that I have had the opportunity to teach and from which to learn. He has been one of our most motivated residents in becoming the best he can be and in trying to learn almost every fact in dermatology that can possibly be learned. Scott has attempted a mastery of the specialty, a goal many of us have hoped to attain but have come to realize, with time, that we will always fall short. Nevertheless, it is a lofty ideal, as stated so well by the poet Robert Browning when he wrote the line "Ah, but a man's reach should exceed his grasp...."

In addition to trying to learn almost every fact he could in dermatology during 3 years of residency training, Scott attempted to teach and transmit that knowledge base to all other residents in the program. He even initiated a weekly game of dermatologic questions for all the residents, a game he called "Jeopardy," complete with different weekly categories for everyone to study. Because of his thirst for knowledge, he made all residents in the program more knowledgeable.

In producing this text, which he worked on for long hours during his residency, and now as a junior faculty member, Scott Jackson has succeeded in a giant undertaking. I applaud his success and know that with each grasp he takes up the ladder of dermatology, he will continue to extend his reach.

Lee T. Nesbitt Jr., M.D.

Acknowledgements

I would like to thank my wife Angie for giving me the time, space, and support I needed to edit this text. I also thank Hannah and Mary for letting me work on this book when they would rather be playing with me. I also thank Dr. Lee Nesbitt for inspiring me to enter the field of clinical dermatology and assisting with the publication of this text. For the love and encouragement they have given me over the years, I thank my parents. Special thanks are given to Dr. Ashley Record, Dr. Steven Klinger, Dr. Kevin Guidry, Dr. Trent Massengale, Dr. Aimee Mistretta, Dr. Matthew Lambert, Dr. Erin Bardin, and Dr. Ann Zedlitz for the contribution of photographs. I also would like to thank those who supported the first edition as they made this second edition possible. Finally, I would like to thank my high school math teacher, Ms. Barbara Stott; for without her guidance, I would not be doing all that I am doing today.

Introduction

The *Handbook of Differential Diagnosis for the Dermatologist* was written for the purpose of providing the reader with quick access to the differential diagnosis of a variety of common and uncommon chief complaints, physical exam findings, dermatopathologic features, diagnoses, and more. An understanding of how this text was organized is essential prior to its use in order to facilitate rapid access to essential information. Firstly, the authors created an exhaustive list of virtually every dermatologic problem, including all important dermatologic diagnoses. Then, these various problems were sorted into chapters based on the key components of the dermatologic workup. All specific diagnoses were placed in the diagnosis chapter. Entities such as pruritus or keratoderma, not being specific diagnoses, were placed in the chief complaint or physical exam chapters, respectively. Useful supporting information was supplied for every problem when appropriate. Finally, each entry is referenced with a recent source article that attempts to increase the reader's understanding of the differential diagnosis of that disease. A summary of the contents of each chapter follows.

Chapter 1

"The Chief Complaint" focuses on complaints that patients make that cannot be more specifically sorted as a diagnosis or physical exam finding. Examples of items included in this brief chapter are pruritus, hyperhidrosis, and flushing.

Chapter 2

"The Past Medical History, Social History, and Review of Systems" highlights the major diagnostic considerations that arise in patients who present with an element of the past medical history, social history, or review of systems that may or may not be relevant to the encounter. In this chapter, one can find the dermatologic manifestations of internal diseases, skin findings in patients reporting certain social activities, and diagnostic considerations in patients revealing key components of the review of systems.

Chapter 3

"The Physical Exam" provides the reader with diagnostic considerations associated with a variety of regional and morphological physical exam findings. Entries included in this chapter are those findings which cannot better be sorted as specific diagnoses.

Chapter 4

"The Biopsy" presents the differential diagnosis of several major histologic reaction patterns or features.

Chapter 5

"The Laboratory Results" focuses on the most important or most common laboratory abnormalities that are encountered by dermatologists and the dermatologic diseases that should be considered in the evaluation of the patient.

Chapter 6

"The Diagnosis" contains an exhaustive alphabetical list of virtually every dermatologic diagnosis. An effort was made to include only the diagnoses that have been reported or discussed in the literature in the past two decades. Under each heading, the reader can find a list of subtypes (if any), the differential diagnosis of the disease and any subtypes, published diagnostic criteria, associations of the disease, associated medications (if any), and recommended initial evaluatory tests, and, new to the second edition, treatment options. When searching this text for the diagnosis in question, it is recommended that the reader search for the most unique term in the name and not descriptive adjectives, such as neutrophilic or superficial or common words such as dermatitis.

Chapter 7

The "Glossary" provides the reader with brief definitions of the rare diagnoses that can be found in the lists of differential diagnoses. These diagnoses were not given special attention in Chap.6 because they are very rare or because they do not have a lengthy differential diagnosis.

Contents

Abdominal Pain and Rash

- Acute graft-vs-host disease
- Acute porphyrias
- Carcinoid syndrome
- Black widow spider bite
- Degos disease
- Dengue fever
- Fabry's disease
- Familial Mediterranean fever
- Henoch–Schonlein purpura
- Inflammatory bowel disease
- Kawasaki disease
- Meningococcemia
- Pancreatic panniculitis
- Parasitic infestation
- Polyarteritis nodosa
- Porphyrias
- Tumor necrosis factor receptor-associated periodic syndrome (TRAPS)
- Viral illness
- Zoster

Further reading:
- Zulian F, Falcini F, Zancan L, Martini G, Secchieri S, Luzzatto C, Zacchello F (2003) Acute surgical abdomen as presenting manifestation of Kawasaki disease. J Pediatr 142(6):731–735

Anhidrosis/Hypohidrosis

Differential Diagnosis (Generalized)

- Acquired idiopathic anhidrosis
- Alcoholism
- Amyloidosis
- Anticholinergic therapy
- Bazex–Dupre–Christol syndrome
- Dehydration
- Diabetes mellitus
- CNS disease or tumor
- Congenital insensitivity to pain with anhidrosis
- Fabry's disease
- Horner's syndrome
- Ectodermal dysplasia, hypohidrotic
- Naegeli–Franceschetti–Jadassohn syndrome
- Pemphigus
- Peripheral nerve disorders (Guillain–Barre syndrome)
- Progressive autonomic failure
- Ross' syndrome
- Scleroderma
- Sjögren's syndrome
- Topiramate therapy
- Total skin electron beam therapy

Differential Diagnosis (Localized)

- Atopic dermatitis
- Burns
- Ectodermal dysplasia, hypohidrotic (carriers)
- Ichthyosis
- Idiopathic segmental anhidrosis
- Incontinentia pigmenti, stage IV

- Leprosy
- Lymphoma
- Postmiliaria
- Psoriasis
- Radiodermatitis
- Syringolymphoid hyperplasia
- Tumors

Further reading:

- Chemmanam T, Pandian JD, Kadyan RS, Bhatti SM (2007) Anhidrosis: a clue to an underlying autonomic disorder. J Clin Neurosci 14(1):94–96
- Haller A, Elzubi E, Petzelbauer P (2001) Localized syringolymphoid hyperplasia with alopecia and anhidrosis. J Am Acad Dermatol 45(1):127–130

Anodynia

- Anal fissure
- Chronic idiopathic anal pain
- Coccydynia
- External hemorrhoids
- Inflammatory bowel disease
- Levator ani syndrome
- Perirectal abscess
- Proctalgia fugax
- Proctitis

Further reading:

- Bharucha AE, Wald A, Enck P, Rao S (2006) Functional anorectal disorders. Gastroenterology 130(5):1510–1518

Arthritis (Arthralgias) with Rash

- Allergic hypersensitivity reaction
- Angioimmunoblastic lymphoma

- Bacterial endocarditis
- Behçet's syndrome
- Blau syndrome
- Bowel bypass dermatosis–arthritis syndrome
- Cryoglobulinemia
- Dermatomyositis
- Disseminated gonococcal infection
- Epstein–Barr virus
- Erythema elevatum diutinum
- Erythema multiforme
- Familial Mediterranean fever
- Gout
- Henoch–Schonlein purpura
- Hepatitis
- Inflammatory bowel disease
- Juvenile rheumatoid arthritis
- Kawasaki disease
- Lofgren's syndrome
- Lyme disease
- Mastocytosis
- Meningococcemia
- Mononucleosis
- Muckle–Wells syndrome
- Multicentric reticulohistiocytosis
- Pancreatic panniculitis
- Parvovirus B19 infection
- Psoriasis
- Pyoderma gangrenosum
- Rat-bite fever
- Reactive arthritis with urethritis and conjunctivitis
- Rheumatic fever, acute
- Rheumatoid arthritis
- Rocky Mountain spotted fever

- Rosai–Dorfman disease
- Sarcoidosis, acute
- Scleroderma
- Serum-sickness-like reaction
- Sjögren's syndrome
- Sweet's syndrome
- Systemic contact dermatitis (joint prosthesis)
- Systemic lupus erythematosus
- Systemic vasculitis syndromes
- TRAPS
- Viral infection

Further reading:
- Jacob SE, Cowen EW, Goldbach-Mansky R, Kastner D, Turner ML (2006) A recurrent rash with fever and arthropathy. J Am Acad Dermatol 54(2):318–321

Bromhidrosis

- Bromidrosiphobia (fear of body odor)
- Garlic, onion, or asparagus ingestion
- Foreign body in nasal passage
- Hepatic failure (fetor hepaticus)
- Hypermethionemia
- Isovaleric acidemia
- Maple syrup urine disease
- Normal apocrine gland sweat
- Oasthouse syndrome
- Olfactory hallucination
- Phenylketonuria
- Plantar hyperhidrosis
- Schizophrenia
- Trimethylaminuria (fish odor syndrome)
- Uremia

Further reading:
- Hasfa S, Schwartz RH (2007) Two 6-year-old twin girls with primary axillary bromhidrosis: discussion, differential diagnosis, and management options. Clin Pediatr 46(8):743–745

Chromhidrosis

- Bleeding disorder
- Clofazimine therapy
- Copper exposure
- *Corynebacterium* infection
- Dyes
- Hyperbilirubinemia
- Intrinsic (lipofucsin)
- Ochronosis
- Paint
- Piedra
- *Pseudomonas* infection
- *Serratia* infection

Further reading:
- Barankin B, Alanen K, Ting PT, Sapijaszko MJ (2004) Bilateral facial apocrine chromhidrosis. J Drugs Dermatol 3(2):184–186

Diarrhea and Rash

- Acute graft-vs-host disease
- Amebiasis
- Amyloidosis
- Bowel bypass dermatitis–arthritis syndrome
- Carcinoid syndrome
- Chemotherapy mucositis
- Crohn's disease
- Dermatitis herpetiformis

- Glucagonoma
- HIV infection
- IPEX syndrome
- Mastocytosis
- Pellagra
- Helminthic infestation
- Reactive arthritis
- Scleroderma
- Ulcerative colitis
- Viral gastroenteritis
- Whipple's disease

Further reading:
- Geusau A, Mooseder G (2002) A maculopapular rash in a patient with severe diarrhea. Arch Dermatol 138(1):117–122

Fever and Rash

- Acute retroviral syndrome
- Bacteremia
- Brucellosis
- Cat-scratch disease
- Deep fungal infection
- Dengue fever
- Dermatomyositis
- Drug hypersensitivity
- Ehrlichiosis
- Endocarditis
- Enterovirus infection
- Erythema migrans
- Erythema multiforme
- Familial Mediterranean fever
- Febrile ulceronecrotic Mucha–Habermann disease
- Gonococcemia

- Hepatitis B virus infection
- Hyper-IgD syndrome
- Juvenile rheumatoid arthritis
- Kawasaki disease
- Kikuchi's disease
- Leptospirosis
- Lymphoma
- Measles
- Meningococcemia
- Mononucleosis
- Muckle–Wells syndrome
- Parvovirus B19 infection
- Pustular psoriasis
- Rat-bite fever
- Reactive arthritis with urethritis and conjunctivitis
- Rickettsial diseases (especially Rocky Mountain spotted fever)
- Roseola infantum
- Rubella
- Sarcoidosis (acute)
- Scarlet fever
- Schnitzler syndrome
- Secondary syphilis
- Sepsis
- Serum-sickness-like reaction
- Smallpox
- Stevens–Johnson syndrome
- Sweet's syndrome
- Systemic lupus erythematosus
- Thrombotic thrombocytopenic purpura
- Toxic shock syndrome
- Toxoplasmosis
- Tularemia
- Typhoid fever
- Typhus

- Varicella
- Viral exanthem
- West Nile virus infection

Further reading:
- McKinnon HD Jr, Howard T (2000) Evaluating the febrile patient with a rash. Am Fam Physician 62(4):804–816

Fever, Periodic

- Borreliosis
- Brucellosis
- Cyclic neutropenia
- Familial cold autoinflammatory syndrome
- Familial Mediterranean fever
- Gonococcemia
- Hyper-IgD syndrome
- Juvenile rheumatoid arthritis
- Lymphoma
- Malaria
- Muckle–Wells syndrome
- NOMID syndrome (CINCA syndrome)
- PFAPA syndrome
- Relapsing fever (tick borne/louse borne)
- Schnitzler's syndrome
- Trench fever
- Tuberculosis
- TRAPS
- Typhoid fever

Further reading:
- Kanazawa N, Furukawa F (2007) Autoinflammatory syndromes with a dermatological perspective. J Dermatol 34(9):601–618

Flushing

- Alcohol ingestion
- Anaphylaxis
- Anxiety
- Autonomic hyperreflexia
- Brain tumors
- Caffeine withdrawal
- Carcinoid syndrome
- Cholinergic drugs
- Cholinergic erythema
- Ciguatera toxin ingestion
- Emotional flushing
- Fever
- Frey syndrome
- Heat-induced flushing
- Horner syndrome
- Mastocytosis
- Medullary thyroid carcinoma
- Menopause
- Migraine
- Monosodium glutamate
- Multiple sclerosis
- Nitrite/sulfite ingestion
- Opiates
- Parkinson's disease
- Pheochromocytoma
- Renal cell carcinoma
- Rifampin
- Rosacea
- Scombroid fish poisoning
- VIPoma

Associated Medications

- ACE inhibitors
- Beta-blockers
- Bromocriptine
- Calcium channel blockers
- Disulfiram (with alcohol)
- Griseofulvin (with alcohol)
- Ketoconazole (with alcohol)
- Metronidazole (with alcohol)
- Niacin
- Nicotinic acid
- Nitroglycerin
- Opioids
- Rifampin
- Sildenafil
- Tacrolimus, topical (with alcohol)
- Tamoxifen
- Vancomycin

Evaluation

- 24-h urine 5-HIAA
- 24-h urine epinephrine
- 24-h urine histamine
- 24-h urine metanephrines
- 24-h urine norepinephrine
- 24-h urine vanillylmandelic acid
- Food diary
- Medication review
- Serum calcitonin
- Serum LH/FSH

- Serum serotonin
- Serum tryptase
- Serum VIP level
- Urinalysis

Further reading:
- Izikson L, English JC III, Zirwas MJ (2006) The flushing patient: differential diagnosis, workup, and treatment. J Am Acad Dermatol 55(2):193–208

Hirsutism

- Adrenal tumor
- Carcinoid tumor
- Choriocarcinoma
- Congenital adrenal hyperplasia
- Cushing's syndrome
- Ectopic hormone production
- Excess ovarian androgen release syndrome
- Familial hirsutism
- Hepatic hirsutism
- Hormonal contraception
- Iatrogenic hirsutism
- Late-onset adrenal hyperplasia
- Metastatic lung carcinoma
- Ovarian hyperthecosis
- Ovarian tumors
- Peripheral failure in converting androgens into estrogens
- Persistent adrenarche syndrome
- Polycystic ovary disease
- Prolactinoma
- Psychogenic drugs
- SAHA syndrome

Evaluation

- 17-OH progesterone
- Cortisol
- Dehydroepiandrosterone sulfate
- Follicle stimulating hormone
- Free and total testosterone
- Luteinizing hormone
- Pelvic examination
- Prolactin
- Sex-hormone-binding globulin

Further reading:
- Rosenfield RL (2005) Clinical practice. Hirsutism. N Engl J Med 15(24):2578–2588

Hyperhidrosis

Differential Diagnosis (Generalized and Localized)

- Alcoholism
- Auriculotemporal syndrome (Frey syndrome)
- Carcinoid syndrome
- CNS tumor or disease
- Cold injury
- Congenital autonomic dysfunction with universal pain loss
- Cortical hyperhidrosis
- Diabetes mellitus
- Drug addiction
- Exercise
- Familial dysautonomia
- Febrile illness/infection
- Gopalan's syndrome

- Heart failure
- Hyperpituitarism
- Hyperthyroidism
- Hypoglycemia
- Lymphoma (especially Hodgkin's disease)
- Menopause
- Meperidine
- Neurologic
- Obesity
- Parkinson's disease
- Phenylketonuria
- Pheochromocytoma
- Physiologic gustatory sweating
- POEMS syndrome
- Porphyria
- Postencephalitis
- Postsympathectomy
- Pregnancy
- Propranolol
- Reflex sympathetic dystrophy
- Rheumatoid arthritis
- Shock
- Spinal injury
- Sympathetic injury
- Syringomyelia
- Tabes dorsalis
- Tricyclic antidepressants
- Tuberculosis

Diagnostic Criteria (Primary Focal)

- Focal, visible, excessive sweating of at least 6 months duration without apparent cause with at least two of the following characteristics:
  - Bilateral and relatively symmetric
  - Impairs daily activities

- Frequency of at least one episode per week
- Age of onset less than 25 years
- Positive family history
- Cessation of focal sweating during sleep

Further reading:

- Hornberger J, Grimes K, Naumann M et al (2004) Recognition, diagnosis, and treatment of primary focal hyperhidrosis. J Am Acad Dermatol 51(2):274–286
- Lear W, Kessler E, Solish N, Glaser DA (2007) An epidemiological study of hyperhidrosis. Dermatol Surg 33:S69–S75

Pruritic Rash, Generalized

- Allergic contact dermatitis
- Aquagenic pruritus
- Arthropod bites
- Asteatotic (xerotic) eczema
- Atopic dermatitis
- Autosensitization dermatitis
- Bullous pemphigoid
- Candidiasis
- Chronic actinic dermatitis
- Cutaneous T cell lymphoma
- Dermatographism
- Dermatitis herpetiformis
- Drug eruption
- Eosinophilic folliculitis of Ofuji
- Eosinophilic, polymorphic, and pruritic eruption associated with radiotherapy
- Fiberglass dermatitis
- Folliculitis
- Grover's disease
- Herpes simplex virus infection
- Itchy purpura
- Irritant contact dermatitis
- Lichen planus

- Lichen simplex chronicus
- Mastocytosis
- Nummular eczema
- Pediculosis
- Polymorphous light eruption
- Pityriasis rubra pilaris
- Prurigo nodularis
- Prurigo pigmentosum
- Pruritic urticarial papules and plaques of pregnancy
- Psoriasis
- Scabies
- Seabather's eruption
- Secondary syphilis
- Subacute prurigo
- Swimmer's itch
- Tinea corporis
- Urticaria
- Varicella
- Viral exanthem

Further reading:

- Yosipovitch G, Fleischer A (2003) Itch associated with skin disease: advances in pathophysiology and emerging therapies. Am J Clin Dermatol 4(9):617–622

Pruritic Scalp

- Acne necrotica
- Allergic contact dermatitis
- Dermatomyositis
- Folliculitis
- Lichen simplex chronicus
- Pediculosis
- Psoriasis
- Renal pruritus
- Scalp dysesthesia

- Seborrheic dermatitis
- Tinea capitis

Further reading:
- Hoss D, Segal S (1998) Scalp dysesthesia. Arch Dermatol 134(3):327–330

Pruritus Ani

- Allergic contact dermatitis
- Anal fissures
- Anal fistulas
- Anosacral amyloidosis
- Candidiasis
- Chronic antibiotic therapy
- Condyloma
- Contact dermatitis
- Excessive coffee intake
- Extramammary Paget's disease
- Fecal incontinence
- Gonococcal proctitis
- Hemorrhoids
- Herpes simplex virus infection
- Inflammatory bowel disease
- Lichen planus
- Lichen sclerosus
- Lichen simplex chronicus
- Lumbosacral radiculopathy
- Pinworm infestation
- Poor hygiene
- Psoriasis
- Radiation dermatitis
- Scabies
- Sexually transmitted diseases
- Spicy food intake
- Squamous cell carcinoma

- Sweating
- Syphilis
- Tinea cruris
- Urinary incontinence

Further reading:
- Zuccati G, Lotti T, Mastrolorenzo A et al (2005) Pruritus ani. Dermatol Ther 18(4):355–362

Pruritus Scroti

- Allergic contact dermatitis
- Candidiasis
- Dermatographism
- Extramammary Paget's disease
- Lichen simplex chronicus
- Lumbosacral radiculopathy
- Pediculosis
- Psoriasis
- Scabies
- Sexually transmitted diseases
- Urinary incontinence

Further reading:
- Cohen AD, Vander T, Medvendovsky E et al (2005) Neuropathic scrotal pruritus: anogenital pruritus is a symptom of lumbosacral radiculopathy. J Am Acad Dermatol 52(1):61–66

Pruritus Without Skin Disease, Generalized

- Carcinoid syndrome
- Cholestatic liver disease
- Chronic renal failure
- CNS tumor

- Cocaine/amphetamine abuse
- Dermatographism
- Dermatomyositis
- Diabetes mellitus
- Drug reaction
- Early bullous pemphigoid or dermatitis herpetiformis
- Hemochromatosis
- Hepatitis C infection
- HIV infection
- Hodgkin's disease
- Hypereosinophilic syndrome
- Hyperparathyroidism
- Hyperthyroidism
- Hypothyroidism
- Iron deficiency
- Lupus erythematosus
- Lymphoma/leukemia
- Mastocytosis
- Multiple endocrine neoplasia, type 2A
- Multiple sclerosis
- Mycosis fungoides (invisible)
- Opioid medications
- Paraproteinemia
- Parasitic infestation
- Polycythemia vera
- Pregnancy
- Psychogenic pruritus
- Sarcoidosis
- Scabies
- Scleroderma
- Systemic lupus erythematosus
- Thrombocytosis
- Transient urticaria
- Xerosis
- Winter itch (Duhring pruritus)

Evaluation

- Antimitochondrial antibodies
- Antinuclear antibodies
- Anti-smooth-muscle antibody
- Antitransglutaminase antibodies
- Bilirubin
- Calcium and phosphate levels
- Chest radiograph
- Complete blood count
- Fasting blood glucose
- Hepatitis panel
- HIV infection
- Iron, ferritin
- Liver function test
- Renal function test
- Sedimentation rate
- Serum histamine
- Serum IgE
- Serum protein electrophoresis
- Serum tryptase
- Stool for occult blood
- Stool for ova, cysts, and parasites
- Thyroid function test
- Urinary 5-HIAA

Further reading:
- Pujol RM, Gallardo F, Llistosella E et al (2002) Invisible mycosis fungoides: a diagnostic challenge. J Am Acad Dermatol 47(2 Suppl):S168–S171
- Zirwas MJ, Seraly MP (2001) Pruritus of unknown origin: a retrospective study. J Am Acad Dermatol 45(6):892–896

Pruritus Vulvae

- Acantholytic dyskeratosis of the vulva
- Allergic contact dermatitis

- Candidiasis
- Condyloma acuminatum
- Extramammary Paget's disease
- Herpes simplex virus infection
- Lichen planus
- Lichen sclerosus
- Lichen simplex chronicus
- Psoriasis
- Scabies
- Sexually transmitted diseases
- Squamous cell carcinoma
- Trichomoniasis
- Urinary incontinence

Further reading:
- Bohl TG (2005) Overview of vulvar pruritus through the life cycle. Clin Obstet Gynecol 48(4):786–807

Xerostomia

- Actinomycosis
- Amyloidosis
- Anticholinergics
- Cirrhosis
- Dermatomyositis
- Diabetes
- Diuretics
- Ectodermal dysplasia
- Graft-vs-host disease
- HIV infection
- Hypoplastic salivary glands
- Hypothyroidism
- Iron deficiency
- Lymphoma
- Mixed connective tissue disease

- Multiple sclerosis
- Mumps
- Nerve injury
- Pernicious anemia
- Radiation to head and neck
- Scleroderma
- Sialolithiasis
- Sjögren's syndrome
- Systemic lupus erythematosus
- Syphilis
- Tuberculosis
- Vitamin deficiency

Further reading:

- Taubert M, Davies EM, Back I (2007) Dry mouth. Br Med J 10(7592):534

The Past Medical History, Social History, and Review of Systems

Acquired Immunodeficiency Syndrome (Potentially Cutaneous AIDS-Defining Illnesses)

- Coccidioidomycosis
- Cytomegalovirus infection
- Herpes simplex viral infection of 1-month duration
- Histoplasmosis
- Kaposi's sarcoma
- *Mycobacterium avium* complex infection
- *Mycobacterium kansasii* infection
- *Mycobacterium tuberculosis* infection

Further reading::
- Rosenberg JD, Scheinfeld NS (2003) Cutaneous histoplasmosis in patients with acquired immunodeficiency syndrome. Cutis 72(6):439–445

Acromegaly

- Acanthosis nigricans
- Coarse facial features
- Cutis verticis gyrata
- Hyperhidrosis
- Fibromas
- Hyperpigmentation
- Hypertrichosis

- Macroglossia
- Thickened nails
- Thickened skin

Further reading:
- Ben-Shlomo A, Melmed S (2006) Skin manifestations in acromegaly. Clin Dermatol 24(4):256–259

Addison's Disease

- Alopecia areata
- Chronic mucocutaneous candidiasis
- Diffuse hyperpigmentation
- Lichen sclerosus
- Vitiligo

Further reading:
- Nieman LK, Chanco Turner ML (2006) Addison's disease. Clin Dermatol 24(4):276–280

AL Amyloidosis

- Alopecia
- Bullous lesions
- Cutis laxa
- Cutis verticis gyrata-like scalp changes
- Macroglossia
- Nail dystrophy
- Peripheral edema
- Pigmentary change
- Purpura (periorificial)
- Sclerodermoid changes
- Waxy papules and nodules

Further reading:
- Silverstein SR (2005) Primary, systemic amyloidosis and the dermatologist: where classic skin lesions may provide the clue for early diagnosis. Dermatol Online J 11(1):5

Alcoholism

- Acquired zinc deficiency
- Erythroderma
- Flushing
- Gout
- Leukoplakia
- Madelung's disease
- Palmar erythema
- Pancreatic panniculitis
- Pellagra
- Porphyria cutanea tarda
- Psoriasis
- Riboflavin deficiency
- Rosacea
- Scurvy
- Spider angiomas

Further reading:
- Kostovic K, Lipozencic J (2004) Skin diseases in alcoholics. Acta Dermatovenerol Croat 12(3):181–190

Aquatic Activity, Recent

- *Aeromonas* infection
- Coral dermatitis
- Erysipeloid
- Jellyfish sting
- *Mycobacterium marinum* infection

- Protothecosis
- *Pseudomonas* folliculitis
- Seabather's eruption
- Sea urchin dermatitis
- *Streptococcus iniae* infection
- Swimmer's itch
- *Vibrio vulnificus* infection

Further reading:

- Burroughs R, Kerr L, Zimmerman B, Elston DM (2005) Aquatic antagonists: sea urchin dermatitis. Cutis 76(1):18–20

Athlete

- Acne mechanica
- Calluses
- Chafing
- Erythrasma
- Exercise-induced anaphylaxis
- Folliculitis
- Friction blister
- Frostbite
- Furunculosis
- Herpes gladiatorum
- Impetigo
- Jogger's nipples
- Molluscum contagiosum
- Otitis externa
- Pitted keratolysis
- Subungual hematoma
- Sunburn
- Talon noir
- Tinea gladiatorum
- Tinea cruris
- Tinea pedis

Further reading:
- Mailler-Savage EA, Adams BB (2006) Skin manifestations of running. J Am Acad Dermatol 55(2):290–301

Bone Pain

- Langerhans cell histiocytosis
- Leukemia
- Lymphoma
- Mastocytosis
- Metastatic disease
- Muckle–Wells syndrome
- Myeloma
- Schnitzler syndrome
- Scurvy
- Sickle cell disease
- Syphilis
- Tuberculosis

Further reading:
- de Koning HD, Bodar EJ, van der Meer JW et al (2007) Schnitzler syndrome. Beyond the case reports: review and follow-up of 94 patients with an emphasis on prognosis and treatment. Semin Arthritis Rheum 37(3):137–148

Cardiovascular Disease

- Behçet's disease
- Carcinoid syndrome
- Cardiofaciocutaneous syndrome
- Carney's complex
- Carvajal syndrome
- Chagas disease
- Cutis laxa
- Dermatomyositis

- Diabetes mellitus
- Ehlers–Danlos syndrome
- Endocarditis
- Exfoliative erythroderma
- Fabry's disease
- Hemochromatosis
- Homocystinuria
- Hyperlipidemia
- Kawasaki disease
- LEOPARD syndrome
- Lyme disease
- Marfan syndrome
- Multicentric reticulohistiocytosis
- Naxos syndrome
- Neonatal lupus erythematosus
- Neurofibromatosis 1
- Noonan's syndrome
- Primary systemic amyloidosis
- Pseudoxanthoma elasticum
- Relapsing polychondritis
- Rheumatic fever
- Sarcoidosis
- Scleroderma
- Systemic lupus erythematosus
- Syphilis
- Takayasu's arteritis
- Tuberous sclerosis
- Werner's syndrome

Further reading:

- Abdelmalek NF, Gerber TL, Menter A (2002) Cardiocutaneous syndromes and associations. J Am Acad Dermatol 46(2):161–183

Cataracts

- Atopic dermatitis (Andogsky syndrome)
- Behçet's disease
- Cockayne's syndrome
- Diabetes mellitus
- Down syndrome
- Dyskeratosis congenita
- Ectodermal dysplasias
- Epidermal nevus syndrome
- Fabry's disease
- Hallermann–Streiff syndrome
- Incontinentia pigmenti
- Neurofibromatosis, type II
- Neutral lipid storage disease
- Psoralen therapy
- Rheumatoid arthritis
- Refsum's disease
- Rothmund–Thomson syndrome
- Sarcoidosis
- Steroids
- Stickler syndrome
- Syphilis
- Vogt–Koyanagi–Harada syndrome
- Werner's disease
- Wilson's disease
- X-linked ichthyosis
- X-linked-dominant chondrodysplasia punctata

Further reading:
- Freiman A, Ting PT, Barankin B, Stanciu M, Rudnisky C (2006) Ophthalmologic manifestations of cutaneous conditions. Ophthalmologica 220(5):281–240

Chemotherapy

- Acneiform eruption
- Acral erythema
- Acral sclerosis
- Anagen effluvium
- Atrophic skin
- Atrophic nails
- Flag sign
- Folliculitis
- Inflamed seborrheic keratoses
- Inflamed actinic keratoses
- Injection site reactions
- Metastatic disease
- Neutrophilic eccrine hidradenitis
- Photosensitivity
- Pruritus
- Radiation enhancement
- Radiation recall
- Raynaud's phenomenon
- Hyperpigmentation
- Stomatitis
- Syringosquamous metaplasia
- Worsening of psoriasis

Further reading:
- Lacouture M et al (2011) Adverse skin reactions to chemotherapeutic agents. Dermatol Ther 24(4):385–442

Cirrhosis (Including Primary Biliary Cirrhosis)

- Caput medusa
- Cirsoid aneurysms
- Gynecomastia
- Hyperpigmentation (PBC)

- Jaundice
- Muehrcke's lines
- Palmar erythema
- Pruritus
- Purpura and ecchymoses (Vitamin K deficiency)
- Scleroderma/morphea (PBC)
- Sparse hair
- Spider angiomas
- Terry's nails
- Xanthomas (PBC)

Further reading:
- Koulentaki M, Ioannidou D, Stefanidou M et al (2006) Dermatological manifestations in primary biliary cirrhosis (PBC) patients: a case control study. Am J Gastroenterol 101(3):541–546

Cleft Lip and/or Palate

- 4p syndrome
- Hay–Wells syndrome
- Beare–Stevenson cutis gyrata syndrome
- Branchio-oculo-facial syndrome
- Cleft lip/palate – ectodermal dysplasia syndrome
- Dermal melanocytosis
- EEC syndrome
- Encephalocele
- Nasal glioma
- Nail–patella syndrome
- Nevoid basal cell carcinoma syndrome
- Oculocerebrocutaneous syndrome
- Oral–facial–digital syndrome
- Popliteal pterygium syndrome
- Rapp–Hodgkin syndrome
- Robert syndrome
- Van der Woude syndrome

- Waardenburg syndrome, type 1 or 3
- Wolf–Hirschhorn syndrome

Further reading:
- Steele JA, Hansen H, Arn P, Kwong PC (2005) Spectrum of phenotypic manifestations from a single point mutation of the p63 gene, including new cutaneous and immunologic findings. Pediatr Dermatol 22(5):415–419

Cold Induced or Cold Exacerbated

- Acrocyanosis
- Asteatotic eczema
- Atopic dermatitis
- Chilblains lupus erythematosus
- Cold panniculitis
- Cold urticaria
- Cold-water foot immersion
- Cryofibrinogenemia
- Cryoglobulinemia
- Cutis marmorata
- Erythrokeratolysis hiemalis
- Familial cold autoinflammatory syndrome
- Frostbite
- Glomus tumor
- Leiomyoma
- Livedo reticularis
- Perniosis
- Raynaud's phenomenon
- Sclerema neonatorum
- Subcutaneous fat necrosis of the newborn

Further reading:
- Aksentijevich ID, Putnam C, Remmers EF et al (2007) The clinical continuum of cryopyrinopathies: novel CIAS1 mutations in North American patients and a new cryopyrin model. Arthritis Rheum 56(4):1273–1285

Cushing's Disease

- Acne
- Candidiasis
- Dermatophytosis
- Facial fullness
- Hirsutism
- Lipoatrophy (arms and legs)
- Lipohypertrophy (especially upper back, abdomen)
- Poor wound healing
- Purpura
- Skin fragility
- Striae distensae
- Tinea versicolor

Further reading:
- Jabbour SA (2003) Cutaneous manifestations of endocrine disorders: a guide for dermatologists. Am J Clin Dermatol 4(5):315–331

Cystic Fibrosis

- Acrodermatitis enteropathica
- Aquagenic wrinkling of the palms and soles
- Clubbing
- Cutaneous vasculitis
- Essential fatty acid deficiency
- Kwashiorkor-like eruption
- Phrynoderma
- Xerosis

Further reading:
- Katz KA, Yan AC, Turner ML (2005) Aquagenic wrinkling of the palms in patients with cystic fibrosis homozygous for the delta F508 CFTR mutation. Arch Dermatol 141(5):621–624

Deafness

- Albinism
- Alezzandrini syndrome
- Alport's syndrome
- Alstrom syndrome
- Bart–Pumphrey syndrome
- Bjornstad's syndrome
- Branchio-oto-renal syndrome
- Cockayne's syndrome
- Congenital rubella
- Congenital syphilis
- Crandall's syndrome
- DOOR syndrome
- Ectodermal dysplasias
- Goldenhar syndrome
- HID syndrome
- Hypomelanosis of Ito
- Johansson–Blizzard
- Johnson–McMillan syndrome
- Keratosis follicularis spinulosa decalvans
- KID syndrome
- LEOPARD syndrome
- Muckle–Wells syndrome
- Neutral lipid storage disease
- NOMID syndrome
- Phylloid hypomelanosis
- Ramsay–Hunt syndrome
- Refsum's disease
- Relapsing polychondritis
- Tietz syndrome
- Townes–Brock syndrome
- Vohwinkel's syndrome
- Waardenburg's syndrome

- Xeroderma pigmentosum
- Ziprkowski–Margolis syndrome

Further reading:
- Richard G, Brown N, Ishida-Yamamoto A, Krol A (2004) Expanding the phenotypic spectrum of Cx26 disorders: Bart–Pumphrey syndrome is caused by a novel missense mutation in GJB2. J Invest Dermatol 123(5):856–863

Diabetes Mellitus

- Acanthosis nigricans (Fig. 2.1)
- Acral gangrene
- Acral erythema
- Bullosis diabeticorum
- Candidiasis
- Clear cell syringoma
- Dermatophytosis
- Diabetic bullae
- Diabetic dermopathy
- Granuloma annulare (especially disseminated type)
- Erythrasma

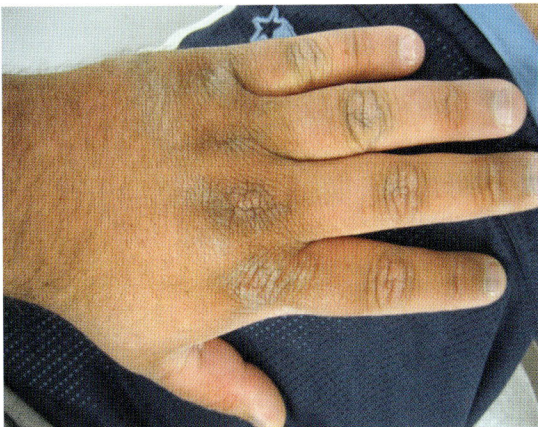

Fig. 2.1 Acral acanthosis nigricans

- Injection lipoatrophy
- Mucormycosis
- Necrobiosis lipoidica
- Neuropathic ulcers
- Partial lipodystrophy
- Perforating disorders
- Pruritus
- Rubeosis
- Scleredema adultorum
- Xerosis

Further reading:
- Ahmed I, Goldstein B (2006) Diabetes mellitus. Clin Dermatol 24(4):237–246

Digital Anomalies

- Adams–Oliver syndrome
- Apert syndrome
- Cleft lip/palate–ectodermal dysplasia
- EEC syndrome
- Epidermal nevus syndrome
- Focal dermal hypoplasia
- Klippel–Trenaunay syndrome
- Limb–mammary syndrome
- Nevoid basal cell carcinoma syndrome
- Oculodentodigital syndrome
- Oral–facial–digital syndrome
- Popliteal pterygium syndrome
- Proteus syndrome
- Trichorhinophalangeal syndrome
- Waardenburg syndrome, type 3

Further reading:
- Kalla G, Garg A (2002) Ectrodactyly. Indian J Dermatol Venereol Leprol 68(3):152–153

Down Syndrome

- Alopecia areata
- Brachycephaly
- Brushfield spots
- Cheilitis
- Collagenomas
- Cutis marmorata
- Dermatophyte infections
- Elastosis perforans serpiginosa
- Folliculitis
- Ichthyosis
- Immunodeficiency
- Leukemia
- Lichen simplex chronicus
- Milia–like calcinosis cutis
- Neonatal transient myeloproliferative disorder
- Norwegian scabies
- Scrotal tongue
- Seborrheic dermatitis
- Single palmar crease
- Syringomas
- Vitiligo

Further reading:
- Daneshpazhooh M, Nazemi TM, Bigdeloo L, Yoosefi M (2007) Mucocutaneous findings in 100 children with Down syndrome. Pediatr Dermatol 24(3):317–320

Dysphagia/Odynophagia

- Behçet's disease
- Candidiasis
- Darier's disease
- Dermatomyositis

- Erosive lichen planus
- Graft-vs-host disease
- Herpes simplex virus infection
- Howell–Evans syndrome
- Inflammatory bowel disease
- Iron deficiency (Plummer–Vinson syndrome)
- Oral–ocular–genital syndrome
- Pemphigus
- Scleroderma
- Stevens–Johnson syndrome
- Zoster

Further reading:

- Espana A, Fernandez S, del Olmo J et al (2007) Ear, nose, and throat manifestations in pemphigus vulgaris. Br J Dermatol 156(4):733–737

Eating Disorder

- Acne
- Acquired zinc deficiency
- Acral coldness
- Acrocyanosis
- Aphthous stomatitis
- Calluses on hands (Russell's sign)
- Carotenemia
- Cheilitis
- Dental caries
- Dermatomyositis-like syndrome (Ipecac)
- Dry hair
- Ecchymoses from vitamin K deficiency
- Edema
- Emesis-related purpura
- Enamel erosion
- Enlarged parotid glands

- Factitial dermatoses
- Finger clubbing
- Fixed drug eruption from phenolphthalein laxative
- Gum recession
- Interdigital intertrigo
- Lanugo-like hair
- Livedo reticularis
- Loss of subcutaneous fat
- Onychorrhexis
- Paronychia
- Pellagra
- Periungual erythema
- Perleche
- Perniosis
- Petechiae and purpura
- Pitting edema
- Poor wound healing
- Prurigo pigmentosa
- Pruritus
- Scurvy
- Seborrheic dermatitis
- Striae distensae
- Telogen effluvium
- Trichotillomania
- Xerosis

Further reading:

- Strumia R (2005) Dermatologic signs in patients with eating disorders. Am J Clin Dermatol 6(3):165–173

Epilepsy

- Anticonvulsant reaction
- Centrofacial lentiginosis

- CNS lupus
- Dupuytren's contracture
- Encephalocraniocutaneous lipomatosis
- Epidermal nevus syndrome
- Focal dermal hypoplasia
- Gingival fibromatosis
- Hypomelanosis of Ito
- Incontinentia pigmenti
- Lhermitte–Duclos disease
- Menkes' kinky-hair syndrome
- Phacomatosis pigmentovascularis
- Sjögren–Larsson syndrome
- Sturge–Weber syndrome
- Tuberous sclerosus
- Wolf–Hirschhorn syndrome
- Wyburn–Mason syndrome

Further reading:

- Hubert JN, Callen JP (2002) Incontinentia pigmenti presenting as seizures. Pediatr Dermatol 19(6):550–552

Gastrointestinal Hemorrhage

- Blue rubber bleb nevus syndrome
- Chronic urticaria (*H. pylori* infection)
- Cowden's disease
- Crohn's disease
- Cronkhite–Canada syndrome
- Diffuse neonatal hemangiomatosis
- Ehlers–Danlos syndrome, type IV
- Gardner's syndrome
- Hemangiomatosis
- Henoch–Schönlein purpura

- Hereditary hemorrhagic telangiectasia
- Kaposi's sarcoma
- Kawasaki disease
- Maffucci's syndrome
- Malignant atrophic papulosis
- Muir–Torre syndrome
- Peutz–Jeghers syndrome
- Polyarteritis nodosa
- Pseudoxanthoma elasticum
- Scurvy
- Ulcerative colitis
- Vasculitis

Further reading:
- Braverman IM (2003) Skin signs of gastrointestinal disease. Gastroenterology 124(6):1595–1614

Gastrointestinal Neoplasia

- Acanthosis nigricans
- Arsenicism
- Carcinoid syndrome
- Cowden's disease
- Cronkhite–Canada syndrome
- Dermatitis herpetiformis
- Dermatomyositis
- Extramammary Paget's disease
- Gardner's syndrome
- Kaposi's sarcoma
- Leser–Trelat sign
- Muir–Torre syndrome
- Necrolytic migratory erythema
- Neurofibromatosis

- Peutz–Jeghers syndrome
- Sister Mary Joseph nodule
- Tylosis (Howell–Evans syndrome)

Further reading:

- Braverman IM (2003) Skin signs of gastrointestinal disease. Gastroenterology 124(6):1595–1614

Hemochromatosis

- Alopecia
- Atrophy
- Generalized hyperpigmentation
- Ichthyosis
- Koilonychia
- Leukonychia
- Onychonychia
- Palmar erythema
- Porphyria cutanea tarda
- Spider telangiectasias
- *Vibrio vulnificus* infection

Further reading:

- Kostler E, Porst H, Wollina U (2005) Cutaneous manifestations of metabolic diseases: uncommon presentations. Clin Dermatol 23(5):457–464

Hemodialysis

- Acquired perforating disease
- Beta-2 microglobulin amyloidosis
- Calciphylaxis/calcinosis cutis
- Lindsay's nails (half-and-half nails)
- Muehrcke's lines

- Nephrogenic fibrosing dermopathy
- Pallor
- Pruritus
- Pseudoporphyria
- Uremic frost
- Xerosis or ichthyosis

Further reading:
- Udayakumar P, Balasubramanian S, Ramalingam KS et al (2006) Cutaneous manifestations in patients with chronic renal failure on hemodialysis. Indian J Dermatol Venereol Leprol 72(2):119–125

Hepatitis B or Hepatitis C Infection

- Cutaneous small vessel vasculitis
- Disseminated superficial porokeratosis (C)
- Erythema multiforme
- Erythema nodosum
- Gianotti–Crosti syndrome (B)
- Lichen planus (C)
- Mixed essential cryoglobulinemia (C > B)
- Necrolytic acral erythema (C)
- Pigmented purpuric dermatosis (C)
- Polyarteritis nodosa (B > C)
- Porphyria cutanea tarda (C)
- Pruritus
- Urticaria
- Urticarial vasculitis
- Xerostomia

Further reading:
- Bonkovsky HL, Mehta S (2001) Hepatitis C: a review and update. J Am Acad Dermatol 44(2):159–182

Hodgkin's Disease

- Cutaneous involvement (rare)
- Eczema
- Erythroderma
- Hyperpigmentation
- Ichthyosis
- Lymphadenopathy
- Mycosis fungoides
- Opportunistic infections
- Pruritus

Further reading:

- Rubenstein M, Duvic M (2006) Cutaneous manifestations of Hodgkin's disease. Int J Dermatol 45(3):251–256

Human Immunodeficiency Virus Infection

- Acanthamebiasis
- Acne vulgaris
- Acquired ichthyosis
- Acute HIV exanthem
- Adrenal insufficiency
- Aphthous ulcer
- Atopic dermatitis
- Atypical mycobacterial infection
- Bacillary angiomatosis
- Bacterial folliculitis
- Basal cell carcinoma
- Botryomycosis
- Bowenoid papulosis
- Bullous impetigo
- Chronic actinic dermatitis
- Condyloma accuminata

- Crusted scabies
- Cryptococcosis
- Cutaneous lymphoma
- Cutaneous pneumocystosis
- Cytomegalovirus
- Demodicidosis
- Dermatophytosis
- Deep fungal infection
- Drug eruption
- Ecthyma
- Ecthyma gangrenosum
- Eosinophilic folliculitis
- Epidermodysplasia verruciformis
- Erythema multiforme
- Erythroderma
- Factitious
- Fungal folliculitis
- Generalized pruritus
- Granuloma annulare
- Herpes simplex infection
- Herpes zoster
- Histoplasmosis
- HTLV-1 leukemia/lymphoma
- Hyperpigmentation
- Insect-bite reaction
- Kaposi's sarcoma
- Kwashiorkor
- Leishmaniasis
- Lymphoma
- Molluscum contagiosum
- Necrotizing fasciitis
- Non-Hodgkin's lymphoma
- Papular eruption of AIDS
- Papular mucinosis

- Papular urticaria
- Penicilliosis
- Perioral dermatitis
- Photosensitive drug eruption
- Pityriasis rubra pilaris (type VI)
- Porphyria cutanea tarda
- Post-inflammatory hyperpigmentation
- Psoriasis (more severe)
- Reactive arthritis with urethritis
- RED syndrome (see toxic shock syndrome)
- Rosacea
- Scabies
- Seborrheic dermatitis
- Smooth muscle tumors (angioleiomyoma)
- Squamous cell carcinoma
- Stevens–Johnson syndrome
- Toxic epidermal necrolysis
- Verruca vulgaris
- Verrucous carcinoma
- Viral exanthem
- Xerosis

Further reading:

- Zancanaro PC, McGirt LY, Mamelak AJ et al (2006) Cutaneous manifestations of HIV in the era of highly active antiretroviral therapy: an institutional urban clinic experience. J Am Acad Dermatol 54(4):581–588

Hyperthyroidism

- Alopecia areata
- Hyperpigmentation
- Koilonychia
- Onycholysis
- Pemphigoid gestationis
- Pretibial myxedema

- Pruritus
- Thyroid acropachy
- Urticaria
- Vitiligo

Further reading:
- Jabbour SA (2003) Cutaneous manifestations of endocrine disorders: a guide for dermatologists. Am J Clin Dermatol 4(5):315–331

Hypothyroidism

- Ascher syndrome
- Carotenoderma
- Chronic urticaria
- Brittle hair
- Easy bruising
- Eruptive and tuberous xanthomas
- Hypohidrosis
- Ichthyosis
- Madarosis
- Myxedema
- Onycholysis
- Palmoplantar keratoderma
- Vitiligo

Further reading:
- Jabbour SA (2003) Cutaneous manifestations of endocrine disorders: a guide for dermatologists. Am J Clin Dermatol 4(5):315–331

Immunosuppressed/Transplant Recipient

- Actinic keratosis
- Basal cell carcinoma
- Candidiasis
- Cryptococcosis

- Cytomegalovirus infection
- Dermatophytosis
- Disseminated aspergillosis
- Disseminated *Fusarium* infection (Fig. 2.2)
- Disseminated zoster
- Ecthyma gangrenosum
- Graft-vs-host disease
- Herpes simplex virus
- Histoplasmosis
- Kaposi's sarcoma
- Malakoplakia
- Melanoma
- Merkel cell carcinoma
- Pneumocystosis
- Post-transplant lymphoproliferative disorder
- Sebaceous hyperplasia (cyclosporine)
- Squamous cell carcinoma
- Tinea versicolor
- Trichodysplasia spinulosa
- Viral warts

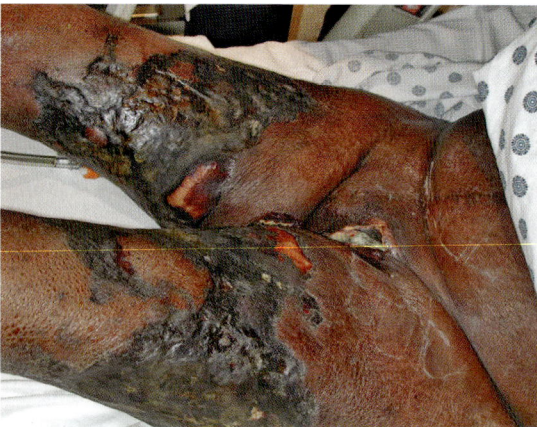

Fig. 2.2 Disseminated Fusarium infection (Courtesy of K. Guidry)

Further reading:

• Hassan G, Khalaf H, Mourad W (2007) Dermatologic complications after liver transplantation: a single-center experience. Transplant Proc 39(4):1190–1194

Inflammatory Bowel Disease

- Acne fulminans
- Acrodermatitis enteropathica-like lesions
- Angular cheilitis
- Annular erythema
- Aphthosis
- Bowel-associated dermatosis–arthritis syndrome
- Clubbing
- Cutaneous polyarteritis nodosa
- Epidermolysis bullosa acquisita
- Erythema elevatum diutinum
- Erythema nodosum
- Granulomatous infiltrates
- Hidradenitis suppurativa
- Lichen planus
- Lichen nitidus
- Malnutrition
- Metastatic Crohn's disease
- Ostomy dermatitis
- Psoriasis
- Pustular vasculitis
- Pyoderma gangrenosum
- Pyostomatitis vegetans
- Small vessel vasculitis
- Urticaria
- Vitiligo

Further reading:

• Ruocco E, Cuomo A, Salerno R et al (2007) Crohn's disease and its mucocutaneous involvement. Skinmed 6(4):179–185

Klinefelter Syndrome

- Gynecomastia
- Leg ulcers
- Tall stature
- Testosterone-induced acne
- Varicose veins

Further reading:
- De Morentin HM, Dodiuk-Gad RP, Brenner S (2004) Klinefelter's syndrome presenting with leg ulcers. Skinmed 3(5):274–278

Leukemia

- Acral ischemia
- Cheilitis
- Chloroma (granulocytic sarcoma)
- Erythema elevatum diutinum
- Erythema multiforme
- Erythema nodosum
- Erythroderma
- Exaggerated arthropod-bite reactions
- Fingertip hypertrophy
- Gingival infiltration
- Grover's disease-like eruption
- Leonine facies
- Neutrophilic dermatosis of the dorsal hands
- Neutrophilic eccrine hidradenitis
- Oral ulcers
- Panniculitis
- Paraneoplastic pemphigus
- Polyarteritis nodosa
- Purpura
- Pyoderma gangrenosum

- Recalcitrant eczema
- Subungual nodule
- Sweet's syndrome (especially bullous)
- Urticaria
- Vasculitis

Further reading:

- Agnew KL, Ruchlemer R, Catovsky D et al (2004) Cutaneous findings in chronic lymphocytic leukaemia. Br J Dermatol 150(6):1129–1135

Lupus Erythematosus, Systemic

- Antiphospholipid antibody syndrome
- Basaloid follicular hamartoma
- Benign hypergammaglobulinemic purpura
- Bullous lesions
- Butterfly (malar) rash
- Calcinosis cutis
- Chilblains-like lesions
- Cryoglobulinemia
- Dermatofibromas (>15)
- Digital infarctions
- Discoid lesions (Fig. 2.3)
- Erythema multiforme-like lesions
- Fractured hairs
- Leg ulcers
- Lichen planus–lupus erythematosus overlap
- Livedo reticularis
- Livedoid vasculopathy
- Lupus panniculitis
- Malignant atrophic papulosis
- Mucinous lesions
- Oral painless ulcers
- Palmar erythema

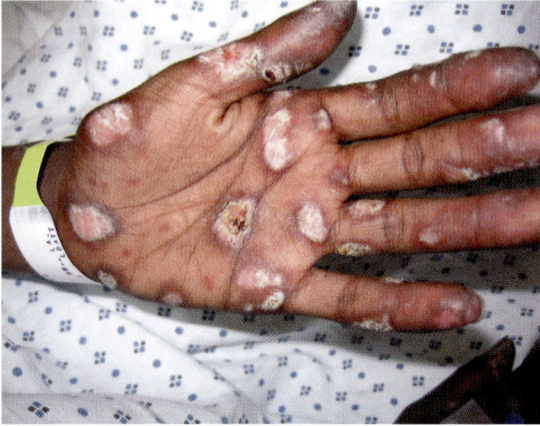

Fig. 2.3 Discoid lupus erythematosus

- Periorbital edema
- Periungual telangiectasias
- Photosensitivity
- Poikilodermatous skin changes
- Purpura
- Raynaud's phenomenon
- Red lunula
- Rheumatoid nodules
- Scarring alopecia
- Sweet's syndrome
- Telogen effluvium
- Toxic epidermal necrolysis-like presentation
- Urticarial vasculitis

Further reading:
- Rothfield N, Sontheimer RD, Bernstein M (2006) Lupus erythematosus: systemic and cutaneous manifestations. Clin Dermatol 24(5):348–362

Malignancy, Internal

- Acanthosis nigricans
- Acquired ichthyosis

- Bazex's syndrome
- Carcinoid syndrome
- Cushing's syndrome
- Cutaneous small vessel vasculitis
- Dermatitis herpetiformis
- Dermatomyositis
- Erythema annulare centrifugum
- Erythema gyratum repens
- Exfoliative erythroderma
- Extramammary Paget's disease
- Hypertrichosis lanuginosa (malignant down)
- Multicentric reticulohistiocytosis
- Mycosis fungoides
- Necrobiotic xanthogranuloma
- Necrolytic migratory erythema
- Paget's disease of the breast
- Paraneoplastic pemphigus
- Porphyria cutanea tarda
- Pyoderma gangrenosum
- Sign of Leser–Trélat
- Sweet's syndrome
- Tripe palms
- Urticaria
- Urticarial vasculitis

Further reading:
- Chung VQ, Moschella SL, Zembowicz A, Liu V (2006) Clinical and pathologic findings of paraneoplastic dermatoses. J Am Acad Dermatol 54(5):745–762

Monoclonal Gammopathy/Multiple Myeloma

- Acquired angioedema
- Acquired cutis laxa
- Amyloidosis
- Atypical scleroderma

- Bullous amyloidosis
- Digital cutis laxa-like changes
- Epidermolysis bullosa acquisita
- Erythema elevatum diutinum
- Extramedullary cutaneous plasmacytomas (Fig. 2.4)
- Follicular hyperkeratosis (spines)
- Hair casts
- IgA pemphigus
- IgM storage papules (cutaneous macroglobulinosis)
- Leukocytoclastic vasculitis
- Necrobiotic xanthogranuloma
- Paraneoplastic pemphigus
- Plane xanthomas
- POEMS syndrome
- Pyoderma gangrenosum
- Schnitzler syndrome
- Scleredema

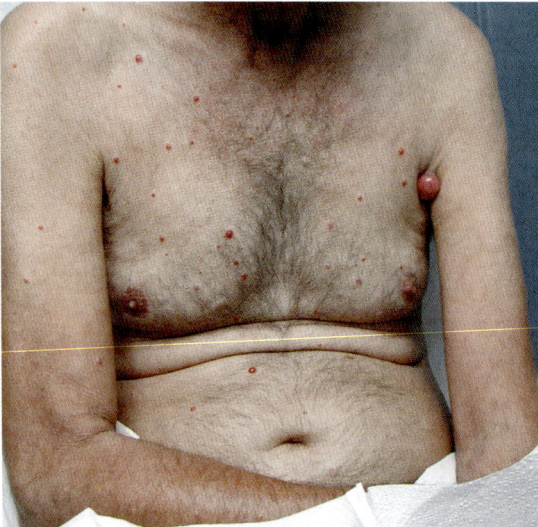

Fig. 2.4 Plasmacytomas (Courtesy of K. Guidry)

- Scleromyxedema
- Subcorneal pustular dermatosis
- Subepidermal bullous dermatosis
- Sweet's syndrome
- Xanthoma disseminatum

Further reading:
- Satta R, Casu G, Dore F, Longinotti M, Cottoni F (2003) Follicular spicules and multiple ulcers: cutaneous manifestations of multiple myeloma. J Am Acad Dermatol 49(4):736–740

Multiple Endocrine Neoplasia, Type I

- Adrenocortical tumors
- Angiofibromas
- Cafe-au-lait macules
- Collagenomas
- Confetti-like hypopigmentation
- Gastrointestinal tumors
- Gingival papules
- Leiomyomas
- Lipomas
- Melanoma
- Parathyroid adenoma
- Pituitary adenoma

Further reading:
- Jabbour SA, Davidovici BB, Wolf R (2006) Rare syndromes. Clin Dermatol 24(4):299–316

Multiple Endocrine Neoplasia, Type IIA

- Lichen amyloidosis
- Medullary thyroid carcinoma

- Parathyroid hyperplasia
- Pheochromocytoma
- Pruritus

Further reading:
- Jabbour SA, Davidovici BB, Wolf R (2006) Rare syndromes. Clin Dermatol 24(4):299–316

Multiple Endocrine Neoplasia, Type IIB

- Cafe-au-lait macules
- Elongated facies
- Marfanoid habitus
- Medullary thyroid carcinoma
- Mucosal neuromas
- Pheochromocytoma

Further reading:
- Jabbour SA, Davidovici BB, Wolf R (2006) Rare syndromes. Clin Dermatol 24(4):299–316

Obesity

- Acanthosis nigricans
- Acrochordons
- Adiposis dolorosa
- Bacterial infections
- Candidiasis
- Dermatophytosis
- Frictional hyperpigmentation
- Gout

- Hidradenitis
- Hyperhidrosis
- Intertrigo
- Keratosis pilaris
- Lipodermatosclerosis
- Plantar hyperkeratosis
- Pseudoacanthosis nigricans
- Psoriasis
- Stasis dermatitis
- Striae distensae
- Venous insufficiency ulcers

Further reading:
- Yosipovitch G, DeVore A, Dawn A (2007) Obesity and the skin: skin physiology and skin manifestations of obesity. J Am Acad Dermatol 56(6):901–916

Pancreatic Disease

- Cullen's sign
- Familial melanoma
- Glucagonoma syndrome
- Jaundice
- Livedo reticularis
- Metastatic disease
- Migratory thrombophlebitis (Trousseau's syndrome)
- Multiple endocrine neoplasia
- Panniculitis
- Systemic lupus erythematosus
- Turner's sign
- Xanthomas (hypertriglyceridemia)

Further reading:
- Kobayashi S, Yoshida M, Kitahara T et al (2007) Autoimmune pancreatitis as the initial presentation of systemic lupus erythematosus. Lupus 16(2):133–136

POEMS Syndrome (Crow–Fukase Syndrome)

- Alopecia
- Cherry angiomas
- Clubbing
- Flushing
- Glomeruloid hemangiomas
- Hyperpigmentation
- Hypertrichosis
- Lymphadenopathy
- Ichthyosis
- Microvenular hemangiomas
- Raynaud's phenomenon
- Sclerodermoid changes

Further reading:
- Phillips JA, Dixon JE, Richardson JB et al (2006) Glomeruloid hemangioma leading to a diagnosis of POEMS syndrome. J Am Acad Dermatol 55(1):149–152

Polyps, Intestinal

- Bannayan–Riley–Ruvalcaba
- Birt–Hogg–Dube syndrome
- Cronkhite–Canada syndrome
- Familial polyposis
- Gardner's syndrome
- Muir–Torre syndrome
- Neurofibromatosis
- Peutz–Jeghers syndrome

Further reading:
- Braverman IM (2003) Skin signs of gastrointestinal disease. Gastroenterology 124(6):1595–1614

Pregnant

- Acne vulgaris
- Atopic dermatitis of pregnancy
- Cholestasis of pregnancy
- Darkening of nevi
- Diffuse hyperpigmentation
- Erythema nodosum
- Folliculitis
- Impetigo herpetiformis
- Melasma
- Palmar erythema
- Pemphigoid gestationis
- Prurigo of pregnancy
- Pruritic urticarial papules and plaques of pregnancy
- Pyogenic granuloma
- Spider telangiectasias
- Striae gravidarum
- Urticaria
- Varicosities

Further reading:
- Ambros-Rudolph CM (2006) Dermatoses of pregnancy. J Dtsch Dermatol Ges 4(9):748–759

Pulmonary Disease

- Antitrypsin deficiency panniculitis
- Arsenicism
- Aspergillosis
- Atopic dermatitis
- Birt–Hogg–Dube syndrome
- Blastomycosis

- Chronic granulomatous disease
- Churg–Strauss syndrome
- Coccidioidomycosis
- CREST syndrome
- Cystic fibrosis
- Dermatomyositis
- Hereditary hemorrhagic telangiectasia
- Histoplasmosis
- Langerhans cell histiocytosis
- Lymphomatoid granulomatosis
- Mycoplasma infection
- Nocardiosis
- Sarcoidosis
- Scleroderma
- Sweet's syndrome
- Tuberculosis
- Wegener's granulomatosis
- Viral infection
- Tuberous sclerosus

Further reading:
- Astudillo L, Sailler L, Launay F et al (2006) Pulmonary involvement in Sweet's syndrome: a case report and review of the literature. Int J Dermatol 45(6):677–680

Renal Disease

- Alport's syndrome
- Birt–Hogg–Dube syndrome
- Cholesterol emboli syndrome
- Fabry's disease
- Goodpasture's syndrome
- Henoch–Schönlein purpura
- Hereditary leiomyomatosis
- Myeloma

- Nail–patella syndrome
- Neurofibromatosis
- Oxalosis
- Polyarteritis nodosa
- Primary systemic amyloidosis
- Pseudoporphyria
- Pseudoxanthoma elasticum
- Renal cell carcinoma
- Sarcoidosis
- Scleroderma
- Small vessel vasculitis
- Systemic lupus erythematosus
- Tuberous sclerosus
- Wegener's granulomatosis

Further reading:
- Abdelbaqi-Salhab M, Shalhub S et al (2003) A current review of the cutaneous manifestations of renal disease. J Cutan Pathol 30(9):527–538

Rheumatoid Arthritis

- Accelerated rheumatoid nodulosis
- Alopecia areata
- Bullous pemphigoid
- Bywaters lesions
- Cicatricial pemphigoid
- Clubbing
- Dermatitis herpetiformis
- Digital pulp nodules
- Epidermolysis bullosa acquisita
- Erythema elevatum diutinum
- Erythema multiforme
- Erythema nodosum
- Erythromelalgia

- Felty's syndrome
- Hyperpigmentation
- Interstitial granulomatous dermatitis with arthritis
- Linear necrobiotic subcutaneous bands
- Localized hyperhidrosis
- Mondor's disease
- Nail-fold telangiectasia
- Onychorrhexis
- Palisaded neutrophilic and granulomatous dermatitis
- Palmar erythema
- Pemphigus
- Pyoderma gangrenosum
- Reactive angioendotheliomatosis
- Rheumatoid neutrophilic dermatitis
- Rheumatoid nodules
- Rheumatoid vasculitis
- Small vessel vasculitis
- Splinter hemorrhages
- Subcorneal pustular dermatosis
- Sweet's syndrome
- Transient macular erythema
- Urticaria
- Vasculitis
- Vitiligo
- Yellow nail syndrome

Further reading:
- Sayah A, English JC III (2005) Rheumatoid arthritis: a review of the cutaneous manifestations. J Am Acad Dermatol 53(2):191–209

Sexually Promiscuous

- Amebiasis
- Candidiasis

- Chancroid
- *Chlamydia*
- Cytomegalovirus
- Giardiasis
- Gonorrhea
- Granuloma inguinale
- Hepatitis A virus
- Hepatitis B virus
- Hepatitis C virus
- Herpes simplex virus
- Human herpes virus, type 8
- Human immunodeficiency virus
- Human papillomavirus virus
- Human T cell lymphotrophic virus
- Lymphogranuloma venereum
- Mobiluncus infection
- Molluscum contagiosum
- Nongococcal urethritis
- Pediculosis pubis
- Scabies
- Syphilis
- Trichomoniasis

Further reading:
- Wang QQ, Mabey D, Peeling RW et al (2002) Validation of syndromic algorithm for the management of genital ulcer diseases in China. Int J STD AIDS 13(7):469–474

Sjögren Syndrome

- Amyloidosis
- Annular erythema
- Benign hypergammaglobulinemic purpura of Waldenstrom
- Erythema multiforme-like lesions
- Erythema nodosum

- Photosensitivity
- Pyoderma gangrenosum
- Sweet's syndrome
- Urticarial vasculitis
- Vaginal dryness
- Vasculitis
- Xerophthalmia
- Xerosis
- Xerostomia

Further reading:
- Soy M, Piskin S (2007) Cutaneous findings in patients with primary Sjogren's syndrome. Clin Rheumatol 26(8):1350–1352

Smoker

- Chronic cutaneous lupus erythematosus
- Favre–Racouchot syndrome
- Hidradenitis suppurativa
- Keratoacanthoma
- Mid dermal elastolysis
- Metastatic lung cancer
- Oral leukoplakia
- Nicotine patch allergy
- Nicotine stomatitis
- Palmoplantar pustulosis
- Psoriasis
- Squamous cell carcinoma
- Thromboangiitis obliterans
- Trench mouth

Further reading:
- Freiman A, Bird G, Metelitsa AI, Barankin B, Lauzon GJ (2004) Cutaneous effects of smoking. J Cutan Med Surg 8(6):415–423

Spinal Dysraphism

- Acrochordons
- Aplasia cutis congenita
- Capillary malformations
- Cobb syndrome
- Congenital melanocytic nevi
- Dermal sinuses
- Dimples
- Ependymomas
- Hemangiomas
- Hyperpigmentation
- Hypertrichosis (faun tail)
- Hypopigmentation
- Lipomas
- Lipomyelomeningoceles
- Meningoceles
- Plexiform neurofibromas
- Pseudotails
- Telangiectasias
- Teratomas
- True tails

Further reading:
- Guggisberg D, Hadj-Rabia S, Viney C et al (2004) Skin markers of occult spinal dysraphism in children: a review of 54 cases. Arch Dermatol 140(9):1109–1115

Stroke

- Antiphospholipid antibody syndrome
- Atrial myxoma
- Behçet's disease
- Cholesterol emboli

- Cryoglobulinemia
- Disseminated intravascular coagulation
- Endocarditis
- Fabry's disease
- Hereditary hypercoagulability
- Intravascular lymphoma
- Malignant atrophic papulosis
- Neurosyphilis
- Septic emboli
- Sneddon syndrome
- Systemic lupus erythematosus
- Thrombotic thrombocytopenic purpura

Further reading:
- Al Aboud D, Broshtilova V, Al Aboud K (2005) Dermatological aspects of cerebrovascular diseases. Acta Dermatovenerol Alp Panonica Adriat 14(1):9–14

Sun Exposure, Chronic

- Actinic granuloma
- Actinic keratosis
- Atypical fibroxanthoma
- Basal cell carcinoma
- Bateman's purpura
- Bullous lesions
- Colloid milium (Fig. 2.5)
- Cutis rhomboidalis nuchae
- Elastotic nodules of the ear
- Favre–Racouchot syndrome
- Fibroelastolytic papulosis
- Keratoacanthoma
- Marginal keratoderma
- Melanoma
- Merkel cell carcinoma
- Poikiloderma of Civatte

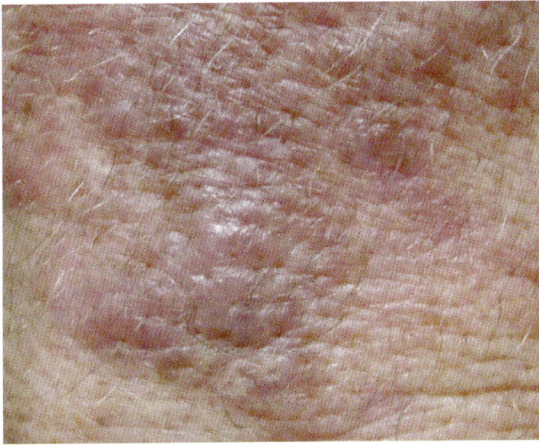

Fig. 2.5 Colloid milium (Courtesy of W. T. Massengale)

- Solar lentigines
- Squamous cell carcinoma
- Stellate pseudoscars
- Telangiectasia
- Weathering nodules
- Venous lake

Further reading:
- Heras JA, Jimenez F, Soguero ML et al (2007) Bullous solar elastosis. Clin Exp Dermatol 32(3):272–274

Tick Bite

- Babesiosis
- Boutonneuse fever
- Colorado tick fever
- Human granulocytic anaplasmosis
- Human monocytic ehrlichiosis
- Lyme disease
- Q fever

- Rocky Mountain spotted fever
- Southern tick-associated rash illness
- Tick-borne relapsing fever
- Tularemia

Further reading:
- McGinley-Smith DE, Tsao SS (2003) Dermatoses from ticks. J Am Acad Dermatol 49(3):363–392

Turner Syndrome

- Alopecia areata
- Cardiovascular defects
- Cystic hygroma
- Gonadal dysgenesis
- Halo nevus
- Keloids
- Lymphedema
- Multiple melanocytic nevi
- Renal malformations
- Short stature
- Thyroid disease
- Webbed neck
- Widely spaced nipples

Further reading:
- Lowenstein EJ, Kim KH, Glick SA (2004) Turner's syndrome in dermatology. J Am Acad Dermatol 50(5):767–776

Virilization

- Abnormal menstrual cycle
- Acne
- Androgenic alopecia
- Clitoral hypertrophy

- Decreased breast size
- Deep voice
- Hirsutism

Further reading:
- Lee AT, Zane LT (2007) Dermatologic manifestations of polycystic ovary syndrome. Am J Clin Dermatol 8(4):201–219

X-Linked Dominant Inheritance Pattern

- Albright hereditary osteodystrophy
- Bazex's syndrome
- CHILD syndrome
- Congenital generalized hypertrichosis
- Conradi–Hunermann syndrome
- Goltz syndrome
- Incontinentia pigmenti
- Oral–facial–digital syndrome

X-Linked Recessive Inheritance Pattern

- Anhidrotic ectodermal dysplasia
- Bruton's agammaglobulinemia
- Chronic granulomatous disease
- Crandall's syndrome
- Duncan's syndrome
- Dyskeratosis congenita
- Fabry's disease
- Hunter syndrome
- Keratosis follicularis spinulosa decalvans
- Lesch–Nyhan disease
- Menkes kinky-hair disease
- Severe combined immunodeficiency
- Wiskott–Aldrich syndrome
- X-linked ichthyosis

Abdomen

- Accessory nipple
- Bowen's disease
- Cherry angioma
- Cutaneous endometriosis
- Desmoid tumor
- Dysplastic nevi
- Fistula
- Hernia
- Larva currens
- Lipoma
- Melanocytic nevus
- Metastatic disease
- Nickel contact dermatitis
- Omphalomesenteric duct remnant
- Pemphigoid gestationis
- Pruritic urticarial papules and plaques of pregnancy
- Scabies
- Seborrheic keratosis
- Striae atrophicans
  - Strongyloidiasis
- Zoster

Acral Necrosis/Purpura (Fig. 3.1)

- Achenbach syndrome
- Acrokeratosis paraneoplastica of Bazex
- Antiphospholipid antibody syndrome
- Arteriosclerosis
- Calciphylaxis
- Carcinoma
- Cholesterol emboli
- Coumadin blue-toe syndrome
- CREST syndrome
- Cryoglobulinemia
- Endocarditis
- Erythema multiforme
- Gonococcemia
- Hepatitis C virus infection
- Hyperglobulinemic purpura
- Left atrial myxoma
- Leukocytoclastic vasculitis
- Lupus erythematosus
- Metastatic disease
- Mixed connective-tissue disease
- Myeloma

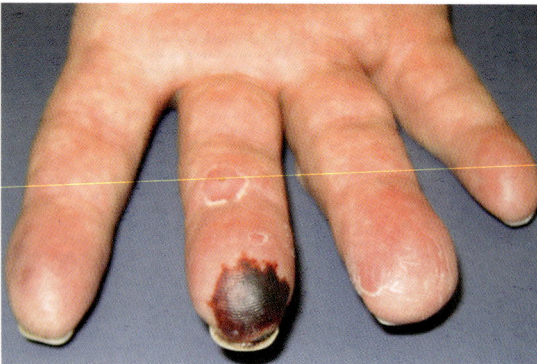

Fig. 3.1 Acral purpura

- Paraneoplastic acral vascular syndrome
- Parvovirus B19 infection
- Perniosis
- Polyarteritis nodosa
- Polycythemia
- Raynaud's phenomenon
- Rocky Mountain spotted fever
- Scleroderma
- Sepsis
- Septic emboli
- Sjögren's syndrome
- Sneddon syndrome
- Wegener's granulomatosis

Further reading:

- Poszepczynska-Guigne E, Viguier M, Chosidow O et al (2002) Paraneoplastic acral vascular syndrome: epidemiologic features, clinical manifestations, and disease sequelae. J Am Acad Dermatol 47(1):47–52

Agminated

- Acquired melanocytic nevi
- Atypical nevi
- Blue nevi
- Collagenomas
- Dermatofibroma
- Dermatofibrosarcoma protuberans
- Elastomas
- Leiomyomata
- Lentigines
- Melanoma metastasis
- Nevus lipomatosus
- Nevus spilus
- Neurilemmomas
- Pyogenic granulomas

- Segmental angiofibromas
- Segmental neurofibromatosis
- Spitz nevi
- Trichoepitheliomas
- Xanthogranuloma

Further reading:
- Torrelo A, Baselga E, Nagore E et al (2005) Delineation of the various shapes and patterns of nevi. Eur J Dermatol 15(6):439–450

Alopecia, Acquired Nonscarring

- Alopecia areata
- Androgenetic alopecia
- Drug-induced alopecia
- Hair-shaft disorders
- Iron deficiency
- Lipedematous alopecia
- Loose anagen hair
- Lupus hair
- Psoriasis
- Seborrheic dermatitis
- Secondary syphilis
- Telogen effluvium
- Temporal arteritis
- Thyroid disease
- Traction alopecia
- Trichorrhexis nodosa
- Trichotillomania

Evaluation

- Antinuclear antibodies
- Complete blood count

- DHEA-S
- Ferritin
- Fungal culture
- Hair mount
- Syphilis serologic test
- Testosterone
- Thyroid function test

Further reading:
- Wiedemeyer K, Schill WB, Loser C (2004) Diseases on hair follicles leading to hair loss part I: nonscarring alopecias. Skinmed 3(4):209–214

Alopecia, Acquired Scarring

- Actinic keratosis
- Alopecia neoplastica
- Aplasia cutis
- Bacterial infection
- Basal cell carcinoma
- Burns
- Central centrifugal cicatricial alopecia
- Cicatricial pemphigoid
- Discoid lupus erythematosus
- Epidermolysis bullosa
- Erosive pustular dermatosis
- Favus
- Folliculitis decalvans
- Frontal fibrosing alopecia
- Keratosis follicularis spinulosa decalvans
- Kerion
- Lichen planopilaris
- Lymphoma
- Metastasis
- Morphea

- Necrobiosis lipoidica
- Nevus sebaceous
- Porphyria cutanea tarda
- Radiation
- Sarcoidosis
- Squamous cell carcinoma
- Scleroderma
- Tinea capitis
- Trauma
- Zoster

Evaluation

- Antinuclear antibodies
- Bacterial culture
- Biopsy with elastic tissue, PAS, and mucin stains
- Direct immunofluorescence
- Fungal culture

Further reading:
- Ross EK, Tan E, Shapiro J (2005) Update on primary cicatricial alopecias. J Am Acad Dermatol 53(1):1–37

Alopecia/Hypotrichosis, Congenital

Localized

- Aplasia cutis congenita
- Dermoid cyst
- Encephalocele
- Epidermal nevus
- Hair follicle hamartoma
- Hallermann–Streiff syndrome (sutural)
- Incontinentia pigmenti (vertex)
- Meningocele

- Nevus sebaceous
- Temporal triangular alopecia

Diffuse

- Acrodermatitis enteropathica
- Atrichia with papular lesions
- Bazex–Dupre–Christol syndrome
- Cartilage–hair hypoplasia
- Citrullinemia
- Coffin–Siris syndrome
- Congenital hypothyroidism
- Conradi–Hunermann syndrome
- Ectodermal dysplasias
- IFAP syndrome
- KID syndrome
- Marie Unna hypotrichosis
- Marinesco–Sjögren syndrome
- Menkes kinky-hair disease
- Monilethrix
- Neonatal telogen effluvium
- Netherton's syndrome
- Nutritional deficiency
- Pili torti
- Progeria
- Roberts syndrome
- Schopf–Schulz–Passarge syndrome
- Trichorhinophalangeal syndrome
- Trichorrhexis invaginata
- Trichorrhexis nodosa
- Trichothiodystrophy

Further reading:
- Lenane P, Pope E, Krafchik B (2005) Congenital alopecia areata. J Am Acad Dermatol 52(2 Suppl 1):8–11

Anesthetic

- Congenital sensory neuropathy
- Leprosy
- Necrotizing fasciitis
- Neuropathic ulcer
- Syringomyelia
- Tabes dorsalis
- Trigeminal trophic syndrome

Further reading:
- Wang YS, Wong CH, Tay YK (2007) Staging of necrotizing fasciitis based on the evolving cutaneous features. Int J Dermatol 46(10):1036–1041

Angioid Streaks

- Acromegaly
- Cowden syndrome
- Ehlers–Danlos syndrome
- Iron deficiency
- Lead poisoning
- Paget's disease of bone
- Pseudoxanthoma elasticum
- Sickle cell disease
- Trauma
- Tuberous sclerosis

Further reading:
- Agarwal A, Patel P, Adkins T et al (2005) Spectrum of pattern dystrophy in pseudoxanthoma elasticum. Arch Ophthalmol 123(7):923–928

Annular

- Actinic granuloma
- Alopecia mucinosa

- Annular erythema of infancy
- Annular lichenoid dermatitis of youth
- Arthropod bite reaction
- Creeping eruption
- Cutaneous T cell lymphoma
- Dermatomyofibroma
- Discoid lupus erythematosus
- Erythema annulare centrifugum (Fig. 3.2)
- Erythema multiforme
- Elastosis perforans serpiginosa
- Erythema marginatum
- Fixed drug eruption
- Granuloma annulare
- Granuloma multiforme
- Ichthyosis linearis circumflexa
- Impetigo
- Jessner's lymphocytic infiltrate
- Leishmaniasis
- Leprosy
- Leukemia and lymphoma cutis

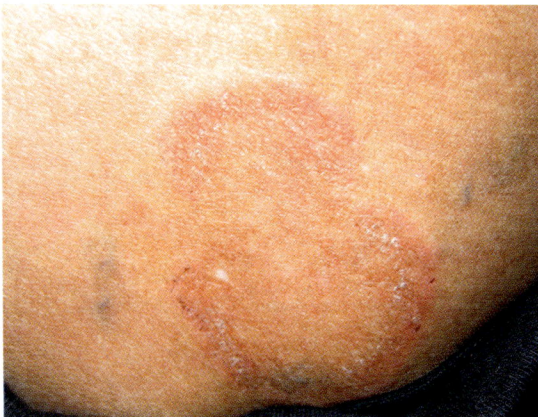

Fig. 3.2 Erythema annulare centrifugum

- Lichen planus
- Linear IgA bullous dermatosis
- Lupus vulgaris
- Lyme disease
- Majocchi's pigmented purpuric dermatosis
- Miescher's granuloma
- Meyerson nevus
- Morphea
- Necrobiosis lipoidica
- Neonatal lupus erythematosus
- Parapsoriasis
- Polymorphous light eruption
- Porokeratosis
- Pityriasis rosea
- Psoriasis
- Sarcoidosis
- Subacute cutaneous lupus erythematosus
- Seborrheic dermatitis
- Secondary and tertiary syphilis
- Systemic lupus erythematosus
- Subcorneal pustular dermatosis
- Sweet's syndrome
- Tertiary yaws
- Tinea corporis
- Tumid lupus
- Urticaria
- Urticarial dermatitis
- Urticarial vasculitis
- Wells syndrome

Further reading:

- Hsu S, Le EH, Khoshevis MR (2001) Differential diagnosis of annular lesions. Am Fam Physician 64(2):289–296

Atrophy

- Acrodermatitis chronica atrophicans
- Anetoderma
- Aplasia cutis congenita
- Atrophoderma of Pasini and Pierini
- Cutaneous T cell lymphoma
- Cutis laxa
- Degos disease
- Dermatomyositis
- Ehlers–Danlos syndrome
- Erosive pustular dermatosis
- Goltz syndrome
- Hallermann–Streiff syndrome
- Kindler syndrome
- Lichen planus
- Lichen sclerosus et atrophicus
- Linear atrophoderma
- Lupus erythematosus
- Medallion-like dermal dendrocyte hamartoma
- Photoaging
- Pityriasis versicolor atrophicans
- Progeria
- Pseudoxanthoma elasticum
- Radiation dermatitis
- Sarcoidosis
- Striae atrophicans
- Steroid atrophy
- Xeroderma pigmentosum

Further reading:
- Aksoy B, Ustün H, Gülbahçe R et al (2009) Confetti-like macular atrophy: a new entity? J Dermatol 36(11):592–597

Axilla

- Acanthosis nigricans
- Apocrine gland neoplasm
- Asymmetric periflexural exanthem
- Axillary granular parakeratosis
- Contact dermatitis
- Crowe's sign of neurofibromatosis
- Cutis laxa
- Dowling–Degos disease
- Drug eruption
- Erythrasma
- Extramammary Paget's disease
- Fox–Fordyce disease
- Granulomatous slack skin
- Hailey–Hailey disease (Fig. 3.3)
- Hidradenitis suppurativa
- Inverse pityriasis rosea
- Inverse psoriasis
- Lymphangiectasias
- Pemphigus
- Plane xanthoma
- Pseudoxanthoma elasticum
- Seborrheic dermatitis
- Tinea versicolor
- Trichomycosis axillaris

Further reading:
- Chagpar AB, Heim K, Carron KR et al (2007) Extramammary Paget's disease of the axilla: an unusual case. Breast J 13(3):291–293

Back, Christmas Tree Pattern

- Erythema dyschromicum perstans
- Lichenoid drug eruption

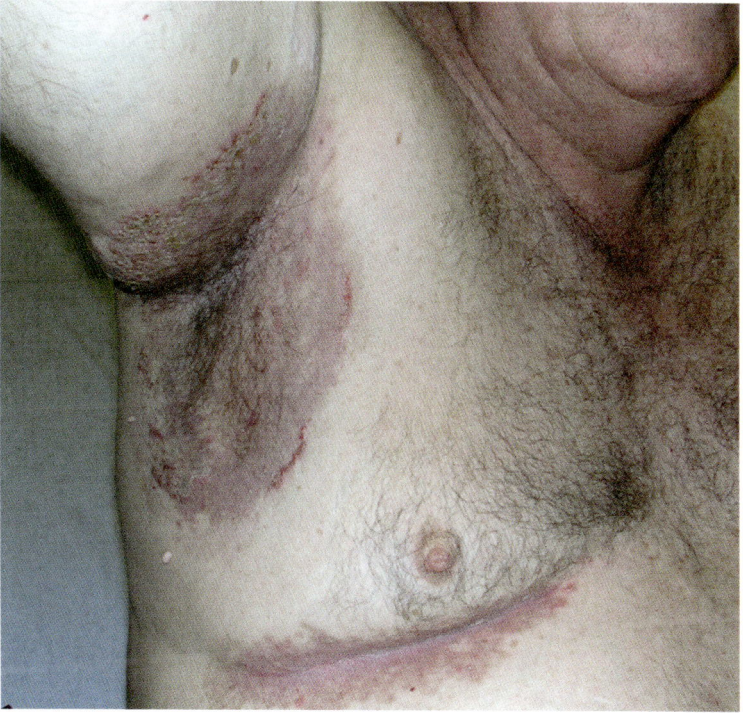

Fig. 3.3 Hailey–Hailey disease (Courtesy of A. Record)

- Kaposi's sarcoma (HIV-associated)
- Pityriasis lichenoides
- Pityriasis rosea
- Sign of Leser–Trelat

Further reading:

- Chuh AA (2002) Rash orientation in pityriasis rosea: a qualitative study. Eur J Dermatol 12(3):253–256

Balanoposthitis

- Allergic contact dermatitis
- Amebiasis
- Candidiasis
- Chlamydia
- Chronic inflammation
- Circinate balanitis of reactive arthritis (Fig. 3.4)
- Condom allergy
- Erythema multiforme
- Extramammary Paget's disease
- Fixed drug eruption
- Foscarnet ulceration
- Herpes simplex virus infection
- Imiquimod
- Inflammatory bowel disease
- Lichen nitidus
- Lichen planus
- Lichen sclerosus

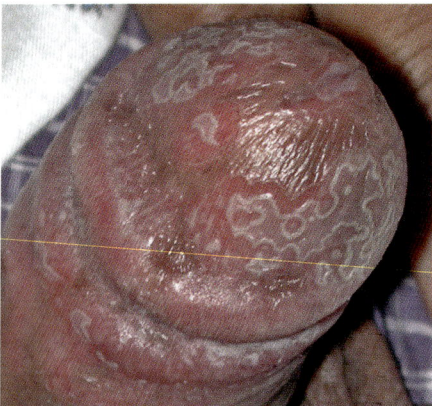

Fig. 3.4 Circinate balanitis (Courtesy of K. Guidry)

- Morphea
- Pilonidal sinus
- Plasma cell balanitis
- Psoriasis
- Scabies
- Seborrheic dermatitis
- Squamous dysplasias
- Streptococcal infection
- Syphilis
- Trauma
- Trichomoniasis

Further reading:

- Banerjee R, Banerjee K, Datta A (2006) Condom leukoderma. Indian J Dermatol Venereol Leprol 72(6):452–453
- Sakuma S, Komiya H (2005) Balanitis caused by *Streptococcus pyogenes*: a report of two cases. Int J STD AIDS 16(9):644–645

Bathing Trunk Distribution

- Angiokeratoma corporis diffusum
- Bathing suit lamellar ichthyosis
- Giant congenital nevus
- Large plaque parapsoriasis
- *Pseudomonas* folliculitis
- Mycosis fungoides
- Seabather's eruption
- Viral exanthem

Further reading:

- Huerta-Brogeras M, Aviles Izquierdo JA, Hernanz Hermosa JM et al (2005) Petechial exanthem in "bathing trunk" distribution caused by parvovirus B19 infection. Pediatr Dermatol 22(5):430–433
- Jacyk WK (2005) Bathing-suit ichthyosis. A peculiar phenotype of lamellar ichthyosis in South African blacks. Eur J Dermatol 15(6):433–436

Beau's Lines/Onychomadesis

- Acrodermatitis enteropathica
- Antibiotic usage
- Chemotherapy
- Coxsackievirus infection
- Cutaneous T cell lymphoma
- Drug reaction
- Epidermolysis bullosa
- Erythroderma
- Febrile illness
- Hypoparathyroidism
- Kawasaki disease
- Paronychia
- Pemphigus
- Radiation
- Retinoid therapy
- Stevens–Johnson syndrome
- Syphilis
- Trauma

Further reading:
- Chen W (2007) Nail changes associated with chemotherapy in children. J Eur Acad Dermatol Venereol 21(2):186–190

Blepharitis

- Cicatricial pemphigoid
- Contact dermatitis
- Demodicosis
- Discoid lupus erythematosus
- Drug eruption
- Herpes simplex virus infection

- Molluscum contagiosum
- Pediculosis
- Rosacea
- Seborrheic dermatitis
- Sjögren's syndrome
- Staphylococcal blepharitis

Further reading:
- Stone DU, Chodosh J (2004) Ocular rosacea: an update on pathogenesis and therapy. Curr Opin Ophthalmol 15(6):499–502

Blue Lesions

- Acrocyanosis
- Amiodarone pigmentation
- Antimalarial pigmentation
- Argyria
- Blue nevus
- Blue tattoo
- Chlorpromazine pigmentation
- Dermal melanocytosis
- Erythema dyschromicum perstans
- Hidrocystoma
- Hyaluronic acid nodule
- Maculae cerulae
- Melanoma
- Minocycline pigmentation
- Ochronosis
- Purpura

Further reading:
- Fernandez-Flores A, Montero MG (2006) Ashy dermatosis, or "Tyndall-effect" dermatosis. Dermatol Online J 12(4):14

Breast

- Acanthosis nigricans
- Bacterial mastitis
- Basal cell carcinoma
- Bowen's disease
- Breast cancer, inflammatory
- Candidiasis
- Contact dermatitis, irritant, or allergic
- Darier's disease
- Factitial
- Hidradenitis suppurativa
- Jogger's nipple
- Leiomyomas
- Lichen simplex chronicus
- Lupus mastitis
- Lupus panniculitis
- Montgomery's tubercles
- Morphea
- Mycosis fungoides
- Neurofibroma
- Nevoid hyperkeratosis
- Nipple eczema (atopic dermatitis)
- Paget's disease
- Papillary adenoma
- Psoriasis
- Radiation dermatitis
- Seborrheic dermatitis
- Seborrheic keratosis
- Tuberculous mastitis
- Warfarin necrosis

Further reading:
- Whitaker-Worth DL, Carlone V, Susser WS et al (2000) Dermatologic diseases of the breast and nipple. J Am Acad Dermatol 43(5 Pt 1):733–751

Bullous Drug Eruption

- Bullous acral erythema
- Bullous leukocytoclastic vasculitis
- Bullous Sweet's syndrome
- Drug-induced linear IgA bullous dermatosis
- Drug-induced pemphigoid
- Drug-induced pemphigus
- Eczematous drug eruptions
- Erythema multiforme
- Fixed drug eruption
- Halogenoderma
- Pseudoporphyria
- Stevens–Johnson syndrome
- Toxic epidermal necrolysis

Further reading:
- Rai R, Jain R, Kaur I, Kumar B (2002) Multifocal bullous fixed drug eruption mimicking Stevens–Johnson syndrome. Indian J Dermatol Venereol Leprol 68(3):175–176

Canities, Premature

- Ataxia–telangiectasia
- Book syndrome
- Hereditary premature canities
- Myotonic dystrophy
- Oasthouse syndrome
- Piebaldism
- Progeria
- Prolidase deficiency
- Rothmund–Thomson syndrome
- Seckel syndrome
- Sudden whitening of hair (alopecia areata)

- Vitiligo
- Waardenburg syndrome
- Werner syndrome

Further reading:
- Tobin DJ, Paus R (2001) Graying: gerontobiology of the hair follicle pigmentary unit. Exp Gerontol 36(1):29–54

Cheilitis

- Acrodermatitis enteropathica
- Actinic cheilitis
- Actinic prurigo cheilitis
- Angular cheilitis
- Atopic dermatitis
- Candidiasis
- Cheilitis exfoliativa
- Cheilitis glandularis
- Cheilitis granulomatosis
- Dental care products
- Cosmetics
- Erythema multiforme
- Herpes simplex virus infection
- Lip licking
- Lipstick allergy
- Photosensitive cheilitis
- Plasma cell cheilitis
- Retinoid cheilitis
- Sarcoidosis
- Stevens–Johnson syndrome
- Sunscreen allergy
- Syphilis
- Toothpaste allergy
- Vitamin deficiency

Further reading:

- Due E, Wulf HC (2006) Cheilitis: the only presentation of photosensitivity. J Eur Acad Dermatol Venereol 20(6):766–767

Clubbing

- Acromegaly
- Aortic aneurysm
- Bacterial endocarditis
- Bronchiectasis
- Bronchogenic carcinoma
- CINCA syndrome (NOMID syndrome)
- Congestive heart failure
- Cyanotic congenital heart disease
- Cystic fibrosis
- HIV infection
- Hyperthyroidism
- Hypertrophic osteoarthropathy (thyroid acropachy)
- Inflammatory bowel disease
- Liver disorders
- Lung abscess
- Lymphoma
- Mesothelioma
- Pachydermoperiostosis
- Parasitic infestations
- POEMS syndrome
- Pulmonary fibrosis
- Sarcoidosis
- Tuberculosis

Further reading:

- Spicknall KE, Zirwas MJ, English JC III (2005) Clubbing: an update on diagnosis, differential diagnosis, pathophysiology, and clinical relevance. J Am Acad Dermatol 52(6):1020–1028

Collarette, Peripheral

- Acquired digital fibrokeratoma
- Clear cell acanthoma
- Pityriasis lichenoides chronica
- Pityriasis rosea
- Pyogenic granuloma
- Secondary syphilis
- Staphylococcal furunculosis
- Subacute cutaneous lupus erythematosus
- Transient neonatal pustular melanosis

Further reading:
- Levy AL, Simpson G, Skinner RB Jr (2006) Medical pearl: circle of desquamation: a clue to the diagnosis of folliculitis and furunculosis caused by *Staphylococcus aureus*. J Am Acad Dermatol 55(6):1079–1080

Collodion Baby

- Conradi–Hünermann–Happle syndrome
- Ectodermal dysplasias
- Hay–Wells syndrome
- Infantile Gaucher disease
- Lamellar ichthyosis
- Netherton syndrome
- Neutral lipid storage disease
- Nonbullous congenital ichthyosiform erythroderma
- Self-healing collodion baby
- Sjögren–Larsson syndrome
- Trichothiodystrophy (IBIDS)

Further reading:
- Van Gysel D, Lijnen RL, Moekti SS et al (2002) Collodion baby: a follow-up study of 17 cases. J Eur Acad Dermatol Venereol 16(5):472–475

Crepitus

- Anaerobic cellulitis
- Clostridial cellulitis
- Clostridial myonecrosis
- Iatrogenic subcutaneous emphysema
- Necrotizing fasciitis
- Streptococcal myositis
- Synergistic necrotizing gangrene
- Traumatic subcutaneous emphysema
- Vascular gangrene

Further reading:
- Fox A, Sheick H, Ekwobi C, Ho-Asjoe M (2007) Benign surgical emphysema of the hand and upper limb: gas is not always gangrene – a report of two cases. Emerg Med J 24(11):798–799

Cutaneous Horn

- Actinic keratosis
- Angiokeratoma
- Angioma
- Arsenical keratosis
- Basal cell carcinoma
- Benign lichenoid keratosis
- Bowen's disease
- Cutaneous leishmaniasis
- Dermatofibroma
- Discoid lupus erythematosus
- Epidermal inclusion cyst
- Epidermal nevus
- Granular cell tumor
- Inverted follicular keratosis
- Kaposi's sarcoma

- Keratoacanthoma
- Melanoma
- Nevus sebaceous
- Paget's disease
- Pilomatrixoma
- Prurigo nodularis
- Pyogenic granuloma
- Renal cell carcinoma
- Sebaceous adenoma
- Sebaceous carcinoma
- Seborrheic keratosis
- Squamous cell carcinoma (Fig. 3.5)
- Trichilemmoma
- Verruca vulgaris

Further reading:

- Cristobal MC, Urbina F, Espinoza A (2007) Cutaneous horn malignant melanoma. Dermatol Surg 33(8):997–999
- Mencia-Gutierrez E, Gutierrez-Diaz E, Redondo-Marcos I et al (2004) Cutaneous horns of the eyelid: a clinicopathological study of 48 cases. J Cutan Pathol 31(8):539–543

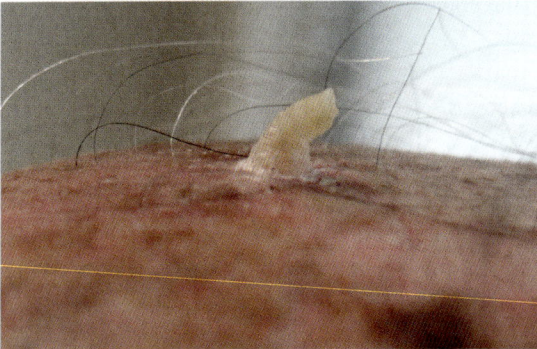

Fig. 3.5 Cutaneous horn

Cyst

- Branchial cleft cyst
- Bronchogenic cyst
- Cutaneous ciliated cyst
- Cutaneous metaplastic synovial cyst
- Cystic basal cell carcinoma
- Dermoid cyst
- Digital mucous cyst
- Ear pit cyst
- Epidermoid cyst
- Ganglion cyst
- Hidrocystoma
- Median raphe cyst
- Milium
- Mucocele
- Omphalomesenteric duct cyst
- Phaeohyphomycotic cyst
- Pigmented follicular cyst
- Pilonidal cyst
- Proliferating epidermoid cyst
- Proliferating trichilemmal cyst
- Pseudocyst of the auricle
- Steatocystoma
- Thyroglossal duct cyst
- Trichilemmal cyst
- Vellus hair cyst
- Verrucous cyst

Further reading:

- Golden BA, Zide MF (2005) Cutaneous cysts of the head and neck. J Oral Maxillofac Surg 63(11):1613–1619

Deck-Chair Sign

- Adult T cell leukemia/lymphoma
- Angioimmunoblastic T cell lymphoma
- Drug-induced erythroderma
- Mycosis fungoides
- Papuloerythroderma of Ofuji
- Waldenstrom's macroglobulinemia

Further reading:
- Ferran M, Gallardo F, Baena V et al (2006) The "deck chair sign" in specific cutaneous involvement by angioimmunoblastic T-cell lymphoma. Dermatology 213(1):50–52

Dermatoglyphics, Absent

- Basan syndrome
- Dermatopathia pigmentosa reticularis
- Naegeli–Franceschetti–Jadassohn syndrome
- Rapp–Hodgkin syndrome
- X-linked hypohidrotic ectodermal dysplasia

Further reading:
- Lugassy J, Itin P, Ishida-Yamamoto A et al (2006) Naegeli–Franceschetti–Jadassohn syndrome and dermatopathia pigmentosa reticularis: two allelic ectodermal dysplasias caused by dominant mutations in KRT14. Am J Hum Genet 79(4):724–730

Diaper Dermatitis

- Acrodermatitis enteropathica
- Allergic contact dermatitis
- Biotin deficiency
- Bullous mastocytosis
- Candidiasis
- Chafing dermatitis
- Child abuse

- Congenital syphilis
- Cystic fibrosis
- Eczema herpeticum
- Epidermolysis bullosa simplex
- Essential fatty acid deficiency
- Granuloma gluteale infantum
- Impetigo
- Irritant contact dermatitis
- Jacquet's erosive diaper dermatitis
- Langerhans cell histiocytosis
- Linear IgA bullous dermatosis
- Miliaria
- Perianal strep infection
- Psoriasis
- Scabies
- Seborrheic dermatitis
- Staphylococcal scalded-skin syndrome

Further reading:

- Scheinfeld N (2005) Diaper dermatitis: a review and brief survey of eruptions of the diaper area. Am J Clin Dermatol 6(5):273–281

Draining/Sinus Tracts

- Actinomycosis
- Amebiasis
- Antitrypsin deficiency panniculitis
- Botryomycosis
- Bronchogenic cyst
- Chromoblastomycosis
- Cutaneous Crohn's disease
- Cutaneous myiasis
- Dental sinus
- Elephantiasis verrucosa
- Enterocutaneous fistula

- Hidradenitis suppurativa
- Hodgkin's disease
- Lymphogranuloma venereum
- Malakoplakia
- Melioidosis
- Mycetoma
- *Mycobacterium fortuitum*, *M. chelonei*, or *M. abscessus* infection
- Nocardiosis
- Nodular vasculitis
- Osteomyelitis
- Pancreatic panniculitis
- Pilonidal sinus
- Preauricular sinus
- Prototheccosis
- Pyoderma faciale
- Scrofuloderma

Further reading:
- Erkilic S, Erbagci Z, Kocer NE et al (2004) Cutaneous involvement in Hodgkin's lymphoma: report of two cases. J Dermatol 31(4):330–334

Dyschromia

- Arsenical pigmentary alteration
- Dyschromatosis symmetrica hereditaria
- Dyschromatosis universalis hereditaria
- Dyschromic amyloidosis cutis
- Epidermolysis bullosa simplex with mottled pigmentation
- Kwashiorkor
- Monobenzyl ether of hydroquinone
- Syphilitic leukoderma
- Tinea versicolor
- Xeroderma pigmentosum
- Ziprkowski–Margolis syndrome

Further reading:

- Ohtoshi E, Matsumura Y, Nishigori C et al (2001) Useful applications of DNA repair tests for differential diagnosis of atypical dyschromatosis symmetrica hereditaria from xeroderma pigmentosum. Br J Dermatol 144(1):162–168

Ear

- Actinic keratosis
- Allergic contact dermatitis
- Amyloidosis
- Angiolymphoid hyperplasia with eosinophilia
- *Aspergillus otomycosis*
- Atypical fibroxanthoma
- Auricular pseudocyst
- Basal cell carcinoma
- Borrelial lymphocytoma
- Calcinosis cutis
- Candidiasis
- Ceruminous gland tumor
- Chondrodermatitis nodularis helicis
- Cocaine-induced vasculopathy (Fig. 3.6)

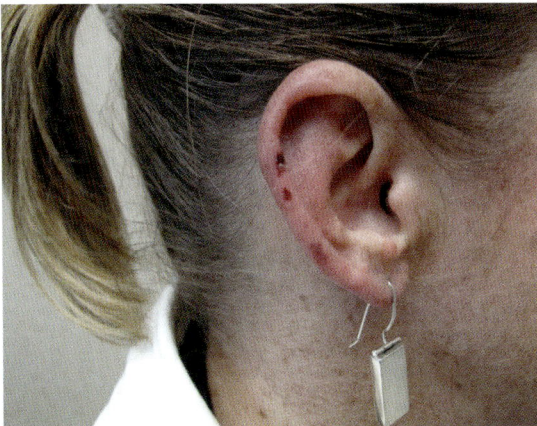

Fig. 3.6 Cocaine-related vasculitis

- Discoid lupus erythematosus
- Eczema
- Elastotic nodule
- Extramammary Paget's disease
- Foreign body
- Gout
- Herpes zoster (Ramsay–Hunt syndrome)
- Infectious eczematoid dermatitis
- Infectious perichondritis
- Juvenile spring eruption
- Keloid
- Langerhans cell histiocytosis
- Leishmaniasis (chiclero ulcer)
- Leprosy
- Lobomycosis
- Lupus pernio
- Milia en plaque
- Multicentric reticulohistiocytosis
- Nickel dermatitis
- Ochronosis
- Otitis externa
- Otomycosis
- Papular mucinosis
- Perniosis
- Pneumocystosis
- Pseudomonas infection
- Psoriasis
- Relapsing polychondritis
- Sarcoidosis
- Seborrheic dermatitis
- Seborrheic keratosis
- Squamous cell carcinoma
- Syphilis
- Traumatic auricular hematoma
- Tuberculosis

- Venous lake
- Weathering nodule

Further reading:
- Mahalingam M, Palko M, Steinberg-Benjes L et al (2002) Amyloidosis of the auricular concha: an uncommon variant of localized cutaneous amyloidosis. Am J Dermatopathol 24(5):447–448

Elbows and Knees

- Calcinosis cutis
- Dermatitis herpetiformis
- Dermatomyositis (Gottron's sign)
- Epidermolysis bullosa
- Erythema elevatum diutinum
- Erythema multiforme
- Eruptive xanthoma
- Frictional lichenoid dermatosis
- Granuloma annulare
- Gonococcemia
- Gout
- Juvenile pityriasis rubra pilaris
- Keratosis circumscripta
- Lichen simplex chronicus
- Lipoid proteinosis
- Papillon–Lefèvre syndrome
- Progressive symmetric erythrokeratodermia
- Prototothecosis
- Psoriasis
- Rheumatoid nodule
- Scabies
- Tuberous xanthoma

Further reading:
- Brumwell EP, Murphy SJ (2007) Keratosis circumscripta revisited: a case report and review of the literature. Cutis 79(5):363–366

Erythronychia, Longitudinal

- Amyloidosis
- Darier's disease (Fig. 3.7)
- Glomus tumor
- Lichen planus
- Onychopapilloma
- Squamous cell carcinoma
- Warty dyskeratoma

Further reading:
- de Berker DA, Perrin C, Baran R (2004) Localized longitudinal erythronychia: diagnostic significance and physical explanation. Arch Dermatol 140(10):1253–1257

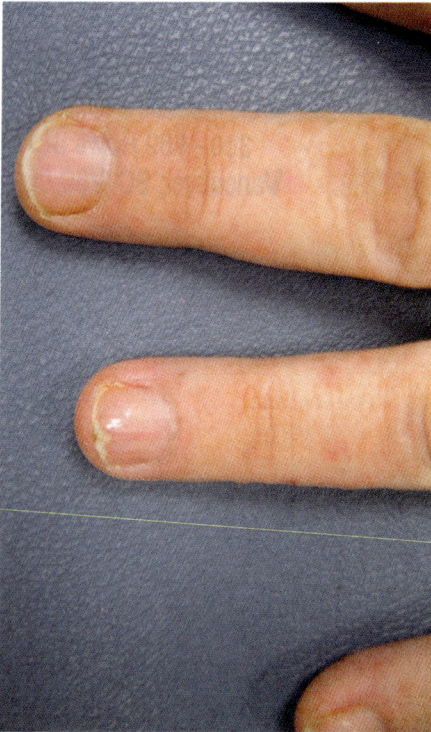

Fig. 3.7 Darier's disease

Esthiomene (Genital Elephantiasis)

- Granuloma inguinale
- Lymphatic filariasis
- Lymphogranuloma venereum
- Lymphoma
- Syphilis
- Tuberculosis

Further reading:
- Sarkar R, Kaur C, Thami GP, Kanwar AJ (2002) Genital elephantiasis. Int J STD AIDS 13(6):427–429

Exanthem

- Acute HIV infection
- Chicken pox
- DRESS syndrome
- Enterovirus infection
- Erythema infectiosum
- Gianotti–Crosti syndrome
- Helminth infestation
- Measles
- Morbilliform drug eruption
- Picornavirus infection
- Pityriasis rosea
- Roseola
- Rubella
- Scarlet fever
- Secondary syphilis
- Toxic shock syndrome
- Toxoplasmosis

Further reading:
- Drago F, Rampini E, Rebora A (2002) Atypical exanthems: morphology and laboratory investigations may lead to an aetiological diagnosis in about 70% of cases. Br J Dermatol 147(2):255–260

Excoriations

- Acne excoriée
- Amphetamine therapy
- Cocaine abuse
- Dermatitis herpetiformis
- Diabetes
- Drug reactions
- Dry skin
- Hyperthyroidism
- Hypothyroidism
- Internal malignancy
- Liver disease
- Lymphoma
- Myeloma
- Neurotic excoriations
- Opiate abuse
- Parasitic infestation
- Polycythemia vera
- Pregnancy
- Renal disease
- Scabies
- Trigeminal trophic syndrome
- Urticaria

Further reading:
- Fried RG, Fried S (2003) Picking apart the picker: a clinician's guide for management of the patient presenting with excoriations. Cutis 71(4):291–298

Erythroderma, Adult

- Atopic dermatitis
- Autosensitization dermatitis

- Bullous pemphigoid
- Chronic actinic dermatitis
- Congenital ichthyosis
- Darier's disease
- Dermatomyositis
- Dermatophyte infection
- Diffuse cutaneous mastocytosis
- Drug reaction
- Erythrodermic mycosis fungoides
- Graft-vs-host disease
- Hypereosinophilic syndrome
- Id reaction
- Idiopathic
- Lichen planus
- Norwegian crusted scabies
- Onchocerciasis
- Papuloerythroderma of Ofuji
- Paraneoplastic erythroderma
- Paraneoplastic pemphigus
- Pemphigus foliaceus
- Pityriasis rubra pilaris
- Psoriasis
- Reiter's syndrome
- Sarcoidosis
- Seborrheic dermatitis
- Sezary syndrome
- Staphylococcal scalded-skin syndrome
- Stasis dermatitis
- Subacute cutaneous lupus erythematosus
- Systemic contact dermatitis
- Tinea corporis
- Viral eruption
- Zinc deficiency

Associated Medications

- Allopurinol
- Amiodarone
- Amitriptyline
- Amoxicillin
- Ampicillin
- Barbiturates
- Beta-blockers
- Bumetanide
- Bupropion
- Carbamazepine
- Chlorpromazine
- Cimetidine
- Ciprofloxacin
- Clofazimine
- Cytarabine
- Dapsone
- Diazepam
- Diclofenac
- Diltiazem
- Doxorubicin
- Doxycycline
- Etodolac
- Fluconazole
- Furosemide
- Gemfibrozil
- Gold
- Griseofulvin
- Hydroxychloroquine
- Indomethacin
- Iodine
- Isoniazid
- Ketoconazole
- Lithium
- Minocycline

- Naproxen
- Nifedipine
- Nitrofurantoin
- Nitroglycerin
- Omeprazole
- Penicillamine
- Penicillin
- Pentobarbital
- Phenobarbital
- Phenytoin
- Piroxicam
- Propranolol
- Rifampin
- Sulfadoxine
- Sulfamethoxazole
- Sulfasalazine
- Sulfonamides
- Sulfonylurea
- Tetracycline
- Tobramycin
- Trazodone
- Vancomycin
- Verapamil

Evaluation

- Antinuclear antibodies
- Appropriate cancer screening
- Chest radiograph
- Complete blood count
- Liver function test
- Lymph node exam and biopsy
- Nutritional evaluation
- Patch testing
- Potassium hydroxide examination of scale
- Sedimentation rate

- Serum chemistry
- Sezary cell preparation
- Stool for occult blood
- T cell gene rearrangement
- Urinalysis

Further reading:
- Akhyani M, Ghodsi ZS, Toosi S et al (2005) Erythroderma: a clinical study of 97 cases. BMC Dermatol 5:5

Erythroderma, Neonatal/Infantile/Childhood

- Atopic dermatitis
- Bullous congenital ichthyosiform erythroderma
- Diffuse cutaneous mastocytosis
- Drug reaction
- Graft-vs-host disease
- KID syndrome
- Netherton syndrome
- Nonbullous congenital ichthyosiform erythroderma
- Omenn syndrome
- Pityriasis rubra pilaris
- Psoriasis
- Refsum disease
- Scarlet fever
- Seborrheic dermatitis
- Severe combined immunodeficiency
- Sjögren–Larsson disease
- Staphylococcal scalded-skin syndrome
- Wiskott–Aldrich syndrome

Further reading:
- Al-Dhalimi MA (2007) Neonatal and infantile erythroderma: a clinical and follow-up study of 42 cases. J Dermatol 34(5):302–307
- Sehgal VN, Srivastava G (2006) Erythroderma/generalized exfoliative dermatitis in pediatric practice: an overview. Int J Dermatol 45(7):831–839

Eyelid/Periorbital

- Amyloidosis
- Angioedema
- Anthrax
- Ascher syndrome
- Atopic dermatitis
- Basal cell carcinoma
- Bites
- Cat-scratch disease (oculoglandular syndrome)
- Cellulitis
- Chagas disease
- Chalazion
- Contact dermatitis
- Cutaneous T cell lymphoma
- Demodicosis
- Dermatomyositis
- Dermatosis papulosa nigra
- Erysipelas
- Extramammary Paget's disease
- Filariasis
- Herpes simplex virus infection
- Hidrocystoma
- Hyperthyroidism
- Hypothyroidism
- Leishmaniasis
- Leukemia cutis
- Lipoid proteinosis
- Lupus erythematosus
- Lupus miliaris disseminata faciei
- Lupus vulgaris
- Microcystic adnexal carcinoma
- Milia
- Mucinous eccrine carcinoma
- Necrobiotic xanthogranuloma

- Ocular rosacea
- Onchocerciasis
- Ophthalmic zoster
- Orbital cellulitis
- Periorbital cellulitis
- Sarcoidosis
- Sebaceous carcinoma
- Seborrheic dermatitis
- Seborrheic keratosis
- Squamous cell carcinoma
- Stye
- Syringomas
- Trauma
- Trichinosis
- Xanthelasma

Further reading:
- Amin KA, Belsito DV (2006) The aetiology of eyelid dermatitis: a 10-year retrospective analysis. Contact Dermatitis 55(5):280–285

Facial Sparing

- Lichen planus
- Mastocytosis
- Parapsoriasis
- Pityriasis rosea
- Psoriasis
- Scabies

Flagellate

- Bleomycin hyperpigmentation
- Dermatographism

- Dermatomyositis
- Excoriation
- Jellyfish sting
- Mushroom ingestion
- Phytophotodermatitis
- Poison ivy dermatitis

Further reading:
- Yamamoto T, Nishioka K (2006) Flagellate erythema. Int J Dermatol 45(5):627–631

Follicular Hyperkeratosis

- Acquired perforating dermatosis
- Atrophoderma vermiculatum
- Ichthyosis follicularis alopecia and photophobia
- Dermatomyositis pityriasis rubra pilaris-like eruption (Wong type)
- Disseminate and recurrent infundibulofolliculitis
- Keratosis pilaris
- Keratosis pilaris atrophicans
- Keratosis follicularis spinulosa decalvans
- Keratotic spicules of myeloma
- Lichen planopilaris
- Lichen scrofulosorum
- Lichen spinulosa
- Phrynoderma
- Pityriasis rubra pilaris
- Scurvy
- Trichostasis spinulosa

Further reading:
- Lupton JR, Figueroa P, Berberian BJ, Sulica VI (2000) An unusual presentation of dermatomyositis: the type Wong variant revisited. J Am Acad Dermatol 43(5 Pt 2):908–912

Gangrenous

- Antiphospholipid antibody syndrome
- Arteriosclerosis
- Buerger's disease
- Calciphylaxis
- Cholesterol emboli syndrome
- Clostridial myonecrosis
- Cryoglobulinemia
- Disseminated aspergillosis
- Ecthyma gangrenosum
- Fournier's gangrene
- Necrotizing fasciitis
- Necrotizing mucormycosis
- Oxalosis
- Paraneoplastic acral vascular syndrome
- Polyarteritis nodosa
- Progressive synergistic gangrene
- *Pseudomonas* cellulitis
- Pyoderma gangrenosum
- Warfarin necrosis
- Vasculitis

Further reading:
- Caputo R, Marzano AV, Benedetto A di et al (2006) Juvenile gangrenous vasculitis of the scrotum: is it a variant of pyoderma gangrenosum? J Am Acad Dermatol 55(2 Suppl):S50–S53

Genital Erosions and Ulcers

- Amebiasis
- Behçet's disease
- Bullous pemphigoid
- Candidiasis
- Chancriform pyoderma
- Chancroid

- Cicatricial pemphigoid
- Crohn's disease
- Epidermolysis bullosa acquisita
- Erosive lichen planus
- Erythema multiforme
- Extramammary Paget's disease
- Factitial disease
- Fixed drug eruption (Fig. 3.8)
- Granuloma inguinale
- Hailey–Hailey disease
- Herpes simplex virus infection
- Histoplasmosis
- Impetigo
- Intraepithelial neoplasia
- Jacquet's erosive diaper dermatitis
- Leishmaniasis
- Lichen sclerosus
- Linear IgA bullous dermatosis
- Lipschutz ulcer
- Lymphogranuloma venereum
- Necrolytic migratory erythema
- Pemphigus vulgaris
- Pyoderma gangrenosum

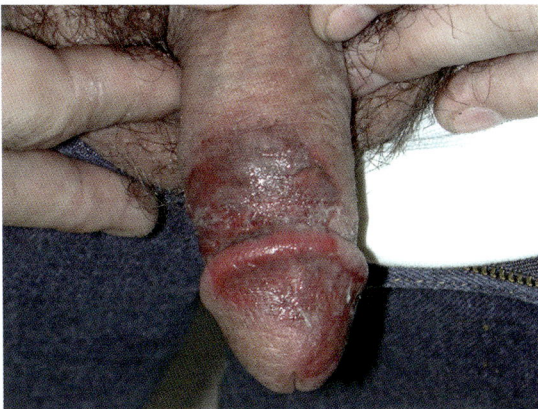

Fig. 3.8 Fixed drug eruption (Courtesy of K. Guidry)

- Squamous cell carcinoma
- Syphilis
- Traumatic ulcer
- Zoon's plasma cell balanitis/vulvitis

Further reading:

- Barnes CJ, Alio AB, Cunningham BB, Friedlander SF (2007) Epstein-Barr virus-associated genital ulcers: an under-recognized disorder. Pediatr Dermatol 24(2):130–134

Gingiva

- Acromegaly
- Addison's disease
- Amalgam tattoo
- Ameloblastoma
- Amyloidosis
- Chronic gingivitis
- Cowden syndrome
- Crohn's disease
- Cross syndrome
- Fibroma
- Giant cell fibroma
- Gingival cyst
- Juvenile hyaline fibromatosis
- Kaposi's sarcoma
- Leukemic infiltration
- Lichen planus
- Lipoid proteinosis
- Lymphoma
- Melanoma
- Metastatic tumors
- Mucosal neuroma
- Mucosal pemphigoid
- Odontogenic cyst

- Papillon–Lefèvre syndrome
- Paraneoplastic pemphigus
- Parulis
- Peripheral ossifying fibroma
- Proliferative verrucous leukoplakia
- Pyogenic granuloma
- Racial pigmentation
- Sarcoidosis
- Scurvy
- Tuberous sclerosis
- Wegener's granulomatosis

Associated Medications (Gingival Hyperplasia)

- Cyclosporine
- Diltiazem
- Nefidipine
- Phenytoin
- Valproate
- Verapamil

Further reading:
- Khera P (2005) Diffuse gingival enlargement. J Am Acad Dermatol 52:491–499

Gingivitis, Desquamative

- Cicatricial pemphigoid
- Epidermolysis bullosa acquisita
- Lichen planus
- Linear IgA disease
- Pemphigus vulgaris

Further reading:
- Castellano Suarez JL (2002) Gingival disorders of immune origin. Med Oral 7(4):271–283

Hair Collar Sign

- Aplasia cutis congenita
- Encephalocele
- Heterotopic brain tissue
- Meningocele
- Rudimentary meningocele

Further reading:
- Harrington BC (2007) The hair collar sign as a marker for neural tube defects. Pediatr Dermatol 24(2):138–140

Hair, Hypomelanotic

- Albinism
- Book syndrome
- Chediak–Higashi syndrome
- Copper deficiency
- Cross syndrome
- Down syndrome
- Elejalde syndrome
- Fanconi syndrome
- Griscelli syndrome
- Hallermann–Streiff syndrome
- Hyperthyroidism
- Menkes kinky-hair syndrome
- Phenylketonuria
- Prolidase deficiency
- Rothmund–Thomson syndrome
- Vitamin B12 deficiency
- Waardenburg's syndrome

- Woolf's syndrome
- Ziprkowski–Margolis syndrome

Further reading:
- Malhotra AK, Bhaskar G, Nanda M et al (2006) Griscelli syndrome. J Am Acad Dermatol 55(2):337–340

Hair-Shaft Tapering

- Alopecia areata
- Anagen effluvium
- Syphilis
- Thallium toxicity
- Tinea capitis

Further reading:
- Bleiker TO, Nicolaou N, Traulsen J, Hutchinson PE (2005) "Atrophic telogen effluvium" from cytotoxic drugs. Br J Dermatol 153(1):103–112

Halo

- Lymphomatoid papulosis
- Melanoma
- Neurofibromas
- Nevus
- Psoriasis
- Sarcoidosis (Fig. 3.9)

Further reading:
- Oguz O, Engin B (2005) Skin lesions of lymphomatoid papulosis with a white halo. J Eur Acad Dermatol Venereol 19(4):517–518

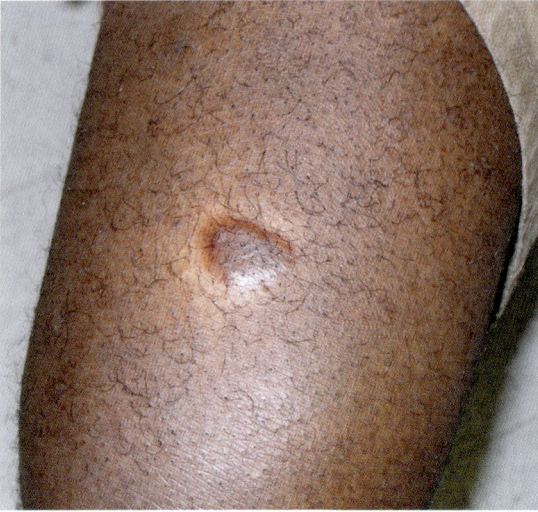

Fig. 3.9 Sarcoidosis

Hand Eczema

- Allergic contact dermatitis
- Chronic contact urticaria
- Dyshidrotic eczema
- Hyperkeratotic hand eczema
- Id reaction
- Irritant contact dermatitis
- Mechanic's hands
- Mycosis fungoides palmaris et plantaris
- Palmoplantar pustulosis
- Porphyria cutanea tarda
- Psoriasis
- Tinea manuum

Further reading:

- Diepgen TL, Agner T, Aberer W et al (2007) Management of chronic hand eczema. Contact Dermatitis 57(4):203–210

Herpetiform

- Aphthous stomatitis, herpetiform subtype
- Bullous impetigo
- Dermatitis herpetiformis
- Epidermolysis bullosa simplex, Dowling–Meara type
- Herpes simplex virus infection
- Impetigo herpetiformis
- Linear IgA disease
- Lymphangioma circumscriptum
- Metastatic lesions
- Pemphigus herpetiformis
- Pustular psoriasis
- Varicella
- Zoster

Further reading:

- Somani BK, Prita D, Grant S et al (2006) Herpetiform cutaneous metastases from transitional cell carcinoma of the urinary bladder: immunohistochemical analysis. J Clin Pathol 59(12):1331–1333

Hyperpigmentation Along Blaschko's Lines

- Café-au-lait macules in McCune–Albright syndrome
- Early epidermal nevus
- Focal dermal hypoplasia
- Incontinentia pigmenti, stage III
- Linear and whorled nevoid hypermelanosis
- Linear atrophoderma of Moulin
- Linear biphasic cutaneous amyloidosis
- Linear fixed drug eruption
- Linear lichen planus
- Progressive cribriform and zosteriform hyperpigmentation
- X-linked chondrodysplasia punctata
- X-linked reticulate pigmentary disorder

Further reading:

- Choi JC, Yang JH, Lee UH et al (2005) Progressive cribriform and zosteriform hyperpigmentation: the late onset linear and whorled nevoid hypermelanosis. J Eur Acad Dermatol Venereol 19(5):638–639

Hyperpigmentation, Diffuse

- Addison's disease
- Adrenoleukodystrophy
- AIDS
- B12 deficiency
- Carbon baby syndrome
- Carcinoid syndrome
- Congenital adrenal hyperplasia
- Cronkhite–Canada syndrome
- Ectopic ACTH-secreting tumor
- Eosinophilia–myalgia syndrome
- Familial diffuse hypermelanosis
- Gaucher's disease
- Hemochromatosis
- Hyperthyroidism
- Malabsorption
- Malaria
- Medications
- Metastatic melanoma
- Nelson's syndrome
- Niemann–Pick disease
- Pellagra
- Pheochromocytoma
- POEMS syndrome
- Porphyria cutanea tarda
- Pregnancy
- Primary biliary cirrhosis
- Progressive systemic sclerosis

- Protein deficiency
- Renal disease
- Still's disease
- Toxic oil syndrome
- Visceral leishmaniasis
- Whipple's disease
- Wilson's disease

Associated Medications

- 5-fluorouracil
- Amiodarone
- Antimalarials
- Arsenic
- AZT
- BCNU
- Bismuth
- Bleomycin
- Busulfan
- Chlorpromazine
- Cyclophosphamide
- Dactimycin
- Desipramine
- Diltiazem
- Dioxins
- Doxorubicin
- Gold
- Hydroquinone
- Hydroxyurea
- Imipramine
- Iron
- Lead
- Mercury
- Methotrexate

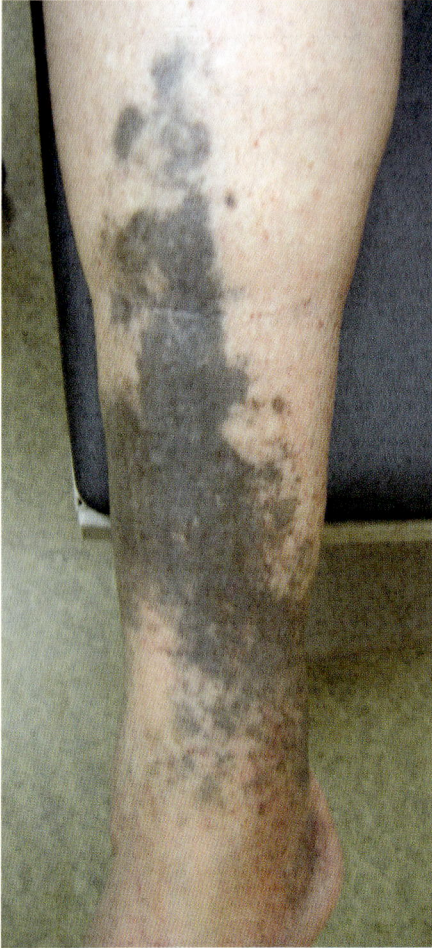

Fig. 3.10 Minocycline hyperpigmentation

- Minocycline (Fig. 3.10)
- Nitrogen mustard
- Oral contraception
- Phenothiazine
- Psoralens
- Silver

Further reading:

- Dereure O (2001) Drug-induced skin pigmentation. Epidemiology, diagnosis and treatment. Am J Clin Dermatol 2(4):253–262
- Filho T, Neto PB, Reis JC et al (2007) Diffuse cutaneous melanosis in malignant melanoma. Dermatol Online J 13(2):9

Hyperpigmentation, Oral

- Addison's disease
- Argyria
- Amalgam tattoo
- Drug-induced pigmentation
- Hemochromatosis
- Laugier–Hunziker syndrome
- Melanocytic nevus
- Melanoma
- Oral melanotic macule
- Peutz–Jeghers syndrome
- Racial pigmentation
- Smoker's melanosis

Further reading:

- Gaeta GM, Satriano RA, Baroni A (2002) Oral pigmented lesions. Clin Dermatol 20(3):286–288

Hyperpigmentation, Reticulated

- Acropigmentation of Dohi
- Congenital diffuse mottling of the skin
- Dermatopathia pigmentosa reticularis
- Dowling–Degos disease
- Dyskeratosis congenita
- Erythema ab igne
- Galli–Galli disease
- Hereditary universal dyschromatosis

- Macular amyloidosis
- Naeg eli–Franceschetti–Jadassohn syndrome
- Prurigo pigmentosa
- Reticulate acropigmentation of Kitamura
- Scleroderma
- X-linked reticulate pigmentary disorder

Further reading:
- Ee HL, Tan SH (2005) Reticulate hyperpigmented scleroderma: a new pigmentary manifestation. Clin Exp Dermatol 30(2):131–133

Hypertrichosis, Generalized

- Ambras syndrome
- Anorexia nervosa
- Barber–Say syndrome
- Cantu syndrome
- Coffin–Siris syndrome
- Congenital generalized hypertrichosis (XLD, AD, XLR)
- Cornelia de Lange syndrome
- Craniofacial dysostosis
- Dermatomyositis (especially juvenile)
- Donahue syndrome
- Drug-induced hypertrichosis
- Distichiasis–lymphedema syndrome
- Dystrophic epidermolysis bullosa
- Fetal alcohol syndrome
- Fetal hydantoin syndrome
- Gingival fibromatosis and hypertrichosis
- Globoid leukodystrophy
- Gorlin's syndrome
- Hypothyroidism
- Lawrence syndrome
- Malnutrition
- Mucopolysaccharidoses

- Osteochondrodysplasia
- POEMS syndrome
- Porphyrias
- Rubinstein–Taybi syndrome
- Waardenburg syndrome
- Winchester syndrome

Associated Medications

- Acetazolamide
- Anabolic steroids
- Benoxaprofen
- Cyclosporine
- Danazol
- Diazoxide
- Glucocorticosteroids
- Hexachlorobenzene
- Minoxidil
- Penicillamine
- Phenytoin
- Psoralens
- Streptomycin

Further reading:
- Wendelin DS, Pope DN, Mallory SB (2003) Hypertrichosis. J Am Acad Dermatol 48(2):161–179

Hypertrichosis, Localized

- Anterior cervical hypertrichosis
- Auricular hypertrichosis
- Becker's nevus
- Chicken pox
- Chronic irritation
- Congenital melanocytic nevi

- Dermatofibroma
- Hairy polythelia
- Hypertrichosis cubiti
- Immunization site
- Lymphedema
- Nevoid hypertrichosis
- Paradoxical hypertrichosis (laser hair removal)
- Plexiform neurofibroma
- Pretibial myxedema
- Reflex sympathetic dystrophy
- Spinal dysraphism-associated hypertrichosis
- Topical steroid induced

Further reading:
- Wendelin DS, Pope DN, Mallory SB (2003) Hypertrichosis. J Am Acad Dermatol 48(2):161–179

Hypopigmentation/Depigmentation, Generalized

- Albinism
- Alezzandrini syndrome
- Arsenical hypomelanosis
- Ataxia–telangiectasia
- Chediak–Higashi syndrome
- Chemical leukoderma
- Cross syndrome
- Darier's disease leukoderma
- Elejalde syndrome
- Griscelli syndrome
- Halo nevus
- Hermansky–Pudlak syndrome
- Hypomelanosis of Ito
- Idiopathic guttate hypomelanosis
- Leprosy

- Melanoma-associated leukoderma
- Menkes' kinky hair disease
- Mycosis fungoides (hypopigmented type)
- Onchocerciasis
- Phenylketonuria
- Piebaldism
- Pinta
- Pityriasis alba
- Pityriasis lichenoides chronica
- Postinflammatory hypopigmentation
- Progressive macular hypomelanosis
- Sarcoidosis
- Scleroderma (Fig. 3.11)
- Steroid-induced hypopigmentation
- Syphilis
- Tinea versicolor
- Tuberous sclerosis
- Vitiligo
- Vogt–Koyanagi–Harada syndrome
- Waardenburg's syndrome

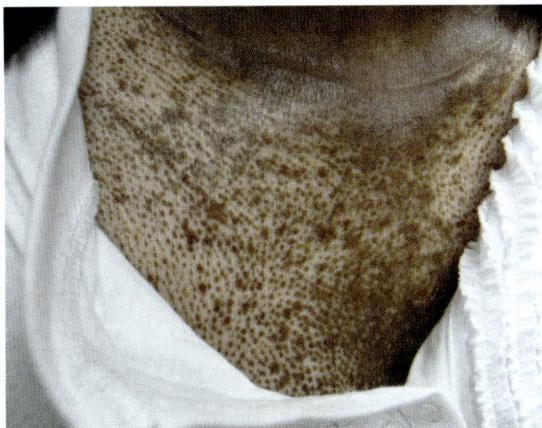

Fig. 3.11 Scleroderma

- Woolf's syndrome
- Yaws
- Ziprkowski–Margolis syndrome

Further reading:
- Mollet I, Ongenae K, Naeyaert JM (2007) Origin, clinical presentation, and diagnosis of hypomelanotic skin disorders. Dermatol Clin 25(3):363–371

Hypopigmentation, Localized

- Annular lichenoid dermatitis of youth
- Chemical leukoderma
- Darier's disease leukoderma
- Discoid lupus erythematosus
- Halo nevus
- Idiopathic guttate hypomelanosis
- Imiquimod hypopigmentation
- Incontinentia pigmenti achromians
- Intralesional steroid hypopigmentation (Fig. 3.12)
- Leprosy (especially tuberculoid)
- Lichen sclerosus
- Morphea
- Mycosis fungoides (hypopigmented type)
- Nevus anemicus
- Nevus depigmentosus
- Onchocerciasis
- Piebaldism
- Pinta
- Postinflammatory hypopigmentation
- Sarcoidosis
- Syphilis
- Tinea versicolor
- Tuberous sclerosis
- Vitiligo

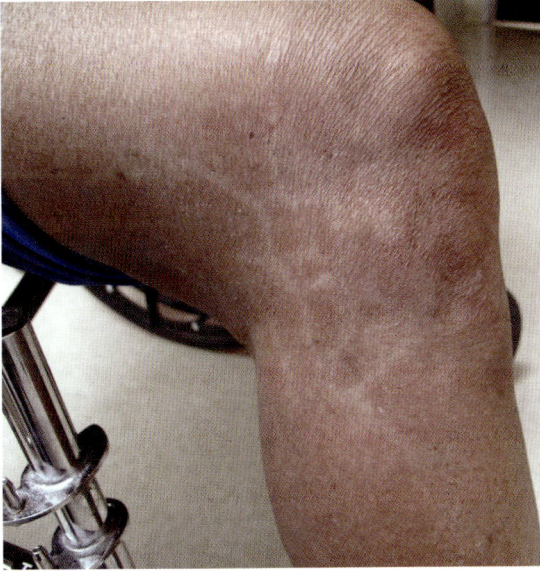

Fig. 3.12 Cortisone injection-induced hypopigmentation

Further reading:

- Mollet I, Ongenae K, Naeyaert JM (2007) Origin, clinical presentation, and diagnosis of hypomelanotic skin disorders. Dermatol Clin 25(3):363–371

Hypomelanosis, Diffuse Neonatal

- Chediak–Higashi syndrome
- Copper deficiency
- Cross syndrome
- EEC syndrome
- Elejalde syndrome
- Griscelli syndrome
- Histidinemia
- Homocystinuria
- Menkes' syndrome

- Oculocutaneous albinism
- Phenylketonuria
- Selenium deficiency
- Sialic acid storage disease
- Waardenburg's syndrome

Further reading:

- Ruiz-Maldonado R (2007) Hypomelanotic conditions of the newborn and infant. Dermatol Clin 25(3):373–382

Ichthyosis, Acquired

- Chronic renal failure
- Graft-vs-host disease
- HIV infection
- HTLV-1 infection
- Hyperparathyroidism
- Hypothyroidism
- Leprosy
- Malnutrition
- Medications
- Mycosis fungoides
- Onchocerciasis
- Sarcoidosis (Fig. 3.13)
- Systemic lupus erythematosus
- Systemic lymphomas
- Tuberculosis

Associated Medications

- Cimetidine
- Clofazimine
- Hydroxyurea

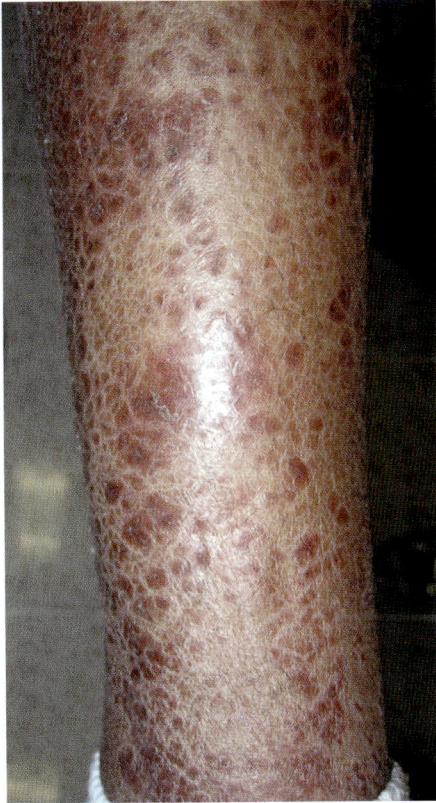

Fig. 3.13 Ichthyosiform sarcoidosis

- Isoniazid
- Nicotinic acid
- Retinoids
- Statins

Further reading:

- Patel N, Spencer LA, English JC III et al (2006) Acquired ichthyosis. J Am Acad Dermatol 55(4):647–656

Ichthyosis, Hereditary

- Cardiofaciocutaneous syndrome
- CHIME syndrome
- Chondrodysplasia punctata
- IBIDS syndrome (Tay syndrome)
- Ichthyosis bullosa of Siemens
- Ichthyosis vulgaris
- Lamellar ichthyosis
- Netherton's syndrome
- Neutral lipid storage disease
- NISCH syndrome
- Nonbullous congenital ichthyosiform erythroderma
- Refsum disease
- Sjögren–Larsson syndrome
- Vohwinkel's with ichthyosis
- X-linked ichthyosis

Further reading:
- DiGiovanna JJ, Robinson-Bostom L (2003) Ichthyosis: etiology, diagnosis, and management. Am J Clin Dermatol 4(2):81–95

Inframammary

- Candidiasis
- Darier's disease
- Hailey–Hailey disease
- Inflammatory breast cancer
- Intertrigo
- Inverse psoriasis
- Paget's disease
- Seborrheic dermatitis
- Tinea corporis

Further reading:

- Cohen PR (2003) Darier disease: sustained improvement following reduction mammaplasty. Cutis 72(2):124–126

Interdigital Web Spaces

- Dermatophytosis
- Erosio interdigitalis blastomycetica
- Erythrasma
- Gram-negative infection
- Interdigital hair sinuses
- Intertrigo
- Scabies
- Soft corn
- Xanthoma

Further reading:

- Schroder CM, Merk HF, Frank J (2006) Barber's hair sinus in a female hairdresser: uncommon manifestation of an occupational dermatosis. J Eur Acad Dermatol Venereol 20(2):209–211

Jarisch–Herxheimer Reaction

- Bacillary angiomatosis
- Leptospirosis
- Lyme disease
- Q fever
- Relapsing fever
- Secondary syphilis
- Trypanosomiasis

Further reading:

- See S, Scott EK, Levin MW (2005) Penicillin-induced Jarisch–Herxheimer reaction. Ann Pharmacother 39(12):2128–2130

Jaundice

- Acute hepatic injury (including drug-induced)
- Cirrhosis
- Crigler–Najjar syndrome
- Drug-induced cholestasis
- Dubin–Johnson syndrome
- Extrahepatic cholestasis
- Familial hyperbilirubinemia
- Gilbert syndrome
- Hemolysis
- Leptospirosis
- Intrahepatic cholestasis
- Physiologic jaundice of the newborn
- Primary biliary cirrhosis
- Rotor's syndrome
- Viral hepatitis

Evaluation

- Abdominal CT scan
- Complete blood count
- Direct and indirect bilirubin
- Endoscopic retrograde cholangiopancreatography
- Hepatitis screening
- Liver function tests
- Liver ultrasound
- Reticulocyte count
- Urine bilirubin
- Urine urobilinogen

Further reading:
- Lewis JH, Ahmed M, Shobassy A, Palese C (2006) Drug-induced liver disease. Curr Opin Gastroenterol 22(3):223–233

Koebner Phenomenon

- Darier's disease
- Dermatographism
- Erythema multiforme
- Lichen nitidus
- Lichen planus
- Lichen sclerosus
- Perforating disorders
- Pityriasis lichenoides et varioliformis acuta
- Porokeratosis of Mibelli
- Psoriasis
- Reactive perforating collagenosis
- Sarcoid
- Sweet syndrome
- Vitiligo

Further reading:
- Thappa DM (2004) The isomorphic phenomenon of Koebner. Indian J Dermatol Venereol Leprol 70(3):187–189

Koilonychia (Fig. 3.14)

- Alopecia areata
- Acanthosis nigricans
- Acrylic nail polishes
- Benign childhood koilonychia
- Coronary artery disease
- Familial koilonychia
- High altitude
- Iron deficiency
- Lichen planus
- Mal de Meleda
- Monilethrix

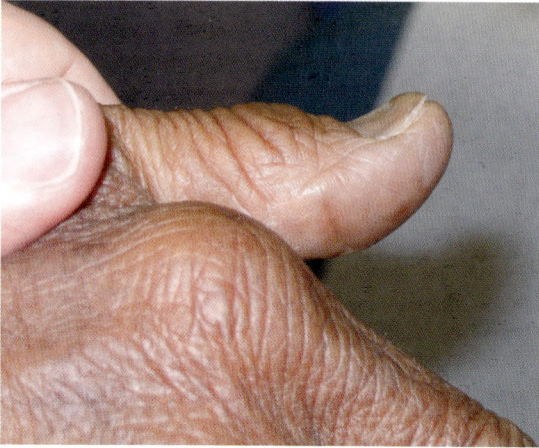

Fig. 3.14 Koilonychia

- Occupational
- Plummer–Vinson syndrome
- Polycythemia vera
- Psoriasis
- Raynaud's phenomenon
- Steatocystoma multiplex
- Syphilis
- Trauma

Further reading:
- Fawcett RS, Linford S, Stulberg DL (2004) Nail abnormalities: clues to systemic disease. Am Fam Physician 69(6):1417–1424

Leonine Facies

- Acromegaly
- Amyloidosis
- Carcinoid
- Cutaneous lymphoid hyperplasia
- Cutaneous T cell lymphoma
- Cutis verticis gyrata

- Follicular mucinosis
- Leishmaniasis
- Leukemia cutis
- Leprosy
- Lipoid proteinosis
- Mastocytosis
- Multicentric reticulohistiocytosis
- Multiple keratoacanthomas
- Multiple trichoepitheliomas
- Pachydermoperiostosis
- Phymatous rosacea
- Progressive nodular histiocytoma
- Sarcoidosis
- Scleromyxedema
- Setleis syndrome

Further reading:
- Kendrick CG, Brown RA, Reina R et al (2004) Cutaneous sarcoidosis presenting as leonine facies. Cutis 73(1):57–62

Leukonychia, Apparent

- Half-and-half nails
- Muehrcke's nails
- Terry's nails

Further reading:
- Weiser JA, Rogers HD, Scher RK et al (2007) Signs of a "broken heart": suspected Muehrcke lines after cardiac surgery. Arch Dermatol 143(6):815–816

Leukonychia Partialis

- Chilblains
- Hodgkin's disease
- Idiopathic

- Leprosy
- Metastatic carcinoma
- Nephritis
- Tuberculosis

Further reading:
- Assadi F (2005) Leukonychia associated with increased blood strontium level. Clin Pediatr 44(6):531–533

Leukonychia Totalis

- Bart–Pumphrey syndrome
- Cirrhosis
- Deafness
- Duodenal ulcer
- Hereditary leukonychia totalis
- LEOPARD syndrome
- Leprosy
- Multiple sebaceous cysts and renal calculi
- Nail biting
- Selenium deficiency
- Trichinosis
- Typhoid fever
- Ulcerative colitis

Further reading:
- Antonarakis ES (2006) Images in clinical medicine. Acquired leukonychia totalis. N Engl J Med 355(2):e2
- De D, Handa S (2007) Hereditary leukonychia totalis. Indian J Dermatol Venereol Leprol 73(5):355–357

Leukonychia, Transverse True

- Acrodermatitis enteropathica
- Chemotherapy
- Febrile illness

- Mees lines
- Stevens–Johnson syndrome
- Trauma

Further reading:
- Fujita Y, Sato-Matsumura KC, Doi I et al (2007) Transverse leukonychia (Mees' lines) associated with pleural empyema. Clin Exp Dermatol 32(1):127–128

Leukoplakia

- Bite keratosis
- Candidiasis
- Darier's disease
- Dyskeratosis congenita
- Frictional keratosis
- Leukoedema
- Lichen planus
- Lichen sclerosus
- Oral florid papillomatosis
- Oral hairy leukoplakia
- Pachyonychia congenita
- Premalignant leukoplakia
- Proliferative verrucous neoplasia
- Squamous cell carcinoma
- Syphilis
- White sponge nevus

Further reading:
- Warnakulasuriya S, Johnson NW, van der Waal I (2007) Nomenclature and classification of potentially malignant disorders of the oral mucosa. J Oral Pathol Med 36(10):575–580

Lichenoid Papules

- Frictional lichenoid dermatosis
- Gianotti–Crosti syndrome

- Keratosis lichenoides chronica
- Lichen amyloidosis
- Lichen aureus
- Lichen myxedematosus
- Lichen nitidus
- Lichen planus
- Lichen scrofulosorum
- Lichen spinulosus
- Lichen striatus
- Lichenoid contact dermatitis
- Lichenoid drug eruption
- Lichenoid graft-vs-host disease
- Lichenoid keratosis
- Lichenoid pigmented purpuric dermatosis
- Lichenoid sarcoidosis
- Lichenoid secondary syphilis

Further reading:

- Tang MB, Yosipovitch G, Tan SH (2004) Secondary syphilis presenting as a lichen planus-like rash. J Eur Acad Dermatol Venereol 18(2):185–187

Linear Hypopigmentation

- Epidermal nevus
- Focal dermal hypoplasia (Goltz syndrome)
- Hypomelanosis of Ito
- Incontinentia pigmenti (stage IV)
- Intralesional steroids
- Lichen striatus
- Menkes' kinky-hair disease (female carrier)
- Morphea
- Nevus depigmentosus
- Postinflammatory hypopigmentation
- Segmental ash-leaf macule
- Segmental vitiligo

Further reading:

- Nanda V, Parwaz MA, Handa S (2006) Linear hypopigmentation after triamcinolone injection: a rare complication of a common procedure. Aesthetic Plast Surg 30(1):118–119

Linear

- Basal cell carcinoma
- Basaloid follicular hamartoma
- Bites and stings (especially jellyfish)
- Blaschkitis
- Bullous ichthyosiform erythroderma
- Chronic graft-vs-host disease
- Connective tissue nevus
- Darier's disease
- Eccrine spiradenomas
- Epidermal nevi
- Factitial disease
- Fibromatosis
- Fixed-drug eruption
- Futcher's lines
- Goltz syndrome
- Hailey–Hailey disease
- Hypomelanosis of Ito
- Incontinentia pigmenti
- Inflammatory linear verrucous epidermal nevus
- Lichen nitidus
- Lichen planus
- Lichen striatus
- Linea alba
- Linea nigra
- Linear Cowden's nevus
- Linear and whorled nevoid hypermelanosis
- Linear atrophoderma of Moulin
- Linear focal elastosis

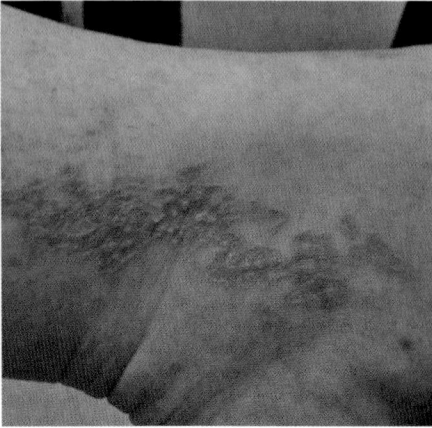

Fig. 3.15 Linear porokeratosis
(Courtesy of A. Mistretta)

- Lupus erythematosus
- Lymphangiitis
- Molluscum contagiosum
- Morphea
- Nevoid telangiectasia
- Nevus comedonicus
- Nevus corniculatus
- Nevus depigmentosus
- Nevus lipomatosus superficialis
- Nevus sebaceous
- Palmoplantar verrucous nevus
- Pemphigus
- Phytophotodermatitis
- Plant contact dermatitis
- Porokeratosis (Fig. 3.15)
- Porokeratotic eccrine ostial and dermal duct nevus
- Psoriasis
- Rope sign of interstitial granulomatous dermatitis
- Segmental angiofibromas
- Segmental leiomyomas

- Segmental neurofibromas
- Segmental vitiligo
- Sporotrichoid lesions
- Striae atrophicans
- Syringomas
- Thrombophlebitis
- Trichoepitheliomas
- Unilateral nevoid telangiectasia
- Verruca
- Zosteriform lentiginous nevus

Further reading:
- Grosshans EM (1999) Acquired blaschkolinear dermatoses. Am J Med Genet 85(4):334–372
- Happle R (2007) Linear Cowden nevus: a new distinct epidermal nevus. Eur J Dermatol 17(2):133–136

Lip Pits

- Branchio-oculo-facial syndrome
- Branchio-oto-renal syndrome
- Oral–facial–digital syndrome, type I
- Popliteal pterygium syndrome
- Van der Woude's syndrome

Further reading:
- Dissemond J, Haberer D, Franckson T et al (2004) The Van der Woude syndrome: a case report and review of the literature. J Eur Acad Dermatol Venereol 18(5):611–613

Lip Swelling

- Amyloidosis
- Angioedema
- Ascher syndrome
- Cheilitis glandularis

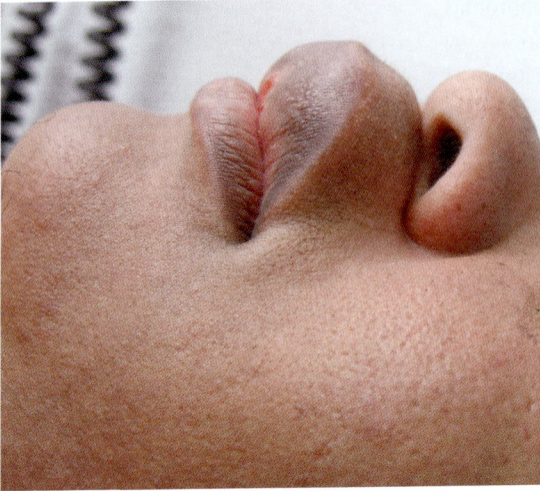

Fig. 3.16 Pleomorphic adenoma

- Cheilitis granulomatosis
- Crohn's disease
- Hemangioma
- Herpes simplex virus infection
- Lupus erythematosus
- Leishmaniasis
- Leprosy
- Lymphangioma
- Lymphatic obstruction
- Melkersson–Rosenthal syndrome
- Microcystic adnexal carcinoma
- Mucosal neuroma
- Neurofibroma
- Normal variant
- Paraffinoma
- Rhinoscleroma
- Salivary gland neoplasm (Fig. 3.16)

- Sarcoidosis
- Squamous cell carcinoma
- Syphilis
- Trauma
- Tuberculosis

Further reading:
- Kauzman A, Quesnel-Mercier A, Lalonde B (2006) Orofacial granulomatosis: 2 case reports and literature review. J Can Dent Assoc 72(4):325–329

Lymphadenitis, Suppurative

- Acne conglobata
- Actinomycosis
- Atypical mycobacterial infection
- Cat-scratch disease
- Chancroid
- Coccidioidomycosis
- Granuloma inguinale
- Hidradenitis suppurativa
- Histoplasmosis
- Lymphogranuloma venereum
- Melioidosis
- Nocardiosis
- Paracoccidioidomycosis
- Plague
- Rat bite fever
- Scrofuloderma
- Syphilis
- Tularemia

Further reading:
- Chlebicki MP, Tan BH (2006) Six cases of suppurative lymphadenitis caused by Burkholderia pseudomallei infection. Trans R Soc Trop Med Hyg 100(8):798–801

Lymphadenopathy

- African trypanosomiasis
- Angioimmunoblastic lymphadenopathy
- Brucellosis
- Bubonic plague
- Castleman's disease
- Chronic lymphocytic leukemia
- CMV infection
- Dermatopathic lymphadenitis
- Drug reaction
- EBV infection
- HIV infection
- Hodgkin's disease
- Kawasaki disease
- Kikuchi's disease
- Kimura's disease
- Langerhans cell histiocytosis
- Leishmaniasis
- Lymphogranuloma venereum
- Lymphoma
- Metastatic disease
- Mononucleosis
- Mycobacterial infection
- Mycosis fungoides
- Nocardiosis
- Non-Hodgkin's lymphoma
- Nonspecific bacterial lymphadenitis
- Salivary gland tumor
- Sarcoidosis
- Scrofuloderma
- Sinus histiocytosis with massive lymphadenopathy
- Streptococcal pharyngitis
- Syphilis
- Systemic mycoses
- Tinea capitis

- Toxoplasmosis
- Tularemia

Further reading:
- Kumar SS, Kuruvilla M, Pai GS et al (2003) Cutaneous manifestations of non-Hodgkin's lymphoma. Indian J Dermatol Venereol Leprol 69(1):12–15

Lymphedema, Primary (Hereditary)

- Aagenaes syndrome
- Distichiasis–lymphedema syndrome
- Hennekam syndrome
- Klippel–Trenaunay syndrome
- Lymphedema ptosis syndrome
- Meige lymphedema (lymphedema praecox or tarda)
- Milroy disease (congenital lymphedema)
- Njolstad syndrome
- Noonan syndrome
- Phakomatosis pigmentovascularis
- Turner syndrome
- Yellow nail syndrome

Further reading:
- Shinawi M (2007) Lymphedema of the lower extremity: is it genetic or nongenetic? Clin Pediatr 46(9):835–841

Lymphedema, Secondary

- Acne vulgaris (midface)
- Factitial disease (Secretan's syndrome)
- Granulomatous infection (especially chromoblastomycosis)
- Lymph node dissection
- Malignant obstruction
- Obesity
- Parasitic infections/filariasis
- Primary amyloidosis

- Radiation injury
- Recurrent lymphangitis and cellulitis
- Rosacea lymphedema
- Surgical excision

Further reading:
- Tiwari A, Cheng KS, Button M et al (2003) Differential diagnosis, investigation, and current treatment of lower limb lymphedema. Arch Surg 138(2):152–161

Macroglossia

- Acromegaly
- Actinomycosis
- Amyloidosis
- Angioedema
- Beckwith–Wiedemann syndrome
- Carcinoma of tongue
- Congenital hypothyroidism
- Down syndrome
- Granular cell tumor
- Hemangioma
- Hunter's syndrome
- Hurler's syndrome
- Hypothyroidism
- Leprosy
- Lipoid proteinosis
- Lymphatic malformation
- Melkersson–Rosenthal syndrome
- Mucosal neuroma syndrome
- Neurofibroma
- Neurofibromatosis
- Sarcoidosis
- Superior vena cava syndrome
- Venous malformation

Further reading:

- van der Waal RI, van de Scheur MR, Huijgens PC et al (2002) Amyloidosis of the tongue as a paraneoplastic marker of plasma cell dyscrasia. Oral Surg Oral Med Oral Pathol Oral Radiol Endod 94(4):444–447

Madarosis

- Alopecia areata
- Alopecia mucinosa
- Amyloidosis
- Atopic dermatitis (Hertoghe's sign)
- Cutaneous T cell lymphoma
- Discoid lupus erythematosus
- Ectodermal dysplasia
- Erythroderma
- Familial eyebrow hypoplasia
- Hyperthyroidism
- Hypothyroidism (Queen Anne's sign)
- Infiltrating tumor
- Lamellar ichthyosis
- Leprosy
- Monilethrix
- Pili torti
- Sarcoidosis
- Scleroderma/"en coup de sabre"
- Scleromyxedema
- Syphilis
- Trichotillomania
- Ulerythema ophryogenes
- Vogt–Koyanagi–Harada syndrome

Further reading:

- Khong JJ, Casson RJ, Huilgol SC, Selva D (2006) Madarosis. Surv Ophthalmol 51(6):550–560

Malar Rash

- Actinic prurigo
- Bloom's syndrome
- Carcinoid syndrome flushing
- Cockayne's syndrome
- Contact dermatitis
- Demodicosis
- Dermatomyositis
- Erythema infectiosum
- Granuloma faciale
- Jessner's lymphocytic infiltrate
- Lupus erythematosus
- Lupus pernio
- Lupus vulgaris
- Pemphigus erythematosus
- Perioral dermatitis
- Phototoxicity
- Polymorphous light eruption
- Rosacea
- Rothmund–Thomson syndrome
- Seborrheic dermatitis
- Telangiectasia macularis eruptiva perstans

Further reading:
- Black AA, McCauliffe DP, Sontheimer RD (1992) Prevalence of acne rosacea in a rheumatic skin disease subspecialty clinic. Lupus 1(4):229–237

Marfanoid Body Habitus

- Congenital contractural arachnodactyly
- Ehlers–Danlos syndrome type VI
- Ehlers–Danlos syndrome type VIII
- Gorlin syndrome
- Homocystinuria

- Marfan syndrome
- Multiple endocrine neoplasia, type IIB
- Stickler syndrome

Further reading:
- Svensson LG, Blackstone EH, Feng J et al (2007) Are Marfan syndrome and marfanoid patients distinguishable on long-term follow-up? Ann Thorac Surg 83(3):1067–1074

Melanonychia, Longitudinal

- Addison's disease
- Antimalarials
- Basal cell carcinoma
- Bowen's disease
- Cancer chemotherapeutic agents
- Chronic radiodermatitis
- Fluconazole
- Friction
- HIV infection
- Hydroxyurea
- Laugier–Hunziker syndrome
- Lichen planus
- Manicures
- Melanocyte hyperplasia
- Myxoid cyst
- Nail matrix melanoma
- Nail matrix nevus
- Onychomycosis
- Onychotillomania
- Peutz–Jeghers syndrome
- Postinflammatory
- Pregnancy
- Psoralens
- Pustular psoriasis

- Racial melanonychia
- *Scytalidium* infection
- Subungual keratosis
- Verrucae
- Zidovudine

Further reading:
- Andre J, Lateur N (2006) Pigmented nail disorders. Dermatol Clin 24(3):329–339

Michelin Tire Baby Appearance

- Congenital cutis laxa
- Diffuse nevus lipomatosus
- Smooth muscle hamartoma

Further reading:
- Palit A, Inamadar AC (2007) Circumferential skin folds in a child: a case of Michelin tire baby syndrome. Indian J Dermatol Venereol Leprol 73(1):49–51

Migratory

- Creeping eruption
- Erythema annulare centrifugum (Fig. 3.17)
- Erythema gyratum repens
- Erythema marginatum
- Erythema migrans
- Erythrokeratodermia variabilis
- Juvenile rheumatoid arthritis
- Necrolytic migratory erythema
- Urticaria

Creeping Eruption

- Cutaneous larva migrans
- Dirofilariasis

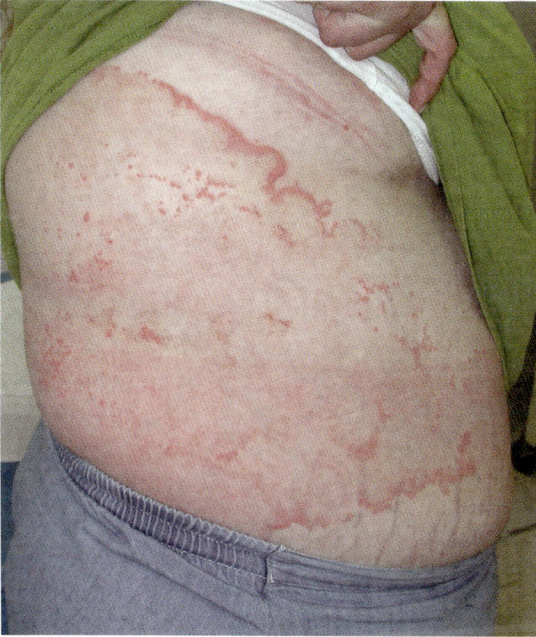

Fig. 3.17 Erythema annulare centrifugum (Courtesy of K. Guidry)

- Fascioliasis
- Gnathostomiasis
- Hookworm infestation
- Loaiasis
- Paragonimiasis
- Scabies
- Sparganosis
- Strongyloidiasis

Further reading:

- Goldsmith LA (2003) Migrating skin lesions: a genetic clue. J Invest Dermatol 121(3):vii–viii

Morbilliform

- Acute graft-vs-host disease
- Acute hepatitis
- Acute HIV infection
- Angioimmunoblastic lymphadenopathy
- Asymmetric periflexural exanthem
- Dengue fever
- Drug eruption
- Ehrlichiosis
- Erythema marginatum
- Guttate psoriasis
- Infectious mononucleosis
- Kawasaki disease
- Kikuchi's disease
- Measles
- Meningococcemia
- Papular pityriasis rosea
- Parvovirus infection
- Pityriasis rosea
- Relapsing fever
- Rocky Mountain spotted fever
- Roseola
- Rubella
- Scabies
- Scarlet fever
- Secondary syphilis
- Serum sickness-like reaction
- Toxic-shock syndrome
- Toxoplasmosis
- Typhus
- Urticaria
- Vaccination reaction
- Viral exanthem

Further reading:

- Furness C, Sharma R, Harnden A (2004) Morbilliform rash. Br Med J 329(7468):719

Nails, Absent/Atrophic (Acquired)

- Epidermolysis bullosa acquisita
- Erythroderma
- Lesch–Nyhan syndrome
- Lichen planus
- Onychotillomania
- Pemphigus
- Scleroderma
- Severe paronychia
- Stevens–Johnson syndrome
- Toxic epidermal necrolysis

Further reading:

- Pall A, Gupta RR, Gulati B et al (2004) Twenty nail anonychia due to lichen planus. J Dermatol 31(2):146–147

Nails, Absent/Atrophic (Congenital)

- Acrodermatitis enteropathica
- Amniotic bands
- Anonychia with ectrodactyly
- Apert syndrome
- Cartilage–hair hypoplasia
- Coffin–Siris syndrome
- Congenital onychodysplasia of the index fingers
- Cook's syndrome
- DOOR syndrome
- Dyskeratosis congenita
- Ectodermal dysplasias
- Ellis–van Creveld syndrome

- Epidermolysis bullosa
- Fetal alcohol syndrome
- Fetal dilantin syndrome
- Fetal warfarin syndrome
- Glossopalantine syndrome
- Goltz syndrome
- Hidrotic ectodermal dysplasia
- Hypohidrotic ectodermal dysplasia
- Incontinentia pigmenti
- KID syndrome
- Lamellar ichthyosis
- Nail–patella syndrome
- Noonan syndrome
- Popliteal web syndrome
- Progeria
- Rothmund–Thomson syndrome
- Trisomy 8
- Turner syndrome

Further reading:
- Rigopoulos D, Petropoulou H, Nikolopoulou M et al (2006) Total congenital anonychia in two children of the same family. J Eur Acad Dermatol Venereol 20(7):894–896

Nails, Brittle (Onychorrhexis)

- Alopecia areata
- Arsenic poisoning
- Biotin deficiency
- Chemicals
- Hand dermatitis
- Iron deficiency
- Lichen planus

- Psoriasis
- Severe chronic illness
- Thyroid disease
- Trauma
- Vitamin deficiency
- Wet work

Further reading:
- van de Kerkhof PC, Pasch MC, Scher RK et al (2005) Brittle nail syndrome: a pathogenesis-based approach with a proposed grading system. J Am Acad Dermatol 53(4):644–651

Nail Pigmentation

- Busulfan
- Cyclophoshamide
- Dermatophytes
- Hair dyes in hairdressers
- Hydroxyurea
- Iron or gold
- Melanocytic hyperplasia
- Melanoma
- Minocycline
- Nevus
- *Proteus* infection
- *Pseudomonas* colonization
- Smokers
- Subungual hematoma
- Zidovudine

Further reading:
- Andre J, Lateur N (2006) Pigmented nail disorders. Dermatol Clin 24(3):329–339

Nail Pitting

- Alopecia areata
- Dermatitis of proximal nail fold
- Eczema
- Lichen planus
- Pityriasis rosea
- Psoriasis
- Reactive arthritis
- Rheumatoid arthritis
- Sarcoidosis
- Syphilis

Further reading:
- Jiaravuthisan MM, Sasseville D, Vender RB et al (2007) Psoriasis of the nail: anatomy, pathology, clinical presentation, and a review of the literature on therapy. J Am Acad Dermatol 57(1):1–27

Nails with Blue Lunula

- Alkaptonuria
- Argyria
- Chemotherapy
- Hemochromatosis
- Minocycline
- Osler–Weber–Rendu disease
- Quinacrine
- Wilson's disease
- Zidovudine

Further reading:
- Cohen PR (1996) The lunula. J Am Acad Dermatol 34(6):943–953

Nails with Red Lunula

- Alopecia areata
- Cardiovascular disease
- Congestive heart failure
- Carbon monoxide poisoning
- Chronic obstructive pulmonary disease
- Glomus tumor
- Lymphogranuloma venereum
- Lichen planus
- Lichen sclerosus
- Psoriasis
- Rheumatoid arthritis

Further reading:
- Cohen PR (1996) The lunula. J Am Acad Dermatol 34(6):943–953

Necrotic

- Amebiasis
- Anthrax
- Arteriosclerosis obliterans
- Aspergillosis
- Basal cell carcinoma
- Blastomycosis
- Calciphylaxis
- Cholesterol emboli
- Chromoblastomycosis
- Coumadin necrosis
- Dermatomyositis
- Disseminated intravascular coagulation
- Ecthyma

- Ecthyma gangrenosum
- Febrile ulceronecrotic Mucha–Habermann disease
- Fusariosis
- Gas gangrene
- Heparin necrosis
- Intravascular lymphoma
- Leishmaniasis
- Livedo vasculitis
- Meningococcemia
- Metastatic lesion
- Necrotic arachnidism
- Necrotizing fasciitis
- Nicolau syndrome
- Panniculitis
- Polyarteritis nodosa
- Pressure ulcer
- Pyoderma gangrenosum
- Sarcoma
- Severe cellulitis
- Squamous cell carcinoma
- Sweet's syndrome
- Vasculitis
- *Vibrio vulnificus* infection
- Zygomycosis

Further reading:

- Luton K, Garcia C, Poletti E, Koester G (2006) Nicolau syndrome: three cases and review. Int J Dermatol 45(11):1326–1328

Neoplasm, Axilla

- Acrochordon
- Apocrine gland carcinoma
- Extramammary Paget's disease
- Fibrous hamartoma

- Lymphangioma circumscriptum
- Macrocystic lymphatic malformation
- Metastatic breast cancer

Neoplasm, Back

- Basal cell carcinoma
- Cellular blue nevus
- Chordoma
- Congenital melanocytic nevus
- Congenital smooth muscle hamartoma
- Cutaneous lymphoid hyperplasia
- Dilated pore
- Elastofibroma dorsi
- Encephalocele/meningocele
- Epidermal inclusion cyst
- Familial cutaneous collagenoma
- Fibroepithelioma of Pinkus
- Hibernoma
- Leiomyoma
- Lipoma
- Lymphoma
- Melanoma
- Meningioma
- Pilonidal sinus
- Pleomorphic lipoma
- Seborrheic keratosis
- Shagreen patch
- Spindle cell lipoma

Neoplasm, Buttock

- Cellular blue nevus
- Dermatofibrosarcoma protuberans

- Malignant fibrous histiocytoma
- Mycosis fungoides
- Nevus lipomatosus superficialis
- Trichoadenoma

Neoplasm, Chest

- Actinic keratosis
- Basal cell carcinoma
- Becker's nevus
- Benign lichenoid keratosis
- Eruptive vellus hair cysts
- Leiomyoma
- Medallion-like dermal dendrocyte hamartoma
- Seborrheic keratosis
- Solar lentigo
- Squamous cell carcinoma
- Steatocystoma

Neoplasm, Digital

- Acquired digital fibrokeratoma
- Acrolentiginous melanoma
- Aggressive digital papillary adenocarcinoma
- Digital mucous cyst
- Enchondroma
- Epidermal inclusion cyst
- Fibroma of the tendon sheath
- Ganglion cyst
- Giant cell tumor of the tendon sheath
- Glomus tumor
- Gouty tophus

- Metastatic lesion
- Multicentric reticulohistiocytosis
- Neurilemmoma
- Neuroma
- Perineuroma
- Poroma
- Pyogenic granuloma
- Sclerotic fibroma
- Squamous cell carcinoma
- Subungual exostosis
- Verruca
- Xanthoma

Neoplasm, Ear

- Acanthoma fissuratum
- Actinic keratosis
- Angiolymphoid hyperplasia with eosinophilia
- Apocrine hidrocystoma
- Atypical fibroxanthoma
- Basal cell carcinoma
- Ceruminoma
- Chondrodermatitis nodular helicis
- Cutaneous lymphoid hyperplasia
- Elastotic nodule
- Keloid
- Kimura's disease
- Lymphoma
- Milia en plaque
- Pseudocyst of the auricle
- Squamous cell carcinoma
- Venous lake

Neoplasm, Extremity (Upper or Lower)

- Angiolipoma
- Angiosarcoma
- Aponeurotic fibroma
- AV fistula
- Benign lichenoid keratosis
- Bowen's disease
- Common blue nevus
- Dermatofibroma
- Eccrine syringofibroadenoma
- Epithelioid hemangioendothelioma
- Epithelioid sarcoma
- Ganglion cyst
- Giant cell tumor of tendon sheath
- Glomeruloid hemangioma
- Hyperkeratosis lenticularis perstans
- Juvenile hyaline fibromatosis
- Lipoblastomatosis
- Melanocytic nevus
- Myxoma
- Neurilemmoma
- Porocarcinoma
- Primary marginal zone lymphoma
- Retiform hemangioendothelioma
- Seborrheic keratosis
- Spindle cell hemangioendothelioma
- Targetoid hemosiderotic hemangioma

Neoplasm, Extremity (Lower)

- Acroangiodermatitis (pseudo-Kaposi's sarcoma)
- Angioma serpiginosum
- Clear cell acanthoma
- Cutaneous ciliated cyst

- Diffuse large B cell lymphoma of the leg
- Fascial hernia
- Inflammatory linear verrucous epidermal nevus
- Liposarcoma
- Kaposi's sarcoma
- Pigmented spindle cell nevus of Reed
- Reactive angioendotheliomatosis
- Solitary angiokeratoma
- Subcutaneous panniculitis-like T cell lymphoma
- Verrucous vascular malformation

Neoplasm, Extremity (Upper)

- Actinic keratosis
- Arteriovenous fistula
- Blue rubber bleb nevus
- Intravascular papillary endothelial hyperplasia
- Juvenile xanthogranuloma
- Keratoacanthoma
- Leiomyoma
- Lipoma
- Maffucci's syndrome
- Microvenular hemangioma
- Neurilemmoma
- Neurothekeoma
- Nodular fasciitis
- Pilomatrixoma
- Solar lentigo

Neoplasm, Face

- Acrochordon
- Angiofibroma
- Angiosarcoma

- Apocrine hidrocystoma
- Basal cell carcinoma
- B cell lymphoma
- Chondroid syringoma
- Cirsoid aneurysm
- Cutaneous lymphoid hyperplasia
- Cylindroma
- Dermatosis papulosa nigra
- Dermoid cyst
- Desmoplastic melanoma
- Dilated pore
- Eccrine hidrocystoma
- Epidermal inclusion cyst
- Inverted follicular keratosis
- Juvenile hyaline fibromatosis
- Keratoacanthoma
- Lipoma
- Melanocytic nevus
- Meningioma
- Microcystic adnexal carcinoma
- Milia
- Myxoma
- Nevus sebaceous
- Palisaded encapsulated neuroma
- Perifollicular fibroma
- Pilomatrixoma
- Sebaceous carcinoma
- Sebaceous hyperplasia
- Seborrheic keratosis
- Solar lentigo
- Spider angioma
- Spitz nevus
- Squamous cell carcinoma
- Steatocystoma
- Subepidermal calcified nodule

- Syringocystadenoma papilliferum
- Syringoma
- Trichilemmoma
- Trichoadenoma
- Trichoblastoma
- Trichodiscoma
- Trichoepithelioma
- Trichofolliculoma
- Warty dyskeratoma

Neoplasm, Genital/Groin

- Angiofibroma of the vulva
- Angiokeratoma of Fordyce
- Bowenoid papulosis
- Bowen's disease
- Ciliated cyst
- Condyloma acuminatum
- Epidermoid cyst
- Extramammary Paget's disease
- Fox–Fordyce disease
- Granular cell tumor
- Hidradenoma papilliferum
- Idiopathic calcinosis of the scrotum
- Leiomyoma
- Lymphangioma
- Median raphe cyst
- Melanoma
- Pearly penile papules
- Sebaceous carcinoma
- Seborrheic keratosis
- Syringomas
- Verrucous carcinoma
- Vestibular papillomatosis

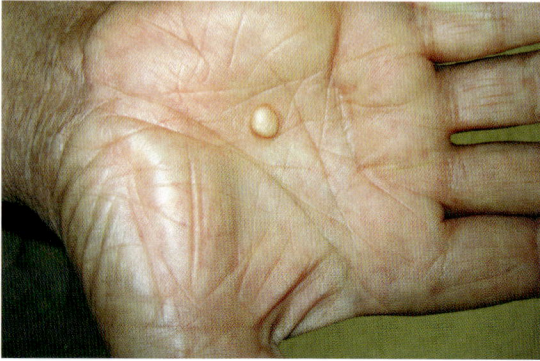

Fig. 3.18 Acquired fibrokeratoma

Neoplasm, Hands and Feet
(Including Dorsal Hands, Digits; Excluding Periungual)

- Acquired digital fibrokeratoma (Fig. 3.18)
- Acral lentiginous melanoma
- Actinic keratosis
- Aggressive digital papillary adenocarcinoma
- Angiokeratoma of Mibelli
- APACHE syndrome
- Arsenical keratosis
- Arteriovenous fistula
- Calcifying aponeurotic fibroma
- Common blue nevus
- Connective tissue nevus of Proteus syndrome
- Digital mucous cyst
- Dupuytren's contracture
- Eccrine angiomatous hamartoma
- Eccrine syringofibroadenoma
- Epidermal inclusion cyst
- Epithelioid sarcoma
- Ganglion cyst
- Giant cell tumor of the tendon sheath

- Glomus tumor
- Infantile digital fibromatosis
- Knuckle pads
- Ledderhose's disease
- Lipoma
- Lymphatic malformation
- Mastocytoma
- Melanocytic nevus
- Neurofibroma
- Piezogenic pedal papules
- Poroma
- Pyogenic granuloma
- Schwannoma
- Squamous cell carcinoma
- Stucco keratoses
- Supernumerary digit
- Traumatic neuroma
- Venous malformation
- Verrucous carcinoma
- Verruca

Neoplasm, Head and Neck (Any Location)

- Actinic keratosis
- Angiolymphoid hyperplasia with eosinophilia
- Angiosarcoma
- Atypical fibroxanthoma
- Clear cell/nodular hidradenoma
- Cutaneous lymphoid hyperplasia
- Granular cell tumor
- Infantile hemangioma
- Intravascular papillary endothelial hyperplasia
- Juvenile xanthogranuloma
- Lentigo maligna melanoma

- Melanoacanthoma
- Merkel cell carcinoma
- Neurothekeoma
- Nodular melanoma
- Palisaded encapsulated neuroma
- Sebaceous adenoma
- Sebaceous carcinoma
- Trichodiscoma
- Trichofolliculoma
- Tumor of the follicular infundibulum
- Venous malformation

Neoplasm, Neck

- Acrochordon
- Atypical fibroxanthoma
- Basal cell carcinoma
- Brachial cleft cyst
- Bronchogenic cyst
- Dilated pore
- Epidermal inclusion cyst
- Fibromatosis colli
- Keloid
- Lipoma
- Macrocystic lymphatic malformation
- Melanocytic nevus
- Nevus sebaceous
- Pigmented follicular cyst
- Pilomatrixoma
- Pleomorphic lipoma
- Spindle cell lipoma
- Squamous cell carcinoma
- Thyroglossal cyst
- Tufted angioma

Neoplasm, Nose

- Acanthoma fissuratum
- Actinic keratosis
- Basal cell carcinoma
- Basaloid follicular hamartoma
- Chondroid syringoma
- Cutaneous lymphoid hyperplasia
- Dermoid cyst
- Encephalocele
- Fibrous papule
- Hidradenoma
- Melanocytic nevus
- Nasal glioma
- Sebaceous hyperplasia
- Solar lentigo
- Squamous cell carcinoma
- Trichilemmoma
- Trichoepithelioma
- Trichofolliculoma

Neoplasm, Oral Cavity

- Benign salivary gland tumor
- Dermoid cyst
- Fibroma (Fig. 3.19)
- Fibrosarcoma
- Fibrous epulis
- Granular cell tumor
- Juvenile hyaline fibromatosis
- Kaposi's sarcoma
- Leukoplakia
- Macrocystic lymphatic malformation
- Malignant fibrous histiocytoma

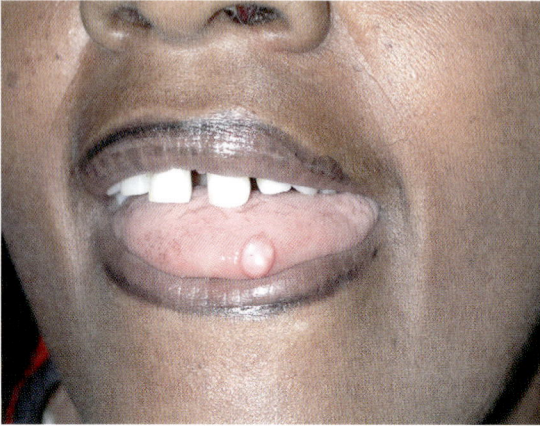

Fig. 3.19 Fibroma (Courtesy of K. Guidry)

- Malignant melanoma
- Malignant salivary gland tumor
- Melanoacanthoma
- Mucosal melanoma
- Odontogenic cyst or tumor
- Oral florid papillomatosis
- Osteomyelitis
- Peripheral giant cell granuloma
- Primary intraosseous carcinoma
- Pyogenic granuloma
- Squamous cell carcinoma
- Submucous fibrosis
- Verrucous carcinoma
- Warty dyskeratoma
- White sponge nevus

Neoplasm, Periocular

- Acrochordon
- Apocrine hidrocystoma

- Eccrine hidrocystoma
- Hidradenoma papilliferum
- Milia
- Mucinous eccrine carcinoma
- Sebaceous carcinoma
- Seborrheic keratosis
- Syringoma

Neoplasm, Perioral

- Basal cell carcinoma
- Epidermization of lip
- Microcystic adnexal carcinoma
- Pilar sheath acanthoma
- Salivary gland tumor
- Squamous cell carcinoma
- Venous lake

Neoplasm, Periungual

- Acral lentiginous melanoma
- Angiokeratoma
- Bowen's disease
- Glomus tumor
- Kaposi's sarcoma
- Keratoacanthoma
- Koenen tumor
- Lentigo
- Melanocytic nevi
- Metastatic disease
- Myxoid cysts
- Neurofibroma
- Onychomatricoma

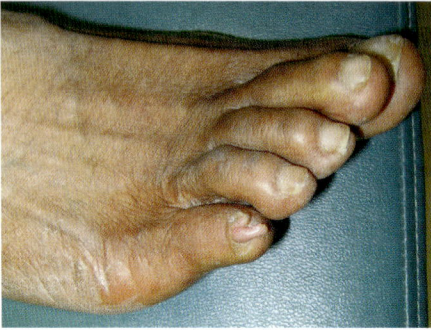

Fig. 3.20 Periungual fibroma

- Periungual fibroma (Fig. 3.20)
- Pyogenic granuloma
- Squamous cell carcinoma
- Subungual exostosis
- Subungual osteochondroma
- Verruca vulgaris
- Verrucous carcinoma

Neoplasm, Scalp

- Angiolymphoid hyperplasia with eosinophilia
- Angiosarcoma
- Atypical fibroxanthoma
- Basal cell carcinoma
- Cirsoid aneurysm
- Cranial fasciitis
- Cylindroma
- Encephalocele/meningocele
- Hibernoma
- Inverted follicular keratosis
- Juvenile hyaline fibromatosis

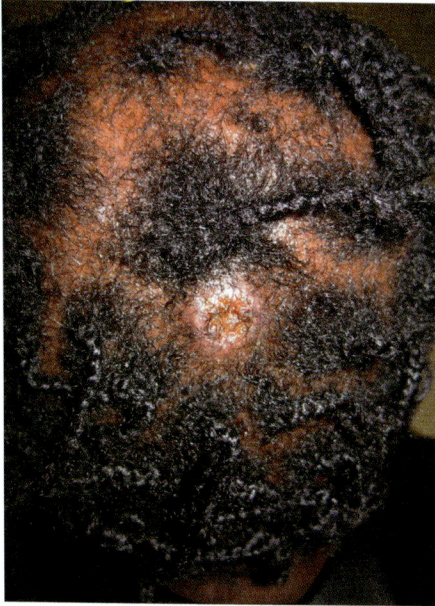

Fig. 3.21 Metastatic breast cancer

- Melanocytic nevus
- Meningioma
- Metastasis (Fig. 3.21)
- Nevus sebaceous
- Pilar cyst
- Proliferating pilar tumor
- Sebaceous carcinoma
- Seborrheic keratosis
- Solar lentigo
- Squamous cell carcinoma
- Syringocystadenoma papilliferum
- Trichoblastoma
- Trichofolliculoma
- Warty dyskeratoma

Neoplasm, Thigh

- Lipoma
- Liposarcoma
- Malignant fibrous histiocytoma
- Nevus lipomatosus superficialis

Neoplasm, Trunk

- B cell lymphoid hyperplasia
- Becker's nevus
- Blue rubber bleb nevus
- Bowen's disease
- Cherry angioma
- Congenital melanocytic nevus
- Dermatofibrosarcoma protuberans
- Dermatofibrosis lenticularis disseminata
- Desmoid tumor
- Dysplastic melanocytic nevus
- Epidermal inclusion cyst
- Fibrous hamartoma
- Glomeruloid hemangioma
- Kaposi's sarcoma
- Keloid
- Lipoma
- Melanocytic nevus
- Metastasis
- Myxoma
- Primary follicular center cell lymphoma
- Primary marginal zone lymphoma
- Sinusoidal hemangioma
- Supernumerary nipple
- Syringocystadenoma papilliferum
- Targetoid hemosiderotic hemangioma
- Tufted angioma

Nodule, Rapidly Growing

- Atypical fibroxanthoma
- Chondrodermatitis nodularis helicis
- Chondroid syringoma
- Hemangioma
- Kaposi's sarcoma
- Keratoacanthoma
- Malignant granular cell tumor
- Merkel cell tumor
- Metastasis
- Nodular fasciitis
- Nodular melanoma
- Pilomatrixoma
- Poroma
- Proliferating pilar tumor
- Pyogenic granuloma

Further reading:
- Liu W, Dowling JP, Murray WK et al (2006) Rate of growth in melanomas: characteristics and associations of rapidly growing melanomas. Arch Dermatol 142(12):1551–1558

Nodule, Red

- Amelanotic melanoma
- Angioma
- Angiolymphoid hyperplasia
- Clear cell acanthoma
- Cutaneous lymphoid hyperplasia
- Eccrine poroma
- Glomus tumor
- Kaposi's sarcoma
- Leukemia cutis
- Lymphoma
- Merkel cell tumor

- Metastasis
- Pyogenic granuloma
- Spitz nevus

Further reading:
- Yazdi AS, Sander CA, Ghoreschi K (2006) Small red nodule of the nose as presenting manifestation of CLL. Eur J Dermatol 16(5):580–581

Nose, Destructive Lesion

- Basal cell carcinoma
- Blastomycosis
- Bejel
- Cocaine abuse
- Leishmaniasis
- Leprosy
- Lupus vulgaris
- NK cell lymphoma
- Mucormycosis
- Noma
- Paracoccidioidomycosis
- Rhabdomyosarcoma
- Rhinoentomophthoromycosis
- Rhinoscleroma
- Rhinosporidiosis
- Sarcoidosis
- Squamous cell carcinoma
- Syphilis
- Trigeminal trophic syndrome
- Wegener's granulomatosis
- Yaws (gangosa)
- Zygomycosis

Further reading:
- Parker NP, Pearlman AN, Conley DB et al (2010) The dilemma of midline destructive lesions: a case series and diagnostic review. Am J Otolaryngol 31(2):104–109

Nose, Midline Mass

- Cephaloceles
- Dermal sinuses
- Dermoid cysts
- Epidermoid cyst
- Hemangioma
- Heterotopic brain tissue (nasal gliomas)
- Leukemia cutis
- Lymphoma
- Rhabdomyosarcoma
- Venous malformation

Further reading:

- Hedlund G (2006) Congenital frontonasal masses: developmental anatomy, malformations, and MR imaging. Pediatr Radiol 36(7):647–662

Onychauxis (Thickening of Nail Plate)

- Acromegaly
- Aging
- Chronic vascular disease
- Darier's disease
- Eczema
- Onychomycosis
- Pachyonychia congenita
- Pityriasis rubra pilaris
- Psoriasis
- Trauma
- Yellow nail syndrome

Further reading:

- Singh G, Haneef NS, Uday A (2005) Nail changes and disorders among the elderly. Indian J Dermatol Venereol Leprol 71(6):386–392

Onycholysis

- Amyloidosis
- Blistering diseases
- Bronchiectasis
- *Candida* infection
- Chemotherapy
- Cyanoacrylates
- Darier's disease
- Diabetes mellitus
- Ectodermal dysplasia
- Eczema
- Erythropoietic porphyria
- Erythropoietic protoporphyria
- Excessive manicuring
- Exposure to irritants or water
- False nails
- Fibroma
- Formaldehyde
- Herpes simplex infection
- Hyperthyroidism
- Hypothyroidism
- Iron deficiency
- Ischemia
- Keratosis lichenoides chronica
- Langerhans cell histiocytosis
- Leprosy
- Lichen planus
- Lichen striatus
- Long nails
- Lupus erythematosus
- Melanoma
- Methyl methacrylate
- Neuritis
- Onychomycosis

- Pachyonychia congenita
- Paclitaxel
- Pellagra
- Pemphigus vulgaris
- Phototoxicity
- Pleural effusion
- Porphyria cutanea tarda
- Pregnancy
- Pseudomonal infection
- Psoriasis
- Psoriatic arthritis
- Reiter's syndrome
- Retinoids
- Sarcoidosis
- Scabies
- Scleroderma
- Squamous cell carcinoma
- Subungual exostosis
- Syphilis
- Trauma
- Verruca
- Yellow nail syndrome

Associated Medications (Photoonycholysis)

- 6-mercaptopurine
- Chloramphenicol
- Fluoroquinolones
- Psoralen
- Tetracyclines

Further reading:
- Daniel CR III, Tosti A, Iorizzo M, Piraccini BM (2005) The disappearing nail bed: a possible outcome of onycholysis. Cutis 76(5):325–327

- Kechijian P (1985) Onycholysis of the fingernails: evaluation and management. J Am Acad Dermatol 12(3):552–560
- Piraccini BM, Iorizzo M, Starace M, Tosti A (2006) Drug-induced nail diseases. Dermatol Clin 24(3):387–391

Oral Cobblestone Appearance

- Cowden syndrome
- Crohn's disease
- Darier's disease
- Heck's disease
- Lipoid proteinosis
- Malignant acanthosis nigricans
- Mucosal neuroma syndrome
- Nicotine stomatitis
- Pseudoxanthoma elasticum

Further reading:
- William T, Marsch WC, Schmidt F et al (2007) Early oral presentation of Crohn's disease. J Dtsch Dermatol Ges 5(8):678–679

Oral Erosions

- Allergic contact stomatitis
- Aphthous stomatitis
- Behçet's disease
- Candidiasis
- Chemotherapy stomatitis
- Cicatricial pemphigoid
- Crohn's disease
- Epidermolysis bullosa acquisita

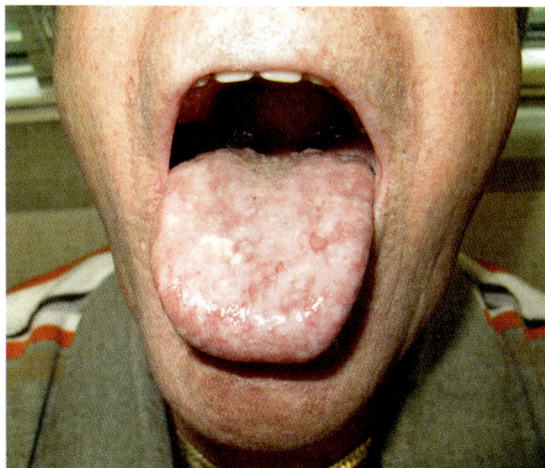

Fig. 3.22 Erosive lichen planus

- Erythema multiforme
- Fixed drug eruption
- Herpes simplex virus infection
- Linear IgA bullous dermatosis
- Lupus erythematosus
- Oral erosive lichen planus (Fig. 3.22)
- Paraneoplastic pemphigus
- Pemphigus vulgaris
- Pyostomatitis vegetans
- Stevens–Johnson syndrome (Fig. 3.23)

Further reading:

- Ayangco L, Rogers RS III (2003) Oral manifestations of erythema multiforme. Dermatol Clin 21(1):195–205

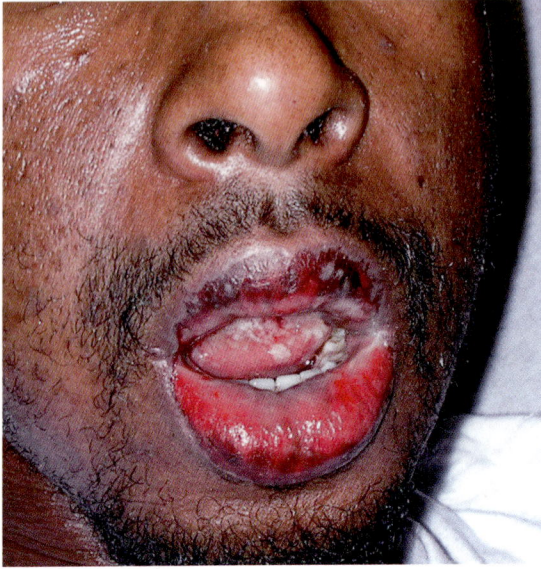

Fig. 3.23 Stevens–Johnson syndrome (Courtesy of A. Record)

Painful and Acral

- Abscess
- Achenbach syndrome
- Acral erythema
- Arthropod bite
- Behçet's disease
- Chilblains
- Chilblains lupus
- Coumadin blue-toe syndrome
- Erythema multiforme
- Erythromelalgia
- Fabry's disease
- Granuloma annulare, acute-onset painful type
- Metastatic lesions
- Neutrophilic eccrine hidradenitis
- Osler's nodes

- Palmar granuloma annulare
- Papular purpuric gloves and socks syndrome
- Piezogenic pedal papules
- Plantar eccrine hidradenitis
- Plantar erythema nodosum
- Pressure urticaria
- *Pseudomonas* hot-foot syndrome
- Raynaud's phenomenon
- Sarcoidosis
- Scleroderma
- Sweet's syndrome
- Traumatic neuroma
- Vasculitis

Further reading:
- Brey NV, Malone J, Callen JP (2006) Acute-onset, painful acral granuloma annulare: a report of 4 cases and a discussion of the clinical and histologic spectrum of the disease. Arch Dermatol 142(1):49–54

Painful Nodule

- Angioleiomyoma
- Angiolipoma
- Blue rubber bleb nevus
- Calciphylaxis
- Chondrodermatitis nodularis helicis
- Dercum's disease
- Eccrine spiradenoma
- Endometriosis
- Erythema nodosum
- Erythema nodosum leprosum
- Furunculosis/abscess
- Glomus tumor
- Granular cell tumor
- Leiomyoma

- Metastatic lesion
- Neurilemmoma
- Osler's nodes
- Piezogenic pedal papules
- Schwannoma
- Sweet's syndrome

Further reading:
- Rothman A, Glenn G, Choyke L et al (2006) Multiple painful cutaneous nodules and renal mass. J Am Acad Dermatol 55(4):683–686

Palmar Erythema

- Acute graft-vs-host disease
- Chemotherapy-induced acral erythema
- Cirrhosis
- CNS tumor
- Dermatomyositis
- Endocarditis
- Erythromelalgia
- Granuloma annulare
- Hyperthyroidism
- Leukemia
- Papular and purpuric gloves and stockings syndrome
- Pregnancy
- Rheumatoid arthritis
- Rocky Mountain spotted fever
- Systemic lupus erythematosus
- Trichinosis
- Topiramate

Further reading:
- Noble JP, Boisnic S, Branchet-Gumila MC et al (2002) Palmar erythema: cutaneous marker of neoplasms. Dermatology 204(3):209–213
- Scheinfeld N, Spahn C (2004) Palmar erythema due to topiramate. J Drugs Dermatol 3(3):321–322

Palmar Pitting/Keratoses

- Arsenical keratoses
- Basal cell nevus syndrome
- Basaloid follicular hamartoma syndrome
- Chronic renal failure
- Cowden syndrome
- Darier's disease
- Pitted keratolysis
- Paraneoplastic filiform hyperkeratosis
- Porokeratosis punctata palmaris et plantaris
- Porokeratotic eccrine ostial and dermal duct nevus
- Punctate keratoderma
- Punctate keratoses of the palmar creases
- Reticulate acropigmentation of Kitamura
- Sarcoidosis
- Spiny "music box" keratoses
- Warts

Further reading:

- Fox GN (2005) Puzzling palmar papules and pits. J Fam Pract 54(3):227–230
- Mehta RK, Mallett RB, Green C, Rytina E (2002) Palmar filiform hyperkeratosis (FH) associated with underlying pathology? Clin Exp Dermatol 27(3):216–219

Palmoplantar Keratoderma, Acquired

- Acral mycosis fungoides
- Acrokeratosis paraneoplastica
- Aquagenic keratoderma
- Arsenical keratoses
- Calluses/corns
- Confluent HPV infection
- Dyshidrotic eczema
- Eczema
- HIV related

- Howell–Evans syndrome
- Hypothyroidism-related keratoderma
- Keratoderma blenorrhagicum
- Keratoderma climactericum (Haxthausen syndrome)
- Leprosy
- Lichen planus
- Norwegian scabies
- Obesity associated
- Paraneoplastic keratoderma
- Pityriasis rubra pilaris
- Psoriasis
- Secondary syphilis
- Sezary syndrome
- Systemic lupus erythematosus
- Tinea manuum/pedis
- Tripe palms
- Tuberculosis verrucosa cutis

Further reading:
- Patel S, Zirwas M, English JC III (2007) Acquired palmoplantar keratoderma. Am J Clin Dermatol 8(1):1–11

Palmoplantar Keratoderma, Inherited

Diffuse

- Bart–Pumphrey syndrome
- Erythrokeratodermia variabilis
- Hidrotic ectodermal dysplasia (Clouston)
- Huriez syndrome with scleroatrophy
- Mal de Meleda
- Naxos disease
- Olmsted syndrome
- Papillon–Lefèvre syndrome
- Palmoplantar keratoderma with sensorineural deafness

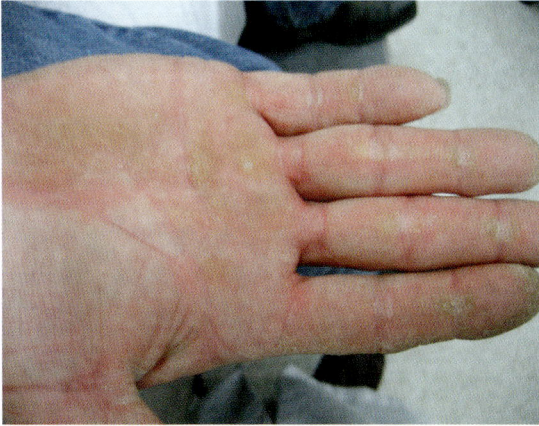

Fig. 3.24 Striate palmoplantar keratoderma

- Sybert type (Greither's type)
- Unna–Thost nonepidermolytic type
- Vohwinkel's syndrome
- Vörner's epidermolytic type

Focal

- Carvajal syndrome
- Hereditary painful callosities
- Howel–Evans syndrome
- Nummular epidermolytic type
- Pachyonychia congenita, type I
- Pachyonychia congenita, type II
- Richner–Hanhart syndrome (tyrosinemia, type II)
- Striate type (Braunauer–Fohs–Siemens; Fig. 3.24)

Punctate

- Acrokeratoelastoidosis
- Focal acral hyperkeratosis
- Punctate keratoses of the palmar creases
- Punctate palmoplantar keratoderma

Transgrediens

- Hidrotic ectodermal dysplasia
- Erythrokeratodermia variabilis
- Sybert (Greither's) type
- Mal de Meleda
- Olmsted syndrome
- Papillon–Lefèvre syndrome
- Vohwinkel syndrome

Further reading:
- Itin PH, Fistarol SK (2005) Palmoplantar keratodermas. Clin Dermatol 23(1):15–22
- Kimyai-Asadi A, Kotcher LB, Jih MH (2002) The molecular basis of hereditary palmoplantar keratodermas. J Am Acad Dermatol 47(3):327–343
- Ratnavel RC, Griffiths WA (1997) The inherited palmoplantar keratodermas. Br J Dermatol 137(4):485–490

Panniculitis

- Antitrypsin deficiency panniculitis
- Behçet's disease
- Calciphylaxis
- Cellulitis
- Cold panniculitis
- Cytophagic histiocytic panniculitis
- Deep granuloma annulare
- Equestrian panniculitis
- Erythema nodosum
- Erythema nodosum leprosum
- Factitial injury
- Infectious panniculitis
- Lipodermatosclerosis
- Lupus panniculitis
- Lymphoma
- Morphea profunda

- Neutrophilic panniculitis of rheumatoid arthritis
- Nicolau syndrome
- Nodular vasculitis
- Oxalosis
- Panniculitis of dermatomyositis
- Polyarteritis nodosa
- Scleroderma
- Subcutaneous fat necrosis
- Subcutaneous T cell lymphoma
- Thrombophlebitis

Evaluation

- ACE level
- Antineutrophil cytoplasmic antibodies
- Antinuclear antibodies
- Antistreptolysin O titer
- Antitrypsin level
- Calcium
- Chest radiograph
- Colonoscopy
- CT scan of chest, abdomen, and pelvis
- Fasting glucose
- Immunohistochemistry stains for lymphoma/leukemia
- Lower extremity Doppler ultrasound
- Pancreatic enzymes
- Parathyroid hormone
- Phosphate
- Polarizing microscopy
- Rheumatoid factor level
- Serum protein electrophoresis
- Tissue culture for bacteria, mycobacteria, and fungus
- Tuberculin skin test
- Uric acid

Further reading:

- Requena L, Yus ES (2001) Panniculitis. Part I. Mostly septal panniculitis. J Am Acad Dermatol 45(2):163–183
- Requena L, Sanchez Yus E (2001) Panniculitis. Part II. Mostly lobular panniculitis. J Am Acad Dermatol 45(3):325–361

Papules, Acneiform

- Acne aestivalis
- Acne conglobata
- Acne cosmetica
- Acne excoriee
- Acne fulminans
- Acne mechanica
- Acne miliaris necrotica
- Acne necrotica
- Acne vulgaris
- Acneiform follicular mucinosis
- Angiofibromas (Fig. 3.25)
- Behçet's disease
- Chloracne
- Cryptococcosis
- Cutaneous Rosai–Dorfman disease
- Disseminate and recurrent infundibulofolliculitis
- Drug reaction
- Drug-induced acne
- Eosinophilic folliculitis
- Eruptive milia
- Eruptive syringomas
- Eruptive vellus hair cysts
- Folliculitis
- Histoplasmosis
- Hormonal acne
- Infantile acne
- Milia

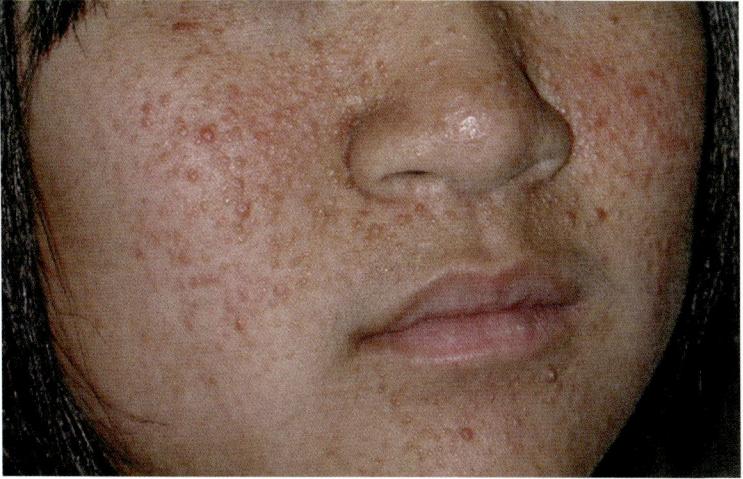

Fig. 3.25 Angiofibromas (Courtesy of K. Guidry)

- Neonatal acne
- Occupational acne
- Papular eruption of HIV
- Papular xanthoma
- Periorificial dermatitis
- Pityrosporum folliculitis
- Pseudofolliculitis barbae
- Radiation acne
- Rosacea
- Secondary syphilis
- Steroid acne
- Trichoepithelioma
- Tropical acne

Associated Medications

- Bromides
- Coal tar

- Cyclosporine
- Dactinomycin
- Daunorubicin
- EGF receptor inhibitors
- Isoniazid
- Iodides
- Lithium
- Methotrexate
- Oral contraceptives
- Phenytoin
- Progesterone-based oral contraception
- Rifampin
- Systemic corticosteroids
- Testosterone
- Topical steroids
- 5-FU

Further reading:
- Passaro EM, Silveira MT, Valente NY (2004) Acneiform follicular mucinosis. Clin Exp Dermatol 29(4):396–398
- Plewig G, Jansen T (1998) Acneiform dermatoses. Dermatology 196(1):102–107

Papules, Flesh Colored

- Acrochordon
- Colloid milium
- Connective tissue nevus
- Eruptive vellus hair cyst
- Follicular mucinosis
- Granuloma annulare
- Granulomatous periorificial dermatitis
- Intradermal nevus
- Leiomyoma
- Lichen nitidus
- Molluscum

- Neurofibroma
- Palisaded encapsulated neuroma
- Papular mucinosis
- Piezogenic pedal papules
- Subcutaneous lesion
- Syringoma
- Trichoepithelioma
- Verruca plana

Further reading:

- Kineston DP, Willard RJ, Krivda SJ (2004) Flesh-colored papules on the wrists of a 61-year-old man. Arch Dermatol 140(1):121–126

Papules, Umbilicated

- Basal cell carcinoma
- Coccidioidomycosis
- Cryptococcosis
- Eczema herpeticum
- Eruptive xanthomas
- Granuloma annulare
- Histoplasmosis
- Keratoacanthoma
- Lichen planus
- Molluscum contagiosum
- Palisaded neutrophilic and granulomatous dermatitis
- Perforating disorders
- Prurigo nodularis
- Sebaceous hyperplasia
- Smallpox

Further reading:

- Karakatsanis G, Patsatsi A, Kastoridou C et al (2007) Palmoplantar lichen planus with umbilicated papules: an atypical case with rapid therapeutic response to cyclosporin. J Eur Acad Dermatol Venereol 21(7):1006–1007

Papules, Vascular

- Acquired elastotic hemangioma
- Acroangiodermatitis
- Atypical fibroxanthoma
- Amelanotic melanoma
- Angina bullosa hemorrhagica
- Angiokeratoma
- Angiolymphoid hyperplasia with eosinophilia
- Angioma serpiginosum
- Angiosarcoma
- APACHE syndrome
- Bacillary angiomatosis
- Blue rubber bleb nevus
- Congenital hemangioma
- Eruptive pseudoangiomatosis
- Eruptive pyogenic granuloma
- Glomus tumor
- Infantile hemangioma
- Intravascular lymphoma
- Kaposi's sarcoma
- Merkel cell carcinoma
- Metastatic renal cell carcinoma
- Multinucleate cell angiohistiocytoma
- Poorly differentiated squamous cell carcinoma
- Pyogenic granuloma (Fig. 3.26)
- Reactive angioendotheliomatosis
- Targetoid hemosiderotic hemangioma
- Telangiectatic metastatic breast cancer
- Venous lake

Further reading:

- Patrizi A, Neri I, D'Acunto C et al (2003) Asymptomatic, smooth, violaceous papules of the thighs. Arch Dermatol 139(7):933–938

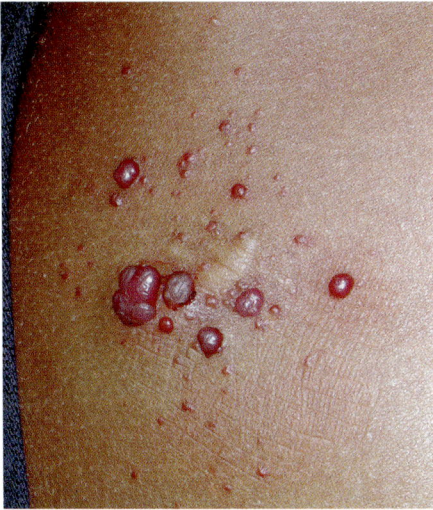

Fig. 3.26 Eruptive pyogenic granulomas

Papules, Verrucous

- Acrokeratosis verruciformis
- Angiokeratoma circumscriptum
- Blastomycosis-like pyoderma
- Bowenoid papulosis
- Condyloma acuminatum
- Condyloma lata
- Confluent and reticulated papillomatosis
- Costello syndrome
- Cowden syndrome
- Darier's disease
- Deep fungal infection
- Eccrine syringofibroadenoma
- Elephantiasis verrucosa nostra
- Epidermal nevus

- Epidermodysplasia verruciformis
- Granular cell tumor
- Halogenoderma
- Hypertrophic lichen planus
- Hypertrophic lupus erythematosus
- Incontinentia pigmenti, second stage
- Keratosis lichenoides chronica
- Lichen amyloidosis
- Lichen striatus
- Lipoid proteinosis
- Lymphangioma circumscriptum
- Nevus sebaceous
- Norwegian scabies
- Porocarcinoma
- Porokeratosis
- Prurigo nodularis
- Sebaceous adenoma
- Seborrheic keratosis
- Syringocystadenoma papilliferum
- Trichilemmoma
- Tuberculosis verrucosa cutis
- Verruca
- Verruciform xanthoma
- Verrucous carcinoma
- Verrucous hemangioma
- Verrucous psoriasis
- Verrucous syphilis
- Warty dyskeratoma

Further reading:

- Gonzalez ME, Blanco FP, Garzon MC (2007) Verrucous papules and plaques in a pediatric patient: cutaneous papillomas associated with Costello syndrome. Arch Dermatol 143(9):1201–1206

Pathergy

- Behçet's disease
- Bowel bypass syndrome
- Eosinophilic pustular folliculitis
- Pyoderma gangrenosum
- Sweet's syndrome
- Wegener's granulomatosis

Further reading:
- Hsu PJ, Huang CJ, Wu MT (2005) Pathergy in atypical eosinophilic pustular folliculitis. Int J Dermatol 44(3):203–205

Peau d'Orange Appearance

- Breast cancer
- Calciphylaxis
- Chronic lymphedema
- Eosinophilic fasciitis
- Eosinophilia–myalgia syndrome
- Granuloma faciale
- Mastocytoma
- Nephrogenic fibrosing dermopathy
- Pretibial myxedema
- Sarcoidosis
- Scleredema

Further reading:
- Nahm WK, Badiavas E, Touma DJ et al (2002) Calciphylaxis with peau d'orange induration and absence of classical features of purpura, livedo reticularis and ulcers. J Dermatol 29(4):209–213
- Solomon GJ, Wu E, Rosen PP (2007) Nephrogenic systemic fibrosis mimicking inflammatory breast carcinoma. Arch Pathol Lab Med 131(1):145–148

Penile Rash

- Behçet's disease
- Circinate balanitis
- Contact dermatitis
- Crohn's disease
- Fixed drug eruption
- Lichen nitidus
- Lichen planus
- Lichen sclerosus
- Necrobiosis lipoidica
- Pediculosis pubis
- Pityriasis rosea
- Plasma cell balanitis
- Pseudoepitheliomatous, keratotic, and micaceous balanitis
- Psoriasis
- Sarcoidosis
- Scabies
- Sexually transmitted disease

Further reading:
- Buechner SA (2002) Common skin disorders of the penis. BJU Int 90(5):498–506

Penile and Scrotal Edema

- Allergic contact dermatitis
- Angioedema
- Bladder cancer
- Colon cancer
- Crohn's disease
- Filariasis
- Hematocele
- Hypoproteinemia
- Incarcerated hernia
- Kawasaki disease

- Pancreatitis
- Parenteral fluid overload
- Paraffinoma
- Penile tourniquet syndrome
- Peritonitis
- Postoperative
- Postradiation
- Priapism
- Prostatic cancer
- Smooth muscle hamartoma of scrotum
- Torsion
- Varicocele
- Venereal disease

Further reading:
- Weinberger LN, Zirwas MJ, English JC III (2007) A diagnostic algorithm for male genital oedema. J Eur Acad Dermatol Venereol 21(2):156–162

Perforating

- Acquired perforating dermatosis
- Calcinosis cutis
- Elastosis perforans serpiginosa
- Perforating calcific elastosis
- Perforating folliculitis
- Perforating granuloma annulare
- Perforating necrobiosis lipoidica
- Perforating periumbilical calcific elastosis
- Pilomatrixoma
- Reactive perforating collagenosis

Further reading:
- Ohnishi T, Nakamura Y, Watanabe S (2003) Perforating pilomatrixoma in a process of total elimination. J Am Acad Dermatol 49(2 Suppl Case Reports):S146–S148
- Vanhooteghem O, Andre J, Brassinne M de la (2005) Epidermoid carcinoma and perforating necrobiosis lipoidica: a rare association. J Eur Acad Dermatol Venereol 19(6):756–758

Perianal

- Acrodermatitis enteropathica
- Anal fissures
- Anosacral amyloidosis
- Baboon syndrome
- Candidiasis
- Contact dermatitis
- Crohn's disease
- Dermatophyte infection
- Early decubitus ulcer
- Extramammary Paget's disease
- Fixed drug eruption
- Fournier's gangrene
- Herpes simplex virus infection
- Intertrigo
- Kawasaki disease
- Necrolytic migratory erythema
- Perianal pyramidal protrusion
- Pilonidal cyst
- Pinworm infestation
- Pruritus ani
- Psoriasis
- Streptococcal perianal eruption
- Syphilis

Further reading:
- Bauer A, Geier J, Elsner P (2000) Allergic contact dermatitis in patients with anogenital complaints. J Reprod Med 45(8):649–654

Periodontitis

- Chediak–Higashi syndrome
- Congenital neutropenias

- Ehlers–Danlos, types IV and VIII
- Haim–Munk syndrome
- Juvenile colloid milium
- Kindler syndrome
- Langerhans cell histiocytosis
- Leukocyte adhesion deficiency
- Papillon–Lefèvre syndrome
- Scurvy

Further reading:
- Hart TC, Atkinson JC (2007) Mendelian forms of periodontitis. Periodontology 45:95–112

Periorbital Edema

- Acute sinusitis
- Amyloidosis
- Angioedema
- Cellulitis
- Contact dermatitis
- Dermatomyositis
- EBV infection
- Imatinib therapy
- Leukemia
- Lupus erythematosus
- Lymphatic malformation
- Melkersson–Rosenthal syndrome
- Mucormycosis
- Sarcoidosis
- Scleredema
- Seasonal allergies
- Superior vena cava syndrome
- Tumor necrosis factor receptor-associated periodic syndrome
- Trichinosis

Further reading:
- Ioannidou DI, Krasagakis K, Stefanidou MP et al (2005) Scleredema adultorum of Buschke presenting as periorbital edema: a diagnostic challenge. J Am Acad Dermatol 52(2 Suppl 1):41–44
- Rafailidis PI, Falagas ME (2007) Fever and periorbital edema: a review. Surv Ophthalmol 52(4):422–433

Petechiae

- Acquired platelet function defects
- Aspirin therapy
- Bone marrow failure
- Congenital platelet function defects
- Dengue hemorrhagic fever
- Disseminated intravascular coagulation
- Drug-induced (see purpura)
- Essential thrombocytosis
- Hypergammaglobulinemic purpura
- Immune thrombocytopenic purpura
- Langerhans cell histiocytosis
- Monoclonal gammopathy
- Parvovirus infection
- Pigmented purpuric dermatoses
- Renal insufficiency
- Rocky Mountain spotted fever
- Scurvy
- Stasis-related
- Thrombocytopenia
- Thrombotic thrombocytopenic purpura
- Trauma
- Valsalva-related
- Wiskott–Aldrich syndrome

Further reading:
- McNeely M, Friedman J, Pope E (2005) Generalized petechial eruption induced by parvovirus B19 infection. J Am Acad Dermatol 52(5 Suppl 1):S109–S113

Phimosis

- Chancroid
- Chronic inflammation/infection
- Histoplasmosis
- Lichen sclerosus
- Squamous cell carcinoma
- Syphilis
- Verrucous carcinoma
- Trauma

Further reading:

- Ariyanayagam-Baksh SM, Baksh FK, Cartun RW et al (2007) Histoplasma phimosis: an uncommon presentation of a not uncommon pathogen. Am J Dermatopathol 29(3):300–302
- Fueston JC, Adams BB, Mutasim DF (2002) Cicatricial pemphigoid-induced phimosis. J Am Acad Dermatol 46(5 Suppl):S128–S129

Photoaggravated

- Acne vulgaris
- Atopic dermatitis
- Bullous pemphigoid
- Carcinoid syndrome
- Contact dermatitis
- Cutaneous T cell lymphoma
- Darier's disease
- Dermatomyositis
- Disseminated superficial actinic porokeratosis
- Erythema multiforme
- Grover's disease
- Hailey–Hailey disease
- Hartnup syndrome
- Herpes simplex virus infection
- Lichen planus

- Lupus erythematosus
- Pellagra
- Pemphigus erythematosus
- Pityriasis rubra pilaris
- Psoriasis
- Reticular erythematous mucinosis
- Rosacea
- Seborrheic dermatitis
- Sweet's syndrome
- Viral exanthem

Further reading:
- Murphy GM (2001) Diseases associated with photosensitivity. J Photochem Photobiol B 64(2–3):93–98

Poikiloderma

- Bloom syndrome
- Cockayne syndrome
- Dermatomyositis
- Dyskeratosis congenita
- Erythema ab igne
- Goltz syndrome
- Lupus erythematosus
- Macular amyloidosis
- Poikiloderma of Civatte
- Poikiloderma atrophicans vasculare
- Poikilodermatous mycosis fungoides
- Radiation dermatitis
- Rothmund–Thomson syndrome
- Topical steroid-induced
- Weary–Kindler syndrome
- Xeroderma pigmentosum

Further reading:
- Lipsker D (2003) What is poikiloderma? Dermatology 207(3):243–245

Poliosis

- Alezzandrini syndrome
- Alopecia areata (regrowth phase)
- Associated with nevus comedonicus
- Halo nevus
- Idiopathic poliosis
- Isolated white forelock
- Marfan syndrome
- Neurofibromatosis
- Nevus depigmentosus
- Piebaldism
- Postinflammatory poliosis
- Posttraumatic poliosis
- Rubinstein–Taybi syndrome
- Tuberous sclerosis
- Vitiligo
- Vogt–Koyanagi–Harada syndrome
- Waardenburg syndrome

Further reading:
- Wu JJ, Huang DB, Tyring SK (2006) Postherpetic poliosis. Arch Dermatol 142(2):250–251

Pseudoainhum

- Actinic reticuloid
- Burn
- Cutaneous T cell lymphoma
- Ehlers–Danlos syndrome
- Erythropoietic protoporphyria
- Factitial disease
- Frostbite
- Hair or thread tourniquet
- Leishmaniasis

- Leprosy
- Mal de Meleda
- Olmstead syndrome
- Pachyonychia congenita
- Parasitic disease
- Porokeratosis of Mibelli
- Pityriasis rubra pilaris
- Psoriasis
- Scleroderma
- Severe palmoplantar keratoderma
- Syphilis
- Syringomyelia
- Vohwinkel syndrome

Further reading:
- Rashid RM, Cowan E, Abbasi SA et al (2007) Destructive deformation of the digits with auto-amputation: a review of pseudo-ainhum. J Eur Acad Dermatol Venereol 21(6):732–737

Pseudo-Hutchinson Sign

- Amlodipine therapy
- Bowen's disease
- Congenital nevus
- Ethnic pigmentation
- Hematoma
- Laugier–Hunziker disease
- Melanocytic nevus
- Minocycline pigmentation
- Nevoid melanosis
- Peutz–Jeghers syndrome
- Radiation
- Zidovudine therapy

Further reading:

- Baran R, Kechijian P (1996) Hutchinson's sign: a reappraisal. J Am Acad Dermatol 34(1):87–90
- Sladden MJ, Mortimer NJ, Osborne JE (2005) Longitudinal melanonychia and pseudo-Hutchinson sign associated with amlodipine. Br J Dermatol 153(1):219–220

Pterygium (Fig. 3.27)

Dorsal

- Atherosclerosis
- Burns
- Cicatricial pemphigoid
- Congenital
- Diabetic vasculopathy
- Dyskeratosis congenita
- Graft-vs-host disease
- Idiopathic
- *Candida* paronychia

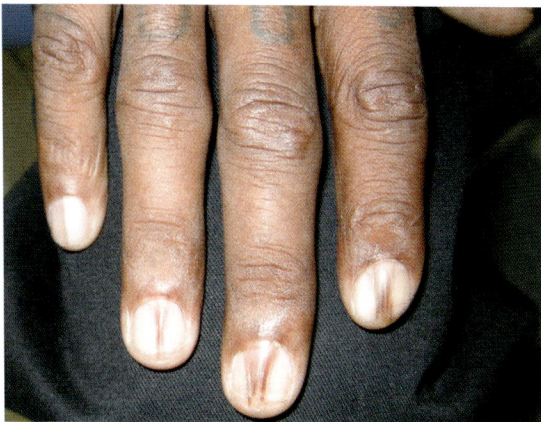

Fig. 3.27 Pterygium

- Lichen planus
- Onychotillomania
- Pemphigus foliaceus
- Radiodermatitis
- Raynaud's phenomenon
- Sarcoidosis
- Systemic lupus erythematosus
- Toxic epidermal necrolysis
- Trauma
- Type II lepra reaction

Ventral

- Congenital
- Formaldehyde-containing hardeners
- Leprosy
- Neurofibromatosis
- Subungual exostosis
- Systemic lupus erythematosus
- Systemic sclerosis

Further reading:
- Richert BJ, Patki A, Baran RL (2000) Pterygium of the nail. Cutis 66(5):343–346

Purpura and Ecchymoses

Flat and Nonbranching

- Anticoagulant use
- Bateman's purpura
- Cullen and Turner signs
- Disseminated intravascular coagulation (Fig. 3.28)
- Ehlers–Danlos syndrome
- Gardner–Diamond syndrome

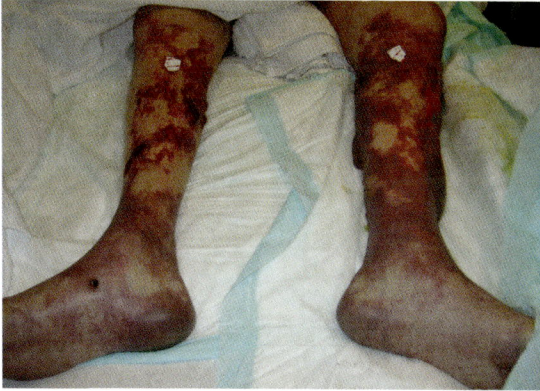

Fig. 3.28 Disseminated intravascular coagulation (Courtesy of H. Gilchrist)

- Hepatic failure
- Hypergammaglobulinemic purpura
- Scurvy
- Steroid purpura
- Systemic AL amyloidosis
- Vitamin K deficiency
- Traumatic

Palpable

- Churg–Strauss syndrome
- Cutaneous small vessel vaculitis
- Henoch–Schonlein purpura
- Livedoid vasculopathy
- Microscopic polyangiitis
- Mixed cryoglobulinemia
- Pustular vasculitis
- Rheumatic vasculitis
- Septic emboli
- Urticarial vasculitis
- Wegener's granulomatosis

Retiform

- Antiphospholipid antibody syndrome
- Aspergillosis
- Atrial myxoma
- Calciphylaxis
- Cholesterol emboli
- Churg–Strauss syndrome
- Cold agglutinins
- Coumadin necrosis
- Cryofibrinogenemia
- Cutaneous polyarteritis nodosa
- Ecthyma gangrenosum
- Endocarditis
- Heparin necrosis
- Livedoid vasculopathy
- Microscopic polyangiitis
- Monoclonal cryoglobulinemia
- Oxalosis
- Paroxysmal nocturnal hemoglobinuria
- Protein-C or protein-S deficiency
- Purpura fulminans
- Rheumatic vasculitis
- Sepsis
- Septic emboli
- Sickle cell disease
- Wegener's granulomatosis

Neonatal

- Alloimmune neonatal thrombocytopenia
- Alport syndrome variants
- Congenital (TORCH) infections
- Drug-related immune thrombocytopenia
- Extramedullary erythropoiesis

- Fanconi anemia
- Giant platelet syndromes (Bernard–Soulier, May–Hegglin)
- Glanzmann thrombasthenia
- Hemorrhagic disease of the newborn
- Hereditary clotting factor deficiencies
- Hermansky–Pudlak syndrome
- HIV infection
- Kasabach–Merritt syndrome
- Maternal autoimmune thrombocytopenia (ITP, lupus)
- Neonatal lupus erythematosus
- Protein-C and protein-S deficiency (neonatal purpura fulminans)
- Sepsis
- Thrombocytopenia with absent radii syndrome
- Trauma
- Trisomy 13 or 18
- Wiskott–Aldrich syndrome
- X-linked recessive thrombocytopenia

Purpura Fulminans

- Acetaminophen overdose
- *Capnocytophaga canimorsus* infection
- Catastrophic antiphospholipid antibody syndrome
- Churg–Strauss syndrome
- Factor-V Leiden mutation
- Gram-negative sepsis (various organisms)
- Idiopathic
- Meningococcemia
- Pneumococcal sepsis
- Protein-C and protein-S deficiency
- Scarlet fever
- Streptococcal infection
- Varicella
- *Vibrio vulnificus* infection

Associated Medications

- Allopurinol
- Aspirin
- Bactrim
- Barbiturates
- Chlorpromazine
- Diltiazem
- Furosemide
- Gold
- Hydantoins
- Isoniazid
- NSAIDs
- Penicillin
- Streptokinase
- Sulfonylureas
- Thiazides
- Thiouracils

Evaluation

- Antinuclear antibodies
- Antiphospholipid antibodies
- Bleeding time
- Blood cultures
- Complete blood count with smear
- Cryoglobulins
- Gamma globulin level
- Liver function test
- Partial thromboplastin time
- Protein-C and protein-S level
- Prothrombin time
- Rheumatoid factor level

- Serum protein electrophoresis
- Urinalysis

Further reading:

- Betrosian AP, Berlet T, Agarwal B (2006) Purpura fulminans in sepsis. Am J Med Sci 332(6):339–345
- Carlson JA, Chen KR (2007) Cutaneous pseudovasculitis. Am J Dermatopathol 29(1):44–55
- Carlson JA, Chen KR (2006) Cutaneous vasculitis update: small vessel neutrophilic vasculitis syndromes. Am J Dermatopathol 28(6):486–506
- Jones A, Walling H (2007) Retiform purpura in plaques: a morphological approach to diagnosis. Clin Exp Dermatol 32(5):596–602

Pustules, Diffuse

- Acute generalized exanthematous pustulosis
- Amicrobial pustulosis
- Disseminated zoster
- Folliculitis
- Generalized pustular psoriasis
- Halogenoderma
- IgA pemphigus
- Infantile acropustulosis
- Monkeypox
- Occupational acne
- Pemphigus foliaceus
- Pustulosis acuta generalisata
- Smallpox
- Subcorneal pustular dermatosis
- Varicella
- Viral exanthem (Fig. 3.29)

Further reading:

- Patrizi A, Savoia F, Giacomini F et al (2007) Diffuse acute pustular eruption after streptococcal infection: a new instance of pustulosis acuta generalisata. Pediatr Dermatol 24(3):272–276

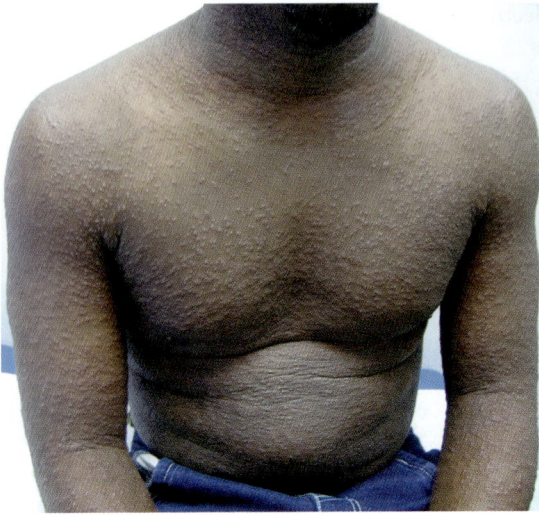

Fig. 3.29 Viral exanthem

Red Man Syndrome, Postinfusion

Associated Medications

- Amphotericin B
- Ciprofloxacin
- Infliximab
- Rifampin
- Teicoplanin
- Vancomycin

Further reading:
- Sivagnanam S, Deleu D (2003) Red man syndrome. Crit Care 7(2):119–120

Reticulated

- Atopic dirty neck
- Cantu syndrome

- Confluent and reticulated papillomatosis
- Cutis marmorata
- Dermatopathia pigmentosa reticularis
- Dowling–Degos disease
- Dyskeratosis congenita
- Eccrine hidradenitis
- Epidermolysis bullosa herpetiformis
- Erythema ab igne
- Erythema infectiosum
- Fanconi's anemia
- Galli–Galli disease
- Keratosis lichenoides chronica
- Livedo reticularis
- Mycosis fungoides
- Naegeli–Franceschetti–Jadassohn syndrome
- Pigmentatio reticularis faciei et colli
- Prurigo pigmentosa
- Reticular erythematous mucinosis
- Reticulate acropigmentation of Kitamura
- Retiform parapsoriasis
- Rothmund–Thomson syndrome
- X-linked reticulate pigmentary disorder
- Tinea versicolor
- Weary–Kindler syndrome

Further reading:
- Martin JM, Jorda E, Monteagudo C et al (2007) Occlusive eccrine hidradenitis presented as a reticulated eruption on the buttocks. Pediatr Dermatol 24(5):561–563

Retroauricular

- Acanthoma fissuratum
- Allergic contact dermatitis
- Basal cell carcinoma
- Chloracne

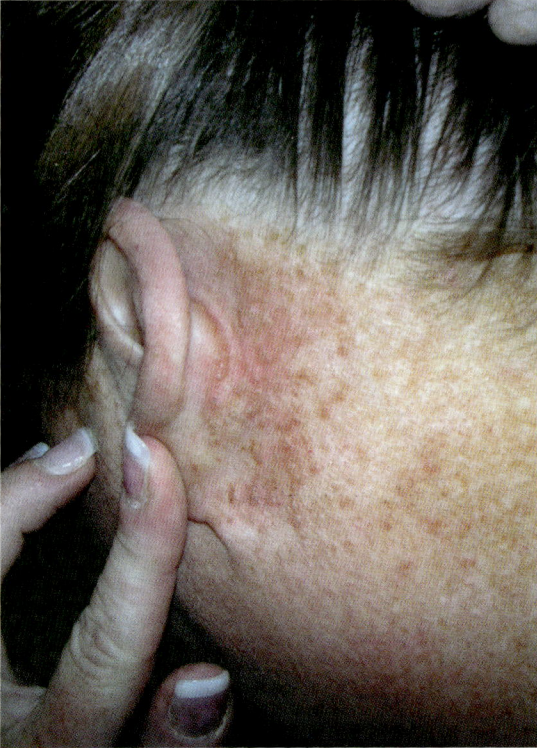

Fig. 3.30 Darier's disease (Courtesy of A. Record)

- Darier's disease (Fig. 3.30)
- Hyperimmunoglobulin E syndrome
- Infectious eczematoid dermatitis
- Infective dermatitis
- Langerhans cell histiocytosis
- Merkel cell carcinoma
- Milia en plaque
- Norwegian scabies
- Psoriasis
- Seborrheic dermatitis
- Squamous cell carcinoma

Further reading:

- Mahe A, Meertens L, Ly F et al (2004) Human T-cell leukaemia/lymphoma virus type I-associated infective dermatitis in Africa: a report of five cases from Senegal. Br J Dermatol 150(5):958–965

Saddle-Nose Deformity

- Anhidrotic ectodermal dysplasia
- Congenital rubella
- Congenital syphilis
- Crohn's disease
- Hurler syndrome
- Leishmaniasis
- Lepromatous leprosy
- Pyoderma gangrenosum
- Relapsing polychondritis
- Trauma
- Wegener's granulomatosis

Further reading:

- Daniel RK, Brenner KA (2006) Saddle nose deformity: a new classification and treatment. Facial Plast Surg Clin North Am 14(4):301–312

Scalp

- Acne necrotica
- Actinic keratosis
- Alopecia areata
- Alopecia neoplastica
- Angiosarcoma
- Atypical fibroxanthoma
- Aplasia cutis congenita
- Basal cell carcinoma
- Brunsting–Perry cicatricial pemphigoid

- Central centrifugal cicatricial alopecia
- Cirsoid aneurysm
- Contact dermatitis
- Cranial fasciitis
- Cutis verticis gyrata
- Cylindroma
- Darier's disease
- Dermatitis herpetiformis
- Discoid lupus erythematosus
- Dissecting cellulitis
- Erosive pustular dermatosis
- Folliculitis
- Kerion
- Langerhans cell histiocytosis
- Leprosy
- Lichen planopilaris
- Lichen simplex chronicus
- Melanoma
- Meningioma
- Merkel cell carcinoma
- Metastatic lesions
- Myiasis
- Nevus sebaceous
- Pediculosis capitis
- Pemphigus foliaceus
- Pilar cyst
- Pityriasis amiantacea
- Proliferating pilar tumor
- Psoriasis
- Pyogenic granuloma
- Sarcoidosis
- Scalp dysesthesia
- Seborrheic dermatitis
- Seborrheic keratosis

- Squamous cell carcinoma
- Syphilis
- Syringocystadenoma papilliferum
- Temporal arteritis
- Tinea capitis
- Tuberculosis
- Warty dyskeratoma
- Zoster

Further reading:

- Hillen U, Grabbe S, Uter W (2007) Patch test results in patients with scalp dermatitis. Contact Dermatitis 56(2):87–93

Scalp Nodule, Child

- Aplasia cutis congenita
- Arteriovenous fistula
- Cephalocele
- Cephalohematoma
- Cranial fasciitis
- Dermoid cyst
- Foreign body granuloma
- Furuncular myiasis
- Hemangioma
- Heterotopic brain tissue
- Langerhans cell histiocytosis
- Lipoma
- Lymphangioma
- Meningioma
- Metastatic disease
- Osteoma
- Pilomatrixoma
- Sarcoidosis
- Schwannoma

- Sinus pericranii
- Subcutaneous granuloma annulare

Further reading:
- Yébenes M, Gilaberte M, Romaní J et al (2007) Cranial fasciitis in an 8-year-old boy: clinical and histopathologic features. Pediatr Dermatol 24(4):E26–E30

Scalp, Scaly

- Actinic keratoses
- Atopic dermatitis
- Crusted scabies
- Dermatomyositis
- Discoid lupus erythematosus
- Erosive pustular dermatosis
- Favus
- Infective dermatitis
- Keratosis follicularis spinulosa decalvans
- Langerhans cell histiocytosis
- Pityriasis amiantacea
- Pityriasis rubra pilaris
- Psoriasis
- Seborrheic dermatitis
- Secondary syphilis
- Tinea capitis

Further reading:
- Kasteler JS, Callen JP (1994) Scalp involvement in dermatomyositis. Often overlooked or misdiagnosed. JAMA 272(24):1939–1941

Scars, Occurs in

- Amyloidosis
- Basal cell carcinoma
- Endometriosis

- Lichen nitidus
- Lichen planus
- Lichen sclerosus
- Metaplastic synovial cyst
- Metastatic Crohn's disease
- Metastatic disease
- Milia
- Necrobiosis lipoidica
- Pityriasis rubra pilaris
- Psoriasis
- Recurrent lesion
- Sarcoidosis
- Squamous cell carcinoma
- Suture granuloma
- Xanthoma

Further reading:
- Rubin AI, Stiller MJ (2002) A listing of skin conditions exhibiting the Koebner and pseudo-Koebner phenomena with eliciting stimuli. J Cutan Med Surg 6(1):29–34

Sclera, Blue

- Argyria
- Ehlers–Danlos syndrome
- Goltz syndrome
- Incontinentia pigmenti
- Marfan syndrome
- Minocycline therapy
- Nevus of Ota
- Ochronosis
- Osteogenesis imperfecta
- Pseudoxanthoma elasticum

Further reading:
- McAllum P, Slomovic A (2007) Scleral and conjunctival pigmentation following minocycline therapy. Can J Ophthalmol 42(4):626–627

Scrotum

- Addicted scrotum (steroids)
- Allergic contact dermatitis
- Angiokeratoma of Fordyce
- Behçet's disease
- Bowenoid papulosis
- Candidiasis
- Condyloma acuminatum
- Condyloma lata
- Crohn's disease
- Extramammary Paget's disease
- Fixed drug eruption
- Fournier's gangrene
- Hailey–Hailey disease
- Idiopathic scrotal calcinosis
- Irritant contact dermatitis
- Leiomyoma
- Lichen nitidus
- Lichen planus
- Lichen sclerosus
- Lichen simplex chronicus
- Metastatic lesions
- Necrolytic migratory erythema
- Porokeratosis of Mibelli
- Pruritus scroti
- Psoriasis
- Riboflavin deficiency
- Seborrheic dermatitis
- Zinc deficiency

Further reading:
- Im M, Kye KC, Kim JM et al (2007) Extramammary Paget's disease of the scrotum with adenocarcinoma of the stomach. J Am Acad Dermatol 57(2 Suppl):S43–S45

Seborrheic Distribution

- Confluent and reticulated papillomatosis
- Darier's disease
- Fogo selvagem
- Grover's disease
- Langerhans cell histiocytosis
- Pemphigus foliaceus
- Pityrosporum folliculitis
- Seborrheic dermatitis
- Tinea versicolor

Further reading:
- Gupta AK, Batra R, Bluhm R et al (2004) Skin diseases associated with Malassezia species. J Am Acad Dermatol 51(5):785–798

Serpiginous

- Epidermal nevus
- Elastosis perforans serpiginosa
- Erythema annulare centrifugum
- Erythema gyratum repens
- Erythrokeratodermia variabilis
- Granuloma annulare
- Hypomelanosis of Ito
- Ichthyosis hystrix
- Incontinentia pigmenti, third stage
- Jellyfish sting
- Larval migrans
- Lichen striatus
- Linear IgA bullous dermatosis
- Porokeratosis
- Subacute cutaneous lupus erythematosus
- Subcorneal pustular dermatosis

- Tertiary syphilis
- Tinea corporis
- Urticaria

Further reading:
- Kaminska-Winciorek G, Pierzchala E et al (2007) Cutaneous larva migrans syndrome: clinical and ultrasonographic picture of the skin lesions. Eur J Dermatol 17(3):246–247

Splinter Hemorrhages

- Antiphospholipid antibody syndrome
- Endocarditis
- High-altitude living
- HIV infection
- Lupus erythematosus
- Meningococcemia
- Onychomycosis
- Psoriasis
- Sarcoidosis
- Septic emboli
- Thyroid disease
- Trauma
- Trichinosis
- Vasculitis

Further reading:
- Saladi RN, Persaud AN, Rudikoff D et al (2004) Idiopathic splinter hemorrhages. J Am Acad Dermatol 50(2):289–292

Sporotrichoid

- Anthrax
- Atypical mycobacteria

- Cat-scratch disease
- Chromoblastomycosis
- Dimorphic fungi
- Leishmaniasis
- Mycetoma
- Nocardiosis
- Pyogenic lesions
- Streptococcal pyoderma
- Sporotrichosis
- Syphilis
- Tuberculosis
- Tularemia

Further reading:

- Madan V, Lear JT (2007) Sporotrichoid streptococcal pyoderma. J Eur Acad Dermatol Venereol 21(4):572–573

Targetoid

- Acute hemorrhagic edema of infancy
- Bullous pemphigoid
- Dermatophytosis
- Erythema multiforme-like contact dermatitis
- Erythema multiforme-like ID reaction
- Erythema migrans
- Erythema multiforme
- Fixed drug eruption
- Granuloma annulare
- Halo nevus
- Lepromatous leprosy
- Linear IgA bullous dermatosis
- Lupus erythematosus tumidus
- Metastatic lesions
- Nevus en cocarde

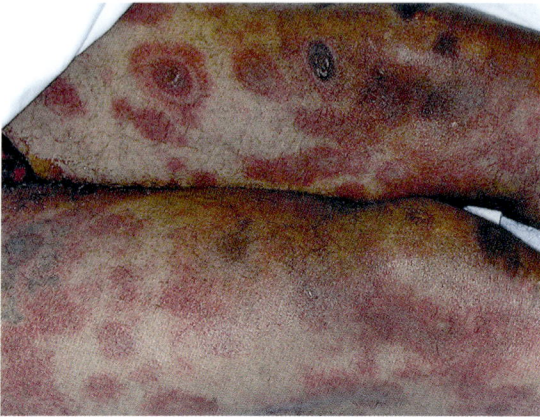

Fig. 3.31 Stevens–Johnson syndrome (Courtesy of A. Record)

- Pigmented purpuric dermatosis
- Pityriasis rosea
- Rowell's syndrome
- Secondary syphilis
- Serum-sickness like drug eruption
- Stevens–Johnson syndrome (Fig. 3.31)
- Subacute cutaneous lupus erythematosus
- Targetoid hemosiderotic hemangioma
- Toxic epidermal necrolysis
- Urticarial vasculitis
- Vasculitis

Further reading:

- Atzori L, Pau M, Aste M (2003) Erythema multiforme ID reaction in atypical dermatophytosis: a case report. J Eur Acad Dermatol Venereol 17(6):699–701
- Dereure O, Guilhou JJ, Guillot B (2003) An unusual clinical pattern of cutaneous metastasis: target-like lesions. Br J Dermatol 148(2):361

Telangiectasias

- Angioma serpiginosum
- Ataxia–telangiectasia
- Bloom syndrome
- Carcinoid syndrome
- Carcinoma telangiectaticum
- Corticosteroids
- CREST syndrome
- Cutis marmorata telangiectatica congenita
- Dermatomyositis
- Dyskeratosis congenita
- Essential telangiectasia
- Goltz syndrome
- Hereditary benign telangiectasia
- HIV infection
- Klippel–Trenaunay syndrome
- Liver disease
- Lupus erythematosus
- Lupus pernio
- Medication-induced telangiectasia
- Mycosis fungoides
- Nevus araneus
- Osler–Weber–Rendu disease
- Photodamage
- Pregnancy
- Radiodermatitis
- Rosacea
- Rothmund–Thomson syndrome
- Scleroderma
- Telangiectasia macularis eruptiva perstans
- Telangiectatic hemangioma
- Trauma

- Unilateral nevoid telangiectasia
- Venous hypertension
- Xeroderma pigmentosum

Associated Medications

- Calcium channel blockers
- Cefotaxime
- Corticosteroids
- Interferons
- Isotretinoin
- Lithium
- Methotrexate
- Oral contraception
- Thiothixene

Further reading:

- MacFarlane DF, Gregory N (1994) Telangiectases in human immunodeficiency virus-positive patients. Cutis 53(2):79–80
- Silvestre JF, Albares MP, Carnero L et al (2001) Photodistributed felodipine-induced facial telangiectasia. J Am Acad Dermatol 45(2):323–324

Tongue

- Amyloidosis
- Angioedema
- Aphthous ulcers
- Atrophic glossitis (Hunter glossitis)
- Beefy red tongue
- Behçet's disease
- Benign papillomas
- Black hairy tongue
- Blue rubber bleb nevus
- Bowen's disease

- Burning-mouth syndrome
- *Candida* infection
- Cowden disease
- Crohn's disease
- Darier's disease
- Eosinophilic ulcer
- Eruptive lingual papillitis
- Fibroma
- Fixed drug eruption
- Geographic tongue
- Granular cell tumor
- Hemangioma
- Herpes simplex
- Heterotopic lingual tonsil
- Histoplasmosis
- Leukoplakia
- Lichen planus
- Lingual thyroid nodule
- Lipoid proteinosis
- Lymphangioma
- Lymphoma
- Macroglossia
- Median rhomboid glossitis
- Metastatic carcinoma
- Multiple mucosal neuromas
- Oral hairy leukoplakia
- Polyarteritis nodosa
- Psoriasis
- Pyogenic granuloma
- Scrotal tongue
- Secondary syphilis
- Squamous cell carcinoma
- Traumatic lesions
- Tuberculosis

- Varicosities
- Venous malformation
- Verruca
- Verruciform xanthoma
- White sponge nevus

Further reading:
- Dalmau J, Alegre M, Sambeat MA et al (2006) Syphilitic nodules on the tongue. J Am Acad Dermatol 54(2 Suppl):S59–S60

Tongue, Atrophic (Glossitis)

- Atrophic candidiasis
- Vitamin B12 deficiency (Hunter glossitis)
- Iron deficiency
- Lichen planus
- Lichen sclerosus
- Malabsorption
- Median rhomboid glossitis
- Pellagra
- Squamous cell carcinoma
- Systemic lupus erythematosus
- Tertiary syphilis

Further reading:
- Terai H, Shimahara M (2007) Partial atrophic tongue other than median rhomboid glossitis. Clin Exp Dermatol 32(4):381

Trachyonychia/20 Nail Dystrophy

- Alopecia areata
- Chronic paronychia
- Eczema

- Graft-vs-host disease
- Ichthyosis vulgaris
- IgA deficiency
- Incontinentia pigmenti
- Lichen planus
- Onychophagia
- Psoriasis
- Trauma
- Vitiligo

Further reading:
- Scheinfeld NS (2003) Trachyonychia: a case report and review of manifestations, associations, and treatments. Cutis 71(4):299–302

Trichomegaly of Eyelashes

- AIDS
- Cetuximab therapy
- Cornelia de Lange syndrome
- Cyclosporine therapy
- Dermatomyositis
- Erlotinib therapy
- Interferon therapy
- Malnutrition
- Metastatic renal cell carcinoma
- Oliver–McFarlane syndrome
- Prostaglandin analogues for glaucoma
- Topiramate
- Visceral leishmaniasis

Further reading:
- Aghaei S, Dastgheib L (2006) Acquired eyelash trichomegaly and generalized hypertrichosis associated with breast anomaly. Dermatol Online J 12(2):19

Tufted Folliculitis

- Actinic keratosis
- Chronic lupus erythematosus
- Chronic staphylococcal infection
- Dissecting cellulitis
- Folliculitis decalvans
- Graham–Little syndrome
- Immunobullous disorders
- Lichen planopilaris

Further reading:
- Farhi D, Buffard V, Ortonne N et al (2006) Tufted folliculitis of the scalp and treatment with cyclosporine. Arch Dermatol 142(2):251–252

Ulcer, Leg

- Artifactual
- Arterial insufficiency
- Atherosclerosis
- Atrophie blanche
- Arteriovenous fistula
- Basal cell carcinoma
- Bites and stings
- Bullous pemphigoid
- Buruli ulcer
- Calciphylaxis
- Cellulitis
- Cholesterol emboli
- Cryoglobulinemia
- Diabetic neuropathic ulcer
- Diffuse large B cell lymphoma of the leg
- Epithelioid sarcoma

- Gummatous ulcer
- Hydroxyurea
- Hypertensive ulcer
- Intravenous drug use
- Kaposi's sarcoma
- Klinefelter syndrome
- Klippel–Trenaunay syndrome
- Leishmaniasis
- Leprosy
- Livedoid vasculopathy
- Malignant fibrous histiocytoma
- Melanoma
- Merkel cell carcinoma
- Metastatic lesion
- Mycobacterial infection
- Mycotic ulcer
- Necrobiosis lipoidica
- Osteomyelitis
- Prolidase deficiency
- Pyoderma gangrenosum
- Radiation
- Rheumatoid ulcers
- Scleroderma
- Sickle cell disease
- Small vessel vasculitis
- Spinal disorders
- Squamous cell carcinoma
- Thalassemia
- Trauma
- Tropical ulcer
- Tuberculous ulcer
- Vascular malformation
- Venous insufficiency
- Yaws

Further reading:
- Labropoulos N, Manalo D, Patel NP et al (2007) Uncommon leg ulcers in the lower extremity. J Vasc Surg 45(3):568–573
- Suss A, Simon JC, Sticherling M (2007) Primary cutaneous diffuse large B-cell lymphoma, leg type, with the clinical picture of chronic venous ulceration. Acta Derm Venereol 87(2):169–170

Ulcer, Painless

- Anthrax
- Lymphogranuloma venereum ulcer
- Lucio phenomenon/leprosy-related ulcers
- Neoplastic ulcers
- Neuropathic ulcers
- Syphilitic chancre
- Syphilitic gumma
- Syringomyelia
- Trigeminal trophic ulcer
- Varicose ulcers

Further reading:
- Hernandez FG, Rosa JN, Serra AJ, Rey JP (1999) Diffuse painless ulcerations. Arch Dermatol 135(8):984–985, 987–988

Ulcer with Lymphadenitis (Ulceroglandular Syndrome)

- Animal bite
- Anthrax
- Atypical mycobacterium
- Brucella
- Bubonic plague
- Cat-scratch disease
- Chancroid
- Glanders
- Lymphogranuloma venereum

- Melioidosis
- Primary inoculation tuberculosis
- Rat-bite fever
- Sporotrichosis
- Streptococcal/staphylococcal adenitis
- Syphilis
- Tularemia

Further reading:
- Boyce S, Pena JR, Davis DA (1999) An ulcerated nodule associated with lymphadenopathy. Arch Dermatol 135(8):985, 988

Umbilicus

- Abscess
- Atopic dermatitis
- Crohn's disease
- Endometriosis
- Fabry's disease
- Hemangioma
- Nickel dermatitis
- Omphalomesenteric duct remnant
- Pemphigoid gestationis
- Perforating calcific elastosis
- Pilonidal sinus
- Pruritic urticarial papules and plaques of pregnancy
- Psoriasis
- Pyogenic granuloma
- Rose spots of typhoid fever
- Scabies
- Seborrheic dermatitis
- Sister Mary Joseph nodule
- Strongyloidiasis
- Tuberculosis
- Vitiligo

Further reading:

- Rencic A, Cohen BA (1999) Prominent pruritic periumbilical papules: a diagnostic sign in pediatric atopic dermatitis. Pediatr Dermatol 16(6):436–438

Vesicles, Vesicopustules, and Bullae

Child

- Acute generalized exanthematous pustulosis
- Dermatitis herpetiformis
- Drug reaction
- Eczema herpeticum
- Erythema multiforme
- Hand, foot, and mouth disease
- Impetigo
- Linear IgA bullous dermatosis
- Pemphigus
- Rickettsialpox
- Scabies
- Smallpox
- TORCH infection
- Varicella
- Vesicular viral exanthem

Localized

- Allergic contact dermatitis
- Blistering distal dactylitis
- Bullous fixed drug eruption
- Bullous insect bites
- Bullous morphea
- Bullous pemphigoid
- Bullous tinea pedis
- Chemical born

- Dermatitis herpetiformis
- Dyshidrotic eczema
- Eczema herpeticum
- Erythema multiforme
- Herpes simplex virus infection
- Herpetic whitlow
- Friction blister
- Pemphigus vulgaris
- Thermal burns
- Staphylococcal scalded-skin syndrome
- Zoster

Generalized

- Bullous drug eruption
- Bullous lichen planus
- Bullous lupus erythematosus
- Bullous Sweet's syndrome (Fig. 3.32)
- Dermatitis herpetiformis

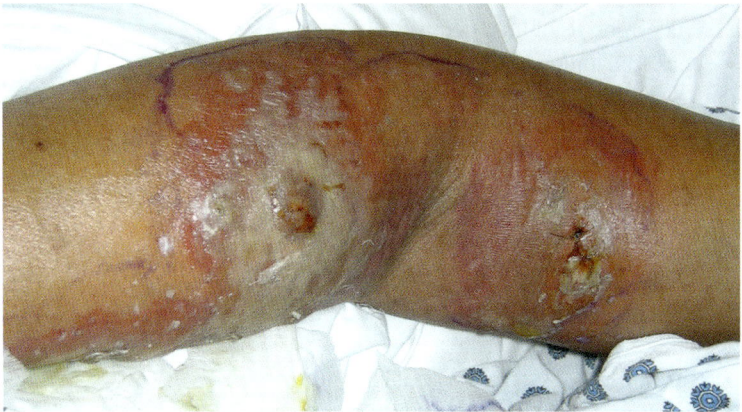

Fig. 3.32 Bullous Sweet's syndrome (Courtesy of S. Klinger)

- Disseminated zoster
- Eczema herpeticum
- Epidermolysis bullosa acquisita
- Lichen planus pemphigoides
- Linear IgA bullous dermatosis
- Pemphigoid
- Pemphigus
- Smallpox
- Staphylococcal scalded-skin syndrome
- Toxic epidermal necrolysis
- Vesicular pityriasis rosea
- Vesicular viral exanthem

Lower Extremity

- Allergic contact dermatitis
- Bullosis diabeticorum
- Bullous drug eruption
- Bullous impetigo
- Bullous insect bites
- Edema bullae
- Epidermolysis bullosa acquisita
- Localized bullous pemphigoid

Neonatal/Infantile

- Acrodermatitis enteropathica
- Acropustulosis of infancy
- Bullous congenital ichthyosiform erythroderma
- Bullous impetigo
- Bullous pemphigoid
- Chronic bullous dermatosis of childhood
- Congenital candidiasis
- Congenital erosive and vesicular dermatosis
- Congenital syphilis

- Eosinophilic pustular folliculitis
- Epidermolysis bullosa
- Erythema toxicum neonatorum
- Herpes simplex virus infection
- Herpes zoster
- Hyperimmunoglobulin E syndrome
- Iatrogenic injury
- Incontinentia pigmenti
- Intrauterine epidermal necrosis
- Intrauterine herpes simplex virus
- Kindler syndrome
- Langerhans cell histiocytosis
- *Listeria monocytogenes* infection
- Mastocytosis
- Maternal autoimmune bullous disease
- Miliaria
- Neonatal cephalic pustulosis
- Neonatal purpura fulminans
- Pemphigoid gestationis
- Porphyrias
- Pustular psoriasis
- Pyoderma gangrenosum
- Scabies
- Staphylococcal scalded-skin syndrome
- Sucking blisters
- Toxic epidermal necrolysis
- Transient bullous dermolysis
- Transient neonatal pustular melanosis
- *Varicella* infection

Noninflammatory

- Bullosis diabeticorum
- Bullous amyloidosis
- Bullous lichen sclerosus

- Bullous pemphigoid
- Drug reaction
- Edema bullae
- Epidermolysis bullosa acquisita
- Friction blister
- Porphyria cutanea tarda
- Suction blister
- Trauma

Further reading:

- Forschner A, Fierlbeck G (2005) Localized pemphigoid on the soles of both feet. Int J Dermatol 44(4):312–314
- Nanda S, Reddy BS, Ramji S et al (2002) Analytical study of pustular eruptions in neonates. Pediatr Dermatol 19(3):210–215
- Vun YY, Malik MM, Murphy GM et al (2005) Congenital erosive and vesicular dermatosis. Clin Exp Dermatol 30(2):146–148

Vulva

- Acantholytic dyskeratosis of the vulva
- Allergic contact dermatitis
- Angiofibroma of the vulva
- Angiokeratoma
- Bartholin gland cyst/abscess
- Basal cell carcinoma
- Behçet's disease
- Bullous pemphigoid
- Candidiasis
- Chancroid
- Cicatricial pemphigoid
- Ciliated cyst
- Condyloma acuminatum
- Condyloma lata
- Crohn's disease

- Dermographism
- Dysesthetic vulvodynia
- Extramammary Paget's disease
- Granular cell tumor
- Hailey–Hailey disease
- Herpes simplex virus infection
- Irritant contact dermatitis
- Lichen planus
- Lichen sclerosus
- Lymphangioma
- Lymphogranuloma venereum
- Melanocytic nevus
- Melanosis
- Melanoma
- Psoriasis
- Seborrheic dermatitis
- Squamous cell carcinoma
- Syphilis
- Syringomas
- Tinea cruris
- Trichomoniasis
- Verruciform xanthoma
- Vulvar vestibulitis syndrome

Further reading:

- Hammock LA, Barrett TL (2005) Inflammatory dermatoses of the vulva. J Cutan Pathol 32(9):604–611

Woolly Hair

- Cardiofaciocutaneous syndrome
- Carvajal syndrome
- CHANDS syndrome

- Familial woolly hair
- Naxos syndrome
- Noonan syndrome
- Woolly hair–skin fragility syndrome

Further reading:

- Chien AJ, Valentine MC, Sybert VP (2006) Hereditary woolly hair and keratosis pilaris. J Am Acad Dermatol 54(2 Suppl):S35–S39

4   The Biopsy

Acantholysis

- Acantholytic dyskeratosis of the vulva
- Actinic keratosis
- Darier's disease
- Galli–Galli disease
- Grover's disease
- Hailey–Hailey disease
- Herpes simplex virus infection
- Impetigo
- Pemphigus
- Squamous cell carcinoma
- Staphylococcal scalded-skin syndrome
- Subcorneal pustular dermatosis
- Warty dyskeratosis

Further reading:
- Mahalingam M (2005) Follicular acantholysis: a subtle clue to the early diagnosis of pemphigus vulgaris. Am J Dermatopathol 27(3):237–239

Asteroid Bodies

- Leprosy
- Sarcoidosis

- Sporotrichosis
- Tuberculosis

Further reading:
- Rodriguez G, Sarmiento L (1998) The asteroid bodies of sporotrichosis. Am J Dermatopathol 20(3):246–249

Basaloid Cells

- Basal cell carcinoma
- Basaloid follicular hamartoma
- Eccrine spiradenoma
- Lymphadenoma
- Merkel cell carcinoma
- Metastatic lesion
- Microcystic adnexal carcinoma
- Nodular hidradenoma
- Poroma
- Sebaceous carcinoma
- Sebaceous epithelioma
- Trichoadenoma
- Trichoblastoma
- Trichoepithelioma

Further reading:
- LeBoit PE (2003) Trichoblastoma, basal cell carcinoma, and follicular differentiation: what should we trust? Am J Dermatopathol 25(3):260–263

Borst–Jadassohn Phenomenon

- Actinic keratosis
- Bowen's disease

- Clonal seborrheic keratosis
- Extramammary Paget's disease
- Intracpidermal junctional nevus
- Melanoma in situ
- Porocarcinoma
- Poroma

Further reading:
- Amichai B, Grunwald MH, Halevy S (1995) A seborrheic keratosis-like lesion. Intraepidermal epithelioma of Borst–Jadassohn. Arch Dermatol 131(11):1331, 1334

Caseation Necrosis

- Demodicosis
- Granulomatous rosacea
- Lupus miliaris disseminata faciei
- Tuberculosis

Further reading:
- Ferrara G, Cannone M, Scalvenzi M et al (2001) Facial granulomatous diseases: a study of four cases tested for the presence of *Mycobacterium tuberculosis* DNA using nested polymerase chain reaction. Am J Dermatopathol 23(1):8–15

CD30+ Lymphocytes

- Anaplastic large cell lymphoma
- Arthropod bites
- Atopic dermatitis
- Drug reactions
- Hidradenitis suppurativa
- Lymphomatoid papulosis
- Molluscum contagiosum

- Mycosis fungoides
- Nodular scabies
- Parapoxvirus infection

Further reading:

- Dummer W, Rose C, Brocker EB (1998) Expression of CD30 on T helper cells in the inflammatory infiltrate of acute atopic dermatitis but not of allergic contact dermatitis. Arch Dermatol Res 290(11):598–602
- Rose C, Starostik P, Brocker EB (1999) Infection with parapoxvirus induces CD30-positive cutaneous infiltrates in humans. J Cutan Pathol 26(10):520–522

Cicatricial Alopecia

Lymphocytic

- Alopecia mucinosa
- Central centrifugal alopecia
- Chronic cutaneous lupus erythematosus
- Classic lichen planus
- Classic pseudopelade (Brocq)
- Frontal fibrosing alopecia
- Graham–Little syndrome
- Keratosis follicularis spinulosa decalvans
- Lichen planopilaris

Neutrophilic

- Dissecting cellulitis
- Folliculitis decalvans

Mixed

- Erosive pustular dermatosis
- Folliculitis (acne) keloidalis
- Folliculitis (acne) necrotica

Further reading:
* Ross EK, Tan E, Shapiro J (2005) Update on primary cicatricial alopecias. J Am Acad Dermatol 53(1):1–37

Clear Cells

* Adipose tumors
* Balloon cell tumors
* Clear cell acanthoma
* Clear cell basal cell carcinoma
* Clear cell hidradenoma
* Clear cell sarcoma
* Clear cell squamous cell carcinoma
* Clear cell syringoma
* Clear cell trichoblastoma
* Metastatic renal cell cancer
* Pilomatrixoma
* Sebaceous carcinoma
* Squamous cell carcinoma
* Trichilemmal carcinoma
* Trichilemmoma

Further reading:
* Forman SB, Ferringer TC (2007) Clear-cell basal cell carcinoma: differentiation from other clear-cell tumors. Am J Dermatopathol 29(2):208–209

Clefts or Crystals

* Amyloidosis (especially nodular)
* Basal cell carcinoma
* Cholesterol emboli syndrome
* Colloid milium
* Factitial disease
* Gout

- Necrobiosis lipoidica
- Necrobiotic xanthogranuloma
- Paraffinoma
- Post-steroid panniculitis
- Scleredema
- Sclerema neonatorum
- Sclerotic fibroma
- Spitz nevus
- Subcutaneous fat necrosis

Further reading:
- Torre C de la, Losada A, Cruces MJ (1999) Necrobiosis lipoidica: a case with prominent cholesterol clefting and transepithelial elimination. Am J Dermatopathol 21(6):575–577

Clonal T Cell Populations

- Atypical lobular lymphocytic panniculitis
- Clonal dermatitis
- Cutaneous lymphoid hyperplasia
- Cutaneous T cell lymphoma
- Idiopathic erythroderma
- Idiopathic follicular mucinosis
- Lichen planus
- Lichen sclerosus et atrophicus
- Lymphomatoid papulosis
- Pigmented purpuric dermatosis (long standing)
- Pityriasis lichenoides
- Syringolymphoid hyperplasia with alopecia

Further reading:
- Guitart J, Magro C (2007) Cutaneous T-cell lymphoid dyscrasia: a unifying term for idiopathic chronic dermatoses with persistent T-cell clones. Arch Dermatol 143(7):921–932

Cornoid Lamella

- Actinic keratosis
- Basal cell carcinoma
- Porokeratosis
- Seborrheic keratosis
- Squamous cell carcinoma
- Verruca vulgaris

Further reading:
- Shen CS, Tabata K, Matsuki M et al (2002) Premature apoptosis of keratinocytes and the dysregulation of keratinization in porokeratosis. Br J Dermatol 147(3):498–502

Direct Immunofluorescence

Basement Membrane Zone

- Bullous pemphigoid
- Chronic active hepatitis
- Dermatitis herpetiformis
- Dermatomyositis
- Epidermolysis bullosa acquisita
- Erythema multiforme
- Leukocytoclastic vasculitis
- Lichen planus
- Linear IgA bullous dermatosis
- Lupus erythematosus
- Paraneoplastic pemphigus
- Pemphigoid gestationis
- Pemphigus erythematosus
- Porphyria cutanea tarda
- Primary biliary cirrhosis
- Pseudoporphyria

- Rheumatoid arthritis
- Rosacea
- Systemic sclerosis

Intercellular Epidermis

- IgA pemphigus
- Paraneoplastic pemphigus
- Pemphigus erythematosus
- Pemphigus foliaceus
- Pemphigus vulgaris

Further reading:
- Mutasim DF, Adams BB (2001) Immunofluorescence in dermatology. J Am Acad Dermatol 45(6):803–822

Dyskeratosis

- Acantholytic dyskeratosis of the vulva
- Acrodermatitis enteropathica
- Arthropod bite
- Darier's disease
- Familial dyskeratotic comedones
- Grover's disease
- Hailey–Hailey disease
- Herpes simplex virus infection
- Incontinentia pigmenti
- Lupus erythematosus
- Lichen planus
- Lichen sclerosis
- Light reactions
- Orf/milker's nodule
- Porokeratosis
- Spitz nevus

- Warts
- Warty dyskeratoma

Further reading:
- Steffen C (1988) Dyskeratosis and the dyskeratoses. Am J Dermatopathol 10(4):356–363

Edema, Papillary Dermal

- Arthropod bite
- Gianotti–Crosti syndrome
- Pernio
- Polymorphous light eruption
- Sweet's syndrome

Further reading:
- Cribier B, Djeridi N, Peltre B et al (2001) A histologic and immunohistochemical study of chilblains. J Am Acad Dermatol 45(6):924–929

Elastic Tissue, Decreased

- Acrokeratoelastoidosis
- Anetoderma
- Cutis laxa
- Fibroelastolytic papulosis
- Granulomatous slack skin
- Middermal elastolysis
- Nevus anelasticus
- Papular elastorrhexis
- Perifollicular elastolysis (acne scars)

Further reading:
- Lewis KG, Bercovitch L, Dill SW et al (2004) Acquired disorders of elastic tissue: part II. Decreased elastic tissue. J Am Acad Dermatol 51(2):165–185

Eosinophils

- Angiolymphoid hyperplasia
- Arthropod bites and stings
- Atopic dermatitis
- Bullous pemphigoid
- Churg–Strauss syndrome
- Cutaneous T cell lymphoma
- Drug reactions
- Eosinophilic folliculitis
- Eosinophilia–myalgia syndrome
- Eosinophilic cellulitis
- Eosinophilic, polymorphic, and pruritic eruption of radiotherapy
- Eosinophilic ulcer of the tongue
- Granuloma faciale
- Hypereosinophilic syndrome
- Mastocytosis
- Parasitic infestation
- Pemphigus
- Pemphigoid gestationis
- Pruritic urticarial papules and plaques of pregnancy
- Toxic oil syndrome
- Urticaria and angioedema
- Urticarial dermatitis
- Wells syndrome

Further reading:
- Bahrami S, Malone JC, Webb KG et al (2006) Tissue eosinophilia as an indicator of drug-induced cutaneous small-vessel vasculitis. Arch Dermatol 142(2):155–161

Eosinophilic Deposits, Amorphous

- Colloid milium
- Erythropoietic protoporphyria
- Gout

- Keratoelastoidosis marginalis
- Lichen sclerosus
- Lipoid proteinosis
- Nodular amyloidosis
- Waldenstrom's macroglobulinemia

Further reading:
- Saeed S, Sagatys E, Morgan MB (2006) Acral keratosis with eosinophilic dermal deposits: a distinctive clinicopatholgic entity or colloid milium redux? J Cutan Pathol 33(10):679–685

Eosinophilic Spongiosis

- Allergic contact dermatitis
- Arthropod bite reaction
- Drug reaction
- Early bullous pemphigoid
- Eosinophilic folliculitis
- Erythema toxicum neonatorum
- Herpes gestationis
- Incontinentia pigmenti
- Pemphigus
- Photoallergic drug reaction

Further reading:
- Machado-Pinto J, McCalmont TH, Golitz LE (1996) Eosinophilic and neutrophilic spongiosis: clues to the diagnosis of immunobullous diseases and other inflammatory disorders. Semin Cutan Med Surg 15(4):308–316

Epidermal Pallor

- Acrodermatitis enteropathica
- Hartnup's disease
- Necrolytic acral erythema
- Necrolytic migratory erythema
- Pellagra

- Psoriasis
- Radiodermatitis
- Syphilis

Epidermolytic Hyperkeratosis

- Bullous congenital ichthyosiform erythroderma
- Epidermal nevus
- Follicular cysts
- Ichthyosis hystrix
- Melanocytic nevus
- Seborrheic keratosis
- Vorner's palmoplantar keratoderma

Further reading:
- Mahaisavariya P, Cohen PR, Rapini RP (1995) Incidental epidermolytic hyperkeratosis. Am J Dermatopathol 17(1):23–28

Epidermotropism

- Epidermotropic CD8+ T cell lymphoma
- Langerhans cell histiocytosis
- Metastatic adenocarcinoma
- Metastatic melanoma
- Metastatic squamous cell carcinoma
- Mycosis fungoides
- Pagetoid reticulosis
- Xanthoma

Further reading:
- Arai E, Shimizu M, Tsuchida T et al (2007) Lymphomatoid keratosis: an epidermotropic type of cutaneous lymphoid hyperplasia: clinicopathological, immunohistochemical, and molecular biological study of 6 cases. Arch Dermatol 143(1):53–59
- Northcutt AD (2000) Epidermotropic xanthoma mimicking balloon cell melanoma. Am J Dermatopathol 22(2):176–178

- Stanko C, Grandinetti L, Baldassano M et al (2007) Epidermotropic metastatic prostate carcinoma presenting as an umbilical nodule – Sister Mary Joseph nodule. Am J Dermatopathol 29(3):290–292

Erythrocyte Extravasation/Hemosiderin

- Allergic contact dermatitis
- Arthropod bite reaction
- Bleeding disorder
- Dermatofibroma
- Discoid lupus erythematosus
- Erythema ab igne
- Granuloma faciale
- Hemochromatosis
- Kaposi's sarcoma
- Leukocytoclastic vasculitis
- Lichen sclerosus et atrophicus
- Lymphomatoid papulosis
- Pigmented purpuric dermatoses
- Pityriasia rosea
- Pityriasis lichenoides et varioliformis acuta
- Porphyria cutanea tarda
- Renal cell carcinoma
- Rickettsial infection
- Scurvy
- Stasis dermatitis
- Targetoid hemosiderotic hemangioma
- Trichotillomania
- Vascular neoplasms
- Vasculitis
- Viral infection

Further reading:

- Carlson JA, Chen KR (2007) Cutaneous pseudovasculitis. Am J Dermatopathol 29(1):44–55

Fat in Dermis

- Goltz syndrome
- Lipedematous alopecia
- Melanocytic nevus
- "Michelin tire baby" syndrome
- Nevus lipomatosus
- Piezogenic pedal papules
- Proteus syndrome

Further reading:
- Martin JM, Monteagudo C, Montesinos E et al (2005) Lipedematous scalp and lipedematous alopecia: a clinical and histologic analysis of 3 cases. J Am Acad Dermatol 52(1):152–156

Flame Figures

- Arthropod bite reaction
- Bullous pemphigoid
- Drug reaction
- Eczema
- Hypereosinophilic syndrome
- Parasitic infestation
- Tinea
- Wells syndrome

Further reading:
- Leiferman KM, Peters MS (2006) Reflections on eosinophils and flame figures: where there's smoke there's not necessarily Wells syndrome. Arch Dermatol 142(9):1215–1218

Foam Cells

- Atypical fibroxanthoma
- Balloon cell melanoma

- Balloon cell nevus
- Dermatofibroma
- Granular cell tumor
- Hibernoma
- Juvenile xanthogranuloma
- Langerhans cell histiocytosis
- Lepromatous leprosy
- Liposarcoma
- Malakoplakia
- Necrobiotic xanthogranuloma
- Pneumocystosis
- Rhinoscleroma
- Sebaceous gland tumors
- Verruciform xanthoma
- Xanthoma disseminatum
- Xanthomas

Further reading:

- Terayama K, Hirokawa M, Shimizu M et al (1999) Balloon melanoma cells mimicking foamy histiocytes. Acta Cytol 43(2):325–326

Giant Cells

- Atypical fibroxanthoma
- Erythema nodosum
- Foreign body
- Giant cell tumor of the tendon sheath
- Juvenile xanthogranuloma
- Keratin granuloma
- Necrobiosis lipoidica
- Pilomatricoma
- Reticulohistiocytoma
- Sarcoidosis

Granulomas

- Actinic granuloma
- Annular elastolytic giant cell granuloma
- Atypical necrobiosis lipoidica
- Blau syndrome
- Chronic granulomatous disease
- Common variable immunodeficiency
- Crohn's disease
- Deep fungal infection
- Foreign body reactions
- Granuloma annulare
- Granuloma multiforme
- Granulomatous mycosis fungoides
- Granulomatous rosacea
- Granulomatous slack skin
- Interstitial granulomatous drug reaction
- Interstitial granulomatous dermatitis with arthritis
- Leishmaniasis
- Lupus miliaris disseminata faciei
- Necrobiosis lipoidica
- Necrobiotic xanthogranuloma
- Prototothecosis
- Rheumatic fever nodule
- Rheumatoid nodule
- Sarcoidosis
- Systemic lymphoma
- Tertiary syphilis
- Tuberculoid leprosy
- Tuberculosis
- Wegener's granulomatosis

Further reading:
- Limas C (2004) The spectrum of primary cutaneous elastolytic granulomas and their distinction from granuloma annulare: a clinicopathological analysis. Histopathology 44(3):277–282

- Rongioletti F, Cerroni L, Massone C et al (2004) Different histologic patterns of cutaneous granulomas in systemic lymphoma. J Am Acad Dermatol 51(4):600–605

Grenz Zone

- B cell lymphoma
- Cutaneous T cell lymphoma
- Granuloma faciale
- Lepromatous leprosy
- Lymphocytoma cutis
- Multicentric reticulohistiocytosis

Further reading:
- Ortonne N, Wechsler J, Bagot M et al (2005) Granuloma faciale: a clinicopathologic study of 66 patients. J Am Acad Dermatol 53(6):1002–1009

Hobnail Endothelium

- Angiolymphoid hyperplasia with eosinophilia
- Hobnail (targetoid hemosiderotic) hemangioma
- Endovascular papillary angioendothelioma
- Retiform hemangioendothelioma

Further reading:
- Franke FE, Steger K, Marks A et al (2004) Hobnail hemangiomas (targetoid hemosiderotic hemangiomas) are true lymphangiomas. J Cutan Pathol 31(5):362–367

Interstitial Inflammation

- Abscess/cellulitis
- Arthropod bite reaction
- Erythema marginatum
- Granuloma annulare
- Granuloma faciale
- Interstitial drug reaction

- Interstitial granulomatous dermatitis with arthritis
- Interstitial mycosis fungoides
- Intertriginous eruptions
- Pyoderma gangrenosum
- Sweet's syndrome
- Urticaria
- Urticarial dermatitis
- Wells syndrome

Further reading:

- Kwon EJ, Hivnor CM, Yan AC et al (2007) Interstitial granulomatous lesions as part of the spectrum of presenting cutaneous signs in pediatric sarcoidosis. Pediatr Dermatol 24(5):517–524

Lichenoid Reaction Pattern/Band-Like Infiltrate

Cell Rich

- Chronic graft-vs-host disease
- Cutaneous lymphoid hyperplasia
- Halo nevus
- Hyperkeratosis lenticularis perstans
- Keratosis lichenoides chronica
- Langerhans cell histiocytosis
- Lichen planus
- Lichen sclerosus et atrophicus
- Lichen striatus
- Lichenoid actinic keratosis
- Lichenoid drug eruption
- Lichenoid keratosis
- Lichenoid pigmented purpuric dermatosis
- Lymphomatoid keratosis
- Lymphomatoid papulosis
- Melanoma

- Mycosis fungoides
- Parapsoriasis
- Pityriasis lichenoides et varioliformis acuta
- Poikiloderma atrophicans vasculare
- Secondary syphilis
- Zoon balanitis

Cell Poor

- Dermatomyositis
- Erythema multiforme
- Fixed drug eruption
- Graft-vs-host disease
- Lupus erythematosus
- Lichen sclerosus et atrophicus
- Morbilliform drug reaction
- Pityriasis lichenoides chronica

Further reading:
- Morgan MB, Stevens GL, Switlyk S (2005) Benign lichenoid keratosis: a clinical and pathologic reappraisal of 1040 cases. Am J Dermatopathol 27(5):387–392

Perivascular Inflammation

Superficial

- Dermatophytosis
- Drug reaction
- Eczematous dermatitis
- Erythema dyschromicum perstans
- Erythema multiforme
- Pigmented purpuric dermatosis
- Post-inflammatory pigmentary alteration

- Telangiectasia macularis eruptiva perstans
- Urticaria
- Viral exanthem

Superficial and Deep

- Arthropod bite reaction
- Cutaneous T cell lymphoma
- Discoid lupus erythematosus
- Erythema annulare centrifugum
- Fixed drug eruption
- Gyrate erythemas
- Jessner's lymphocytic infiltrate
- Leukemia/lymphoma
- Lichen striatus
- Lichenoid drug
- Lupus erythematosus
- Lymphocytoma cutis
- Lymphomatoid papulosis
- Pityriasis lichenoides et varioliformis acuta
- Polymorphous light eruption
- Reticular erythematous mucinosis
- Syphilis

Further reading:
- Carlson JA, Chen KR (2007) Cutaneous vasculitis update: neutrophilic muscular vessel and eosinophilic, granulomatous, and lymphocytic vasculitis syndromes. Am J Dermatopathol 29(1):32–43

Lymphocytic Vasculitis

- Angiocentric lymphoma
- Degos' disease

- Erythema annulare centrifugum
- Insect bite reactions
- Kawasaki disease
- Livedoid vasculopathy
- Lupus erythematosus
- Perniosis
- Pigmented purpuric dermatosis
- Pityriasis lichenoides
- Polymorphous light eruption
- Rickettsial infection
- Sjögren's syndrome
- Viral exanthem

Further reading:
- Kossard S (2000) Defining lymphocytic vasculitis. Australas J Dermatol 41(3):149–155

Lymphoid Follicles

- Actinic prurigo cheilitis
- Angiolymphoid hyperplasia with eosinophilia
- Branchial cleft cyst
- Bronchogenic cyst
- Insect bite reaction
- Lupus profundus
- Lymphocytoma cutis
- Lymphoma cutis
- Necrobiosis lipoidica
- Necrobiotic xanthogranuloma

Further reading:
- Herrera-Geopfert R, Magana M (1995) Follicular cheilitis. A distinctive histopathologic finding in actinic prurigo. Am J Dermatopathol 17(4):357–361

Mucin

Primary

- Acral persistent papular mucinosis
- Cutaneous focal mucinosis
- Cutaneous lupus mucinosis
- Cutaneous mucinosis of infancy
- Digital mucous cyst
- Mycosis fungoides-associated follicular mucinosis
- Generalized myxedema
- Lichen myxedematosus
- Mucinous nevus
- Pinkus' follicular mucinosis
- Pretibial myxedema
- Reticular erythematous mucinosis
- Scleredema
- Scleromyxedema
- Self-healing cutaneous mucinosis
- Urticaria-like follicular mucinosis

Secondary

- Actinic elastosis
- Angiolymphoid hyperplasia with eosinophilia
- Basal cell carcinoma
- Chronic graft-vs-host disease
- Cutaneous leukemia
- Degos' disease
- Dermatomyositis
- Epithelial tumors
- Familial reticuloendotheliosis

- Follicular mucinosis
- Granuloma annulare
- Hodgkin's disease
- Hypertrophic lichen planus
- Hypertrophic scar
- Insect bites
- Keratoacanthoma
- Lichen striatus
- Lupus erythematosus
- Lymphoma
- Mesenchymal tumors
- Mycosis fungoides
- Neural tumors
- Pachydermoperiostosis
- Cutaneous lymphoid hyperplasia
- Sarcoidosis
- Scleroderma
- Spongiotic dermatitis
- Squamous cell carcinoma
- UV radiation and PUVA
- Verruca vulgaris

Further reading:

- Rongioletti F, Rebora A (2001) Cutaneous mucinoses: microscopic criteria for diagnosis. Am J Dermatopathol 23(3):257–267

Neutrophils

- Acropustulosis of infancy
- Acute generalized exanthematous pustulosis
- Atypical mycobacteria
- Behçet's disease
- Bowel bypass syndrome

- Bullous pemphigoid
- Bullous systemic lupus erythematosus
- Candidiasis
- Clear cell acanthoma
- Dermatitis herpetiformis
- Dermatophytosis
- Epidermolysis bullosa acquisita
- Erythema elevatum diutinum
- Fire ant bites
- Geographic tongue
- Gonococcemia
- Granuloma faciale
- Halogenoderma
- IgA pemphigus
- Impetigo
- Infectious diseases
- Leukocytoclastic vasculitis
- Linear IgA bullous dermatosis
- Necrolytic migratory erythema
- Neutrophilic eccrine hidradenitis
- Neutrophilic urticaria
- Palisaded neutrophilic and granulomatous dermatitis
- Pemphigus foliaceus
- Pityriasis lichenoides et varioliformis acuta
- Prurigo pigmentosa
- Psoriasis
- Pustular vasculitis
- Pyoderma gangrenosum
- Pyogenic granuloma
- Rheumatoid neutrophilic dermatosis
- Ruptured cysts/follicles
- Scabies
- Sneddon–Wilkinson disease

- Sweet's syndrome
- Transient neonatal pustular melanosis
- Ulceration

Further reading:
- Nischal KC, Khopkar U (2007) An approach to the diagnosis of neutrophilic dermatoses: a histopathological perspective. Indian J Dermatol Venereol Leprol 73(4):222–230

Normal Appearance (Subtle Histologic Abnormalities)

- Amyloidosis
- Anetoderma
- Connective tissue nevus
- Cutis laxa
- Dermatophytosis
- Ichthyosis
- Morbilliform drug
- Morphea
- Myxedema
- Post-inflammatory pigmentary alteration
- Tinea versicolor
- Telangiectasia macularis eruptive perstans
- Urticaria
- Urticaria pigmentosa
- Viral exanthem
- Vitiligo

Pagetoid Cells

- Acral melanocytic nevus
- Borst–Jadassohn phenomenon
- Bowen's disease

- Epidermotropic adnexal carcinoma
- Epidermotropic CD8+ T cell lymphoma
- Langerhans' cell histiocytosis
- Lymphomatoid papulosis
- Melanoma
- Merkel cell carcinoma
- Mycosis fungoides
- Paget's disease
- Sebaceous carcinoma

Further reading:
- Kohler S, Rouse RV, Smoller BR (1998) The differential diagnosis of pagetoid cells in the epidermis. Mod Pathol 11(1):79–92

Palisading

- Churg-Strauss syndrome
- Granuloma annulare
- Interstitial granulomatous dermatitis
- Necrobiosis lipoidica
- Rheumatoid nodule
- Wegener's granulomatosis

Papillomatosis, Hyperkeratosis, and Acanthosis

- Acanthosis nigricans
- Acrokeratosis verruciformis
- Confluent and reticulated papillomatosis
- Epidermal nevus
- Seborrheic keratosis
- Verruca

Further reading:
- Ersoy-Evans S, Sahin S, Mancini AJ et al (2006) The acanthosis nigricans form of epidermal nevus. J Am Acad Dermatol 55(4):696–698

Parakeratosis

- Actinic keratosis
- Axillary granular parakeratosis
- Benign lichenoid keratosis
- Darier's disease
- Dermatophytosis
- Discoid lupus erythematosus
- Eczematous dermatitis
- Erythema annulare centrifugum
- Grover's disease
- Inflammatory linear verrucous epidermal nevus
- Lichenoid drug eruption
- Mycosis fungoides, plaque stage
- Necrolytic migratory erythema
- Pityriasis lichenoides
- Pityriasis rosea
- Pityriasis rubra pilaris
- Porokeratosis
- Psoriasis
- Seborrheic dermatitis
- Small and large plaque parapsoriasis
- Verruca vulgaris

In Mounds

- Dermatophytosis
- Erythema annulare centrifugum
- Guttate psoriasis
- Pityriasia rosea
- Seborrheic dermatitis
- Small plaque parapsoriasis

Further reading:
- Brady SP (2004) Parakeratosis. J Am Acad Dermatol 50(1):77–84

Parasitized Histiocytes

- Ehrlichiosis
- Granuloma inguinale
- Histoplasmosis
- Leishmaniasis
- *Penicillium marneffei* infection
- Rhinoscleroma
- Toxoplasmosis

Pigment in Dermis

- Alkaptonuria
- Amiodarone
- Chlorpromazine
- Gold
- Hemosiderin
- Imipramine
- Lipofuscin
- Melanin
- Minocycline
- Silver
- Tattoo

Further reading:
- Suzuki H, Baba S, Uchigasaki S et al (1993) Localized argyria with chrysiasis caused by implanted acupuncture needles. Distribution and chemical forms of silver and gold in cutaneous tissue by electron microscopy and X-ray microanalysis. J Am Acad Dermatol 29(5 Pt 2):833–837

Plasma Cells

- Acne keloidalis nuchae
- Actinic keratosis

- Basal cell carcinoma
- Borrelial infection
- Cutaneous plasmacytosis
- Folliculitis
- Foreign body reaction
- HIV infection
- Morphea
- Mucosal surfaces
- Mycosis fungoides
- Necrobiosis lipoidica
- Plasmacytoma
- Rhinoscleroma
- Secondary syphilis
- Squamous cell carcinoma
- Syringocystadenoma papilliferum

Further reading:
- Jayaraman AG, Cesca C, Kohler S (2006) Cutaneous plasmacytosis: a report of five cases with immunohistochemical evaluation for HHV-8 expression. Am J Dermatopathol 28(2):93–98

Pseudoepitheliomatous Hyperplasia

- Blastomycosis
- Chromoblastomycosis
- Chronic ulcer
- Granular cell tumor
- Halogenoderma
- Hypertrophic lichen planus
- Keratoacanthoma
- Melanoma
- Mycobacterial infections
- Orf
- Pemphigus vegetans

- Pyoderma gangrenosum
- Sporotrichosis
- Syphilis
- Tattoo
- T cell lymphoma
- Venous stasis ulcer
- Verrucous lupus erythematosus

Further reading:
- Zayour M, Lazova R (2011) Pseudoepitheliomatous hyperplasia: a review. Am J Dermatopathol 33(2):112–122; quiz 123–126

Spindle Cells

- Atypical fibroxanthoma
- Blue nevus
- Dermatofibrosarcoma protuberans
- Fibrous proliferations
- Kaposi's sarcoma
- Leiomyoma
- Leiomyosarcoma
- Melanoma
- Metastatic sarcoma
- Neural neoplasms
- Spindle cell hemangioendothelioma
- Spindle cell lipoma
- Spindle cell squamous cell carcinoma
- Spindle cell xanthogranuloma
- Spitz nevus

Further reading:
- Folpe AL, Cooper K (2007) Best practices in diagnostic immunohistochemistry: pleomorphic cutaneous spindle cell tumors. Arch Pathol Lab Med 131(10):1517–1524

Splendore–Hoeppli Phenomenon

- Actinomycosis
- Botryomycosis
- Mycetoma
- Nocardiosis
- Sporotrichosis

Further reading:
- Rodig SJ, Dorfman DM (2001) Splendore–Hoeppli phenomenon. Arch Pathol Lab Med 125(11):1515–1516

Spongiosis

- Atopic dermatitis
- Bullous pemphigoid
- Contact dermatitis
- Dyshidrotic eczema
- Eczematoid purpura of Doucas and Kapetanakis
- Erythema annulare centrifugum
- Erythema multiforme
- Gianotti–Crosti syndrome
- Herpes gestationis
- Id reaction
- Incontinentia pigmenti
- Insect bite reactions
- Lichen striatus
- Miliaria rubra
- Mycosis fungoides
- Nummular eczema
- Photoallergic contact dermatitis
- Pityriasis rosea

- Seborrheic dermatitis
- Small plaque parapsoriasis
- Spongiotic drug eruption

Square Specimen

- Lichen myxedematosus
- Keloid
- Morphea
- Necrobiosis lipoidica
- Nephrogenic systemic fibrosis
- Normal back
- Radiation dermatitis
- Scleredema

Transepidermal Elimination

- Acquired perforating dermatosis
- Calcinosis cutis
- Elastosis perforans serpiginosa
- Granuloma annulare
- Gout
- Melanoma
- Nevus
- Pilomatrixoma
- Pseudoxanthoma elasticum
- Reactive perforating collagenosis

Further reading:
- Ohnishi T, Nakamura Y, Watanabe S (2003) Perforating pilomatricoma in a process of total elimination. J Am Acad Dermatol 49(2 Suppl Case Reports):S146–S147

Vesicles

Intraepidermal

- Acrodermatitis enteropathica
- Darier's disease
- Epidermolysis bullosa simplex
- Friction blister
- Grover's disease
- Hailey–Hailey disease
- Herpes simplex virus infection
- IgA pemphigus, intraepidermal type
- Incontinentia pigmenti
- Palmoplantar pustulosis
- Paraneoplastic pemphigus
- Pemphigus vegetans
- Pemphigus vulgaris
- Varicella-zoster virus infection

Subcorneal or Intracorneal

- Acute generalized exanthematous pustulosis
- Candidiasis
- Dermatophytosis
- Erythema toxicum neonatorum
- IgA pemphigus, subcorneal type
- Impetigo
- Infantile acropustulosis
- Miliaria crystallina
- Pemphigus foliaceus
- Pustular psoriasis
- Subcorneal pustular dermatosis
- Staphylococcal scalded-skin syndrome

Subepidermal with Eosinophils

- Arthropod bite reaction
- Bullous eosinophilic cellulitis
- Bullous pemphigoid
- Drug eruption
- Pemphigoid gestationis

Subepidermal with Lymphocytes

- Erythema multiforme
- Fixed drug eruption
- Lichen planus, bullous type
- Lichen sclerosus et atrophicus
- Paraneoplastic pemphigus
- Polymorphous light eruption

Subepidermal with Neutrophils

- Bullous cellulitis
- Bullous leukocytoclastic vasculitis
- Bullous pemphigoid
- Bullous Sweet's syndrome
- Bullous systemic lupus erythematosus
- Cicatricial pemphigoid
- Dermatitis herpetiformis
- Inflammatory epidermolysis bullosa acquisita
- Linear IgA bullous dermatosis
- Pyoderma gangrenosum

Subepidermal and Noninflammatory

- Bullous amyloidosis
- Bullous diabetes
- Bullous drug eruption

- Bullous lichen sclerosus
- Bullous morphea
- Bullous pemphigoid, cell-poor type
- Burns
- Coma bullae
- Cryotherapy bullae
- Noninflammatory epidermolysis bullosa acquisita
- Porphyria cutanea tarda
- Pseudoporphyria
- Suction blister
- Toxic epidermal necrolysis

ACE Level Elevated

- Alpha1-antitrypsin deficiency
- Amyloidosis
- Asbestosis
- Asthma
- Gaucher's disease
- Hypertension
- Kaposi's sarcoma
- Leprosy
- Liver disease
- Melkersson–Rosenthal syndrome
- Myeloma
- Primary biliary cirrhosis
- Renal failure
- Sarcoidosis
- Silicosis
- Small cell lung cancer
- Smoker
- Tuberculosis
- Type I diabetes mellitus

Further reading:

- Uçar G, Yildirim Z, Ataol E et al (1997) Serum angiotensin converting enzyme activity in pulmonary diseases: correlation with lung function parameters. Life Sci 61(11):1075–1182

Anemia

- Aplastic anemia
- Bone marrow infiltration
- Chronic infection
- Chronic inflammatory disease (RA, SLE, etc.)
- Chronic liver disease
- Chronic renal disease
- Congenital anemia
- Fanconi anemia
- Folate deficiency
- Hemoglobinopathy
- Hemolysis
- Internal malignancy
- Iron deficiency
- Leukemia
- Lymphoma
- Malabsorption
- Pregnancy
- Vitamin B12 deficiency

Further reading:
- Tefferi A (2003) Anemia in adults: a contemporary approach to diagnosis. Mayo Clin Proc 78(10):1274–1280

Antineutrophilic Cytoplasmic Antibodies

- Churg–Strauss syndrome (P > C)
- Cocaine-associated vasculopathy
- Drug-induced vasculitis (P)
- Hydralazine therapy
- Microscopic polyangiitis (P > C)
- Minocycline therapy

- Primary biliary cirrhosis (P)
- Propylthiouracil therapy
- Rheumatoid arthritis (P)
- Sclerosing cholangitis (P)
- Systemic lupus erythematosus (P)
- Ulcerative colitis (P)
- Wegener's granulomatosis (C > P)

Further reading:
- Colglazier CL, Sutej PG (2005) Laboratory testing in the rheumatic diseases: a practical review. South Med J 98(2):185–191

Antinuclear Antibodies

- Addison's disease
- Autoimmune hemolytic anemia
- Autoimmune hepatitis
- Autoimmune urticaria
- Cocaine-associated vasculopathy
- Dermatomyositis
- Hashimoto's thyroiditis
- Immune thrombocytopenic purpura
- Mixed connective tissue disease
- Primary biliary cirrhosis
- Rheumatoid arthritis
- Scleroderma
- Sjögren syndrome
- Systemic lupus erythematosus

Further reading:
- Kavanaugh A, Tomar R, Reveille J et al (2000) Guidelines for clinical use of the antinuclear antibody test and tests for specific autoantibodies to nuclear antigens. Arch Pathol Lab Med 124:71–81

Eosinophilia

- Addison's disease
- Allergic bronchopulmonary aspergillosis
- Allergic contact dermatitis
- Atheroembolic disease
- Atopic dermatitis
- Bullous pemphigoid
- Churg–Strauss vasculitis
- Coccidioidomycosis
- Dermatitis herpetiformis
- Dermatomyositis
- Drug hypersensitivity
- Drug-induced interstitial nephritis
- Eosinophilia–myalgia syndrome
- Eosinophilic cellulitis
- Eosinophilic fasciitis
- Eosinophilic pneumonia
- Episodic angioedema with eosinophilia
- Exfoliative erythroderma
- Hypereosinophilic syndrome
- Hyper-IgE syndrome
- Internal malignancy
- Interstitial nephritis
- Leukemia
- Lymphomas
- Mastocytosis
- Omenn syndrome
- Parasitic infestation
- Pemphigus
- Rheumatoid arthritis
- Sarcoidosis
- Scabies

- Scleroderma
- Sezary syndrome
- Systemic lupus erythematosus
- Urticaria

Further reading:
- Sade K, Mysels A, Levo Y et al (2007) Eosinophilia: a study of 100 hospitalized patients. Eur J Intern Med 18(3):196–201

Hypergammaglobulinemia

- Angioimmunoblastic lymphadenopathy with dysproteinemia
- Chronic infection
- Chronic inflammatory diseases
- HIV infection
- Monoclonal gammopathy of undetermined significance
- Myeloma
- Sarcoidosis
- Waldenstrom's hypergammaglobulinemia

Further reading:
- Kyle RA, Rajkumar SV (2006) Monoclonal gammopathy of undetermined significance. Br J Haematol 134(6):573–589

Hypogammaglobulinemia

- Bruton's agammaglobulinemia
- Common variable immunodeficiency
- Glucocorticosteroids and other immunosuppressants
- Hyper-IgM syndrome
- Lymphoma
- Nephrotic syndrome

- Protein-losing enteropathy
- Severe combined immunodeficiency
- Thymoma (Good syndrome)

Further reading:
- Grimbacher B, Schäffer AA, Peter HH (2004) The genetics of hypogammaglobulinemia. Curr Allergy Asthma Rep 4(5):349–358

Liver Enzymes Elevated

- Alcoholic hepatitis
- Amebic lever abscess
- Antitrypsin deficiency
- Autoimmune hepatitis
- Bacterial sepsis
- Cholestatic liver disease
- Disseminated fungal infection
- Drug-induced hepatotoxicity
- Gonococcal infection
- Leptospirosis
- Heart failure
- Liver ischemia
- Mononucleosis
- Pancreatic disease
- Sarcoidal hepatitis
- Steatohepatitis
- Tuberculosis
- Viral hepatitis
- Wilson's disease

Further reading:
- Pratt DS, Kaplan MM (2000) Evaluation of abnormal liver-enzyme results in asymptomatic patients. N Engl J Med 342(17):1266–1271

Lymphocytosis

- Drug reaction (especially anticonvulsants)
- Lymphocytic leukemia
- Pertussis
- Syphilis
- Tuberculosis
- Viral infection (especially mononucleosis)

Further reading:
- Yetgin S, Kuskonmaz B, Aytaç S, Tavil B (2007) An unusual case of reactive lymphocytosis mimicking acute leukemia. Pediatr Hematol Oncol 24(2):129–135

Lymphopenia

- Chemotherapy
- Chronic renal failure
- Glucocorticosteroids
- Hereditary immunodeficiency syndromes
- HIV infection
- Idiopathic CD4+ lymphopenia
- Internal malignancy
- Lymphoma
- Methotrexate
- Sarcoidosis
- Systemic lupus erythematosus
- Tuberculosis

Further reading:
- Walker UA, Warnatz K (2006) Idiopathic CD4 lymphocytopenia. Curr Opin Rheumatol 18(4):389–395

Neutropenia

- Aplastic anemia
- Bacteremia
- Bone marrow infiltration
- Chemotherapy
- Cyclic neutropenia
- Felty's syndrome
- Hereditary (benign) neutropenia
- HIV infection
- Leukemia
- Lupus erythematosus
- Lymphoma
- Nutritional deficiency
- Viral infection

Further reading:
- Kyono W, Coates TD (2002) A practical approach to neutrophil disorders. Pediatr Clin North Am 49(5):929–971

Neutrophilia

- Bone marrow infiltration
- Connective tissue disease
- Cushing's syndrome
- Down syndrome
- Glucocorticosteroids
- Inflammatory diseases
- Internal malignancy
- Leukemia
- Myeloproliferative diseases
- Pregnancy
- Systemic infection
- Vasculitis syndromes

Further reading:
- Kyono W, Coates TD (2002) A practical approach to neutrophil disorders. Pediatr Clin North Am 49(5):929–971

Rheumatoid Factor Elevated

- EBV infection
- Endocarditis
- Hepatitis C infection
- Hypergammaglobulinemic purpura of Waldenstrom
- Leukemia
- Lyme disease
- Mixed cryoglobulinemia
- Rheumatoid arthritis
- Scleroderma
- Sjögren syndrome
- Syphilis
- Systemic lupus erythematosus
- Waldenstrom's macroglobulinemia

Further reading:
- Colglazier CL, Sutej PG (2005) Laboratory testing in the rheumatic diseases: a practical review. South Med J 98(2):185–191

Thrombocytopenia

- Aplastic anemia
- B12 deficiency
- Bone marrow infiltration
- Disseminated intravascular coagulation
- Folate deficiency
- Hemolytic uremic syndrome
- Hereditary thrombocytopenia
- HIV infection

- Immune thrombocytopenic purpura
- Leukemia
- Lymphoma
- Medications
- Systemic lupus erythematosus
- Thrombotic thrombocytopenic purpura
- Viral infection

Further reading:
- Sekhon SS, Roy V (2006) Thrombocytopenia in adults: a practical approach to evaluation and management. South Med J 99(5):491–498

Thrombocytosis

- Chronic infection
- Chronic inflammatory disease (RA, etc.)
- Essential thrombocytosis
- Internal malignancy
- Iron deficiency
- Leukemia
- Polycythemia vera
- Splenectomy

Further reading:
- Dame C, Sutor AH (2005) Primary and secondary thrombocytosis in childhood. Br J Haematol 129(2):165–177

Triglycerides and/or Cholesterol Elevated

- Alcohol abuse
- Cyclosporine therapy
- Diabetes mellitus
- Dietary excess

- Estrogen therapy
- Familial dysbetalipoproteinemia (type III hyperlipidemia)
- Familial hypercholesterolemia (type II hyperlipidemia)
- Familial hypertriglyceridemia (type IV hyperlipidemia)
- Familial lipoprotein lipase deficiency (type I hyperlipidemia)
- Glucocorticosteroid therapy
- Hypothyroidism
- Isotretinoin therapy
- Lipodystrophy syndromes
- Monoclonal gammopathies
- Nephrotic syndrome
- Obesity
- Pancreatic disease
- Thiazide therapy
- Type V hyperlipidemia

Further reading:
- Eaton CB (2005) Hyperlipidemia. Prim Care 32(4):1027–1055
- Yuan G, Al-Shali KZ, Hegele RA (2007) Hypertriglyceridemia: its etiology, effects and treatment. Can Med Assoc J 176(8):1113–1120

VDRL Positive

- Antiphospholipid syndrome
- Borreliosis
- Drug abuse
- Endemic treponematoses
- Hepatic cirrhosis
- Idiopathic, familial
- Infectious mononucleosis
- Lepromatous leprosy
- Leptospirosis
- Lymphomas
- Malaria

- Pregnancy
- Syphilis
- Systemic lupus erythematosus

Further reading:

- Geusau A, Kittler H, Hein U et al (2005) Biological false-positive tests comprise a high proportion of Venereal Disease Research Laboratory reactions in an analysis of 300,000 sera. Int J STD AIDS 16(11):722–726

Acanthoma Fissuratum (Spectacle Granuloma)

Flesh-colored or erythematous, focal thickening of the skin of the retroauricular fold or nasal sidewall that results from frictional trauma induced by eyeglasses

Differential Diagnosis

- Actinic keratosis
- Adnexal neoplasm
- Basal cell carcinoma
- Chondrodermatitis nodularis helicis
- Foreign body reaction
- Keloid/hypertrophic scar
- Melanocytic nevus
- Seborrheic dermatitis
- Seborrheic keratosis
- Squamous cell carcinoma

Treatment Options

- Change to better fitting eyewear
- Cryosurgery
- Electrosurgery

Further reading:
- Betti R, Inselvini E, Pozzi G et al (1994) Bilateral spectacle frame acanthoma. Clin Exp Dermatol 19(6):503–504

Acanthosis Nigricans

Acquired skin disease associated with a variety of internal diseases that is characterized by velvety, papillomatous, hyperpigmented plaques usually localized to the intertriginous areas, especially the neck, but also in a periorificial distribution in patients with an underlying malignancy

Subtypes/Variants

- Acral
- Drug induced
- Facial (Fig. 6.1)
- Familial
- Insulin-resistance related
- Malignancy related
- Nevoid
- Oral
- Syndromic

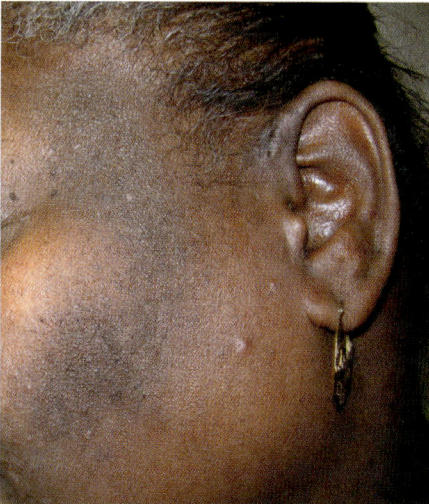

Fig. 6.1 Facial acanthosis nigricans

Differential Diagnosis

Cutaneous

- Acanthosis-nigricans-like lesions associated with pemphigus
- Addison's disease
- Atopic dermatitis (dirty neck)
- Becker's nevus
- Berloque dermatitis
- Chronic phototoxicity
- Confluent and reticulated papillomatosis
- Dermatosis neglecta
- Diabetic finger pebbles
- Dowling–Degos disease
- Florid cutaneous papillomatosis
- Granular parakeratosis
- Haber syndrome
- Hemochromatosis
- Ichthyosis hystrix
- Intertrigo
- Kitamura's acropigmentation
- Linear epidermal nevus
- Mycosis fungoides (especially papillomatous type)
- Parapsoriasis en plaque
- Pellagra
- Pemphigus vegetans
- Pseudoatrophoderma colli
- Riehl's melanosis
- Seborrheic keratoses
- <u>Terra firma–forme dermatosis</u>

Oral

- Oral florid papillomatosis
- Cowden's syndrome
- Dyskeratosis congenita
- Lipoid proteinosis

- Pachyonychia congenita
- Wegener's granulomatosis

Associations

- Acromegaly
- Addison's disease
- Adenocarcinoma
- Alstrom syndrome
- Ataxia–telangiectasia
- Autoimmune disease
- Bannayan–Riley–Ruvalcaba syndrome
- Bardet–Biedl syndrome
- Beare–Stevenson cutis verticis gyrata syndrome
- Bloom syndrome
- Cohen syndrome
- Costello syndrome
- Crouzon's syndrome
- Diabetes
- Down syndrome
- HAIR–AN syndrome
- Hermansky–Pudlak syndrome
- Hypothyroidism
- Insulin resistance
- Lelis syndrome
- Leprechaunism
- Lipodystrophy syndromes
- Malignancy (especially gastric carcinoma)
- Marfan syndrome
- Obesity
- Phenylketonuria
- Pinealoma
- Pituitary tumor
- Prader–Willi syndrome

- Renal transplant
- Stein–Leventhal disease
- Werner syndrome
- Wilson's disease

Associated Medications

- Diethylstilbestrol
- Glucocorticoids
- Niacinamide
- Nicotinic acid
- Oral contraceptives
- Triazineate

Evaluation

- Appropriate cancer screening (malignant type)
- Endocrine evaluation for hyperandrogenism (HAIR–AN)
- Fasting blood glucose/insulin levels
- Review medications

Treatment Options

- Treat underlying cause
- Topical retinoids
- Topical vitamin D analogues
- Ammonium lactate
- Metformin
- Oral contraceptive pills
- Systemic retinoids

Further reading:

- Sinha S, Schwartz RA (2007) Juvenile acanthosis nigricans. J Am Acad Dermatol 57(3):502–508

Achenbach Syndrome (Paroxysmal Finger Hematomas)

Acquired, idiopathic vascular disorder that occurs predominantly in females and that is characterized by tender, burning, purpuric hematoma-like nodules or plaques on the volar aspect of the fingers

Differential Diagnosis

- Acrocyanosis
- Buerger's disease
- Dermatitis artefacta
- Gardner–Diamond syndrome
- Osler's nodes
- Palmoplantar hidradenitis
- Perniosis
- Pressure urticaria
- Raynaud's phenomenon
- Trauma

Treatment Options

- Observation and reassurance

Further reading:
- Robertson A, Liddington MI, Kay SP (2002) Paroxysmal finger haematomas (Achenbach's syndrome) with angiographic abnormalities. J Hand Surg [Br] 27(4):391–393

Acne Aestivalis (Mallorca Acne, Actinic Folliculitis)

Subtype of acne characterized by a sunlight-induced, pruritic, ery-thematous, papulopustular eruption affecting sun-exposed areas (Fig. 6.2)

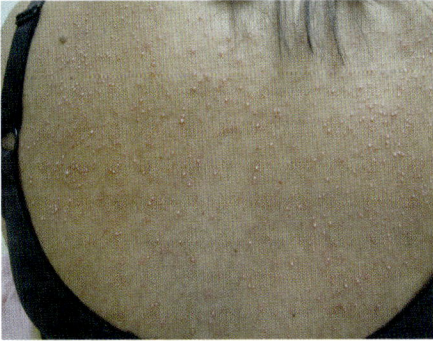

Fig. 6.2   Acne aestivalis

Differential Diagnosis

- Acne cosmetica
- Acne vulgaris (photoexacerbated)
- Folliculitis
- Insect-bite reactions
- Photoallergic contact dermatitis (especially sunscreen)
- Photosensitive drug eruption
- Polymorphous light eruption
- Rosacea
- Steroid acne

Treatment Options

- Topical corticosteroids
- Sunscreen
- Topical antibiotics
- Oral tetracycline antibiotics
- Systemic corticosteroids

Further reading:

- Veysey EC, George S (2005) Actinic folliculitis. Clin Exp Dermatol 30(6):659–661

Acne Conglobata

Severe, disfiguring nodulocystic variant of acne that is often resistant to therapy and that is characterized by comedones, inflammatory pustules, nodules, and sinus tracts on the face, chest, back, and buttocks

Differential Diagnosis

- Acne fulminans
- Furunculosis
- Hidradenitis suppurativa
- Chloracne
- Halogenoderma
- PAPA syndrome
- Tropical acne

Associations

- Dissecting cellulitis of the scalp
- Hidradenitis suppurativa
- PAPA syndrome
- Pilonidal sinus
- SAPHO syndrome

Treatment Options

- Isotretinoin
- Systemic corticosteroids
- Azithromycin
- Sulfamethoxazole–trimethoprim

Further reading:
- Shirakawa M, Uramoto K, Harada FA (2006) Treatment of acne conglobata with infliximab. J Am Acad Dermatol 55(2):344–346

Acne Fulminans

Severe variant of acne characterized by necrotizing inflammatory nodules, leukocytosis, bony lesions, and systemic symptoms

Differential Diagnosis

- Acne conglobata
- Halogenoderma
- PAPA syndrome
- Pyoderma faciale
- Pyoderma gangrenosum
- SAPHO syndrome
- Sweet's syndrome

Associations

- Arthritis
- Crohn's disease
- Erythema nodosum
- Osteolytic bone lesions
- PAPA syndrome
- SAPHO syndrome
- Pyoderma gangrenosum

Evaluation

- Bone scan/radiographs
- Complete blood count
- Sedimentation rate

Treatment Options

- Isotretinoin
- Systemic corticosteroids

- Azithromycin
- Sulfamethoxazole–trimethoprim

Further reading:
- Mehrany K, Kist JM, Weenig RH et al (2005) Acne fulminans. Int J Dermatol 44(2):132–133

Acneiform Drug Eruption (Acne Medicamentosa)

Type of follicular drug eruption characterized by monomorphous erythematous papules and pustules without comedones that are located predominantly on the face and upper trunk

Differential Diagnosis

- Acne aestivalis
- Acne vulgaris
- Gram-negative folliculitis
- Halogenoderma
- Miliaria
- Pityrosporum folliculitis

Associated Medications

- Aripiprazole
- Corticosteroids
- Cyclosporine
- Epidermal growth factor receptor inhibitors
- Haloperidol
- Isoniazid
- Lamotrigine
- Lithium
- Phenytoin
- Progesterone

- Testosterone
- Trazodone

Further reading:

- Du-Thanh A, Kluger N, Bensalleh H et al (2011) Drug-induced acneiform eruption. Am J Clin Dermatol 12(4):233–245

Acne, Infantile

Type of comedonal acne affecting infants 3–6 months old and related to intrinsic hormonal imbalances

Differential Diagnosis

- Acne cosmetica
- Apert's syndrome
- Benign cephalic histiocytosis
- Candidiasis
- Eosinophilic folliculitis
- Eruptive milia
- Gianotti–Crosti syndrome
- Miliaria
- Molluscum contagiosum
- Pityrosporum folliculitis
- Plane warts
- Sebaceous hyperplasia
- Tinea faciei
- Tuberous sclerosis
- Zinc deficiency

Associations

- Adrenocortical tumor
- Congenital adrenal hyperplasia
- Cushing syndrome

Treatment Options

- Topical retinoids
- Benzoyl peroxide
- Topical erythromycin
- Topical clindamycin

Further reading:
- Mann MW, Ellis SS, Mallory SB (2007) Infantile acne as the initial sign of an adrenocortical tumor. J Am Acad Dermatol 56(2 Suppl):S15–S18

Acne Keloidalis Nuchae

Chronic folliculitis of the nape of the neck characterized early by inflammatory papules and pustules and later by keloidal papules, nodules, or plaques

Differential Diagnosis

- Acne necrotica
- Dissecting cellulitis
- Favus
- Folliculitis decalvans
- Pediculosis capitis
- Pseudofolliculitis barbae
- Scalp folliculitis
- Tinea capitis
- Nevus sebaceus

Associations

- Anticonvulsants
- Cyclosporine
- Follicular occlusion triad

- Lithium
- Pseudofolliculitis barbae
- Testosterone

Treatment Options

- Avoidance of close hair trimming
- Intralesional steroids
- Topical steroids
- Topical antibiotics
- Oral antibiotics
- Excisional surgery
- Electrosurgery
- Isotretinoin

Further reading:
- Kelly AP (2003) Pseudofolliculitis barbae and acne keloidalis nuchae. Dermatol Clin 21(4):645–653

Acne Necrotica (Necrotizing Lymphocytic Folliculitis)

Uncommon form of folliculitis with superficial (acne necrotica miliaris) and deep (acne necrotica varioliformis) subtypes that is characterized by erythematous papules and pustules on the head, neck, and upper trunk of middle-aged men, which later progress to necrosis and scarring (in the deep form only)

Differential Diagnosis

- Actinic keratosis
- Bacterial folliculitis
- Erosive pustular dermatosis
- Hydroa vacciniforme
- Metastatic lesions

- Papulonecrotic tuberculid
- Pediculosis capitis
- Pityriasis lichenoides et varioliformis acuta
- <u>Pityrosporum folliculitis</u>
- Tinea capitis
- Vasculitis
- Squamous cell carcinoma

Treatment Options

- <u>Oral tetracycline antibiotics</u>
- Topical corticosteroids
- Topical antibiotics
- Topical retinoids
- Zinc pyrithione shampoo
- Ketoconazole shampoo
- Isotretinoin

Further reading:
- Zirn JR, Scott RA, Hambrick GW (1996) Chronic acneiform eruption with crateriform scars. Acne necrotica (varioliformis) (necrotizing lymphocytic folliculitis). Arch Dermatol 132(11):1367, 1370

Acne, Neonatal (Neonatal Cephalic Pustulosis)

Acneiform eruption caused by *Malassezia* spp. that affects newborns up to 3 months of age and that is characterized by inflammatory papules on the cheeks and nose

Differential Diagnosis

- Benign cephalic histiocytosis
- <u>Candidiasis</u>

- Eosinophilic folliculitis
- Erythema toxicum neonatorum
- Infantile acne
- Langerhans cell histiocytosis
- Miliaria
- Neonatal herpes
- Staphylococcal infection
- Transient neonatal pustular melanosis

Evaluation

- Bacterial culture
- Fungal culture
- Viral culture (HSV infection)
- Wright stain of pustule

Treatment Options

- Ketoconazole cream
- Selenium sulfide lotion
- Benzoyl peroxide

Further reading:
- Ayhan M, Sancak B, Karaduman A et al (2007) Colonization of neonate skin by *Malassezia* species: relationship with neonatal cephalic pustulosis. J Am Acad Dermatol 57(6):1012–1018

Acne Vulgaris

Inflammatory condition involving abnormal keratinization and plugging of follicles of the face and upper trunk, leading to the formation of comedones which subsequently rupture and give rise to inflammatory papules, pustules, and nodules

Differential Diagnosis

- Acne aestivalis
- Acne cosmetica
- Acne medicamentosa
- Angiofibromas
- Colloid milia
- Contact acne
- Demodex folliculitis
- Dilated pore of Winer
- Eosinophilic folliculitis
- Eruptive vellus hair cysts
- Favre–Racouchot disease
- Fibrofolliculomas
- Verruca plana
- Furuncle/carbuncle
- Gram-negative folliculitis
- Granulomatous periorificial dermatitis
- Insect bites
- Keratosis pilaris
- Lupus miliaris disseminatus faciei
- Milia
- Molluscum contagiosum
- Nevus comedonicus
- Occupation acne
- Osteoma cutis
- Perioral dermatitis
- Pityrosporum folliculitis
- Pseudofolliculitis barbae
- Rosacea
- Sebaceous hyperplasia
- Spitz nevi
- Staphylococcal folliculitis
- Steroid acne
- Syringomas

- Tinea barbae
- Tinea faciei
- Trichodiscomas
- Trichoepitheliomas
- Trichostasis spinulosa

Associations

- Adrenal tumor
- Androgen-induced alopecia
- Apert's syndrome
- Congenital adrenal hyperplasia
- Cushing's syndrome
- Hirsutism
- Ovarian tumor
- PAPA syndrome
- Polycystic ovary disease
- SAHA syndrome
- SAPHO syndrome

Evaluation (if Hyperandrogenism Is Suspected)

- DHEA-S
- LH/FSH
- SHBG
- Testosterone (total and free)
- 17-OH progesterone level

Treatment Options

- Benzoyl peroxide
- Topical retinoids
- Topical antibiotics
- Topical dapsone

- Azelaic acid
- Tetracycline antibiotics
- Sulfamethoxazole–trimethoprim
- Azithromycin
- Oral contraceptive pills
- Spironolactone
- Isotretinoin
- Oral dapsone
- Photodynamic therapy
- Pulsed dye laser

Further reading:

- Gebauer K (2000) Acne variants. Am J Clin Dermatol 1(3):187–189

Acroangiodermatitis of Mali

Acquired vascular disorder, and type of pseudo-Kaposi's sarcoma, that is associated with chronic venous insufficiency and is characterized by violaceous patches and plaques on the dorsal feet and anterior lower legs with sparing of the soles

Differential Diagnosis

- Kaposi's sarcoma
- Lichen amyloidosis
- Lichen planus
- Lichen simplex chronicus
- Multinucleate cell angiohistiocytoma
- Pigmented purpuric dermatosis
- Psoriasis
- Vasculitis

Associations

- Arteriovenous malformation
- Venous stasis

Treatment Options

- Observation and reassurance
- Compression and elevation
- Pentoxifylline
- Aspirin
- Dapsone

Further reading:
- Rongioletti F, Rebora A (2003) Cutaneous reactive angiomatoses: patterns and classification of reactive vascular proliferation. J Am Acad Dermatol 49(5):887–896

Acrochordon (Skin Tag)

Benign, fleshy, pedunculated lesion frequently observed in the flexures

Differential Diagnosis

- Basal cell carcinoma (Gorlin's syndrome)
- Dermatosis papulosa nigra
- Fibroepithelioma of Pinkus
- Melanocytic nevus
- Melanoma (including metastatic)
- Neurofibroma
- Seborrheic keratosis
- Wart
- Tick

Associations

- Diabetes
- Nevoid basal cell carcinoma syndrome
- <u>Obesity</u>

Further reading:
- Chiritescu E, Maloney ME (2001) Acrochordons as a presenting sign of nevoid basal cell carcinoma syndrome. J Am Acad Dermatol 44(5):789–794
- Rasi A, Soltani-Arabshahi R, Shahbazi N (2001) Skin tag as a cutaneous marker for impaired carbohydrate metabolism: a case-control study. Int J Dermatol 46(11):1155–1159

Acrocyanosis

Bluish discoloration of the hands and feet that is persistent, associated with hyperhidrosis, exacerbated by a cold environment, and most commonly benign in nature, but that can be a marker of internal disease

Differential Diagnosis

- Achenbach syndrome
- Chilblains (perniosis)
- Erythromelalgia
- Livedo reticularis
- Lupus erythematosus
- <u>Raynaud phenomenon</u>
- Scleroderma

Associations

- Anorexia
- Butyl nitrate
- Cold agglutinin hemolytic anemia

- Connective tissue disease
- Cryoglobulinemia
- Heart failure
- Interferon alpha
- Lymphoma
- Paraneoplastic acral vascular syndrome
- Thromboangiitis obliterans
- Tricyclic antidepressants

Evaluation

- Antinuclear antibodies
- Cold agglutinins
- Complete blood count
- Cryoglobulins
- CT scan
- Echocardiogram

Treatment Options

- Avoidance of cold
- Observation and reassurance

Further reading:
- Strumia R (2005) Dermatologic signs in patients with eating disorders. Am J Clin Dermatol 6(3):165–173

Acrodermatitis Chronica Atrophicans (Herxheimer Disease)

Cutaneous manifestation of late-stage Lyme disease that predominantly affects the extremities, that is seen more commonly in Europe, that is associated with *Borrelia afzelii* infection, and that is characterized by an edematous phase which progresses slowly to cutaneous atrophy and/or scleroderma-like skin changes

Differential Diagnosis

- Acrogeria (Gottron syndrome)
- Cold injury
- Eczematous dermatitis
- Eosinophilic fasciitis
- Erysipelas/cellulitis
- Lichen sclerosus et atrophicus
- Morphea
- Normal aging
- Pernio
- Severe photodamage
- Stasis dermatitis
- Steroid atrophy
- Systemic sclerosis
- Venous insufficiency

Evaluation

- Joint-fluid aspiration (if Lyme arthritis is suspected)
- Lumbar puncture (if CNS Lyme disease is suspected)
- Lyme ELISA and Western blot

Treatment Options

- See "Lyme Disease"

Further reading:
- Zalaudek I, Leinweber B, Kerl H et al (2005) Acrodermatitis chronica atrophicans in a 15-year-old girl misdiagnosed as venous insufficiency for 6 years. J Am Acad Dermatol 52(6):1091–1094

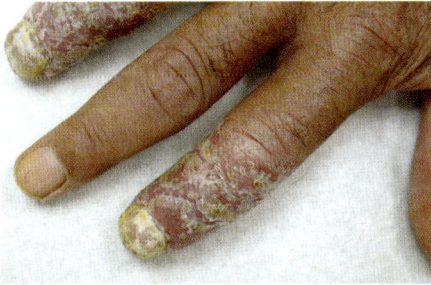

Fig. 6.3 Acrodermatitis continua

Acrodermatitis Continua of Hallopeau (Dermatitis Repens)

Localized, often refractory variant of psoriasis that affects the distal aspect of the digits and that is characterized by sterile pustules, crusting, and hyperkeratosis of the nail bed and periungual area (Fig. 6.3)

Differential Diagnosis

- Acute paronychia
- Blistering distal dactylitis
- Contact dermatitis
- <u>Dyshidrotic eczema</u>
- Herpetic whitlow
- Onychomycosis
- Pompholyx

Evaluation

- Bacterial culture

Treatment Options

- Topical corticosteroids
- Intralesional corticosteroids
- Topical vitamin D analogues
- Acitretin
- Methotrexate
- Etanercept
- Infliximab
- Adalimumab
- Cyclosporine
- Ustekinumab

Further reading:
- Waller JM, Wu JJ, Murase JE et al (2007) Chronically painful right thumb with pustules and onycholysis. Diagnosis: acrodermatitis continua of Hallopeau. Clin Exp Dermatol 32(5):619–620

Acrodermatitis Enteropathica (Brandt's Disease)

Autosomal-recessive disorder caused by a defect in the SLC39A4 gene which leads to decreased absorption of zinc in the gut and a resulting periorificial and acral erythematous, scaly, and fissuring rash, alopecia, candidiasis, and diarrhea with onset shortly after cessation of breast-feeding

Differential Diagnosis

Acrodermatitis Enteropathica
- Atopic dermatitis
- Biotin deficiency
- Chronic mucocutaneous candidiasis
- Cystic fibrosis
- Epidermolysis bullosa
- Essential fatty acid deficiency

- Glucagonoma syndrome
- Hartnup's syndrome
- Langerhans cell histiocytosis
- Maple syrup urine disease
- Multiple carboxylase deficiency
- Necrolytic acral erythema
- Netherton's syndrome
- Olmsted syndrome
- Ornithine transcarbamylase deficiency
- Psoriasis
- Seborrheic dermatitis

Acquired Zinc Deficiency

- Biotin deficiency
- Essential fatty acid deficiency
- Hailey–Hailey disease
- Necrolytic migratory erythema
- Pellagra
- Pemphigus foliaceus
- Seborrheic dermatitis

Associations

- Alcoholism
- Anorexia nervosa
- Chronic renal failure
- Cirrhosis
- Crohn's disease
- Cystic fibrosis
- Decreased intake of zinc
- Dialysis
- Dietary zinc deficiency
- Gastric bypass surgery
- High-fiber diet

- HIV infection
- Malabsorption syndromes
- Lymphoma
- Nephrotic syndrome
- Pregnancy
- Total parenteral nutrition

Evaluation

- Alkaline phosphatase level (low)
- Serum zinc level

Treatment Options

- Zinc supplementation

Further reading:
- Maverakis E, Fung MA, Lynch PJ et al (2007) Acrodermatitis enteropathica and an overview of zinc metabolism. J Am Acad Dermatol 56(1):116–124

Acrodynia

Cutaneous manifestation of mercury poisoning that affects children predominantly and that is characterized by painful, erythematous, swollen hands and feet along with hyperhidrosis, photophobia, and anorexia

Differential Diagnosis

- Acrocyanosis
- Acrodermatitis chronica atrophicans
- Acrodermatitis enteropathica
- Acrogeria (Gottron syndrome)
- Acute generalized exanthematous pustulosis

- Arsenic toxicity
- Chilblains
- Cockayne syndrome
- Copper toxicity
- Erythromelalgia
- Glucagonoma syndrome
- Gold toxicity
- Kawasaki disease
- Progeria
- Steroid atrophy
- Thallium toxicity
- Werner's syndrome

Evaluation

- 24-h urine mercury level
- Serum mercury level

Further reading:
- Boyd AS, Seger D, Vannucci S et al (2000) Mercury exposure and cutaneous disease. J Am Acad Dermatol 43(1 Pt 1):81–90

Acrokeratoelastoidosis of Costa

Inherited (AD) or sporadic type of palmoplantar keratoderma caused by fragmentation of elastic fibers that is characterized by translucent, grouped papules in a linear array at the lateral margins of the palms and soles

Differential Diagnosis

- Acrokeratosis verruciformis of Hopf
- Focal acral hyperkeratosis
- Keratoelastoidosis marginalis
- Verruca

Further reading:
- Hu W, Cook TF, Vicki GJ et al (2002) Acrokeratoelastoidosis. Pediatr Dermatol 19(4):320–322

Acrokeratosis Paraneoplastica of Bazex

Uncommon paraneoplastic disorder affecting older patients with under-lying aerodigestive squamous cell carcinoma that is characterized by nail dystrophy, violaceous hyperkeratotic plaques on the acral areas, including the nose and ears, and palmoplantar keratoderma

Differential Diagnosis

- Acquired zinc deficiency
- Chilblains
- Contact dermatitis
- Dermatophytosis
- Dermatomyositis
- Lupus erythematosus
- Medication reaction
- Necrolytic acral erythema
- Onycholysis
- Onychomycosis
- Photosensitivity reaction
- Psoriasis

Evaluation

- Appropriate cancer screening
- Otorhinolaryngologic evaluation

Further reading:
- Taher M, Grewal P, Gunn B et al (2007) Acrokeratosis paraneoplastica (Bazex syndrome) presenting in a patient with metastatic breast carcinoma: possible etiologic role of zinc. J Cutan Med Surg 11(2):78–83

Acrokeratosis Verruciformis of Hopf

Inherited (AD) disorder allelic with Darier's disease that is caused by mutation of the ATP2A2 gene encoding the SERCA2 calcium pump and that is characterized by verrucous papules on the dorsal hands and occasionally the feet

Differential Diagnosis

- Acrokeratoelastoidosis of Costa
- Actinic keratosis
- Arsenical keratoses
- Colloid milium
- Cowden's disease keratoses
- Darier's disease
- Epidermodysplasia verruciformis
- Verruca plana
- Granuloma annulare
- Lichen planus
- Seborrheic keratosis
- Stucco keratoses

Treatment Options

- Cryosurgery
- Topical retinoids
- Acitretin
- CO_2 laser

Further reading:
- Rallis E, Economidi A, Papadakis P et al (2005) Acrokeratosis verruciformis of Hopf (Hopf disease): case report and review of the literature. Dermatol Online J 11(2):10

Acrokeratotic Poikiloderma (of Kindler and Weary)

Inherited blistering disorder (AR) caused by defect in the gene encoding the KIND1 gene that is characterized by neonatal-onset trauma-induced blistering on the hands and feet, photosensitivity, diffuse and progressive poikiloderma, and periodontal disease

Differential Diagnosis

- Ataxia–telangiectasia
- Bloom's syndrome
- Bullous congenital ichthyosiform erythroderma
- Cockayne syndrome
- Dyskeratosis congenita
- Epidermolysis bullosa
- Erythrokeratodermia variabilis
- Rothmund–Thomson syndrome
- Xeroderma pigmentosum

Further reading:
- Ashton GH (2004) Kindler syndrome. Clin Exp Dermatol 29(2):116–121

Acropigmentation of Dohi (Dyschromatosis Symmetrica Hereditaria)

Inherited dyschromatosis (AD) of unknown cause that has been predominantly reported in Japan, and this is characterized by onset in childhood of hyperpigmented and hypopigmented macules on the dorsal hands and feet

Differential Diagnosis

- Acquired brachial cutaneous dyschromatosis
- Dyschromatosis universalis hereditaria

- Erythema ab igne
- <u>Reticulate acropigmentation of Kitamura</u>

Treatment Options

- Camouflage

Further reading:
- Obieta MP (2006) Familial reticulate acropigmentation of Dohi: a case report. Dermatol Online J 12(3):16

Acropustulosis of Infancy

Pruritic dermatosis affecting infants and young children that is character-ized by crops of pustules and papulovesicles situated on the hands, feet, ankles, and forearms that may represent a persistent cutaneous reaction to scabies infestation

Differential Diagnosis

- <u>Arthropod-bite reaction</u>
- Cutaneous candidiasis
- Dyshidrotic eczema
- Eosinophilic pustular folliculitis
- Erythema toxicum neonatorum
- Hand–foot–mouth disease
- <u>Impetigo, bullous</u>
- Pustular psoriasis
- <u>Scabies</u>
- Subcorneal pustular dermatosis
- Transient neonatal pustular melanosis

Evaluation

- Mineral oil examination for scabies

Treatment Options

- Topical corticosteroids

Further reading:
- Mancini AJ, Frieden IJ, Paller AS (1998) Infantile acropustulosis revisited: history of scabies and response to topical corticosteroids. Pediatr Dermatol 15(5):337–341

Actinic Granuloma (Annular Elastolytic Giant Cell Granuloma)

Uncommon granulomatous disorder predominantly affecting middle-aged women that is probably triggered by actinic injury of the dermis and is characterized by annular, erythematous plaques with hypopigmented atrophic centers on the face, neck, or arms (Fig. 6.4)

Differential Diagnosis

- Anetoderma
- Annular lichen planus
- Cutis laxa
- Elastosis perforans serpiginosa
- Erythema annulare centrifugum
- Granuloma annulare
- Granuloma multiforme
- Granulomatous infections
- Granulomatous slack skin
- Leprosy (especially tuberculoid type)
- Lupus erythematosus
- Morphea
- Necrobiosis lipoidica

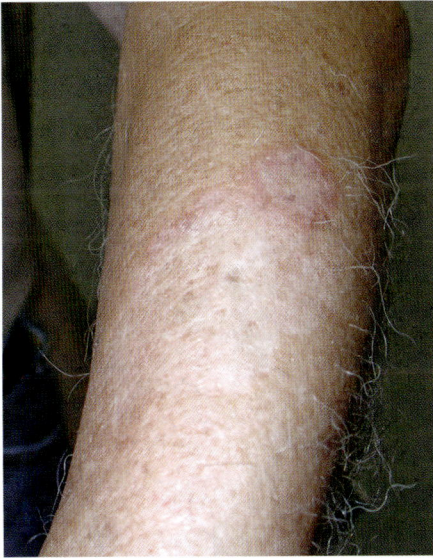

Fig. 6.4 Actinic granuloma (Courtesy of K. Guidry)

- Necrobiotic xanthogranuloma
- Sarcoidosis
- Syphilis
- Tinea corporis

Associations

- Temporal arteritis

Treatment Options

- Sunscreen
- Topical corticosteroids
- Intralesional corticosteroids
- Observation
- Pentoxifylline

- Systemic retinoids
- <u>Antimalarials</u>
- Cyclosporine

Further reading:
- Coelho R, Viana I, Rijo H (2010) Annular lesions on the forehead of a 44-year-old woman. Annular elastolytic giant cell granuloma (AEGCG). Clin Exp Dermatol 35(3):e48–e49

Actinic Keratosis (Solar Keratosis)

Precancerous neoplasm with the potential to progress to squamous cell carcinoma that is caused by ultraviolet-light-induced DNA mutations and characterized by hyperkeratotic, erythematous papules and plaques on the chronically sun-exposed areas of the body

Subtypes/Variants

Clinical
- Actinic cheilitis
- Conjunctival
- Hypertrophic
- Lichenoid
- Pigmented
- Proliferative
- Spreading pigmented

Histological
- Acantholytic
- Atrophic
- Bowenoid
- Hypertrophic
- Lichenoid
- Pigmented

Differential Diagnosis

- Acne necrotica
- Acrokeratosis verruciformis
- Atypical fibroxanthoma
- Arsenical keratosis
- Basal cell carcinoma
- Benign lichenoid keratosis
- Bowen's disease
- Chondrodermatitis nodularis helicis
- Cowden's disease keratoses
- Disseminated superficial actinic porokeratosis
- Epidermodysplasia verruciformis
- Erosive pustular dermatosis
- Gouty tophus
- Keratoacanthoma
- Large cell acanthoma
- Lichen simplex
- Lupus erythematosus
- Lentigo maligna
- Lichenoid keratosis
- Nummular dermatitis
- Picker's nodule
- Psoriasis
- Seborrheic dermatitis
- Seborrheic keratosis
- Squamous cell carcinoma
- Solar lentigo
- Wart

Treatment Options

- Cryotherapy
- Curettage
- Topical 5-FU

- <u>Imiquimod cream</u>
- Ingenol mebutate
- Topical retinoids
- Topical diclofenac
- <u>Photodynamic therapy</u>
- Chemical peels
- Ablative lasers
- Dermabrasion

Further reading:
- Scheinfeld NS (2007) Actinic keratoses. Skinmed 6(4):188–190

Actinic Prurigo (Hutchinson Prurigo)

Chronic dermatosis affecting children that is caused by an abnormal reaction to ultraviolet light and characterized by pruritic, photodistributed, papules, vesicles, and plaques with cheilitis and conjunctivitis

Differential Diagnosis

- <u>Atopic dermatitis (especially photoexacerbated type)</u>
- Chronic actinic dermatitis
- Hydroa vacciniforme
- Insect bites
- Jessner's lymphocytic infiltrate
- Lupus erythematosus
- Photoallergic contact dermatitis
- <u>Polymorphous light eruption</u>
- Porphyrias (especially erythropoietic protoporphyria)
- Prurigo nodularis
- Scabies
- Solar urticaria

Evaluation

- Antinuclear antibodies
- HLA DRB1*0407 (HLA DR-4) testing
- Phototesting
- Porphyrin studies

Treatment Options

- <u>Sun avoidance measures</u>
- Narrowband UVB phototherapy
- <u>Systemic corticosteroids</u>
- Antimalarials
- Pentoxifylline
- <u>Azathioprine</u>
- Thalidomide

Further reading:

- Hojyo-Tomoka MT, Vega-Memije ME, Cortes-Franco R et al (2003) Diagnosis and treatment of actinic prurigo. Dermatol Ther 16(1):40–44

Actinomycosis (Rivalta Disease)

Chronic infection most commonly caused by *Actinomyces israelii* and characterized by a deep infectious focus (usually the mandible in the setting of poor dentition) with an overlying sinus tract which exudes yellow colony-containing sulfur granules

Subtypes/Variants

- Abdominal
- Cervicofacial

- Pelvic (with intrauterine device)
- Thoracic

Differential Diagnosis

- Abscess
- Aerobic bacterial infections
- Appendicitis
- Blastomycosis
- Botryomycosis
- Crohn's disease
- Deep fungal infections
- Dental sinus
- Eumycetoma
- Leishmaniasis
- Lymphoma (especially Hodgkin's disease)
- Neoplasm
- Nocardiosis
- Osteomyelitis
- Pelvic inflammatory disease
- Pneumonia
- Tinea barbae (deep type)
- Tuberculosis (especially scrofuloderma)

Evaluation

- Gram stain and culture of granules
- Immunoperoxidase studies
- CT or MRI scan

Further reading:
- Fazeli MS, Bateni H (2005) Actinomycosis: a rare soft tissue infection. Dermatol Online J 11(3):18

Acute Generalized Exanthematous Pustulosis

Generalized pustular eruption caused most commonly by drugs (with rapid resolution typical after stopping the offending agent) but also by viruses or mercury toxicity that is characterized by rapid-onset eruption of small, superficial nonfollicular pustules on a background of erythema first on the face and flexures and later on the trunk

Differential Diagnosis

- Acute febrile neutrophilic dermatosis
- Amicrobial pustulosis with autoimmunity
- Candidiasis
- Drug reaction with eosinophilia and systemic symptoms (DRESS)
- Erythema multiforme
- Exanthematous drug eruption
- Impetigo herpetiformis
- Pemphigus foliaceus
- Pustular bacterid
- Pustular psoriasis
- Reiter syndrome
- Staphylococcal scalded-skin syndrome
- Subcorneal pustular dermatosis
- Toxic epidermal necrolysis

Associated Medications

- Acetaminophen
- Allopurinol
- Beta-lactam antibiotics
- Carbamazepine
- Celecoxib
- Chloramphenicol

- Clindamycin
- Co-trimoxazole
- Cytarabine
- Diltiazem
- Famotidine
- Furosemide
- Hydrochlorothiazide
- Hydroxychloroquine
- Ibuprofen
- Imatinib
- Imipenem
- Isoniazid
- Itraconazole
- IV contrast dye
- Macrolides
- Mercury
- Metronidazole
- Morphine
- Naproxen
- Nifedipine
- Olanzapine
- Phenytoin
- Pseudoephedrine
- Ranitidine
- Rifampin
- Sertraline
- Simvastatin
- Terbinafine
- Vancomycin

Evaluation

- Bacterial culture
- Complete blood count

- Direct immunofluorescence
- Liver function test

Treatment Options

- Discontinue causative medication
- Systemic corticosteroids

Further reading:
- Knowles SR, Shear NH (2007) Recognition and management of severe cutaneous drug reactions. Dermatol Clin 25(2):245–253

Acute Hemorrhagic Edema of Childhood (Finkelstein's Disease)

Type of cutaneous small vessel vasculitis that affects children under the age of 2 years and that is characterized by preceding infection or medication use in some patients and typical brightly erythematous to purpuric cockade or targetoid plaques on the face and extremities with edema of the hands and feet

Differential Diagnosis

- Acrodynia
- Child abuse/contusions
- Erythema multiforme
- Henoch–Schonlein purpura
- Kawasaki disease
- Leukemia cutis
- Meningococcemia
- Septic vasculitis
- Sweet's syndrome
- Urticaria
- Urticarial vasculitis

Evaluation

- Serum chemistry
- Complete blood cell count
- Complement levels
- Sedimentation rate
- Urinalysis

Treatment Options

- <u>Observation and reassurance</u>
- Systemic corticosteroids

Further reading:
- Sites LY, Woodmansee CS, Wilkin NK et al (2008) Acute hemorrhagic edema of infancy: case reports and a review of the literature. Cutis 82(5):320–324

Acute Necrotizing Gingivitis (Trench Mouth)

Acute infectious form of gingivitis seen in patients with extremely poor oral hygiene that is caused by bacterial infection of the gingiva with *Prevotella*, *Actinomyces*, spirochetes, and streptococcal species and that is characterized by fever, gingival swelling, foul odor, and ulceration

Differential Diagnosis

- Aphthous stomatitis (major type)
- Behçet's disease
- Desquamative gingivitis
- Erosive lichen planus
- Medication toxicity
- Pemphigus vulgaris
- Wegener's granulomatosis

Further reading:
- Buchanan JA, Cedro M, Mirdin A et al (2006) Necrotizing stomatitis in the developed world. Clin Exp Dermatol 31(3):372–374

Adams–Oliver Syndrome

Developmental disorder (AD) characterized by a large, stellate type of aplasia cutis congenita on the scalp, transverse limb defects, cutis marmorata telangiectatica congenita, and cardiac and CNS anomalies

Differential Diagnosis

- Amniotic band syndrome
- Focal dermal hypoplasia (Goltz)
- Intrauterine varicella or herpes simplex infection
- Johanson–Blizzard syndrome
- Methimazole teratogenicity
- MIDAS syndrome
- Misoprostol
- Oculocerebrocutaneous syndrome
- Oculoectodermal syndrome
- Setleis syndrome (focal facial dermal dysplasia)
- Trisomy 13
- Wolf-Hirschhorn syndrome

Further reading:
- Rajabian MH, Aghaei S (2006) Adams–Oliver syndrome and isolated aplasia cutis congenita in two siblings. Dermatol Online J 12(6):17

Adult T Cell Leukemia/Lymphoma

Type of T cell lymphoproliferative disorder associated with HTLV-1 infection of lymphocytes that is characterized by skin lesions that are clinically indistinguishable from other forms of cutaneous T cell lymphoma, along with occasional lymphadenopathy, hepatosplenomegaly, lytic bone lesions, and hypercalcemia

Differential Diagnosis

- Atopic dermatitis
- Contact dermatitis
- HIV infection
- <u>Mycosis fungoides</u>
- Non-Hodgkin's lymphoma

Evaluation

- Blood smear for floret lymphocytes
- Complete blood count
- HIV test
- HTLV-1 ELISA and Western blot
- Lactate dehydrogenase level
- Radiographic studies
- Serum calcium
- Serum chemistry

Further reading:
- Yamaguchi T, Ohshima K, Karube K et al (2005) Clinicopathological features of cutaneous lesions of adult T-cell leukaemia/lymphoma. Br J Dermatol 152(1):76–81

Ainhum (Dactylolysis Spontanea)

Gradual autoamputation of the fifth toe that primarily affects patients in Africa who walk barefoot, that is caused by repeated trauma, and that is characterized by progressive constriction of the digit with thin fibrous band formation and eventual amputation

Differential Diagnosis

- Arterial insufficiency
- Congenital constricting bands
- Endemic syphilis
- Leprosy
- Morphea
- Pachyonychia congenita
- Pityriasis rubra pilaris
- Porokeratosis
- Pseudoainhum
- Systemic sclerosis
- Syphilis
- Tourniquet syndrome
- Tuberculosis
- Yaws

Further reading:

- Olivieri I, Piccirillo A, Scarano E, Ricciuti F, Padula A, Molfese V (2005) Dactylolysis spontanea or ainhum involving the big toe. J Rheumatol 32(12):2437–2439

Alezzandrini Syndrome

Rare syndrome of unknown cause that is characterized by facial vitiligo and poliosis with ipsilateral loss of visual acuity and deafness

Differential Diagnosis

- Piebaldism
- Vitiligo
- Vogt–Koyanagi–Harada syndrome
- Waardenburg syndrome

Further reading:
- Shamsadini S, Meshkat MR, Mozzafarinia K (1994) Bilateral retinal detachment in Alezzandrini's syndrome. Int J Dermatol 33(12):885–886

Alkaptonuria (Ochronosis)

Hereditary metabolic disorder (AR) caused by deficiency of homogentisic acid oxidase which is characterized by the accumulation of a black pigment in tissues, including the cartilage, skin, and sclera, as well as accumulation in the urine, which is often the first identifiable feature of this disease in infants

Differential Diagnosis

- Argyria
- Calcific aortic stenosis
- Chrysiasis
- Drug-induced hyperpigmentation
- Exogenous ochronosis
- Hemochromatosis
- Minocycline hyperpigmentation
- Nevus of Ota
- Osteoarthritis
- Rheumatoid arthritis

Evaluation

- Urinary homogentisic acid level (elevated)
- Sodium hydroxide test (NaOH darkens urine)

Further reading:
- Spenny ML, Suwannarat P, Gahl WA et al (2005) Blue pigmentation and arthritis in an elderly man. J Am Acad Dermatol 52(1):122–124

Alopecia Areata/Totalis/Universalis

Type of alopecia that is potentially self-limited, probably autoimmune in etiology, and characterized by circumscribed (areata) nonscarring alopecia, total scalp alopecia (totalis), or total body alopecia (universalis)

Subtypes/Variants

- Acute diffuse and total alopecia of the scalp
- Circumscribed
- Diffuse
- Gray overnight
- Ophiasis
- Reticular
- Sisaipho
- Totalis
- Universalis

Differential Diagnosis

- Alopecia neoplastica
- Anagen effluvium
- Androgenetic alopecia
- Aplasia cutis
- Atrichia with papular lesions
- Ectodermal dysplasia
- Frontal fibrosing alopecia
- Loose anagen syndrome
- Lupus erythematosus
- Monilethrix
- Pressure alopecia
- Syphilitic alopecia
- Telogen effluvium
- Temporal triangular alopecia

- Tinea capitis
- Traction alopecia
- Trichotillomania
- Vitamin-D-resistant rickets

Associations

- Addison's disease
- Atopic dermatitis
- Autoimmune polyglandular syndromes
- Autoimmune thyroid disease
- Celiac disease
- Diabetes
- Down syndrome
- HIV infection
- Lichen planus
- Loose anagen hair syndrome
- Lupus erythematosus
- Pernicious anemia
- Stress
- Vitiligo
- Trachyonychia
- Turner's syndrome

Evaluation

- AM serum cortisol level
- Antithyroid antibodies
- Complete blood count
- Thyroid function tests

Treatment Options

- Intralesional corticosteroids
- Topical corticosteroids

- Topical tacrolimus
- Topical minoxidil
- Anthralin cream
- Topical squaric acid dibutyl ester
- Systemic steroids
- Sulfasalazine
- Methotrexate
- Mycophenolate mofetil
- Cyclosporine

Further reading:

- Dudda-Subramanya R, Alexis AF, Siu K, Sinha AA (2007) Alopecia areata: genetic complexity underlies clinical heterogeneity. Eur J Dermatol 17(5):367–374

Alpha-1 Antitrypsin Deficiency Panniculitis

Type of panniculitis that is most severe in patients with homozygous deficiency of alpha-1 antitrypsin (PiZZ phenotype) and is characterized by trauma-induced erythematous and tender subcutaneous nodules on the trunk or extremities which ulcerate and drain an oily brown fluid

Differential Diagnosis

- Erythema induratum (nodular vasculitis)
- Infectious panniculitis
- Pancreatic panniculitis
- Pyoderma gangrenosum
- Sweet's syndrome
- Traumatic panniculitis (including factitial)

Associations

- Severe psoriasis

Evaluation

- Bacterial and fungal cultures
- Chest radiograph
- Liver function tests
- Phenotyping (PiMM is normal; PiZZ indicates severe deficiency)
- Plasma alpha-1 antitrypsin level

Treatment Options

- Intravenous replacement of alpha-1 antitrypsin

Further reading:
- Walling H, Geraminejad P (2005) Determine alpha-1 antitrypsin level and phenotype in patients with neutrophilic panniculitis. J Am Acad Dermatol 52(2):373–374

Amalgam Tattoo

Iatrogenic tattoo that is caused by traumatic implantation or diffusion of dental amalgam into surrounding tissues of a restored tooth and that is characterized by a dark gray or blue macule on the gingival or buccal mucosa

Differential Diagnosis

- Heavy-metal intoxication
- Hemangioma
- Hemochromatosis
- Laugier–Hunziker syndrome
- Medication reaction
- Melanoma
- Mucosal melanosis

- Nevus
- Oral melanoacanthoma
- Peutz–Jeghers syndrome
- Venous lake

Further reading:
- Pigatto PD, Brambilla L, Guzzi G (2006) Amalgam tattoo: a close-up view. J Eur Acad Dermatol Venereol 20(10):1352–1353

Amebiasis, Cutaneous

Cutaneous infection most often seen in the perianal area or abdominal area that is caused by the intestinal protozoa *Entamoeba histolytica* and characterized by a painful ulcer with little tendency for spontaneous healing

Differential Diagnosis

- Chancriform pyoderma
- Chancroid
- CMV infection
- Condyloma acuminata
- Deep fungal infection
- Granuloma inguinale
- Herpes simplex virus infection
- Inflammatory bowel disease
- Leishmaniasis
- Lymphogranuloma venereum
- Tropical phagedenic ulcer
- Pyoderma gangrenosum
- Squamous cell carcinoma
- Streptococci
- Syphilis

Evaluation

- Enzyme immunoassay test for *E. histolytica* antibodies

Further reading:
- Kenner BM, Rosen T (2006) Cutaneous amebiasis in a child and review of the literature. Pediatr Dermatol 23(3):231–234

Amicrobial Pustulosis with Autoimmune Disease

Uncommon pustular dermatosis affecting predominantly female patients with autoimmune diseases such as systemic lupus erythematosus and Sjögren's syndrome that is characterized by a chronic course of pustules on the cutaneous folds, scalp, and periorificial regions of the head and neck

Differential Diagnosis

- Acute generalized exanthematous pustulosis
- Behçet's disease
- Bowel-associated dermatosis–arthritis syndrome
- Bromoderma
- Dermatitis herpetiformis
- Eosinophilic pustular folliculitis
- Erosive pustular dermatosis
- Folliculitis
- Furunculosis
- IgA pemphigus
- Impetigo contagiosa
- Iododerma
- Pemphigus
- Pustular psoriasis

- <u>Subcorneal pustular dermatosis</u>
- Sweet's syndrome

Evaluation

- Antinuclear antibodies
- Bacterial culture of pustules
- Erythrocyte sedimentation rate
- Serum protein electrophoresis
- Specific tests for connective tissue diseases
- Urinalysis

Further reading:

- Boms S, Gambichler T (2006) Review of literature on amicrobial pustulosis of the folds associated with autoimmune disorders. Am J Clin Dermatol 7(6):369–374

Amyloidosis, Primary Cutaneous

Localized cutaneous form of amyloidosis which is probably induced by scratching and rubbing, associated with deposition of keratin-derived amyloid in the dermis, and that is characterized by pruritic, waxy hyperkeratotic papules located most commonly on the anterior lower extremities (lichen) or pruritic, hyperpigmented macules and patches most commonly on the upper back (macular)

Subtypes/Variants

- Anosacral
- Lichen (Fig. 6.5)
- Macular (Fig. 6.6)
- Poikiloderma-like
- Vitiliginous

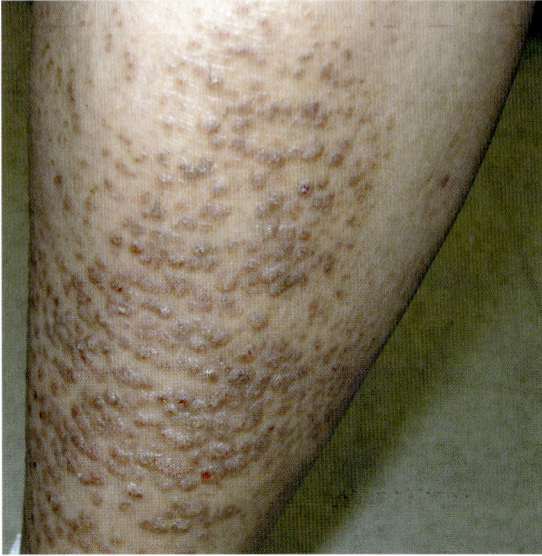

Fig. 6.5 Lichen amyloidosis

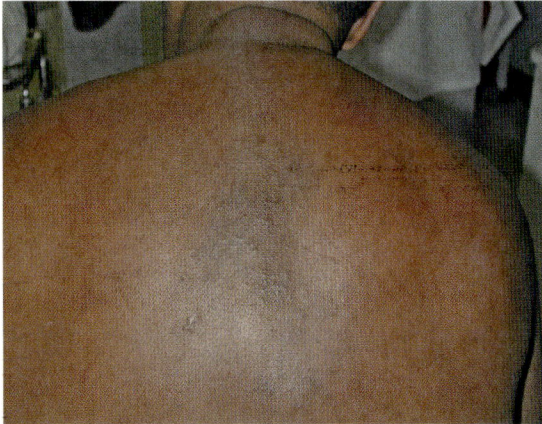

Fig. 6.6 Macular amyloidosis (Courtesy of K. Guidry)

Differential Diagnosis

Lichen

- Contact dermatitis
- Epidermolysis bullosa pruriginosa
- Hypertrophic lichen planus
- Lichen myxedematosus
- <u>Lichen simplex chronicus</u>
- Lichenoid drug eruption
- Mycosis fungoides
- Necrobiosis lipoidica
- Papular mucinosis
- Pemphigoid nodularis
- Postinflammatory hyperpigmentation
- Pretibial myxedema
- Prurigo nodularis

Macular

- Atopic dermatitis
- Atrophic lichen planus
- Dermatomyositis
- Drug-induced pigmentation
- Erythema dyschromicum perstans
- <u>Lichen simplex chronicus</u>
- Mycosis fungoides
- Phototoxic contact dermatitis
- Pityriasis versicolor
- Postinflammatory hyperpigmentation
- Prurigo pigmentosum
- Tinea corporis

Associations

- Multiple endocrine neoplasia, type IIa
- <u>Notalgia paresthetica</u>

Treatment Options

- Topical corticosteroids
- Phototherapy
- Systemic retinoids
- Dermabrasion

Further reading:
- Salim T, Shenoi SD, Balachandran C, Mehta VR (2005) Lichen amyloidosus: a study of clinical, histopathologic and immunofluorescence findings in 30 cases. Indian J Dermatol Venereol Leprol 71(3):166–169

Amyloidosis, Nodular

Localized cutaneous form of amyloidosis which is caused by deposition of light-chain-derived amyloid from plasma cells nearby the deposit and characterized by pink to hyperpigmented firm nodules located anywhere on the body

Differential Diagnosis

- Basal cell carcinoma
- Colloid milium
- Cutaneous lymphoid hyperplasia
- Epidermal inclusion cyst
- Granuloma annulare
- Granuloma faciale
- Leiomyoma
- Lipoma
- Lupus vulgaris
- Lymphoma
- Nodular mucinosis
- Plasmacytoma
- Pretibial myxedema

- Sarcoidosis
- Xanthoma

Associations

- Plasmacytoma
- Monoclonal gammopathy
- Multiple myeloma
- Sjögren's syndrome

Evaluation

- Serum/urine protein electrophoresis

Treatment Options

- Intralesional corticosteroids
- Excision

Further reading:
- Kalajian AH, Waldman M, Knable AL (2007) Nodular primary localized cutaneous amyloidosis after trauma: a case report and discussion of the rate of progression to systemic amyloidosis. J Am Acad Dermatol 57(2 Suppl):S26–S29

Amyloidosis, Primary Systemic AL (Lubarsch–Pick Disease)

Systemic form of amyloidosis with a high mortality that is caused by an occult overproduction of light chains by plasma cells (with or without overt multiple myeloma) and is characterized by systemic deposition of light-chain-derived amyloid in the internal organs, as well the skin, with waxy periorbital papules, macroglossia, and purpura being the most common skin findings

Differential Diagnosis

- Amyloidosis, secondary systemic (AA)
- Condyloma acuminatum
- Histiocytoses
- Familial amyloidosis syndromes
- Kaposi's sarcoma
- Lichen myxedematosus
- Lipoid proteinosis
- Metastatic disease
- Mucinoses
- Multiple trichofolliculomas
- Necrobiotic xanthogranuloma
- Purpura
- Scleromyxedema
- Syringomas
- Xanthelasma
- Xanthoma disseminatum

Evaluation

- Abdominal fat pad or rectal biopsy
- Bone marrow biopsy
- Echocardiogram
- Serum/urine protein electrophoresis
- Urinalysis

Treatment Options

- Melphalan
- Systemic corticosteroids
- Interferon therapy
- Lenalidomide
- Bortezomib

Further reading:

- Gul U, Soylu S, Kilic A et al (2007) Monoclonal gammopathy of undetermined significance diagnosed by cutaneous manifestations of AL amyloidosis. Eur J Dermatol 17(3):255–256

Amyloidosis, Secondary Systemic (AA)

Systemic form of amyloidosis associated with several chronic inflammatory conditions that is caused by deposition of serum amyloid A protein in various organs and that is usually not associated with skin lesions

Differential Diagnosis

- Hemodialysis-related amyloidosis
- Hereditary amyloidosis syndromes
- Membranoproliferative glomerulonephritis
- Primary systemic AL amyloidosis

Associations

- Chronic infection
- Chronic inflammatory diseases
- Dystrophic epidermolysis bullosa
- Familial Mediterranean fever
- Hidradenitis suppurativa
- Hodgkin's disease
- Inflammatory bowel disease
- Leprosy
- Muckle–Wells disease
- Osteomyelitis
- Psoriatic arthritis
- Rheumatoid arthritis

Evaluation

- Rectal biopsy
- Renal biopsy
- Renal function tests
- Renal ultrasound
- Serum/urinary protein electrophoresis
- Urinalysis

Treatment Options

- Treat the underlying cause

Further reading:
- Lachmann HJ, Goodman HJ, Gilbertson JA et al (2007) Natural history and outcome in systemic AA amyloidosis. N Engl J Med 356(23):2361–2371

Anagen Effluvium

Type of reversible, nonscarring, diffuse hair loss occurring in the setting of chemotherapy in which the tapering of the hair shaft (Pohl–Pinkus constrictions) occurs as a response to injury to the hair matrix

Differential Diagnosis

- <u>Alopecia totalis</u>
- Alopecia mucinosa
- Androgenetic alopecia
- Loose anagen syndrome
- Lupus erythematosus
- Malnutrition
- Sezary syndrome
- Syphilitic alopecia
- <u>Telogen effluvium</u>

- Thallium toxicity
- Thyroid disease
- Traction alopecia

Further reading:
- Tosti A, Pazzaglia M (2007) Drug reactions affecting hair: diagnosis. Dermatol Clin 25(2):223–231

Androgenetic Alopecia

Common and inherited form of nonscarring alopecia affecting men and women that is caused by a gradual, androgen-dependent reduction in the size of hair follicles affecting the frontal hairline and vertex in men and the crown in women (with widened partline)

Differential Diagnosis

- Alopecia areata (diffuse type)
- Anagen effluvium
- Androgen-induced alopecia (virilizing disorder)
- Iron deficiency
- Lupus erythematosus
- Senile alopecia
- Telogen effluvium
- Thyroid disease

Associations

- Coronary artery disease
- X-linked ichthyosis

Evaluation

- Complete blood count
- Endocrine evaluation if suspicious hyperandrogenism

- Iron studies
- Thyroid studies

Treatment Options

- <u>Finasteride</u>
- <u>Spironolactone</u>
- Dutasteride
- Topical minoxidil
- Hair transplantation

Further reading:
- Sehgal VN, Aggarwal AK, Srivastava G, Rajput P (2006) Male pattern androgenetic alopecia. Skinmed 5(3):128–135

Anetoderma

Focal loss of elastic tissue due to a variety of causes, associated with a variety of underlying diseases, and characterized by protrusions or depressions of lax skin (Fig. 6.7)

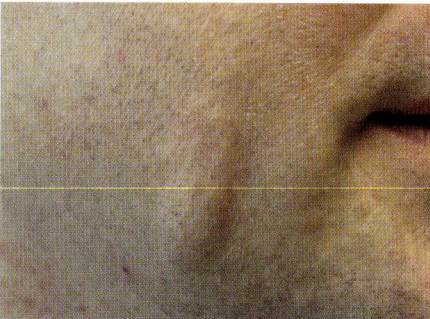

Fig. 6.7 Anetoderma

Subtypes/Variants

- Primary
  - With prior inflammation (Jadassohn–Pellizzari)
  - Without prior inflammation (Schweninger–Buzzi)
- Secondary (to an underlying disease)

Differential Diagnosis

- Arthropod bites
- Atrophic dermatofibroma
- Atrophic scar
- Cutis laxa
- Fascial hernia
- Focal dermal hypoplasia
- Lipoatrophy
- Middermal elastolysis
- Neurofibroma
- Nevus lipomatosus superficialis
- Papular elastorrhexis
- Perifollicular elastolysis (acne scars)
- Pityriasis versicolor atrophicans
- Pseudoxanthoma elasticum
- Postinflammatory elastolysis and cutis laxa (Marshall's syndrome)
- Steroid atrophy
- Striae distensae
- Urticaria

Associations (Secondary)

- Acne vulgaris
- Acrodermatitis chronica atrophicans
- Alopecia areata

- Antiphospholipid antibody syndrome
- Autoimmune hemolytic anemia
- Dermatofibroma
- Folliculitis
- Granuloma annulare
- Graves' disease
- Hepatitis B immunization
- HIV infection
- Hypergammaglobulinemia
- Hypocomplementemia
- Immunocytoma
- Juvenile xanthogranuloma
- Lepromatous leprosy
- Lichen planus
- Lupus erythematosus
- Lymphocytoma cutis
- Mastocytosis
- Melanocytic nevi
- Molluscum contagiosum
- Nodular amyloidosis
- Penicillamine therapy
- Pilomatrixoma
- Plasmacytoma
- Prematurity
- Prurigo nodularis
- Sarcoidosis
- Syphilis
- Systemic sclerosis
- Thyroiditis
- Tuberculosis
- Urticaria pigmentosum
- Varicella
- Vitiligo
- Xanthomas

Evaluation

- Antinuclear antibodies
- Antiphospholipid antibodies syndrome
- Complete blood count
- Sedimentation rate
- HIV test
- Lyme ELISA and Western blot
- Syphilis serologies

Further reading:

- De Souza EM, Daldon PE, Cintra ML (2007) Anetoderma associated with primary antiphospholipid syndrome. J Am Acad Dermatol 56(5):881–882

Angioedema

Subcutaneous or submucosal edema with a variety of causes that is characterized by asymptomatic or painful swelling of the face, lips, eyelids, genitals, and/or hands

Subtypes/Variants

- Acquired C1-INH deficiency/dysfunction
- ACE inhibitor induced
- Contrast media induced
- Chronic urticaria associated
- Cold urticaria related
- Episodic angioedema with eosinophilia
- Food related
- Hereditary C1-INH deficiency/dysfunction
- NERDS syndrome
- NSAID induced
- IgE mediated (allergic)
- Opiate related

- Serum sickness related
- Sunlight induced
- Vibratory

Differential Diagnosis

- Acute contact dermatitis
- Ascher syndrome
- Capillary leak syndrome
- Cellulitis/erysipelas
- Contact urticaria
- Delayed pressure urticaria
- Dermatomyositis
- EBV infection
- Extravasation
- Iatrogenic edema
- Loaiasis (Calabar swelling)
- <u>Lymphedema</u>
- Melkersson–Rosenthal syndrome
- Nephrotic syndrome
- Orofacial granulomatosis
- Rosacea
- Secretan's syndrome (factitial edema)
- Superior vena cava syndrome
- Tumid lupus
- Venous edema

Associations

Hereditary
- Glomerulonephritis
- Pernicious anemia
- Rheumatoid arthritis
- Sjögren's syndrome

- Systemic lupus erythematosus
- Thyroiditis

Acquired

- Anti-C1-INH antibodies (acquired, type II)
- Autoimmunity
- Chronic lymphocytic leukemia
- Cryoglobulinemia
- IgA myeloma
- Lymphosarcoma
- Monoclonal gammopathy
- Non-Hodgkin's lymphoma
- Waldenstrom's macroglobulinemia

Evaluation (if Hereditary or Acquired Are Suspected)

- C1 inhibitor functional assay
- C1 inhibitor level
- C1q level
- C2 level
- C4 level
- Total complement (CH50) level

Treatment Options

- Discontinue any offending medications
- Antihistamines
- Systemic corticosteroids
- Epinephrine
- Intravenous replacement of C1-INH
- Danazol
- Fresh frozen plasma
- Tranexamic acid
- Aminocaproic acid

Further reading:

- Kaplan A et al (2005) Angioedema. J Am Acad Dermatol 53:373–388

Angiofibromas

Benign proliferation of fibrous and vascular tissue with variable clinical presentation

Subtypes/Variants

- Cellular angiofibroma of the vulva
- Facial (adenoma sebaceum)
- Fibrous papule
- Koenen tumors
- Pearly penile papules
- Segmental angiofibromas

Differential Diagnosis (Facial)

- Acne vulgaris
- Adnexal tumors
- Basal cell carcinoma
- Cherry angioma
- Fibrofolliculoma
- Folliculitis
- Granuloma annulare
- Melanocytic nevus
- Molluscum contagiosum
- Multinucleate cell angiohistiocytoma
- Perifollicular fibroma
- Rosacea
- Sarcoidosis
- Trichodiscoma

- <u>Trichoepitheliomas</u>
- Verruca plana

Associations

- Birt–Hogg–Dube syndrome
- Multiple endocrine neoplasia, type I
- <u>Tuberous sclerosis</u>

Further reading:
- Trauner MA, Ruben BS, Lynch PJ (2003) Segmental tuberous sclerosis presenting as unilateral facial angiofibromas. J Am Acad Dermatol 49(2 Suppl Case Reports):S164–S166

Angioimmunoblastic Lymphadenopathy with Dysproteinemia

Type of T cell lymphoproliferative disorder that affects the elderly and is associated with fever, lymphadenopathy, anemia, hepatosplenomegaly, and a morbilliform exanthem

Differential Diagnosis

- Castleman disease
- <u>DRESS syndrome</u>
- Kikuchi disease
- Lymphoma
- Morbilliform drug eruption
- Myeloma
- Viral exanthem

Associations

- Drugs
- Viral infections

Evaluation

- Antinuclear antibodies
- Bone marrow biopsy
- Complete blood count
- CT scan of neck, chest, abdomen, and pelvis
- Lactate dehydrogenase level
- Lymph node biopsy
- Rheumatoid factor
- Serum/urinary protein electrophoresis
- T cell immunophenotyping

Further reading:
- Martel P, Laroche L, Courville P et al (2000) Cutaneous involvement in patients with angioimmunoblastic lymphadenopathy with dysproteinemia: a clinical, immunohistological, and molecular analysis. Arch Dermatol 136(7):881–886

Angiokeratoma

Type of vascular ectasia with a hyperkeratotic surface that can be solitary, localized, circumscribed, or diffusely located in a bathing-trunk distribution (angiokeratoma corporis diffusum)

Subtypes/Variants

- Angiokeratoma circumscriptum (extremities) (Fig. 6.8)
- Angiokeratoma corporis diffusum
- Angiokeratoma of Fordyce (scrotum or labia)
- Angiokeratoma of Mibelli (distal extremities)
- Solitary angiokeratoma (extremities)

Differential Diagnosis

- Angiokeratoma-like pseudolymphoma
- Angioma serpiginosum

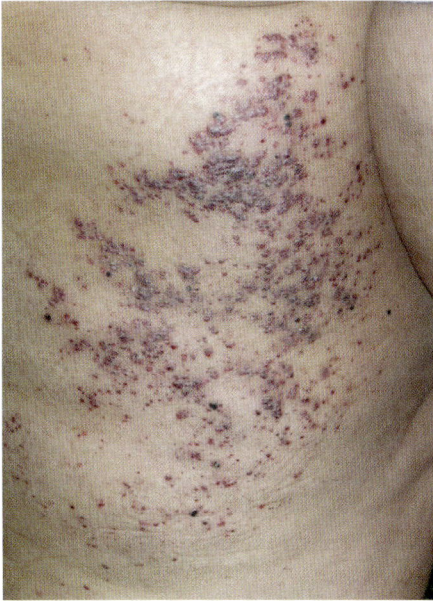

Fig. 6.8 Angiokeratomas
(Courtesy of A. Record)

- APACHE syndrome
- Bacillary angiomatosis
- Blue rubber bleb nevus
- Cherry angioma
- Clear cell acanthoma
- Elastosis perforans serpiginosa
- Hemangioma
- Hobnail (targetoid hemosiderotic) hemangioma
- Lymphangioma circumscriptum
- Melanoma
- Pyogenic granuloma
- Seborrheic keratosis
- Venous lake
- Verrucous hemangioma
- Wart

Associations

Angiokeratoma Circumscriptum
- Cobb syndrome
- Klippel–Trenaunay syndrome
- Nevus flammeus

Angiokeratoma Corporis Diffusum
- Alpha-L-fucosidase deficiency
- Beta-galactosidase deficiency
- Beta-mannosidase deficiency
- Fabry's disease
- Neuraminidase deficiency
- Sialidosis

Evaluation (Angiokeratoma Corporis Diffusum)

- Echocardiogram
- MRI of the brain
- Ophthalmologic exam for cornea verticillata
- Renal function test
- Serum alpha-galactosidase level (if negative, consider other causes)
- Urinalysis (maltese cross-lipid globules)

Further reading:
- Mittal R, Aggarwal A, Srivastava G (2005) Angiokeratoma circumscriptum: a case report and review of the literature. Int J Dermatol 44(12):1031–1034

Angiolymphoid Hyperplasia with Eosinophilia

Type of cutaneous lymphoid hyperplasia of unknown cause that affects young- to middle-aged adults and is characterized by erythematous, single, or grouped papules and nodules most commonly located on the head and neck

Differential Diagnosis

- Amelanotic melanoma
- Angiosarcoma
- Bacillary angiomatosis
- Basal cell carcinoma
- Cutaneous lymphoid hyperplasia
- Cylindromas
- Epidermal inclusion cyst
- Granuloma faciale
- Hemangioma
- Infective perichondritis
- Insect-bite reaction
- Kaposi's sarcoma
- Kimura's disease
- Lymphoma cutis
- Metastatic disease
- Pseudocyst of the auricle
- Pyogenic granuloma
- Relapsing polychondritis
- Sarcoidosis

Treatment Options

- Surgical excision
- Topical corticosteroids
- Intralesional corticosteroids
- Systemic corticosteroids
- Electrosurgery
- Isotretinoin

Further reading:

- Chong WS, Thomas A, Goh CL (2006) Kimura's disease and angiolymphoid hyperplasia with eosinophilia: two disease entities in the same patient: case report and review of the literature. Int J Dermatol 45(2):139–145

Angioma Serpiginosum (Hutchinson Disease)

Uncommon, often inherited vascular ectasia that predominantly affects women and is characterized by grouped punctate vascular macules and papules most commonly on the lower extremity

Differential Diagnosis

- Angiokeratoma circumscriptum
- Carcinoma telangiectaticum
- Nevus flammeus
- Pigmented purpuric dermatosis
- Unilateral nevoid telangiectasia

Treatment Options

- Electrosurgery
- Pulsed dye laser

Further reading:
- Sandhu K, Gupta S (2005) Angioma serpiginosum: report of two unusual cases. J Eur Acad Dermatol Venereol 19(1):127–128

Angiosarcoma

Malignant endothelial tumor that can arise in a variety of clinical settings but is most commonly characterized by a slow-growing violaceous and erythematous plaque with or without ulceration on the head and neck of the elderly

Subtypes/Variants

- Dabska tumor (endovascular papillary angioendothelioma)
- Epithelioid angiosarcoma
- Idiopathic angiosarcoma of the head and neck

- Irradiation related
- Retiform hemangioendothelioma
- Stewart–Treves syndrome (lymphedema related)

Differential Diagnosis

General

- Acquired progressive lymphangioma
- Angioedema
- Angiolymphoid hyperplasia with eosinophilia
- Benign lymphangiomatosis
- Cutaneous lymphoid hyperplasia
- Epithelioid sarcoma
- Hemangiopericytoma
- Kaposi's sarcoma
- Malignant schwannoma
- Masson's intravascular papillary endothelial hyperplasia
- Melanoma
- Merkel cell carcinoma
- Metastatic lesion
- Reactive angioendotheliomatosis
- Recurrent breast cancer
- Retiform hemangioendothelioma
- Rhinophyma
- Tufted angioma
- Venous malformation

Stewart–Treves Syndrome

- Angioendotheliomatosis
- Angiolymphoid hyperplasia
- Hemangioendothelioma
- Hemangiopericytoma
- Kaposi's sarcoma
- Melanoma
- Recurrent or metastatic breast cancer

Associations

- Breast cancer irradiation
- <u>Chronic solar damage</u>
- Congenital lymphedema
- <u>Iatrogenic lymphedema</u>
- Immunosuppression
- Vinyl chloride exposure

Further reading:
- Mendenhall WM, Mendenhall CM, Werning JW et al (2006) Cutaneous angiosarcoma. Am J Clin Oncol 29(5):524–528

Annular Erythema of Infancy

Uncommon annular eruption that arises early in infancy, typically resolves within the first year of life, and is characterized by a cyclic eruption of urticarial papules that evolve to annular erythematous plaques on the head, trunk, and extremities

Differential Diagnosis

- Acute hemorrhagic edema of infancy
- Dermatophytosis
- Erythema annulare centrifugum
- Erythema marginatum
- Erythema toxicum neonatorum
- Granuloma annulare
- <u>Neonatal lupus</u>
- <u>Serum-sickness-like reaction</u>
- Urticaria

Evaluation

- Antinuclear antibodies (including SS-A and SS-B)
- Electrocardiography

Treatment Options

- <u>Observation and reassurance</u>
- Topical corticosteroids

Further reading:
- Wong LC, Kakakios A, Rogers M (2002) Congenital annular erythema persisting in a 15-year-old girl. Australas J Dermatol 43(1):55–61

Annular Lichenoid Dermatitis of Youth

Uncommon lichenoid dermatitis that affects children and is characterized by persistent, annular erythematous plaques with central hypopigmentation in the groin, periumbilical areas, and flanks

Differential Diagnosis

- Annular erythema
- Annular atrophic lichen planus
- Lichen sclerosus et atrophicus
- Granuloma annulare
- Leprosy (especially tuberculoid type)
- Lupus erythematosus
- <u>Morphea</u>
- Mycosis fungoides
- Tinea cruris
- <u>Vitiligo</u>

Treatment Options

- Narrowband UVB phototherapy
- Topical corticosteroids
- Tacrolimus ointment

Further reading:
- Annessi G, Paradisi M, Angelo C et al (2003) Annular lichenoid dermatitis of youth. J Am Acad Dermatol 49(6):1029–1036

Anthrax

Bacterial infection caused by the Gram-positive *Bacillus anthracis* that can be acquired through contact with sheep or cows or by acts of bioterrorism and is characterized by a painless, edematous nodule with a black eschar on the extremities (malignant pustule)

Differential Diagnosis

- Antiphospholipid antibody syndrome
- *Aspergillus* infection
- Atypical mycobacterial infection
- Blastomycosis
- Cat-scratch disease
- Coumadin necrosis
- Cutaneous diphtheria
- Ecthyma gangrenosum
- Glanders
- Leishmaniasis
- Mucormycosis
- Orf/Milker's nodule
- Plague
- Pyoderma gangrenosum
- Rat-bite fever

- Spider bite
- Sporotrichosis
- Staphylococcal pyoderma
- Syphilis
- Tache noir
- Tropical ulcer
- Tularemia

Evaluation

- Gram stain and culture of tissue
- Gram stain, culture, and PCR of blood

Further reading:
- Hart CA, Beeching NJ (2002) A spotlight on anthrax. Clin Dermatol 20(4):365–375

Antiphospholipid Antibody Syndrome

Hypercoagulable disorder associated with the presence of antiphospholipid antibodies that is characterized by arterial or venous thrombosis, multiple miscarriages, livedo reticularis, retiform purpura, and cutaneous necrosis

Differential Diagnosis

- Cholesterol emboli syndrome
- Cocaine-associated vasculopathy
- Cryoglobulinemia/cryofibrinogenemia
- Disseminated intravascular coagulation
- Endocarditis
- Factor V Leiden mutation
- Malignancy
- Oxalate embolism
- Protein-C or protein-S deficiency

- Seronegative antiphospholipid antibody syndrome (SNAPS)
- Systemic vasculitis
- Thrombotic thrombocytopenic purpura
- Waldenstrom's macroglobulinemia

Diagnostic Criteria (Simplified)

- Clinical (1/2)
  - Thrombosis of arterial, venous, or small vessel circulation confirmed with imaging
  - Three unexplained spontaneous abortions or one fetal death after 10 weeks or premature birth due to placental insufficiency or preeclampsia
- Laboratory (1/2)
  - Anticardiolipin antibody IgG and/or IgM positive on two or more occasions 6 weeks apart
  - Lupus anticoagulant positive on two or more occasions 6 weeks apart

Associations

- Atrophie blanche
- Autoimmune disease
- Bullous pemphigoid
- Celiac disease
- HIV infection
- Hydralazine
- Internal malignancy
- Lymphoma
- Malignant atrophic papulosis
- Phenytoin
- Primary anetoderma
- Procainamide
- Rheumatoid arthritis

- Sneddon syndrome
- Sulfonamides
- <u>Systemic lupus erythematosus</u>
- Systemic vasculitis syndromes
- Ulcerative colitis
- Viral illness

Evaluation

- Anticardiolipin IgG and IgM antibodies
- Antinuclear antibodies
- Beta-2-glycoprotein antibodies
- Blood cultures
- Complete blood count
- Cryofibrinogens
- Cryoglobulins
- D-dimer
- Factor V Leiden mutation
- Lupus anticoagulant
- Protein C and protein S
- Prothrombin time and partial thromboplastin time
- Rheumatoid factor

Treatment Options

- Heparin
- <u>Warfarin</u>
- Aspirin
- Hydroxychloroquine
- <u>Systemic corticosteroids</u>
- Intravenous immunoglobulin
- Cyclophosphamide
- Plasmapheresis

Further reading:
- Wilson WA, Gharavi AE, Koike T et al (1999) International consensus statement on preliminary classification criteria for definite antiphospholipid syndrome: report of an international workshop. Arthritis Rheum 42(7):1309–1311

APACHE Syndrome (Acral Pseudolymphomatous Angiokeratoma of Children)

Rare, idiopathic type of cutaneous lymphoid hyperplasia that affects children (and, less commonly, adults) and is characterized by angiokeratoma-like red papules predominantly affecting the acral areas and, less commonly, the trunk

Differential Diagnosis

- Angiokeratoma circumscriptum
- Angiolymphoid hyperplasia with eosinophilia
- Arthropod-bite reaction
- Eruptive pseudoangiomatosis
- Eruptive pyogenic granulomas
- Lymphomatoid papulosis
- Reactive angioendotheliomatosis

Further reading:
- Kim Y, Dawes-Higgs E, Mann S, Cook DK (2005) Acral cutaneous lymphoid hyperplasia angiokeratoma of children (APACHE). Australas J Dermatol 46(3):177–180

Aphthous Stomatitis (Aphthous Ulcers)

Common painful, self-limited superficial mucosal ulcerations of uncertain etiology that typically last 7–14 days and affect the nonkeratinized portions of the mouth

Subtypes/Variants

- Minor
- Major (periadenitis mucosa necrotica recurrens, Sutton's disease)
- Herpetiform

Differential Diagnosis

- Acatalasemia
- Angina bullosa hemorrhagica
- Behçet's disease
- Candidiasis
- Chemotherapy stomatitis
- Contact dermatitis
- Crohn's disease
- Cyclic neutropenia
- Eosinophilic ulcer
- Erythema multiforme
- Fixed drug eruption
- Hand–foot–mouth disease
- Herpangina
- Herpes simplex virus infection
- Lupus erythematosus
- Lichen planus
- Oral cancer
- Paraneoplastic pemphigus
- Pemphigus vulgaris
- Pyoderma gangrenosum
- Reiter syndrome
- Syphilis
- Trauma
- Vitamin deficiency

Associations

- <u>Behçet's disease</u>
- Celiac disease
- Cyclic neutropenia
- HIV infection
- PFAPA syndrome

Evaluation

- Antinuclear antibodies
- Complete blood count
- Iron, B12, and folate studies
- Sedimentation rate
- Viral culture

Treatment Options

- <u>Topical corticosteroids</u>
- Intralesional corticosteroids
- <u>Tacrolimus ointment</u>
- Chlorhexidine oral rinse
- Sucralfate
- Pentoxifylline
- Systemic corticosteroids
- Colchicine
- Dapsone
- Azathioprine
- TNF inhibitors

Further reading:

- Letsinger JA, McCarty MA, Jorizzo JL (2005) Complex aphthosis: a large case series with evaluation algorithm and therapeutic ladder from topicals to thalidomide. J Am Acad Dermatol 52(3 Pt 1):500–508

Aplasia Cutis Congenita

Developmental anomaly representing focal loss of skin in utero that is due to a variety of developmental, traumatic, or ischemic causes and characterized by a well-demarcated stellate or circular, atrophic, smooth, or ulcerated scar-like patch most commonly on the scalp

Subtypes/Variants

- Group 1 – without anomalies
- Group 2 – with Adams–Oliver syndrome
- Group 3 – with epidermal and organoid nevi
- Group 4 – with embryologic malformations
- Group 5 – with fetus papyraceus, placental infarcts, or other ischemic events
- Group 6 – with epidermolysis bullosa (Bart's syndrome)
- Group 7 – extremities without blistering
- Group 8 – teratogenic medications or intrauterine infections
- Group 9 – with malformation syndromes

Differential Diagnosis

- Congenital erosive and vesicular dermatosis
- Congenital varicella
- Encephalocele
- Epidermolysis bullosa
- Focal dermal hypoplasia
- Heterotopic neural tissue
- Iatrogenic injury
- Neonatal herpes simplex virus infection
- Nevus sebaceus
- Scalp pyoderma
- Transient bullous dermolysis

Associations

- Adams–Oliver syndrome
- Amniotic band syndrome
- Cranial or spinal defect
- Focal dermal hypoplasia (Goltz)
- Intrauterine varicella
- Intrauterine herpes simplex infection
- Johanson–Blizzard syndrome
- Methimazole
- MIDAS syndrome
- Misoprostol
- Oculocerebrocutaneous syndrome
- Oculoectodermal syndrome
- Setleis syndrome (focal facial dermal dysplasia)
- Trisomy 13
- Valproic acid
- Wolf–Hirschhorn syndrome

Evaluation

- CT/MRI scan of skull or spine if underlying defect is suspected

Further reading:
- Frieden IJ (1986) Aplasia cutis congenita: a clinical review and proposal for classification. J Am Acad Dermatol 14(4): 646–660

Aquagenic Syringeal Acrokeratoderma

Acquired condition affecting the palms that is characterized by painful, bilateral, white, translucent papules and wrinkling after the palms are exposed to moisture and resolution after drying

Differential Diagnosis

- Pompholyx
- Punctate keratoderma
- Tripe palms
- Warm water immersion syndrome
- Warts

Associations

- Cystic fibrosis

Further reading:
- Luo DQ, Zhao YK, Zhang WJ, Wu LC (2010) Aquagenic acrokeratoderma. Int J Dermatol 49(5):526–531

Argyria

Type of mucocutaneous pigmentary disturbance caused by ingestion or contact with silver characterized by blue, gray, or black hyperpigmentation most prominent on the mucosal surfaces and sun-exposed areas

Differential Diagnosis

- Amiodarone photosensitivity
- Arsenical pigmentation
- Blue nevus (localized as in acupuncture)
- Chloracne
- Chrysiasis
- Cyanosis
- Diffuse melanosis from metastatic melanoma
- Hemochromatosis

- Minocycline hyperpigmentation
- Ochronosis
- Phenothiazine photosensitivity
- Polycythemia vera

Further reading:
- White JM, Powell AM, Brady K, Russell-Jones R (2003) Severe generalized argyria secondary to ingestion of colloidal silver protein. Clin Exp Dermatol 28(3):254–256

Arsenical Keratoses

Premalignant hyperkeratotic papules associated with chronic arsenic exposure that are characteristically located on the palms and soles and develop many years after arsenic exposure

Differential Diagnosis

- Clavus/callus
- Darier disease
- Lichen planus
- Nevoid basal cell carcinoma syndrome
- Palmoplantar psoriasis
- Pityriasis rubra pilaris
- Porokeratosis palmaris et plantaris
- Punctate keratoderma
- Verruca vulgaris

Evaluation

- Cancer screening (if history or physical exam suggests)

Further reading:
- Yerebakan O, Ermis O, Yilmaz E, Basaran E (2002) Treatment of arsenical keratosis and Bowen's disease with acitretin. Int J Dermatol 41(2):84–87

Arteriovenous Malformation

Uncommon vascular malformation in which there is a direct connection between the arterial and venous circulation and that is characterized by an erythematous, violaceous, or flesh-colored, pulsatile nodule most commonly on the head

Subtypes/Variants

- Acquired (trauma)
- Cirsoid aneurysm
- Congenital
- Iatrogenic (hemodialysis)

Differential Diagnosis

- Epidermal inclusion cyst
- Hemangioma
- Infantile hemangiopericytoma
- Kaposi's sarcoma
- Lipoma
- Pilar cyst
- Venous malformation

Staging

- I – dormant
- II – expanding/thrill
- III – necrotic
- IV – cardiac decompensation

Associations

- Cobb syndrome
- Osler–Weber–Rendu disease

- Parkes Weber syndrome
- Stewart–Bluefarb syndrome
- Wyburn–Mason syndrome

Further reading:
- Garzon MC, Huang JT, Enjolras O, Frieden IJ (2007) Vascular malformations: part I. J Am Acad Dermatol 56(3):353–370

Arthropod-Bite Reaction

Cutaneous reaction to the bite or sting of a variety of arthropods that has variable cutaneous presentation and can both mimic and lead to a variety of cutaneous and systemic diseases (Fig. 6.9)

Differential Diagnosis

- Bullous impetigo
- Bullous pemphigoid
- Cutaneous lymphoid hyperplasia

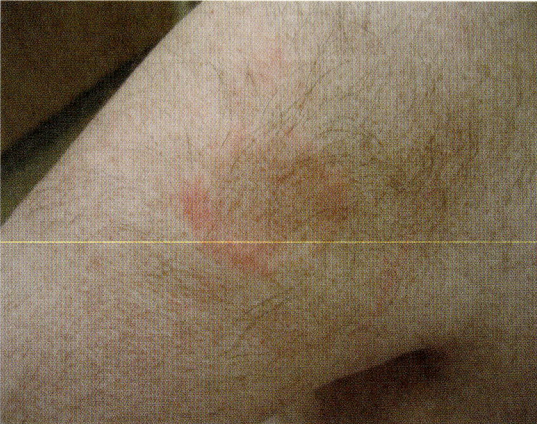

Fig. 6.9 Arthropod-bite reaction

- Dermatitis artefacta
- Erythema migrans
- Fixed drug eruption
- Furunculosis
- Granuloma annulare
- Jessner's lymphocytic infiltrate
- Idiopathic facial aseptic granuloma
- Leukemia
- Lupus erythematosus tumidus
- Lymphoma cutis
- Lymphomatoid papulosis
- Metastatic lesion
- Nodulocystic acne
- Papular urticaria
- Pityriasis lichenoides et varioliformis acuta
- Pyoderma gangrenosum
- Solitary mastocytoma
- Subacute prurigo
- Urticaria
- Urticarial dermatitis
- Wells syndrome

Treatment Options

- <u>Topical corticosteroids</u>
- Intralesional corticosteroids
- Topical anesthetics
- <u>Systemic antihistamines</u>
- Systemic corticosteroids

Further reading:

- Terhune MH, Stibbe J, Siegle RJ (1999) Nodule on the cheek of an 81-year-old woman.
  Persistent arthropod-bite reaction (cutaneous T-cell pseudolymphoma). Arch
  Dermatol 135(12):1543–1544, 1546–1547

Aspergillosis

Respiratory mycosis with the vessel-invasive fungus, *Aspergillus* spp., that predominantly affects immunosuppressed (especially neutropenic) patients, can be localized (most commonly, *A. flavus*) or disseminated from an initial pulmonary focus (most commonly, *A. fumigatus*), and is characterized by hemorrhagic lesions and necrotic black eschars

Differential Diagnosis

- Candidiasis, disseminated
- Cryptococcosis
- Ecthyma
- Ecthyma gangrenosum
- Fusarium infection
- Histoplasmosis
- Mucormycosis
- Phaeohyphomycosis
- Pyoderma gangrenosum
- Septic vasculitis
- Sweet syndrome
- Zygomycosis

Evaluation

- Tissue, sputum, and blood cultures

Further reading:
- Mays SR, Bogle MA, Bodey GP (2006) Cutaneous fungal infections in the oncology patient: recognition and management. Am J Clin Dermatol 7(1):31–43

Asteatotic Eczema (Eczema Craquele)

Type of eczema that most commonly affects the elderly, is caused by increased transepidermal water loss as it relates to decreased barrier-forming lipids of the skin, and is characterized by pruritic, xerotic, erythematous plaques most commonly located on the anterior legs and trunk

Differential Diagnosis

- Atopic dermatitis
- Allergic contact dermatitis
- Autoeczematization
- Erythrokeratolysis hiemalis
- Ichthyosis vulgaris
- Irritant contact dermatitis
- Mycosis fungoides
- Nummular eczema
- Scabies
- Subacute prurigo
- Stasis dermatitis

Associations

- Diuretic therapy
- Fatty acid deficiency
- Internal malignancy
- Radiation
- Statin therapy
- Thyroid disease
- Winter season
- Zinc deficiency

Treatment Options

- <u>Moisturizers</u>
- <u>Topical steroids</u>
- Phototherapy
- Systemic corticosteroids
- Methotrexate

Further reading:
- Norman RA (2003) Xerosis and pruritus in the elderly: recognition and management. Dermatol Ther 16(3):254–259

Ataxia–Telangiectasia

Autosomal-recessive disorder caused by a defect in the ATM gene which is characterized by early childhood onset of cerebellar ataxia, conjunctival and cutaneous telangiectasias, café-au-lait macules, pigmentary changes, noninfectious granulomatous lesions, defective cellular and humoral immunity, recurrent sinopulmonary infections, increased sensitivity to radiation, and lymphoreticular malignancies

Differential Diagnosis

- Benign essential telangiectasia
- <u>Bloom syndrome</u>
- Coats' disease
- Congenital immunodeficiency
- Congenital syphilis
- Friedreich's ataxia
- Generalized essential telangiectasia
- HIV infection
- Hereditary hemorrhagic telangiectasia
- Infectious conjunctivitis
- <u>Nijmegen breakage syndrome</u>

Evaluation

- Alpha-fetoprotein level (elevated)
- Complete blood count
- CT/MRI scan of brain
- Genetic studies
- HIV test
- Immunoglobulin panel

Further reading:
- Mitra A, Pollock B, Gooi J, Darling JC, Boon A, Newton-Bishop JA (2005) Cutaneous granulomas associated with primary immunodeficiency disorders. Br J Dermatol 153(1):194–199

Atopic Dermatitis (Besnier Disease)

Multifactorial, chronic, and relapsing disorder associated with impaired skin barrier function, environmental hypersensitivity, and asthma that may begin in infancy and is characterized by very pruritic, eczematous skin lesions in age-specific patterns

Differential Diagnosis

Infantile
- Acrodermatitis enteropathica
- Ataxia–telangiectasia
- Biotin deficiency
- Chronic mucocutaneous candidiasis
- Congenital syphilis
- Contact dermatitis
- Dermatophytosis
- DiGeorge syndrome
- Ectodermal dysplasias
- Essential fatty acid deficiency
- Hartnup disease

- HTLV-1 infection
- Hyperimmunoglobulin E syndrome
- Ichthyosis vulgaris
- Impetigo
- Infective dermatitis
- Keratosis pilaris
- Langerhans cell histiocytosis
- Netherton's syndrome
- Niacin deficiency
- Phenylketonuria
- Psoriasis
- Pyridoxine deficiency
- Scabies
- <u>Seborrheic dermatitis</u>
- Severe combined immunodeficiency
- Wiskott–Aldrich syndrome

Older Children and Adults

- Acquired ichthyosis
- <u>Asteatotic eczema</u>
- Chronic actinic dermatitis
- <u>Contact dermatitis</u>
- Dermatitis herpetiformis
- Dermatomyositis
- Drug eruption
- Graft-vs-host disease
- Infective dermatitis
- Lichen nitidus
- Lichen simplex chronicus
- Lupus erythematosus
- Mycosis fungoides
- Nummular eczema
- Pemphigus foliaceus
- Photoallergic dermatitis

- Pityriasis rubra pilaris
- Psoriasis
- Scabies
- Seborrheic dermatitis
- Sezary syndrome
- Vesicular pemphigoid

Diagnostic Criteria

AAD Consensus Criteria

- Essential features: must be present and, if complete, are sufficient for diagnosis:
  - Pruritus
  - Eczematous changes
  - Typical and age-specific patterns
    - Facial, neck, and extensor involvement in infants and children
    - Current or prior flexural lesions in adults/any age
    - Sparing of groin and axillary regions
  - Chronic or relapsing course
- Important features: seen in most cases for support of the diagnosis:
  - Early age of onset
  - Atopy (IgE reactivity)
  - Xerosis
- Associated features: help in suggesting the diagnosis:
  - Keratosis pilaris, ichthyosis vulgaris, and palmar hyperlinearity
  - Atypical vascular responses
  - Perifollicular accentuation/lichenification/prurigo
  - Ocular/periorbital changes

Hanifin and Rajka Criteria

- Major criteria (3/4)
  - Chronic or relapsing dermatitis
  - Personal or family history of atopy

- Pruritus
- Typical morphology and distribution
- Minor criteria (3/23)
  - Anterior neck folds
  - Anterior subcapsular cataract
  - Cheilitis
  - Course influenced by environmental/emotional factors
  - Dennie–Morgan infraorbital fold
  - Early age of onset
  - Elevated serum IgE
  - Facial pallor/erythema
  - Food intolerance
  - Ichthyosis/palmar hyperlinearity/keratosis pilaris
  - Immediate (type I) skin test reactivity
  - Intolerance to wool and lipid solvents
  - Keratoconus
  - Nipple eczema
  - Orbital darkening
  - Perifollicular accentuation
  - Pityriasis alba
  - Pruritus when sweating
  - Recurrent conjunctivitis
  - Tendency toward cutaneous infections/impaired cell-mediated immunity
  - Tendency toward nonspecific hand or foot dermatitis
  - White dermatographism
  - Xerosis

Treatment Options

- <u>Moisturizers</u>
- <u>Topical corticosteroids</u>

- <u>Topical calcineurin inhibitors</u>
- Systemic corticosteroids
- Systemic antibiotics
- <u>UVB phototherapy</u>
- Azathioprine
- Mycophenolate mofetil
- Methotrexate
- Cyclosporine

Further reading:
- Krol A, Krafchik B (2006) The differential diagnosis of atopic dermatitis in childhood. Dermatol Ther 19(2):73–82

Atrichia with Papular Lesions

Type of infancy-onset atrichia with autosomal-recessive inheritance that is caused by a defect in either the hairless gene or the vitamin D receptor gene and is characterized by shedding of all hair in the first few months of life followed by the development in early childhood of a milia-like papular eruption on the scalp, face, elbows, and knees (which later involutes to leave pitted scars)

Differential Diagnosis

- <u>Alopecia universalis</u>
- Anagen effluvium
- Ectodermal dysplasias
- IFAP syndrome
- Monilethrix
- Netherton syndrome
- Trichothiodystrophy
- Ulerythema ophryogenes

Diagnostic Criteria

- Family history with pattern of inheritance established as autosomal recessive.
- Patients are sometimes born without hair, and none ever grows. More typically, patients are born with normal hair that is shed after several months and never regrows.
- Papules that start to appear during the first year of life, particularly under the midline of the eye, on the face, and on the extremities.
- Few to many papules distributed over some or all of the following areas: scalp, cheeks, arms, elbows, thighs, and knees.
- Normal nails and teeth, normal sweating, and no growth or developmental problems.
- Sparse eyebrows and eyelashes.
- Lack of secondary axillary, pubic, or body hair.
- Whitish hypopigmented streaks on the scalp.
- Lack of response to any treatment modality.
- Biopsy–absence of mature hair follicle structures, cysts filled with cornified material.
- Mutation in the hairless gene.

Associations

- Vitamin-D-resistant rickets

Further reading:
- Bergman R, Schein-Goldshmid R, Hochberg Z et al (2005) The alopecias associated with vitamin D-dependent rickets type IIA and with hairless gene mutations: a comparative clinical, histologic, and immunohistochemical study. Arch Dermatol 141(3):343–351
- Zlotogorski A, Panteleyev AA, Aita VM, Christiano AM (2002) Clinical and molecular diagnostic criteria of congenital atrichia with papular lesions. J Invest Dermatol 118(5):887–890

Atrophoderma of Pasini and Pierini

Acquired, benign atrophoderma of unknown cause that is characterized by hyperpigmented, depressed plaques most commonly on the back with a typical shelf-like or cliff-like border

Differential Diagnosis

- Anetoderma
- Connective tissue nevus
- Erythema dyschromicum perstans
- Fixed drug eruption
- Lichen sclerosus at atrophicus
- Linear atrophoderma of Moulin
- Lupus profundus
- Morphea
- Nevus anelasticus
- Steroid atrophy
- Striae atrophicans
- Postinflammatory hyperpigmentation

Associations

- Lyme borreliosis

Treatment Options

- Topical corticosteroids
- Doxycycline
- Hydroxychloroquine
- Methotrexate

Further reading:
- Amano H, Nagai Y, Ishikawa O (2007) Multiple morphea coexistent with atrophoderma of Pasini–Pierini (APP): APP could be abortive morphea. J Eur Acad Dermatol Venereol 21(9):1254–1256

Atrophoderma Vermiculatum

Disorder of follicular keratinization (and type of keratosis pilaris atrophicans) that can occur sporadically or as a feature of a syndrome and is characterized by inflammatory keratotic papules on the cheeks that evolve to worm-eaten atrophic pitted scars

Differential Diagnosis

- <u>Acne scars (perifollicular elastolysis)</u>
- <u>Atrophia maculosa varioliformis cutis</u>
- Chloracne
- Erythromelanosis faciei
- Infantile acne
- Keratosis pilaris
- Nevus comedonicus
- Varicella scars

Associations

- Keratosis pilaris atrophicans
- Nicolau–Balus syndrome
- Rombo syndrome

Further reading:
- Van Steensel MA, Jaspers NG, Steijlen PM (2001) A case of Rombo syndrome. Br J Dermatol 144(6):1215–1218

Autoeczematization (Autosensitization) Reaction

Type of immune-mediated cutaneous reaction associated with various types of dermatitis that is characterized by symmetric, erythematous papules, vesicles, and eczematous changes in areas distant to the initial, triggering dermatitis (often stasis dermatitis or allergic contact dermatitis)

Differential Diagnosis

- Airborne contact dermatitis
- Atopic dermatitis
- Contact dermatitis
- Dermatitis herpetiformis
- Drug reaction
- Dyshidrotic eczema
- Erysipelas
- Folliculitis
- Gianotti–Crosti syndrome
- Id reaction
- Mycosis fungoides
- Photoallergic contact dermatitis
- Pityriasis lichenoides
- Prurigo nodularis
- Scabies

Treatment Options

- Address the underlying cause
- Systemic corticosteroids

Further reading:
- Williams J, Cahill J, Nixon R (2007) Occupational autoeczematization or atopic eczema precipitated by occupational contact dermatitis? Contact Dermatitis 56(1):21–26

Baboon Syndrome

A distinct presentation of either systemic contact dermatitis (especially nickel or mercury related) or drug reaction (especially amoxicillin, also known as symmetrical drug-related intertriginous and flexural exanthema (SDRIFE)) that is characterized by an erythematous, dermatitic eruption with well-defined borders in the flexures, especially the perineal area and buttocks

Differential Diagnosis

- <u>Allergic contact dermatitis</u>
- Erythrasma
- Fixed drug eruption
- Intertrigo
- Inverse psoriasis
- Tinea cruris
- Streptococcal perianal eruption

Diagnostic Criteria (SDRIFE)

- Exposure to a systemically administered drug, first or repeated doses (contact allergens excluded)
- Sharply demarcated erythema of the gluteal/perianal area and/or V-shaped erythema of the inguinal/perigenital area
- Involvement of at least one other intertriginous/flexural fold
- Symmetry of affected areas
- Absence of systemic symptoms and signs

Associations

- Amoxicillin
- Ampicillin
- Erythromycin

- Food additives
- Mercury
- Nickel

Treatment Options

- Systemic corticosteroids

Further reading:
- Hausermann P, Harr T, Bircher AJ (2004) Baboon syndrome resulting from systemic drugs: is there strife between SDRIFE and allergic contact dermatitis syndrome? Contact Dermatitis 51(5–6):297–310

Bacillary Angiomatosis

Cutaneous manifestation of *Bartonella* infection seen most commonly in the profoundly immunosuppressed HIV patient that is caused by *Bartonella henselae* or *Bartonella quintana* and is characterized by angiomatous or violaceous papules or nodules, fever, lymphadenopathy, and hepatic lesions (peliosis hepatis)

Differential Diagnosis

- Angiokeratoma
- Angiolymphoid hyperplasia with eosinophilia
- Angiosarcoma
- Atypical mycobacterial infection
- Cherry hemangioma
- Eruptive pseudoangiomatosis
- Glomangioma
- Kaposi sarcoma
- Melanoma
- Pyogenic granuloma
- Verruga peruana

Evaluation

- HIV test
- CD4 count
- ELISA for *Bartonella* antibodies
- Complete blood count
- Liver function test
- CT scan of abdomen

Further reading:
- Rigopoulos D, Paparizos V, Katsambas A (2004) Cutaneous markers of HIV infection. Clin Dermatol 22(6):487–498

Balanitis Xerotica Obliterans (Penile Lichen Sclerosus et Atrophicus)

Fibrosing process affecting the foreskin of the penis that is classically associated with lichen sclerosus et atrophicus; is characterized by white, atrophic, sclerotic plaques on the glans or prepuce; and may present as phimosis

Differential Diagnosis

- Candidiasis
- Erythroplasia of Queyrat
- Lichen planus
- Phimosis due to chronic inflammation and poor hygiene
- Plasma cell balanitis
- Postinflammatory hypopigmentation
- Psoriasis
- Pseudoepitheliomatous, keratotic, and micaceous balanitis
- Reiter syndrome

- Squamous cell carcinoma
- <u>Vitiligo</u>

Treatment Options

- <u>Topical corticosteroids</u>
- Topical calcineurin inhibitors
- Circumcision

Further reading:

- Kiss A, Kiraly L, Kutasy B, Merksz M (2005) High incidence of balanitis xerotica obliterans in boys with phimosis: prospective 10-year study. Pediatr Dermatol 22(4):305–308

Bannayan–Riley–Ruvalcaba Syndrome

Inherited malformation disorder (AD) with onset in childhood that is associated with mutation of the PTEN gene and is characterized by genital lentigines, lipomas, capillary malformations, intestinal polyps, macrocephaly, and mental retardation

Differential Diagnosis

- <u>Cowden disease</u>
- Gardner's syndrome
- Multiple lentigines
- Peutz–Jeghers syndrome
- Proteus syndrome

Further reading:

- Erkek E et al (2005) Clinical and histopathological findings of Bannayan–Riley–Ruvalcaba syndrome. J Am Acad Dermatol 53:639–643

Bartonellosis (Oroya Fever, Verruga Peruana)

Bartonella infection diagnosed predominantly in South America that is caused by *Bartonella bacilliformis*, transmitted by the *Lutzomyia verrucarum* sandfly, and characterized by an acute febrile syndrome with severe hemolytic anemia and septicemia (oroya fever) and a chronic form with hemorrhagic, erythematous papules and nodules on the head and extremities (verruga peruana)

Differential Diagnosis

- AIDS
- Babesiosis
- <u>Bacillary angiomatosis</u>
- Deep fungal infection
- Dengue fever
- Eruptive pyogenic granulomas
- Leukemia
- Lymphogranuloma venereum
- Lymphoma
- Malaria
- Molluscum contagiosum
- Syphilis
- Tuberculosis
- Warts
- Yaws

Evaluation

- ELISA and Western blot for *Bartonella* antibodies

Further reading:
- Chian CA, Arrese JE, Pierard GE (2002) Skin manifestations of *Bartonella* infections. Int J Dermatol 41(8):461–466

Basal Cell Carcinoma

Malignant neoplasm mostly affecting older patients that arises from pluripotent cells of the epidermis or follicle and is characterized as an erythematous, pearly nodule with a rolled border, pigmentation, central umbilication, and/or ulceration most commonly located on the face, neck, and trunk

Subtypes/Variants

Clinical

- Fibroepithelioma of Pinkus
- Giant
- Keloidal
- Linear
- Morpheaform
- Nodular/ulcerative
- Pigmented
- Polypoid
- Superficial

Histological

- Adamantinoid (ameloblastoma-like)
- Adenoid
- Apocrine
- Basosquamous
- Clear cell
- Cystic
- Eccrine
- Fibroepithelioma of Pinkus
- Follicular
- Granular
- Infiltrative
- Infundibulocystic

- Keloidal
- Keratotic
- Matrical
- Metaplastic
- Micronodular
- Myoepithelial
- Neuroendocrine
- Nodular
- Pigmented
- Pleomorphic (giant cell)
- Sclerosing
- Sebaceous
- Signet ring cell
- Superficial multifocal

Differential Diagnosis

- Acrochordon (Gorlin's syndrome)
- Actinic keratosis
- Ameloblastoma
- Angioma
- Apocrine hidrocystoma
- Atypical fibroxanthoma
- Basaloid follicular hamartoma
- Bowen's disease
- Chalazion
- Chronic lymphocytic leukemia
- Cryptococcosis
- Dermatofibroma
- Fibrous papule
- Hidroacanthoma simplex
- Keloid
- Lymphadenoma
- Merkel cell carcinoma

- Metastatic disease
- Molluscum contagiosum
- Neurofibroma
- Nevus
- Sebaceoma
- Sebaceous adenoma
- Sebaceous carcinoma
- Sebaceous hyperplasia
- <u>Seborrheic keratoses</u>
- Spectacle granuloma
- <u>Squamous cell carcinoma</u>
- Trichoblastoma
- Trichoepithelioma
- Wart

Associations

- Albinism
- Arsenic exposure
- Bazex–Dupre–Christol syndrome
- Dyskeratosis congenita
- Myotonic dystrophy
- <u>Nevoid basal cell carcinoma syndrome</u>
- Nevus sebaceus
- Rombo syndrome
- Vaccination scars
- Xeroderma pigmentosum

Treatment Options

- <u>Surgical excision</u>
- <u>Mohs micrographic surgery</u>
- Electrodessication and curettage
- Radiation

- Topical 5-FU
- Imiquimod
- Photodynamic therapy

Further reading:
- Hutcheson A et al (2005) Basal cell carcinomas with unusual histologic patterns. J Am Acad Dermatol 53:833–837

Basaloid Follicular Hamartoma

Rare adnexal hamartoma that can be solitary and sporadic or multiple and familial as a part of the basaloid follicular hamartoma syndrome, which is characterized by flesh-colored facial papules, hypotrichosis, hypohidrosis, and palmoplantar pitting

Subtypes

- Generalized (familial)
- Generalized (acquired)
- Linear type
- Plaque type
- Papular

Differential Diagnosis

- Angiofibromas of tuberous sclerosis
- Basal cell carcinoma (especially infundibulocystic type)
- Bazex–Dupre–Christol syndrome
- Birt–Hogg–Dube syndrome
- Cowden's disease
- Melanocytic nevi
- Multiple trichoepitheliomas
- Nevoid basal cell carcinoma syndrome
- Rombo syndrome

- Sebaceous hyperplasia
- Seborrheic keratoses
- Trichoepitheliomas

Associations

Generalized Acquired
- Cystic fibrosis
- Myasthenia gravis
- Systemic lupus erythematosus

Further reading:
- Lee PL, Lourduraj LT, Palko MJ III et al (2006) Hereditary basaloid follicular hamartoma syndrome. Cutis 78(1):42–46

Bazex–Dupre–Christol Syndrome

X-linked dominant disorder associated with multiple facial basal cell carcinomas, hypotrichosis, hypohidrosis, and follicular atrophoderma on the face, dorsal hands, and dorsal feet

Differential Diagnosis

- Anhidrotic ectodermal dysplasia
- Basaloid follicular hamartoma syndrome
- Familial trichoepitheliomas
- Nevoid basal cell carcinoma syndrome
- Nicolau–Balus syndrome
- Rombo syndrome

Further reading:
- Torrelo A, Sprecher E, Mediero IG, Bergman R et al (2006) What syndrome is this? Bazex–Dupre–Christol syndrome. Pediatr Dermatol 23(3):286–290

Becker's Nevus

Nevoid lesion possibly induced by androgens that most commonly affects males, has onset around puberty, and is characterized by a large unilateral, hyperpigmented patch with hypertrichosis and acne that is located on the chest (with the possible breast hypoplasia), shoulder, or upper arm

Differential Diagnosis

- Café-au-lait macule
- Congenital melanocytic nevus
- Epidermal nevus
- Localized hypertrichosis
- Melanoma
- Nevus of Ito
- Nevus spilus
- Postinflammatory hyperpigmentation
- Segmental lentiginosis

Associations

- Breast and limb hypoplasia
- Pigmented hairy epidermal nevus syndrome
- Renal cysts
- Spina bifida
- Supernumerary nipples

Treatment Options

- Ruby laser
- Nd:YAG laser

Further reading:
- Danarti R, Konig A, Salhi A et al (2004) Becker's nevus syndrome revisited. J Am Acad Dermatol 51(6):965–969

Beckwith–Wiedemann Syndrome

Sporadic syndrome associated with mutation of the p57 gene that is characterized by macrosomia, hemihypertrophy, neonatal hypoglycemia, facial port-wine stain, omphalocele, macroglossia, exophthalmos, and an increased risk of Wilms tumor

Differential Diagnosis

- Congenital hypothyroidism
- Down syndrome
- Mucopolysaccharidoses
- Proteus syndrome
- Sturge–Weber syndrome

Evaluation

- Blood glucose (low)
- Renal ultrasound to evaluate for Wilms tumor

Further reading:
- Millington GW (2006) Genomic imprinting and dermatological disease. Clin Exp Dermatol 31(5):681–688

Bed Bug Bites (Cimicosis)

Cutaneous reaction to the early morning bite of the insect, *Cimex lectularius*, that occurs anywhere on the skin surface and that is characterized by an itchy erythematous papule or nodule, often in groups of three, representing the classic "breakfast, lunch, and dinner" sign

Differential Diagnosis

- Acute urticaria
- Furuncle

- Mosquito bites
- Nodular scabies
- Papular urticaria

Treatment Options

- Topical corticosteroids
- Antihistamines
- Eradication from the living quarters
- Heat treatment
- Insecticide treatment

Further reading:
- Fallen RS, Gooderham M (2011) Bedbugs: an update on recognition and management. Skin Therapy Lett 16(6):5–7

Behçet's Disease

Systemic immune-mediated disease that most commonly affects patients of Mediterranean or Middle Eastern descent and is characterized by oral and genital ulcers, ocular inflammation, erythema nodosum-like skin lesions, and pathergy, among many other systemic and cutaneous manifestations

Differential Diagnosis

- Artifactual ulceration
- B12 deficiency
- Bowel-associated dermatosis–arthritis syndrome
- Erythema nodosum
- Erosive lichen planus
- Folliculitis
- Herpes simplex virus infection
- Inflammatory bowel disease

- Iron deficiency
- Lupus erythematosus
- MAGIC syndrome
- <u>Major aphthous ulcers (Sutton's disease)</u>
- Pemphigus vulgaris
- Pyridoxine deficiency
- Reactive arthritis
- Riboflavin deficiency
- SAPHO syndrome
- Sexually transmitted disease
- Stevens–Johnson syndrome
- Sweet's syndrome
- Thiamine deficiency
- Zinc deficiency

Diagnostic Criteria

- Required: aphthous oral ulceration observed by physician or patient recurring at least three times in a 12-month period
- Two or more of:
  - Aphthous genital ulceration or scarring
  - Anterior or posterior uveitis, cells in the vitreous by slit-lamp examination, or retinal vasculitis
  - Erythema-nodosum-like lesions, papulopustular lesions, or acneiform nodules while not on steroids
  - Positive pathergy test at 24–48 h

Evaluation

- Antinuclear antibodies
- Complete blood cell count
- Iron, B12, and folate levels
- Ophthalmologic exam
- Pathergy test
- Sedimentation rate

Treatment Options

- Topical corticosteroids
- Systemic corticosteroids
- Topical calcineurin inhibitors
- <u>Colchicine</u>
- <u>Dapsone</u>
- Methotrexate
- Azathioprine
- Cyclophosphamide
- Cyclosporine
- Plasmapheresis
- Intravenous immunoglobulin
- TNF inhibitors
- Thalidomide

Further reading:
- Alpsoy E, Donmez L, Onder M et al (2007) Clinical features and natural course of Behçet's disease in 661 cases: a multicentre study. Br J Dermatol 157(5):901–906

Bejel (Endemic Syphilis)

Treponemal infection caused by *Treponema pallidum* spp. *endemicum* that primarily affects children in impoverished areas of the world and is characterized by rare primary lesions and more common secondary mucous patches of the oral cavity and, if untreated, tertiary gummatous lesions of the mucosal areas, skin, and bone.

Differential Diagnosis

- Aphthous stomatitis
- Atopic dermatitis
- Condyloma acuminatum
- Dermatophytosis

- Herpes simplex virus infection
- Leprosy
- Lupus erythematosus
- Lupus vulgaris
- <u>Mucocutaneous leishmaniasis</u>
- Paracoccidioidomycosis
- Perleche
- Pinta
- Psoriasis
- Rhinoscleroma
- Squamous cell carcinoma
- <u>Tuberculosis</u>
- <u>Venereal syphilis</u>
- Vitamin deficiencies
- Yaws

Further reading:

- Antal GM, Lukehart SA, Meheus AZ (2002) The endemic treponematoses. Microbes Infect 4(1):83–94

Berloque Dermatitis (Freund Dermatitis)

Type of phototoxic reaction caused by the application of furocoumarin-containing perfume, such as oil of bergamot, to the skin that is characterized by erythema, vesiculation, and hyperpigmentation on the central chest, neck, and face

Differential Diagnosis

- Acanthosis nigricans
- Contact dermatitis
- Erythromelanosis follicularis faciei et colli
- Fixed drug eruption
- Melasma

- <u>Photosensitive drug eruption</u>
- Phytophotodermatitis
- <u>Postinflammatory hyperpigmentation</u>
- <u>Riehl's melanosis</u>
- Rhus dermatitis

Further reading:

- Wang L, Sterling B, Don P (2002) Berloque dermatitis induced by "Florida water". Cutis 70(1):29–30

Bier Spots (Physiologic Anemic Macules)

Benign skin finding affecting young adults that is characterized by hypopigmented macules on the arms and legs (Fig. 6.10)

Differential Diagnosis

- Cutis marmorata
- Idiopathic guttate hypomelanosis
- Livedo reticularis
- Nevus anemicus

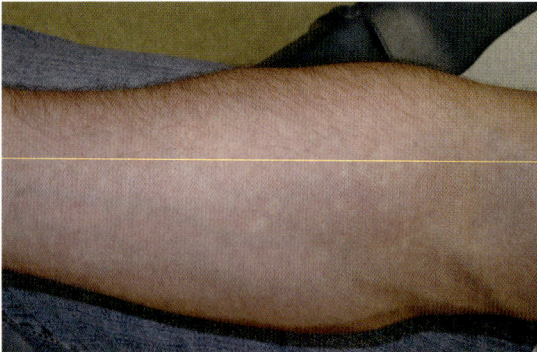

Fig. 6.10 Bier spots

- Postinflammatory hypopigmentation
- Tinea versicolor
- Vitiligo

Further reading:
- Fan YM, Yang YP, Li W et al (2009) Bier spots: six case reports. J Am Acad Dermatol 61(3):e11–e12

Biotin Deficiency

Uncommon vitamin deficiency that can be acquired or inherited and can be characterized by neonatal erythroderma, periorificial erosions, alopecia, conjunctivitis, organic aciduria, lethargy, and depression

Differential Diagnosis

- Acrodermatitis enteropathica
- Congenital syphilis
- Cystic fibrosis
- Epidermolysis bullosa, Dowling–Meara type
- Essential fatty acid deficiency
- Hartnup's disease
- Leiner's disease
- Neonatal erythrodermas
- Organic acidurias

Associations

- Avidin ingestion (raw egg white)
- Biotinidase deficiency (infantile type)
- Holocarboxylase deficiency (neonatal type)
- Malabsorption
- Parenteral nutrition
- Valproic acid therapy

Further reading:
- Arbuckle HA, Morelli J (2006) Holocarboxylase synthetase deficiency presenting as ichthyosis. Pediatr Dermatol 23(2):142–144

Birt–Hogg–Dube Syndrome

Autosomal-dominant syndrome associated with a defect in folliculin that is characterized by facial fibrofolliculomas and trichodiscomas, as well as a tendency to develop renal oncocytoma (an uncommon type of renal cell carcinoma) and pulmonary cysts, which may manifest as spontaneous pneumothorax

Differential Diagnosis

- Basaloid follicular hamartoma syndrome
- Brooke–Spiegler syndrome
- Cowden's disease
- Multiple trichoepitheliomas
- Rombo syndrome
- Tuberous sclerosis

Evaluation

- CT scan of chest, abdomen, and pelvis

Further reading:
- Welsch MJ, Krunic A, Medenica MM (2005) Birt–Hogg–Dube syndrome. Int J Dermatol 44(8):668–673

Black Hairy Tongue

Disorder affecting the tongue that is caused by inadequate mechanical desquamation of the filiform papillae and is characterized by a thickened surface of the dorsal tongue with dark discoloration

Differential Diagnosis

- Argyria
- Candidiasis
- Chrysiasis
- <u>Oral hairy leukoplakia</u>
- Oral lichen planus
- Melanoma
- <u>Stain/pigments</u>

Associations

- Antibiotics
- Coffee or tea consumption
- Oxidizing mouthwashes
- <u>Mouth breathing</u>
- Poor oral hygiene
- Radiation therapy
- Smoking

Treatment Options

- Tongue scraping
- <u>Topical retinoids</u>
- Nystatin

Further reading:
- Taybos G (2003) Oral changes associated with tobacco use. Am J Med Sci 326(4):179–182

Blastomycosis, North American (Gilchrist's Disease)

Type of respiratory mycosis that is caused by the broad-based bud-ding yeast *Blastomyces dermatitidis* and is characterized by a primary pulmonary infection with secondary dissemination to the bones,

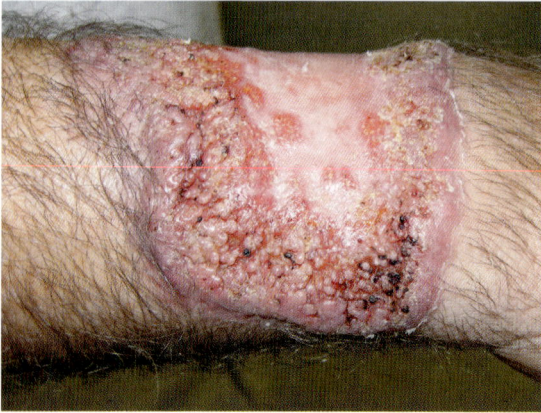

Fig. 6.11 Blastomycosis

genitourinary tract, and skin, giving rise to circumscribed verrucous, crusted, and purulent plaques anywhere on the skin surface (Fig. 6.11)

Differential Diagnosis

- Anthrax
- Atypical mycobacterial infection
- Blastomycosis-like pyoderma
- Cutaneous tuberculosis (especially tuberculosis verrucosa)
- Granuloma inguinale
- Halogenoderma
- Keratoacanthoma
- Leishmaniasis
- Nocardiosis
- Paracoccidioidomycosis
- Pemphigus vegetans
- Pyoderma gangrenosum, vegetative type
- Sarcoidosis
- Squamous cell carcinoma
- Tertiary syphilis
- Trichophytic granuloma

- Verrucae
- Verrucous carcinoma
- Verrucous mycosis fungoides

Evaluation

- Chest radiograph
- Tissue and blood cultures
- Potassium hydroxide wet mount of purulent material

Treatment Options

- <u>Itraconazole</u>
- Ketoconazole

Further reading:
- Lupi O, Tyring SK, McGinnis MR (2005) Tropical dermatology: fungal tropical diseases. J Am Acad Dermatol 53(6):931–951

Blastomycosis-Like Pyoderma

Type of pyoderma caused by several different bacteria including *Staphylococcus aureus* and *Pseudomonas aeruginosa* that is characterized by a large verrucous, crusted plaque studded with pustules

Differential Diagnosis

- Atypical mycobacterium infection
- <u>Blastomycosis</u>
- Botryomycosis
- Deep fungal infections
- Halogenoderma
- Keratoacanthoma
- Majocchi granuloma

- Pemphigus vegetans
- <u>Pyoderma gangrenosum, vegetative type</u>
- Squamous cell carcinoma
- Tuberculosis

Treatment Options

- Antistaphylococcal antibiotics
- Antipseudomonal antibiotics

Further reading:
- Sawalka SS, Phiske MM, Jerajani HR (2007) Blastomycosis-like pyoderma. Indian J Dermatol Venereol Leprol 73(2):117–119

Blau Syndrome

Autosomal-dominant disorder caused by mutation of the NOD2/CARD15 gene that is characterized by an early-onset sarcoidosis-like presentation with granulomatous papules and plaques, noncaseating granulomatous arthritis, uveitis, and camptodactyly without lung or other visceral involvement

Differential Diagnosis

- Crohn's disease
- Familial Mediterranean fever
- Granuloma annulare
- <u>Immunodeficiency-related cutaneous granulomas</u>
- Interstitial granulomatous dermatitis with arthritis
- Juvenile rheumatoid arthritis
- Muckle–Wells syndrome
- NOMID syndrome
- PAPA syndrome

- <u>Sarcoidosis</u>
- Tumor necrosis factor receptor-associated periodic fever syndrome

Further reading:
- Schaffer JV, Chandra P, Keegan BR et al (2007) Widespread granulomatous dermatitis of infancy: an early sign of Blau syndrome. Arch Dermatol 143(3):386–391

Blistering Distal Dactylitis

Streptococcal infection of the skin of the distal aspect of the digits that is characterized by a tender superficial blister

Differential Diagnosis

- Acute contact dermatitis
- <u>Acute paronychia</u>
- Bullous diabeticorum
- Bullous tinea
- Burn
- Epidermolysis bullosa
- Friction blister
- <u>Herpetic whitlow</u>
- Parakeratosis pustulosa
- Suction blister

Treatment Options

- <u>Incision and drainage</u>
- Topical antibiotics
- <u>Systemic antibiotics</u>

Further reading:
- Scheinfeld NS (2007) Is blistering distal dactylitis a variant of bullous impetigo? Clin Exp Dermatol 32(3):314–316

Bloom's Syndrome

Autosomal-recessive disorder caused by a defect in the DNA repair helicase, RECQL3 that is characterized by photosensitivity, photodistributed telangiectasias, café-au-lait macules, growth retardation, recurrent sinopulmonary infections, and tendency to development leukemia and lymphoma

Differential Diagnosis

- Ataxia–telangiectasia
- Childhood dermatomyositis
- Cockayne syndrome
- Erythropoietic protoporphyria
- Kindler syndrome
- Lupus erythematosus
- Rothmund–Thomson syndrome
- Trichothiodystrophy
- Xeroderma pigmentosum

Evaluation

- Antinuclear antibodies
- Chest radiograph
- Complete blood count

Further reading:
- Sahn EE, Hussey RH III, Christmann LM (1997) A case of Bloom syndrome with conjunctival telangiectasia. Pediatr Dermatol 14(2):120–124

Blue Nevus, Common and Cellular (Jadassohn–Tieche Nevus)

Benign neoplasm of dermal melanocytes that is characterized by a uniform blue to black-colored dome-shaped papule on the head and neck, dorsal hands, buttocks, or sacral area

Differential Diagnosis

- Angiokeratoma
- Apocrine hidrocystoma
- Argyria (acupuncture)
- Basal cell carcinoma (pigmented type)
- Dermatofibroma
- Glomus tumor
- Lentigo
- Melanocytic nevus
- Melanoma (including metastatic)
- Pigmented spindle cell nevus
- Sclerosing hemangioma
- Traumatic tattoo
- Venous lake

Associations

- Carney complex (epithelioid type)

Further reading:
- Bogart MM, Bivens MM, Patterson JW, Russell MA (2007) Blue nevi: a case report and review of the literature. Cutis 80(1):42–44

Blueberry Muffin Baby (Congenital Extramedullary Hematopoiesis)

Cutaneous manifestation of extramedullary hematopoiesis that affects newborns with a variety of underlying diseases and is characterized by small, purpuric macules predominantly on the head, neck, and trunk

Differential Diagnosis

- Blue rubber bleb nevus syndrome
- Congenital leukemia cutis

- Congenital self-healing reticulohistiocytosis
- Cutaneous metastatic neuroblastoma
- Neonatal hemangiomatosis

Associations

- ABO incompatibility
- Congenital rhabdomyosarcoma
- Congenital leukemia cutis
- Congenital rubella
- Congenital spherocytosis
- Coxsackie virus infection
- Cytomegalovirus infection
- Hemolytic disease of newborn
- Langerhans cell histiocytosis
- Parvovirus B19 infection
- TORCH infections
- Toxoplasmosis
- Twin–twin transfusion

Evaluation

- Abdominal ultrasound/CT scan
- Complete blood count
- Metaiodobenzylguanidine scan
- Skeletal survey
- TORCH infections serologic tests
- Urinary catecholamines

Further reading:
- Shaffer MP, Walling HW, Stone MS (2005) Langerhans cell histiocytosis presenting as blueberry muffin baby. J Am Acad Dermatol 53(2 Suppl 1):S143–S146

Blue Rubber Bleb Nevus Syndrome

Sporadic condition associated with numerous venous malformations of the skin and gastrointestinal tract that is characterized by blue, soft, compressible, cutaneous nodules with nocturnal pain and gastrointestinal hemorrhage if extensive mucosal lesions are present

Differential Diagnosis

- AV malformation
- Blueberry muffin baby
- Glomangiomas
- Kaposi's sarcoma
- Klippel–Trenaunay–Weber syndrome
- Maffucci syndrome
- Venous lakes

Evaluation

- Stool occult blood studies
- Complete blood count
- Endoscopy to identify gastrointestinal lesions

Further reading:
- Lu R, Krathen RA, Sanchez RL et al (2005) Multiple glomangiomas: potential for confusion with blue rubber bleb nevus syndrome. J Am Acad Dermatol 52(4):731–732

Borrelial Lymphocytoma

Term for type of cutaneous lymphoid hyperplasia that is seen in Europe, is caused by *Borrelia afzelii* or *Borrelia garinii*, and is characterized by a solitary violaceous nodule most commonly on the ear in children

Differential Diagnosis

- <u>Arthropod-bite reaction</u>
- <u>Foreign body granuloma (especially tick parts)</u>
- Granuloma annulare
- Granuloma faciale
- Granulomatous contact dermatitis
- Keloid
- Lupus erythematosus
- <u>Lymphoma cutis</u>
- Metastatic disease
- Perichondritis
- Polymorphous light eruption
- Sarcoidosis

Evaluation

- ELISA and Western blot for Lyme disease

Treatment Options

- Doxycycline
- Intralesional corticosteroids

Further reading:
- Mullegger RR (2004) Dermatological manifestations of Lyme borreliosis. Eur J Dermatol 14(5):296–309

Botryomycosis

Chronic bacterial infection affecting patients with neutrophil dysfunction that is caused most commonly by *Staphylococcus aureus* and is characterized by a crusted, purulent plaque or nodule with draining sinuses that contain granules

Differential Diagnosis

- <u>Actinomycosis</u>
- Atypical mycobacterial infections
- <u>Deep fungal infection</u>
- Kaposi's sarcoma
- Kerion
- Lymphoma
- <u>Mycetoma</u>
- Orf
- Ruptured epidermoid cyst
- Subcutaneous granuloma annulare
- Tuberculosis
- Tinea barbae

Evaluation

- Gram stain and culture of granules

Treatment Options

- Antistaphylococcal antibiotics

Further reading:
- Machado CR, Schubach AO, Conceicao-Silva F et al (2005) Botryomycosis. Dermatology 211(3):303–304

Bowel-Associated Dermatosis–Arthritis Syndrome

Complication of jejunoileal bypass surgery that is likely caused by immune complexes related to bacterial overgrowth in the blind loop of bowel and is characterized by pustular vasculitic skin lesions on the upper trunk and extensor extremities, along with episodic, migratory polyarthritis involving the digits

Differential Diagnosis

- Arthropod bites
- Behçet's disease
- Crohn's disease
- Cutaneous small vessel vasculitis
- Dermatitis herpetiformis
- Erythema multiforme
- Folliculitis
- Gonococcemia
- Henoch–Schonlein purpura
- PAPA syndrome
- Pyoderma gangrenosum
- Reiter's syndrome
- SAPHO syndrome
- Subacute bacterial endocarditis
- Sweet's syndrome
- Systemic candidiasis
- Urticarial vasculitis

Evaluation

- Antinuclear antibodies
- Complement levels
- Complete blood count
- Renal function test
- Rheumatoid factor
- Tissue and blood cultures
- Urinalysis

Treatment Options

- Surgical excision of blind loop
- Metronidazole
- Tetracyclines

- Clindamycin
- Systemic corticosteroids
- Dapsone
- Cyclosporine
- Azathioprine
- Mycophenolate mofetil

Further reading:

- Kawakami A, Saga K, Hida T et al (2006) Fulminant bowel-associated dermatosis–arthritis syndrome that clinically showed necrotizing fasciitis-like severe skin and systemic manifestations. J Eur Acad Dermatol Venereol 20(6):751–753

Bowen's Disease

Distinct type of squamous cell carcinoma in situ that affects older patients and is characterized by an circumscribed erythematous, scaly, superficial, slowly growing plaque on sun-exposed or, commonly, sun-protected areas (Fig. 6.12)

Differential Diagnosis

- Actinic keratosis
- Amelanotic melanoma
- Basal cell carcinoma, superficial type
- Epidermotropic metastasis

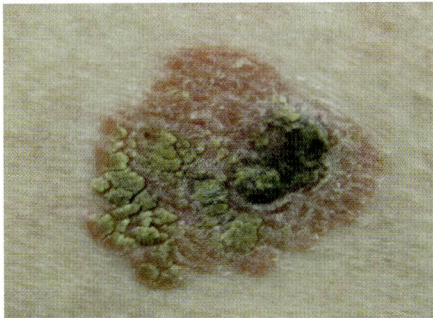

Fig. 6.12 Bowen's disease

- Extramammary Paget's disease
- Hidroacanthoma simplex
- Lichen planus
- Lichenoid keratosis
- Lupus erythematosus
- Nummular eczema
- Pagetoid reticulosis
- Psoriasis
- Seborrheic keratosis, clonal type
- Tinea corporis
- Viral warts

Treatment Options

- Electrodessication and curettage
- 5-FU cream
- Imiquimod cream
- Surgical excision

Further reading:
- Cox NH, Eedy DJ, Morton CA (2007) Therapy guidelines and Audit Subcommittee, British Association of Dermatologists. Guidelines for management of Bowen's disease: 2006 update. Br J Dermatol 156(1):11–21

Bowenoid Papulosis

Dysplastic epidermal disorder affecting the sexually active and induced by HPV subtypes 16 and 18 (among others) that is characterized by hyper-pigmented verrucous papules and plaques in the genital or perianal areas

Differential Diagnosis

- Condyloma acuminatum
- Extramammary Paget's disease

- Lichen planus
- Molluscum contagiosum
- Nevi
- Squamous cell carcinoma
- <u>Seborrheic keratoses</u>

Treatment Options

- <u>Cryosurgery</u>
- Electrodessication and curettage
- <u>Imiquimod</u>
- 5-FU cream
- Podophyllin
- Tazarotene cream

Further reading:

- Papadopoulos AJ, Schwartz RA, Lefkowitz A et al (2002) Extragenital bowenoid papulosis associated with atypical human papillomavirus genotypes. J Cutan Med Surg 6(2):117–121

Brachioradial Pruritus

Localized, neurogenic, pruritic disorder caused by cervical nerve compression and characterized by itching or burning of the brachioradial area which the patient will often attempt to soothe by placing an ice pack on the affected area (ice-pack sign)

Differential Diagnosis

- Acquired brachial cutaneous dyschromatosis
- <u>Asteatotic eczema</u>
- <u>Dermatitis herpetiformis</u>
- Lichen simplex chronicus
- Postherpetic neuralgia

- Tinea corporis
- Scabies

Evaluation

- CT scan of cervical spine

Treatment Options

- Capsaicin cream
- Doxepin cream
- Topical lidocaine cream or patch
- Topical corticosteroids
- Gabapentin
- Amitriptyline

Further reading:
- Barry R, Rogers S (2004) Brachioradial pruritus: an enigmatic entity. Clin Exp Dermatol 29(6):637–638

Branchial Cleft Cyst

Developmental anomaly caused by failure of closure of the second branchial cleft that is characterized by a solitary cyst or mass located most commonly on the lateral neck (Fig. 6.13)

Differential Diagnosis

- Carotid body tumor
- Cystic hygroma
- Ectopic salivary tissue
- Ectopic thyroid tissue
- Epidermal inclusion cyst
- Hemangioma

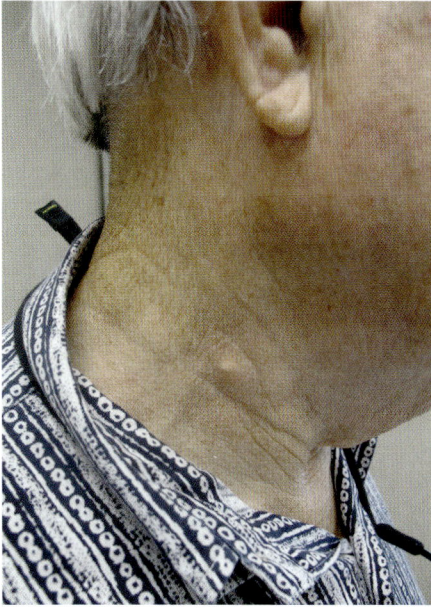

Fig. 6.13   Branchial cleft cyst

- Lymphadenopathy
- Pilomatricoma
- Vascular malformation

Associations

- Branchio-oto-renal syndrome

Evaluation

- Hearing test
- Renal ultrasound

Further reading:
- Acierno SP, Waldhausen JH (2007) Congenital cervical cysts, sinuses and fistulae. Otolaryngol Clin North Am 40(1):161–176

Bronchogenic Cyst

Developmental anomaly representing a remnant of the lung bud of the foregut that is characterized by a cutaneous cyst arising early in life and which is located in the midline superior to the sternal notch

Differential Diagnosis

- Branchial cleft cyst
- Epidermal inclusion cyst
- Lipoma
- Pilomatricoma
- Steatocystoma
- Thymic cyst
- Thyroglossal duct cyst

Further reading:
- Ustundag E, Iseri M, Keskin G et al (2005) Cervical bronchogenic cysts in head and neck region. J Laryngol Otol 119(6):419–423

Brown Recluse Spider Bite (Necrotic Arachnidism)

Injury caused by *Loxosceles reclusa* with a potential for a severe, toxin-mediated necrotic reaction that is characterized by a painless bite, followed by erythema and edema, and eventual necrosis, bullae, and severe pain over 48–72 h in some patients

Differential Diagnosis

- Aspergillosis
- Chancriform pyoderma
- Coumarin necrosis

- Ecthyma
- Erythema migrans
- Factitial ulceration
- Herpes simplex infection
- <u>Insect-bite reaction</u>
- Mucormycosis
- Necrotizing fasciitis
- <u>Pyoderma gangrenosum</u>
- Squamous cell carcinoma
- <u>Staphylococcal infection</u>
- Sweet's syndrome
- Thromboangiitis obliterans
- Thromboembolic event
- Tularemia
- Vasculitis

Treatment Options

- <u>Debridement and wound care</u>
- Elevation
- Immobilization
- Cool compresses
- Dapsone
- Colchicine
- <u>Systemic corticosteroids</u>
- Surgical excision
- Nitroglycerin
- Hyperbaric oxygen

Further reading:

- Dyachenko P, Ziv M, Rozenman D (2006) Epidemiological and clinical manifestations of patients hospitalized with brown recluse spider bite. J Eur Acad Dermatol Venereol 20(9):1121–1125

Brucellosis (Undulant Fever)

Zoonotic bacterial infection caused by the Gram-negative *Brucella* spp. that is acquired by contact with infected animals or by ingestion of unpasteurized milk and is characterized by fever, headache, malaise, and variable cutaneous findings, including erythema nodosum, vasculitis, or a violaceous papular eruption

Differential Diagnosis

- Endocarditis
- Henoch–Schonlein purpura
- Hodgkin's disease
- Influenza
- Listeriosis
- Malaria
- Meningococcemia
- Mononucleosis
- Sarcoidosis
- Salmonellosis
- Tuberculosis
- Tularemia
- Typhoid fever
- Typhus
- Vasculitis

Evaluation

- Anti-O polysaccharide antibodies
- Blood cultures
- Complete blood count

Further reading:
- Metin A, Akdeniz H, Buzgan T, Delice I (2001) Cutaneous findings encountered in brucellosis and review of the literature. Int J Dermatol 40(7):434–438

Fig. 6.14 Bullosis
diabeticorum

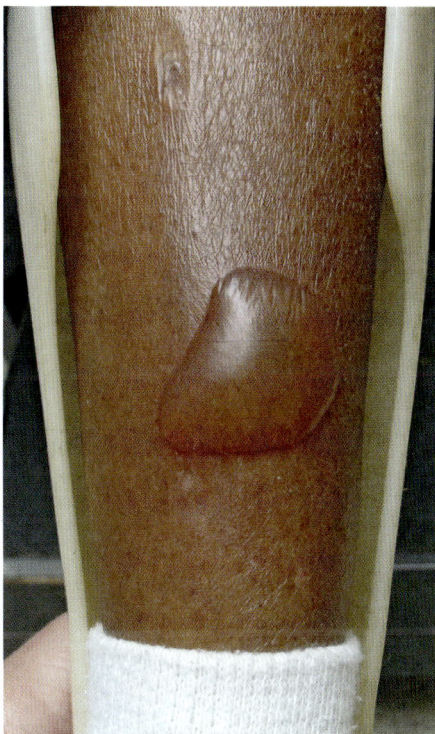

Bullosis Diabeticorum

Uncommon, noninflammatory bullae possibly related to trauma that
arises in patients with a long history of diabetes mellitus and is characterized by tense blisters arising on the distal extremities (Fig. 6.14)

Differential Diagnosis

- Blistering distal dactylitis
- Bullous cellulitis
- Bullous drug eruptions

- <u>Bullous pemphigoid (localized type)</u>
- Burn
- Epidermolysis bullosa acquisita
- <u>Edema bullae</u>
- Friction blister
- Pompholyx
- Porphyria cutanea tarda
- Pseudoporphyria

Evaluation

- Direct immunofluorescence

Treatment Options

- Observation and reassurance

Further reading:
- Aye M, Masson EA (2002) Dermatological care of the diabetic foot. Am J Clin Dermatol 3(7):463–474

Burning Mouth Syndrome (Burning Tongue Syndrome)

Neurocutaneous disorder without any identifiable underlying cause that predominantly affects postmenopausal women and is characterized by a burning sensation of the tongue, mouth, or lips

Differential Diagnosis

- <u>Allergic contact stomatitis</u>
- Atrophic glossitis
- <u>B12 deficiency</u>

- <u>Candidiasis</u>
- Diabetes
- Hypothyroidism
- Iron deficiency
- Leukemia
- Lichen planus
- Malignant lesion
- Medication reaction
- Menopause
- Poorly fitting dentures
- Sjögren's syndrome
- Tobacco abuse
- Uremia
- Xerostomia

Evaluation

- Iron, B12, and folate levels
- Culture for *Candida*
- Sialometry
- Patch testing

Treatment Options

- <u>Amitriptyline</u>
- <u>Gabapentin</u>
- Nystatin
- B vitamins
- <u>SSRIs</u>
- <u>Cognitive therapy</u>

Further reading:

- Savage NW, Boras VV, Barker K (2006) Burning mouth syndrome: clinical presentation, diagnosis and treatment. Australas J Dermatol 47(2):77–81

Buruli Ulcer

Type of tropical ulcer affecting young children in Africa that is caused by a mycolactone toxin released by *Mycobacterium ulcerans* and characterized by extensive and deep cutaneous necrotic ulceration most commonly affecting the extremities

Differential Diagnosis

- Cutaneous tuberculosis
- Deep fungal infection
- Foreign body granuloma
- Fungal infections
- Leishmaniasis
- Necrotizing fasciitis
- Panniculitis
- Pyoderma gangrenosum
- Squamous cell carcinoma
- Suppurative panniculitis
- Tropical phagedenic ulcer
- Vasculitis

Further reading:
- Wansbrough-Jones M, Phillips R (2006) Buruli ulcer: emerging from obscurity. Lancet 367(9525):1849–1858

Buschke–Ollendorf Syndrome

Autosomal-dominant disorder of elastic tissue possibly caused by a defect in the LEMD3 lamin-binding protein that is characterized by elastic tissue nevi most commonly localized to the back and buttocks (dermatofibrosis lenticularis disseminata) and osteopoikilosis

Differential Diagnosis

- <u>Connective tissue nevus</u>
- Eruptive collagenoma
- Familial cutaneous collagenoma
- Juvenile elastoma
- Mastocytosis
- Metastatic disease
- Morphea
- Papular elastorrhexis
- Pseudoxanthoma elasticum
- Tuberous sclerosis

Evaluation

- Radiographs of the hands, lumbosacral spine, tibia, and radius

Further reading:

- Assmann A, Mandt N, Geilen CC, Blume-Peytavi U (2001) Buschke-Ollendorff syndrome: differential diagnosis of disseminated connective tissue lesions. Eur J Dermatol 11(6):576–579

Café-au-Lait Macule

Circumscribed hypermelanotic lesion that is present at birth or develops in early childhood and is characterized by solitary or multiple uniformly hyperpigmented oval macules or patches

Differential Diagnosis

- Becker's nevus
- <u>Congenital melanocytic nevus</u>
- Freckles

- Melasma
- Nevus sebaceus
- Nevus spilus
- Phytophotodermatitis
- Postinflammatory hyperpigmentation
- Solar lentigo

Associations

- Ataxia–telangiectasia
- Bannayan–Riley–Ruvalcaba syndrome
- Bloom syndrome
- Cardiofaciocutaneous syndrome
- Cowden's disease
- Fanconi's anemia
- Gastrocutaneous syndrome
- LEOPARD syndrome
- Jaffe–Campanacci syndrome
- Johnson–McMillin syndrome
- Juvenile xanthogranulomas
- Legius syndrome
- McCune–Albright syndrome
- Multiple endocrine neoplasia 1
- Multiple endocrine neoplasia 2B
- Epidermal nevi
- Neurofibromatosis
- Noonan syndrome
- Piebaldism
- Silver–Russell syndrome
- Tay syndrome
- Tuberous sclerosis
- Watson syndrome

Further reading:

- Landau M, Krafchik BR (1999) The diagnostic value of café-au-lait macules. J Am Acad Dermatol 40(6 Pt 1):877–890

Calcinosis Cutis

Refers to cutaneous calcium deposition due to a variety of causes that is characterized by hard subcutaneous papules, nodules, or plaques with or without overlying ulceration and perforation of a white, chalky material

Subtypes/Variants

- Dystrophic
- Iatrogenic
- Idiopathic
- Metastatic

Differential Diagnosis

- Foreign body granuloma
- Gouty tophus
- Granuloma annulare
- Milium
- Molluscum contagiosum
- Osteoma cutis
- Rheumatoid nodule
- Xanthoma

Associations

Dystrophic
- Acne vulgaris
- Atypical fibroxanthomas
- Basal cell carcinomas
- Burns
- Chondroid syringomas
- CREST syndrome
- Cutaneous tumors
- Dermatomyositis

- Ehlers–Danlos syndrome
- Heel stick injury
- Infections
- Keloids
- Melanocytic nevi
- Panniculitis
- Parasitic infestation
- Pilar cysts
- Pilomatrixoma
- Porphyria cutanea tarda
- Pseudoxanthoma elasticum
- Pyogenic granuloma
- Rothmund–Thompson syndrome
- <u>Scleroderma</u>
- Seborrheic keratoses
- Surgical scars
- <u>Systemic lupus erythematosus</u>
- Trauma
- Trichoepitheliomas
- Werner syndrome

Iatrogenic

- Alginate dressing
- Electrode paste
- Extravasation of intravenous fluid containing calcium
- Liver transplantation
- Tumor lysis syndrome

Idiopathic

- Idiopathic scrotal calcinosis
- Milia-like calcinosis (Down syndrome)
- Subepidermal calcified nodule
- Tumoral calcinosis

Metastatic

- Benign nodular calcification
- Calciphylaxis
- <u>Chronic renal failure</u>
- Hyperparathyroidism
- Hypervitaminosis D
- Paraneoplastic hypercalcemia
- Sarcoidosis

Evaluation

- Serum calcium level (with albumin level)
- Serum phosphate level
- Renal function test
- Parathyroid hormone level
- Antinuclear antibodies
- Vitamin D level

Treatment Options

- Aluminum hydroxide
- <u>Diltiazem</u>
- Probenecid
- <u>Excision</u>
- Colchicine
- Intralesional corticosteroids
- Bisphosphonates
- Warfarin
- Parathyroidectomy

Further reading:

- Becuwe C, Roth B, Villedieu MH et al (2004) Milia-like idiopathic calcinosis cutis. Pediatr Dermatol 21(4):483–485

Fig. 6.15 Calciphylaxis
(Courtesy of M. Lambert)

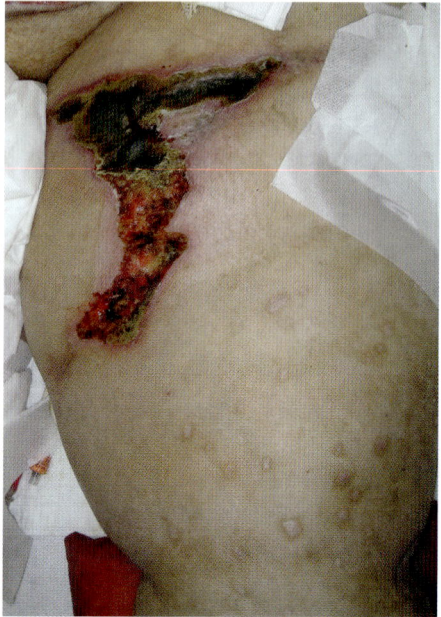

Calciphylaxis

Type of metastatic calcification associated with end-stage renal disease
that is caused by calcification of subcutaneous arterioles and characterized by hard, purpuric, painful subcutaneous plaques with overlying
necrosis and surrounding livedo reticularis which are most commonly
located on the lower extremities (Fig. 6.15)

Differential Diagnosis

- Antiphospholipid antibody syndrome
- Benign nodular calcification
- Cholesterol emboli

- Coumarin necrosis
- Cryofibrinogenemia
- Cryoglobulinemia
- Dermatomyositis
- Disseminated intravascular coagulation
- Lupus erythematosus
- Oxaluria
- Polyarteritis nodosa
- Pancreatic panniculitis
- Pyoderma gangrenosum
- Protein-C or protein-S deficiency
- Tumoral calcinosis
- Wegener's granulomatosis

Evaluation

- Serum calcium level (with albumin level)
- Serum phosphate level
- Renal function test
- Parathyroid hormone level

Treatment Options

- <u>Surgical debridement</u>
- <u>Sodium thiosulfite</u>
- Bisphosphonates
- Cinacalcet
- Hyperbaric oxygen
- Systemic corticosteroids
- Parathyroidectomy

Further reading:
- Guldbakke KK, Khachemoune A (2007) Calciphylaxis. Int J Dermatol 46(3):231–238

Calcifying Aponeurotic Fibroma

Benign proliferation of fibrous tissue with stippled calcifications on radiograph that predominantly affects children and is characterized by a slow-growing subcutaneous nodule or cyst-like lesion on the hand or foot

Differential Diagnosis

- Dupuytren's contracture
- Fibroma of the tendon sheath
- Giant cell tumor of the tendon sheath
- Gouty tophus
- Neuroma
- Plantar fibromatosis
- Rheumatoid nodule
- Sarcoma

Further reading:
- Parker WL, Beckenbaugh RR, Amrami KK (2006) Calcifying aponeurotic fibroma of the hand: radiologic differentiation from giant cell tumors of the tendon sheath. J Hand Surg [Am] 31(6):1024–1028

Candidiasis, Mucocutaneous

Mucocutaneous infection caused by various *Candida* spp. and characterized by confluent, bright-red erythematous plaques with pustules, white exudate, and/or satellite lesions affecting predominantly the warm, moist intertriginous areas

Subtypes/Variants

Cutaneous
- Balanitis
- Diaper dermatitis
- Disseminated/systemic

- Erosio interdigitalis blastomycetica
- Intertrigo
- Paronychia
- Vulvovaginitis

Oral

- Acute atrophic
- Acute pseudomembranous
- Angular cheilitis (perleche)
- Chronic atrophic
- Chronic hyperplastic
- Median rhomboid glossitis

Differential Diagnosis

Cutaneous

- Contact dermatitis
- Dermatophyte infection
- Hailey–Hailey disease
- Intertrigo
- Lichen planus
- Psoriasis
- Pseudomonal infection
- Seborrheic dermatitis
- Subcorneal pustular dermatosis

Oral

- Aphthous stomatitis
- Fordyce spots
- Hairy leukoplakia
- Herpes simplex virus infection
- Leukoplakia
- Lichen planus
- Pemphigus vulgaris
- White sponge nevus

Associations

- Acrodermatitis enteropathica
- Chediak–Higashi syndrome
- Chronic granulomatous disease
- <u>Chronic mucocutaneous candidiasis</u>
- Corticosteroids
- Cushing syndrome
- Diabetes mellitus
- DiGeorge syndrome
- Down syndrome
- Endocrinopathies
- HIV infection
- Hyper-IgE syndrome
- Nezelof syndrome
- Nutritional deficiency
- Severe combined immunodeficiency
- Thymoma

Treatment Options

- Anticandidal antifungals

Further reading:
- Aly R (2001) Producing experimental lesions of cutaneous candidiasis. Cutis 67(5 Suppl):24

Candidiasis, Chronic Mucocutaneous

Group of disorders associated with an inability to mount an effective immunologic response to *Candida* spp. and characterized by severe, recalcitrant candidal infections, including perleche, candida onychomycosis, and hyperkeratotic candidal granulomas

Subtypes/Variants

- APECED syndrome
- Familial
- Late onset
- Localized
- With keratitis
- With other immunodeficiency
- With other syndromes

Differential Diagnosis

- Acrodermatitis enteropathica
- DiGeorge syndrome
- Good syndrome
- HIV infection
- Nezelof syndrome
- Severe combined immunodeficiency
- Tuberculosis
- Twenty-nail dystrophy

Associations

- Acrodermatitis enteropathica
- Adrenal insufficiency
- Alopecia areata
- Autoimmune hepatitis
- Diabetes mellitus
- Ectodermal dysplasias
- Hyper-IgE syndrome
- Hypoparathyroidism
- Keratoconjunctivitis
- KID syndrome

- Iron deficiency
- Malabsorption
- Multiple carboxylase deficiency
- Myasthenia gravis
- Pernicious anemia
- Pulmonary fibrosis
- Thymoma
- Vitiligo

Treatment Options

- Anticandidal antifungals

Further reading:
- Collins SM, Dominguez M, Ilmarinen T et al (2006) Dermatological manifestations of autoimmune polyendocrinopathy–candidiasis–ectodermal dystrophy syndrome. Br J Dermatol 154(6):1088–1093

Capillary Leak Syndrome, Idiopathic (Clarkson's Disease)

Term for an idiopathic syndrome associated with recurrent episodes of shock due to leakage of plasma, generalized edema, hemoconcentration, and hypoalbuminemia, along with sclerosis, livedo, and purpura

Differential Diagnosis

- Hereditary angioedema
- Hypoalbuminemia
- Liver disease
- Medication reaction
- Nephrogenic fibrosing dermopathy
- Nephrotic syndrome
- Septic shock

- Systemic mastocytosis
- Toxic shock syndrome

Associations (Capillary Leak)

- Acitretin therapy
- Carbon monoxide poisoning
- GCSF therapy
- Gemcitabine therapy
- Hemophagocytic syndrome
- IL-2 therapy
- Interferon therapy
- Multiple myeloma/monoclonal gammopathy
- Postpartum state
- Pustular psoriasis
- Sezary syndrome

Evaluation

- Renal function
- Albumin level
- Urinalysis
- 24-h urine protein
- Liver function test
- Complete blood count
- Chest radiograph
- Echocardiogram
- Serum/urinary protein electrophoresis

Further reading:

- Dhir V, Arya V, Malav IC et al (2007) Idiopathic systemic capillary leak syndrome (SCLS): case report and systematic review of cases reported in the last 16 years. Intern Med 46(12):899–904
- Fardet L, Kerob D, Rybojad M et al (2004) Idiopathic systemic capillary leak syndrome: cutaneous involvement can be misleading. Dermatology 209(4):291–295

Carcinoid Syndrome (Thorson–Biorck Syndrome)

Syndrome associated with the presence of a bronchial carcinoid tumor or hepatic metastasis of a gastrointestinal tract carcinoid tumor that is characterized by episodic flushing of the head and neck, telangiectasias, pellagra-like skin changes, abdominal pain, diarrhea, wheezing, and valvular heart disease

Differential Diagnosis

- Anaphylaxis
- Angioedema
- Carcinoma telangiectaticum
- Islet cell tumors
- Mastocytosis
- Multiple endocrine neoplasia
- Pellagra
- Pheochromocytoma
- Renal cell carcinoma
- Urticaria
- VIPoma

Associations

- Bronchoconstriction
- Diarrhea
- Pruritus
- Rosacea
- Sclerodermatous skin changes
- Valvular heart disease

Evaluation

- CT scan of chest, abdomen, and pelvis
- Radiolabeled octreotide scintigraphy scan
- Urinary 5-HIAA

Treatment Options

- <u>Resection of causative tumor</u>
- <u>Octreotide</u>
- Chemotherapy

Further reading:

- Bell HK, Poston GJ, Vora J, Wilson NJ (2005) Cutaneous manifestations of the malignant carcinoid syndrome. Br J Dermatol 152(1):71–75

Cardiofaciocutaneous Syndrome

Genodermatosis of unknown cause that is characterized by heart defects, characteristic facial appearance, sparse woolly hair, café-au-lait macules, keratosis pilaris, and ichthyosis

Differential Diagnosis

- <u>Costello syndrome</u>
- Down syndrome
- LEOPARD syndrome
- <u>Noonan syndrome</u>
- Pallister–Killian syndrome
- Turner syndrome

Further reading:

- Nanda S, Rajpal M, Reddy BS (2004) Cardio-facio-cutaneous syndrome: report of a case with a review of the literature. Int J Dermatol 43(6):447–450

Carney Complex (NAME Syndrome, LAMB Syndrome)

Autosomal-dominantly inherited syndrome caused by a defect in the PRKAR1A gene that is characterized by lentiginosis, blue nevi, atrial and cutaneous myxomas, pigmented nodular adrenocortical disease, acromegaly, and various other tumors

Differential Diagnosis

- Inherited patterned lentiginosis
- LEOPARD syndrome
- McCune–Albright syndrome
- Multiple endocrine neoplasia
- Neurofibromatosis

Diagnostic Criteria (2/7)

- Cardiac myxomas
- Cutaneous myxomas
- Mammary myxoid fibromas
- Lentiginoses and blue nevi
- Pigmented nodular adrenocortical disease
- Testicular tumors
- Pituitary GH-secreting tumors

Evaluation

- Transesophageal echocardiography
- Testicular ultrasound
- CT/MRI scan of the brain, chest, abdomen, and pelvis
- Endocrine evaluation (thyroid, pituitary, adrenal)

Further reading:
- Hachisuka J, Ichikawa M, Moroi Y et al (2006) A case of Carney complex. Int J Dermatol 45(12):1406–1407

Carotenoderma

Inconsequential alteration in cutaneous color caused by excessive consumption of or decreased metabolism of carotene and characterized by yellow skin discoloration accentuated over the palms, soles, and nasolabial folds

Differential Diagnosis

- Addison's disease
- Hypopituitarism
- Hypothyroidism
- Jaundice
- Lycopenemia
- Palmar crease xanthoma
- Quinacrine therapy
- Riboflavinemia

Associations

- Amenorrhea
- Anorexia
- Diabetes
- Hypothyroidism
- Liver disease
- Vegetarian diet

Evaluation

- Serum beta-carotene level

Further reading:
- Tung EE, Drage LA, Ghosh AK (2006) Carotenoderma and hypercarotenemia: markers for disordered eating habits. J Eur Acad Dermatol Venereol 20(9):1147–1148

Casts, Hair

Refers to nit-like keratinous sheaths that arise in hyperkeratotic dermatoses of the scalp, encircle the hair shaft, and, unlike nits, are freely mobile along the hair shaft

Differential Diagnosis

- <u>Pediculosis capitis</u>
- Piedra
- Trichomycosis axillaris

Associations

- Multiple myeloma
- Pityriasis amiantacea
- Psoriasis
- <u>Seborrheic dermatitis</u>

Further reading:
- Miller JJ, Anderson BE, Ioffreda MD et al (2006) Hair casts and cutaneous spicules in multiple myeloma. Arch Dermatol 142(12):1665–1666

Cat-Scratch Disease (Debre Syndrome)

Infection with *Bartonella henselae* that usually affects children, is transmitted by cat scratch, and is characterized by an erythematosus papule or pustule at the scratch site with regional lymphadenopathy; oculoglandular syndrome of Parinaud refers to conjunctival inoculation with granulomatous conjunctivitis and preauricular lymphadenopathy

Differential Diagnosis

- Castleman's disease
- Drug reactions

- Leishmaniasis
- Lymphogranuloma venereum
- Lymphoma
- <u>Malignancy</u>
- *Mycobacterium marinum* infection
- Nocardiosis
- Plague
- Primary inoculation tuberculosis
- Sarcoidosis
- <u>Staphylococcal or streptococcal infection</u>
- Syphilis
- <u>Sporotrichosis</u>
- Tularemia
- Viral infections

Evaluation

- Lymph node biopsy
- Serologic test for *Bartonella* antibodies

Further reading:
- Mehmi M, Lim SP, Tan CY (2007) An unusual cutaneous presentation of cat-scratch disease. Clin Exp Dermatol 32(2):219–220

Cellulitis and Erysipelas

Types of acute bacterial infection involving the skin and subcutaneous layer (cellulitis) or the lymphatics (erysipelas) that are most commonly caused by *Streptococcus* or *Staphylococcus* and are characterized by pain, erythema, warmth, and swelling that is diffuse, poorly defined, and deep (cellulitis) or well circumscribed and superficial (erysipelas) and most typically localized to the lower extremity

Differential Diagnosis

- Angioedema
- <u>Arthropod-bite reaction</u>
- Dermatitis artefacta
- Calciphylaxis
- Carcinoma erysipelatoides
- Chemical burn
- Compartment syndrome
- Contact dermatitis
- <u>Deep venous thrombosis</u>
- <u>Eosinophilic cellulitis</u>
- Eosinophilic fasciitis
- Erysipelas melanomatosum
- Erysipeloid
- Erythema infectiosum
- Erythema migrans
- Erythema nodosum
- Extramammary Paget's disease
- Familial Mediterranean fever
- <u>Fixed drug eruption</u>
- Foreign body reaction
- Gas gangrene
- Hidradenitis suppurativa
- Infectious perichondritis
- Leukemia cutis
- <u>Lipodermatosclerosis</u>
- <u>Lymphedema</u>
- Lymphoma
- <u>Necrotizing fasciitis</u>
- Neutrophilic eccrine hidradenitis
- Nodular vasculitis
- Osteomyelitis
- Paget's disease
- Panniculitis
- Pyoderma gangrenosum (especially subcutaneous type)

- Pyomyositis
- Relapsing polychondritis
- Seal finger
- Secretan syndrome
- Septic arthritis
- Solid facial edema
- Stasis dermatitis
- Subcutaneous panniculitis-like T cell lymphoma
- Superficial thrombophlebitis
- Sweet's syndrome
- Urticaria
- Urticarial vasculitis
- Vasculitis
- Venous edema
- *Vibrio vulnificus* infection
- Zoster

Treatment Options

- Incision and drainage
- Systemic antibiotics
- Systemic corticosteroids

Further reading:

- Falagas ME, Vergidis PI (2005) Narrative review: diseases that masquerade as infectious cellulitis. Ann Intern Med 142(1):47–55
- Torok L (2004) Uncommon manifestations of erysipelas. Clin Dermatol 23(5):515–518

Central Centrifugal Cicatricial Alopecia

Type of scarring alopecia that predominantly affects women of African descent, is probably caused by repeated follicular injury due to a variety of mechanical and chemical stimuli, and is characterized by noninflammatory cicatricial alopecia that involved the central scalp

Differential Diagnosis

- Alopecia mucinosa
- Alopecia neoplastica
- Discoid lupus erythematosus
- Dissecting cellulitis of the scalp
- Folliculitis decalvans
- Lichen planopilaris
- Tinea capitis
- Traction alopecia
- Trichotillomania

Treatment Options

- Avoidance of chemicals and traction
- Topical corticosteroids
- Intralesional corticosteroids
- Tetracycline antibiotics
- Topical minoxidil
- Hair prosthesis

Further reading:

- Ross EK, Tan E, Shapiro J (2005) Update on primary cicatricial alopecias. J Am Acad Dermatol 53(1):1–37

Chalazion/Hordeolum

Inflammatory lesions of the eyelid that are caused by painless granulomatous inflammation of the meibomian glands (chalazion) or painful acute inflammation of the eyelash follicles (external hordeolum) or meibomian glands (internal hordeolum)

Differential Diagnosis

- Basal cell carcinoma
- Foreign body granuloma
- Hidrocystoma
- Leishmaniasis
- Merkel cell carcinoma
- Microcystic adnexal carcinoma
- Milia
- Molluscum contagiosum
- Mucocele
- Periorbital cellulitis
- Sarcoidosis
- Sebaceous neoplasm
- Tuberculosis

Associations

- Chronic blepharitis
- Diabetes
- Hyperlipidemia
- Rosacea

Treatment Options

- Warm compresses
- Incision and drainage
- Topical antibiotics
- Intralesional corticosteroids
- Ophthalmology referral

Further reading:
- Ozdal PC, Codere F, Callejo S et al (2004) Accuracy of the clinical diagnosis of chalazion. Eye 18(2):135–138

Chancriform Pyoderma

A solitary, chronic, necrotizing ulcer on the genitals, tongue, or face that is caused by common bacteria such as *Staphylococcus* or *Pseudomonas*

Differential Diagnosis

- Blastomycosis
- Cat-scratch disease
- Chancroid
- Dermatitis artefacta
- Ecthyma
- Granuloma inguinale
- Inoculation tuberculosis
- Leishmaniasis
- Lymphogranuloma venereum
- Milker's nodule
- Orf
- Pyoderma gangrenosum
- Sporotrichosis
- Syphilis
- Ulcerative basal cell carcinoma
- Ulcerative squamous cell carcinoma

Treatment Options

- Topical antibiotics
- Systemic antibiotics

Further reading:
- Celic D, Lipozencic J, Budimcic D et al (2010) Chancriform pyoderma: a forgotten disease. Skinmed 8(2):119–120

Chancroid (Ducrey Disease)

Sexually transmitted disease caused by *Haemophilus ducreyi* and characterized by a soft, painful ragged ulcer with a dirty base on the genitalia along with painful suppurative lymphadenopathy

Differential Diagnosis

- Behçet's disease
- Bubonic plaque
- Chancriform pyoderma
- Crohn's disease
- Donovanosis
- Fixed drug eruption
- Genital herpes
- Lymphogranuloma venereum
- Squamous cell carcinoma
- Primary syphilis
- Pyoderma gangrenosum
- Traumatic ulcer

Evaluation

- Gram stain of purulent exudate
- Viral culture
- Bacterial culture (with vancomycin-containing special media)
- HIV test
- Syphilis serologic tests
- PCR

Further reading:

- Sehgal VN, Srivastava G (2003) Chancroid: contemporary appraisal. Int J Dermatol 42(3):182–190

Chédiak–Higashi Syndrome

Autosomal-recessive disorder caused by a defect in the LYST lysosomal trafficking gene that is characterized by oculocutaneous albinism, recurrent pyogenic infections, platelet dysfunction, neurologic dysfunction, and an accelerated lymphoproliferative phase

Differential Diagnosis

- Chronic granulomatous disease
- Elejalde syndrome
- Griscelli syndrome
- Hermansky–Pudlak syndrome
- Leukemia
- Oculocutaneous albinism
- Piebaldism
- Pyoderma gangrenosum
- Waardenburg syndrome

Evaluation

- Complete blood cell count and smear
- Bone marrow biopsy and smear
- CT or MRI scan of the brain

Further reading:
- Maari CH, Eichenfield LF (2007) Congenital generalized hypomelanosis and immunodeficiency in a black child. Pediatr Dermatol 24(2):182–185

Cheilitis, Actinic

Type of cheilitis caused by chronic sun exposure that is characterized by a whitish, hyperkeratotic, fissured plaque on the lower lip that obscures the vermilion border and that can evolve to squamous cell carcinoma

Differential Diagnosis

- <u>Cheilitis exfoliativa</u>
- Cheilitis glandularis
- Contact dermatitis
- Lichen planus
- Lupus erythematosus
- Polymorphous light eruption
- Smoker's leukoplakia
- <u>Squamous cell carcinoma</u>

Treatment Options

- Cryosurgery
- Imiquimod cream
- Diclofenac gel
- 5-FU cream
- Vermilionectomy
- CO_2 laser
- TCA peel

Further reading:
- Markopoulos A, Albanidou-Farmaki E, Kayavis I (2004) Actinic cheilitis: clinical and pathologic characteristics in 65 cases. Oral Dis 10(4):212–216

Cheilitis/Stomatitis, Allergic Contact

Inflammation of the lips or oral cavity caused by delayed-type hypersensitivity to a variety of cosmetic preparations, foods, or dental products that is characterized by dryness, fissuring, crusting of the lips (cheilitis) or edema, erythema, erosions, lichen-planus-like changes, or ulcers in the oral cavity (stomatitis)

Differential Diagnosis

Cheilitis

- Actinic cheilitis
- Angular cheilitis
- Atopic dermatitis
- <u>Candidiasis</u>
- <u>Cheilitis exfoliativa</u>
- Cheilitis glandularis
- Lichen planus
- <u>Lip-licker dermatitis</u>
- Lupus erythematosus
- Pemphigus
- Perioral dermatitis
- Plasma cell cheilitis
- Retinoid cheilitis
- Stevens–Johnson syndrome
- Vitamin deficiency

Stomatitis

- Aphthous stomatitis
- Behçet's disease
- <u>Candidiasis</u>
- Chemotherapy-related stomatitis
- Drug reaction
- Erythema multiforme
- <u>Lichen planus</u>
- Pemphigus
- Pemphigoid
- Periorificial tuberculosis
- Stevens–Johnson syndrome
- Viral enanthem

Associations

- Acrylic monomers
- Bismuth
- Chewing gum
- Cosmetics
- Dentifrices
- Epoxy resins
- Food preservatives
- Hardeners
- Lip balms
- Lipsticks
- Mango
- Mercury
- Metals
- Nail polish
- Rubber
- Topical medications

Further reading:
- Torgerson RR, Davis MD, Bruce AJ et al (2007) Contact allergy in oral disease. J Am Acad Dermatol 57(2):315–321

Cheilitis, Angular (Perleche)

Type of intertrigo predominantly affecting the elderly that is caused by excessive moisture and occlusion of the labial commissures which leads to secondary infection with *Candida*, erythema, maceration, and fissuring

Differential Diagnosis

- Acquired zinc deficiency
- Allergic contact cheilitis

- Glucagonoma syndrome
- Iron deficiency
- Lip-licker dermatitis
- Rhagades
- Seborrheic dermatitis
- Split papule
- Vitamin deficiency

Associations

- Chronic mucocutaneous candidiasis
- Diabetes
- Down syndrome
- Sjögren's syndrome
- Vitamin deficiency
- Zinc deficiency

Treatment Options

- <u>Topical corticosteroids</u>
- <u>Nystatin cream</u>
- Mupirocin ointment
- Fluconazole
- Tacrolimus ointment

Further reading:

- Terai H, Shimahara M (2006) Cheilitis as a variation of *Candida* associated lesions. Oral Dis 12(3):349–352

Cheilitis Glandularis (Baelz Syndrome)

Inflammatory disorder of uncertain cause that affects the minor salivary glands of the lower lip and that is characterized by inflammation, swelling, eversion, and occasional clear or purulent discharge from the lower lip

Differential Diagnosis

- Actinic cheilitis
- Allergic cheilitis
- Angioedema
- Cheilitis granulomatosis
- Lip lickers
- Lymphedema
- Plasma cell cheilitis
- Sarcoidosis
- Smoker's lips
- Xerostomia

Treatment Options

- Topical corticosteroids
- Topical antibiotics
- Oral corticosteroids
- Tetracycline
- Intralesional corticosteroids
- 5-FU cream

Further reading:

- Carrington PR, Horn TD (2006) Cheilitis glandularis: a clinical marker for both malignancy and/or severe inflammatory disease of the oral cavity. J Am Acad Dermatol 54(2):336–337

Cheilitis Granulomatosa

Chronic inflammatory disorder affecting the lips that is caused by granulomatous infiltration, is characterized by swelling and induration of the upper lip (more commonly than the lower lip), and is associated with scrotal tongue and facial nerve palsy in the Melkersson–Rosenthal syndrome

Differential Diagnosis

- Angioedema
- Ascher syndrome
- Cheilitis glandularis
- Crohn's disease
- Dental abscess
- Insect-bite reaction
- Leprosy
- Lip trauma
- Sarcoidosis
- Sjögren's syndrome
- Wegener's granulomatosis

Treatment Options

- Intralesional corticosteroids
- Minocycline
- Methotrexate
- Dapsone
- Clofazimine
- Azathioprine
- Systemic corticosteroids

Further reading:
- Van der Waal RI, Schulten EA, van der Meij EH et al (2002) Cheilitis granulomatosa: overview of 13 patients with long-term follow-up: results of management. Int J Dermatol 41(4):225–229

Chemotherapy-Related Acral Erythema (Hand–Foot Syndrome, Palmoplantar Erythrodysesthesia)

Adverse effect of chemotherapy that is characterized by numbness and tingling of the palms and soles that evolves to painful, erythematous, and edematous confluent plaques which later blister and desquamate

Differential Diagnosis

- Contact dermatitis
- Dyshidrotic eczema
- Erythema multiforme
- Erythromelalgia
- Fixed drug eruption
- Graft-vs-host disease
- Lupus erythematosus
- Necrolytic acral erythema
- Palmoplantar hidradenitis
- Perniosis
- Polymorphous light eruption
- Sweet's syndrome

Associated Medications

- 5-FU
- Adriamycin
- Cytosine arabinoside
- Doxorubicin
- Etoposide
- Hydroxyurea
- Mercaptopurine
- Methotrexate
- Sorafenib
- Sunitinib

Treatment Options

- Pain control
- Reduction of dose of chemotherapy
- Substitution of chemotherapy
- Systemic corticosteroids

Further reading:
- Cetkovska P, Pizinger K, Cetkovsky P (2002) High-dose cytosine arabinoside-induced cutaneous reactions. J Eur Acad Dermatol Venereol 16(5):481–485

Cherry Angioma (Senile Angioma, Campbell de Morgan Spot)

Benign vascular proliferation affecting older patients that is characterized by solitary or multiple small, red dome-shaped papule(s) most commonly located on the trunk

Differential Diagnosis

- Angiokeratoma
- Angioma serpiginosum
- Bacillary angiomatosis
- Blue rubber bleb nevus
- Eruptive pseudoangiomatosis
- Glomeruloid hemangiomas
- Insect-bite reaction
- Intravascular lymphoma
- Kaposi's sarcoma
- Melanoma
- Petechiae
- Targetoid hemosiderotic hemangioma

Further reading:
- Motegi S, Tamura A, Takeuchi Y, Ishikawa O (2004) Senile angioma-like eruption: a skin manifestation of intravascular large B-cell lymphoma. Dermatology 209(2):135–137

Child Abuse

Various cutaneous disorders can be confused with child abuse

Differential Diagnosis

- <u>Accidental bruising</u>
- <u>Acute hemorrhagic edema of infancy</u>
- Crohn's disease
- Condyloma acuminatum
- Dermatitis artefacta
- Diaper dermatitis
- Epidermolysis bullosa
- <u>Ehlers–Danlos syndrome</u>
- Genital psoriasis
- Henoch–Schonlein purpura
- Immune thrombocytopenic purpura
- Jellyfish stings
- Kawasaki disease
- Lichen planus
- <u>Lichen sclerosus</u>
- Linear epidermal nevus
- Vulvar pemphigoid
- Millipede burn
- Molluscum contagiosum
- Mongolian spot
- Phytophotodermatitis
- Pinworm infestation
- Plant contact dermatitis
- Pityriasis lichenoides et varioliformis acuta
- Staphylococcal scalded-skin syndrome
- Streptococcal perianal dermatitis

Evaluation

- Skin biopsy
- Skeletal survey
- Platelet count
- PT/PTT

Further reading:
- Swerdlin A, Berkowitz C, Craft N (2007) Cutaneous signs of child abuse. J Am Acad Dermatol 57(3):371–392

CHILD Syndrome

X-linked dominant disorder caused by mutation of the NSDHL gene involved in cholesterol metabolism that is characterized by a large unilateral, inflammatory epidermal nevus involving nearly half of the body but sparing the face, ipsilateral limb defects, and ipsilateral internal organ hemidysplasia

Differential Diagnosis

- Congenital ichthyosiform erythroderma
- Conradi–Hunermann syndrome
- Epidermal nevus syndrome
- Harlequin color change
- Inflammatory linear verrucous epidermal nevus
- Nevus unius lateris
- Phacomatosis pigmentokeratotica
- Phacomatosis pigmentovascularis

Further reading:
- Kaminska-Winciorek G, Brzezinska-Wcislo L, Jezela-Stanek A et al (2007) CHILD syndrome: clinical picture and diagnostic procedures. J Eur Acad Dermatol Venereol 21(5):715–716

Chloracne

Occupational type of acne caused by exposure to chlorinated hydrocarbons that is characterized by small follicular papules, comedones, and cysts on the cheeks, retroauricular areas, neck, shoulders, and scrotum

Differential Diagnosis

- Acne cosmetica
- <u>Acne vulgaris</u>
- Dowling–Degos disease
- Favre–Racouchot syndrome
- Gram-negative folliculitis
- Pomade acne
- Radiation acne
- Steroid acne
- Tropical acne

Associations

- Porphyria cutanea tarda

Evaluation

- Serum dioxin level

Treatment Options

- Isotretinoin

Further reading:
- Passarini B, Infusino SD, Kasapi E (2010) Chloracne: still cause for concern. Dermatology 221(1):63–70

Cholesterol Emboli Syndrome

Systemic syndrome with cutaneous manifestations that results from embolization of cholesterol crystals from an atherosclerotic plaque as a complication of intra-arterial instrumentation that is characterized by livedo reticularis, purpura, gangrene, and cyanosis

Differential Diagnosis

- <u>Antiphospholipid antibody syndrome</u>
- Arteriosclerosis obliterans
- Atrial myxoma
- Buerger disease
- <u>Coumadin necrosis</u>
- Cryoglobulinemia
- <u>Heparin necrosis</u>
- Oxalate embolus
- Polyarteritis nodosa
- Polycythemia vera
- Raynaud phenomenon
- Septic emboli
- Subacute bacterial endocarditis
- Vasculitis
- Waldenstrom's macroglobulinemia
- Wegener's granulomatosis

Evaluation

- Urinalysis
- Renal function
- Complete blood count
- Biopsy of affected organs
- Transesophageal echocardiography

Treatment Options

- Statins
- Discontinue warfarin if causative
- Heparin
- Pentoxifylline
- Iloprost

- Systemic corticosteroids
- <u>Vasodilators such as nifedipine</u>

Further reading:
- Jucgla A, Moreso F, Muniesa C et al (2006) Cholesterol embolism: still an unrecognized entity with a high mortality rate. J Am Acad Dermatol 55(5):786–793

Chondrodermatitis Nodularis Helicis (Winkler Disease)

Painful disorder affecting the helix (men) or antihelix (women) that is possibly caused by a combination of actinic damage and pressure-related trauma and is characterized by a tender, erythematous papule or nodule with central ulceration or crust

Differential Diagnosis

- Acanthoma fissuratum
- <u>Actinic keratosis</u>
- Atypical fibroxanthoma
- Basal cell carcinomas
- Calcinosis cutis
- Colloid milium
- Cutaneous horn
- Darwinian tubercle
- Elastotic nodule
- Gouty tophi
- Granuloma annulare
- Keloid
- Keratoacanthomas
- Reactive perforating collagenosis
- <u>Squamous cell carcinoma</u>
- Verrucae
- Weathering nodule

Treatment Options

- Topical corticosteroids
- Intralesional corticosteroids
- <u>Shave excision</u>
- <u>Punch excision</u>
- Wedge excision
- Cryotherapy

Further reading:
- Magro CM, Frambach GE, Crowson AN (2005) Chondrodermatitis nodularis helicis as a marker of internal disease [corrected] associated with microvascular injury. J Cutan Pathol 32(5):329–333

Chromoblastomycosis

Chronic deep fungal infection predominantly located on the lower extremities that is caused by traumatic inoculation of a dematiaceous fungus of the *Phialophora*, *Fonsecaea*, *Cladosporium*, or *Rhinocladiella* genera and is characterized by a slow-growing verrucous, sclerotic, or keloid-like plaque or plaques with associated lymphedema (Fig. 6.16)

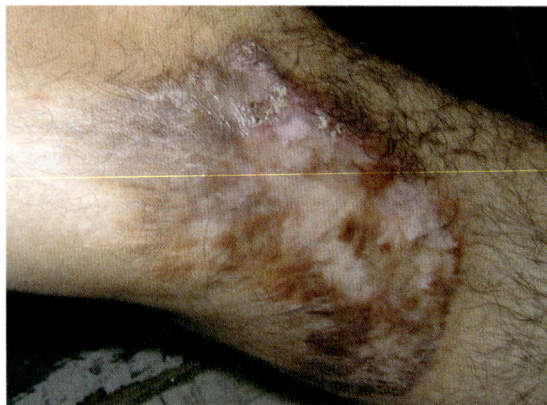

Fig. 6.16 Chromo-blastomycosis (Courtesy of S. Klinger)

Differential Diagnosis

- Atypical mycobacterial infection
- Blastomycosis
- Cutaneous tuberculosis
- Elephantiasis
- <u>Filariasis</u>
- Leishmaniasis
- Leprosy
- <u>Lobomycosis</u>
- <u>Mycetoma</u>
- Nocardiosis
- Paracoccidioidomycosis
- <u>Podoconiosis</u>
- Squamous cell carcinoma
- Sporotrichosis
- Tertiary syphilis
- Verrucous carcinoma
- Yaws

Evaluation

- KOH examination of lesional tissue
- Fungal cultures

Treatment Options

- <u>Itraconazole</u>
- Terbinafine
- <u>Surgical excision</u>
- Local heat therapy
- Cryotherapy

Further reading:
- Lopez Martinez R, Mendez Tovar LJ (2007) Chromoblastomycosis. Clin Dermatol 25(2):188–194

Chronic Actinic Dermatitis (Actinic Reticuloid)

Idiopathic photosensitivity disorder that affects elderly men and is characterized by chronic, thickened, often hypopigmented, eczematous plaques on the sun-exposed areas. Actinic reticuloid is a severe subtype that is characterized by a Sezary-syndrome-like eruption with marked cutaneous infiltration, lymphoma-like histology, and leonine facies

Differential Diagnosis

- Actinic prurigo
- Airborne contact dermatitis
- Atopic dermatitis
- Contact dermatitis
- Cutaneous T cell lymphoma
- Pellagra
- Photosensitive drug eruption
- Photoallergic contact dermatitis
- Lupus erythematosus
- Polymorphous light eruption
- Solar urticaria

Diagnostic Criteria

- Persistent eczematous eruption of infiltrated papules and plaques that predominantly affected exposed skin although sometimes extended to covered areas
- Biopsy consistent with chronic eczema with or without lymphoma-like changes
- Reduction in the minimal erythema dose test to ultraviolet B (UVB) irradiation and often also longer wavelengths

Evaluation

- Phototesting
- Patch testing

Treatment Options

- <u>Sun avoidance measures</u>
- Topical corticosteroids
- <u>Systemic corticosteroids</u>
- <u>Azathioprine</u>
- Cyclosporine
- Hydroxychloroquine
- Mycophenolate mofetil
- Phototherapy

Further reading:

- Hawk JL (2004) Chronic actinic dermatitis. Photodermatol Photoimmunol Photomed 20(6):312–314
- Lim HW et al (1994) Chronic actinic dermatitis: an analysis of 51 patients evaluated in the United States and Japan. Arch Dermatol 130:1284

Chronic Granulomatous Disease (Quie Syndrome)

Inherited (XLR or AR) immunodeficiency syndrome that is caused by a mutation in one of several genes (gp91phox, most commonly) involved in the NADPH oxidase system that is responsible for killing catalase positive organisms and is characterized by recurrent skin and respiratory infections, osteomyelitis, eczema, and granulomatous skin lesions

Differential Diagnosis

- Bruton agammaglobulinemia
- Candidiasis, Chronic mucocutaneous
- Chediak–Higashi syndrome
- Common variable immunodeficiency
- HIV infection
- Hyperimmunoglobulinemia E syndrome
- Hypogammaglobulinemia
- Job syndrome
- Leukocyte adhesion deficiency
- Myeloperoxidase deficiency
- Sarcoidosis
- Seborrheic dermatitis
- Severe combined immunodeficiency
- Wiskott–Aldrich syndrome
- Tuberculosis

Associations

- *Aspergillus* infection
- Chronic cutaneous lupus-like lesions (adult female carriers)
- *Serratia* osteomyelitis
- Staphylococcal infection

Evaluation

- Complete blood count
- Nitroblue tetrazolium assay
- Immunoglobulin levels
- Chest radiograph

Further reading:

- Luis-Montoya P, Saez-de Ocariz Mdel M, Vega-Memije ME (2005) Chronic granulomatous disease: two members of a single family with different dermatologic manifestations. Skinmed 4(5):320–322

Chrysiasis

Hyperpigmentation associated with gold therapy that is characterized by blue-gray pigmentation of the sun-exposed areas

Differential Diagnosis

- Addison's disease
- Amiodarone photosensitivity
- Argyria
- Arsenicism
- Chlorpromazine photosensitivity
- Diffuse melanosis of metastatic melanoma
- Drug-induced pigmentation
- Hemochromatosis
- Hemosiderosis
- Jaundice
- Minocycline hyperpigmentation

Further reading:
- Geist DE, Phillips TJ (2006) Development of chrysiasis after Q-switched ruby laser treatment of solar lentigines. J Am Acad Dermatol 55(2 Suppl):S59–S60

Churg–Strauss Syndrome

Systemic vasculitis syndrome that is possibly allergic in etiology and that is characterized by asthma, tissue and circulating eosinophilia, and p-ANCA(+) vasculitis, which presents with palpable purpura and inflammatory cutaneous papules and nodules and a variety of systemic features

Differential Diagnosis

- Allergic bronchopulmonary aspergillosis
- Asthma

- Atopic dermatitis
- Henoch–Schonlein purpura
- Hypereosinophilic syndrome
- Hypersensitivity pneumonitis
- Lupus erythematosus
- Loeffler syndrome
- Lymphoma
- Lymphomatoid granulomatosis
- Microscopic polyangiitis
- Polyarteritis nodosa
- Rheumatoid arthritis
- Sarcoidosis
- Urticaria
- Wegener granulomatosis

Diagnostic Criteria (ACR; 4/6)

- Asthma
- Eosinophilia (>10%)
- Neuropathy
- Pulmonary infiltrates (nonfixed)
- Sinusitis
- Extravascular eosinophils on biopsy

Evaluation

- Antinuclear antibodies
- c-ANCA and p-ANCA test
- Chest radiograph
- Complement levels
- Complete blood count
- Renal function test

- Rheumatoid factor
- Urinalysis

Treatment Options

- <u>Systemic corticosteroids</u>
- Cyclophosphamide
- Methotrexate
- Azathioprine
- Mycophenolate mofetil
- Infliximab
- Chlorambucil
- Plasma exchange

Further reading:
- Fiorentino DF (2003) Cutaneous vasculitis. J Am Acad Dermatol 48(3):311–340

Ciliated Cyst

Ciliated type of cutaneous cyst with possible Müllerian origin that predominantly affects women and that is characterized by a solitary cutaneous cyst of the vulva, perineum, or lower extremity

Differential Diagnosis

- <u>Bartholin's gland cyst</u>
- <u>Endometriosis</u>
- <u>Epidermal inclusion cyst</u>
- Mature cystic teratoma

Further reading:
- Chong SJ, Kim SY, Kim HS et al (2007) Cutaneous ciliated cyst in a 16-year-old girl. J Am Acad Dermatol 56(1):159–160

Clavus/Callus

Focal hyperkeratosis and thickening of friction-prone or pressure-prone surfaces that are plaque-like (callus) or inverted cone-like (clavus) and most commonly located on the foot

Differential Diagnosis

- Arsenical keratosis
- Crab yaws
- Ectopic nail
- <u>Focal palmoplantar keratoderma</u>
- Gout
- Keratosis punctata
- Lichen planus
- Lichen simplex chronicus
- Melanocytic nevus
- Neuroma
- Nodular amyloidosis
- Porokeratosis plantaris
- Poroma
- Syphilitic clavus
- <u>Wart</u>

Associations

- Bulimia (Russell's sign – knuckles)
- Diabetes
- Focal and punctate hereditary palmoplantar keratodermas
- Hereditary painful callosities
- <u>Ill-fitting shoes</u>
- Kneeling
- <u>Manual labor</u>
- Obesity

- Peripheral neuropathy
- Sucking (newborns)
- Weight lifting

Further reading:
- Pavicic T, Korting HC (2006) Xerosis and callus formation as a key to the diabetic foot syndrome: dermatologic view of the problem and its management. J Dtsch Dermatol Ges 4(11):935–941

Clear Cell Acanthoma (Degos Acanthoma)

Benign epidermal neoplasm arising in middle-aged adults that is characterized by an erythematous, moist nodule with a peripheral collarette most commonly located on the lower extremity

Differential Diagnosis

- Amelanotic melanoma
- Basal cell carcinoma
- Dermatofibroma
- Hidroacanthoma simplex
- Inflamed seborrheic keratosis
- Lichenoid keratosis
- Poroma
- Psoriasis
- Pyogenic granuloma
- Squamous cell carcinoma
- Traumatized hemangioma
- Wart

Associations

- Ichthyosis
- Psoriasis

Further reading:
- Zedek DC, Langel DJ, White WL (2007) Clear-cell acanthoma versus acanthosis: a psoriasiform reaction pattern lacking tricholemmal differentiation. Am J Dermatopathol 29(4):378–384

Clear Cell Sarcoma (Melanoma of the Soft Parts)

Type of malignant tumor of uncertain relationship to melanoma that arises in the soft tissue of young adults, especially on the lower extremity, and that is characterized by a painful subcutaneous tumor which is fixed to tendons and fascia

Differential Diagnosis

- Clear cell myomelanocytic tumor
- Clear cell squamous cell carcinoma
- Dermatofibroma
- Dermatofibrosarcoma
- Epithelioid sarcoma
- Lipoma
- Myxoid liposarcoma
- Neurothekeoma
- Malignant fibrous histiocytoma
- Malignant peripheral nerve sheath tumor
- Malignant schwannoma
- Metastatic melanoma
- Myxoma
- Synovial sarcoma

Further reading:
- Malchau SS, Hayden J, Hornicek F, Mankin HJ (2007) Clear cell sarcoma of soft tissues. J Surg Oncol 95(6):519–522

Cobb Syndrome

Sporadic congenital syndrome characterized by spinal arteriovenous malformations or angiomas along with overlying or closely located cutaneous port-wine stains, angiomas, or other vascular lesions

Differential Diagnosis

- Angiokeratoma circumscriptum
- Infantile hemangioma
- Klippel–Trenaunay syndrome
- Nevus flammeus
- Sturge–Weber syndrome
- Wyburn–Mason syndrome

Evaluation

- MRI scan of the spine

Further reading:
- Clinton TS, Cooke LM, Graham BS (2003) Cobb syndrome associated with a verrucous (angiokeratomalike) vascular malformation. Cutis 71(4):283–287

Cocaine-Associated (Levamisole-Induced) Vasculopathy (Vasculitis)

Vasculopathic disease induced by levamisole, an additive to cocaine, that is characterized by retiform purpura (characteristically on the helices as well as generalized), skin necrosis, arthralgias, leukopenia, antiphospholipid antibodies, and antineutrophil cytoplasmic antibodies (Fig. 6.17)

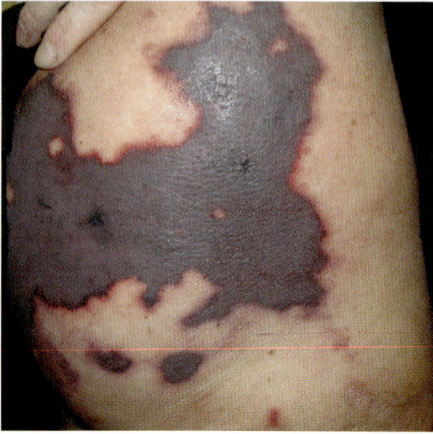

Fig. 6.17 Cocaine-related vasculitis

Differential Diagnosis

- <u>Antiphospholipid antibody syndrome</u>
- Cryoglobulinemia
- Disseminated intravascular coagulation
- <u>Idiopathic ANCA + vasculitis</u>
- Polyarteritis nodosa
- <u>Systemic lupus erythematosus</u>
- Wegener's granulomatosis

Evaluation

- Urine drug screen
- Complete blood cell count
- Cryoglobulins
- Anticardiolipin antibodies
- Beta 2 glycoprotein 1 antibodies
- Lupus anticoagulant
- Antinuclear antibodies
- PT/PTT

- Antineutrophil cytoplasmic antibodies
- Rheumatoid factor

Treatment Options

- <u>Discontinuation of cocaine use</u>
- <u>Wound debridement</u>
- <u>Systemic corticosteroids</u>
- Colchicine
- NSAIDs
- Anticoagulation

Further reading:

- Mouzakis J, Somboonwit C, Lakshmi S et al (2011) Levamisole induced necrosis of the skin and neutropenia following intranasal cocaine use: a newly recognized syndrome. J Drugs Dermatol 10(10):1204–1207

Coccidioidomycosis

Respiratory fungal infection associated with cutaneous dissemination that is caused by the dimorphic *Coccidioides immitis* and characterized by cutaneous abscesses, nodules, and verrucous lesions, predominantly on the face

Differential Diagnosis

- Actinomycosis
- Aspergillosis
- Basal cell carcinoma
- Behçet disease
- <u>Blastomycosis</u>
- Chromoblastomycosis
- Erysipelas
- Granuloma faciale
- Herpes simplex

- <u>Histoplasmosis</u>
- Kaposi's sarcoma
- Leishmaniasis
- Leprosy
- Lichen planus
- Lichen sclerosus et atrophicus
- Lichen simplex chronicus
- Lupus miliaris disseminatus faciei
- Lyme disease
- Malignant melanoma
- Metastatic carcinoma of the skin
- Morphea
- Mycosis fungoides
- Nocardiosis
- Parapsoriasis
- Pityriasis lichenoides
- Rosacea
- Sarcoidosis
- Sporotrichosis
- Syphilis
- Tinea faciei
- <u>Tuberculosis</u>
- Vasculitis
- Wegener's granulomatosis

Associations

- Erythema multiforme
- Erythema nodosum

Evaluation

- ELISA followed by IgG complement-fixing antibody test
- Fungal culture (notify lab)
- Chest radiograph

Further reading:
* Dicaudo DJ (2006) Coccidioidomycosis: a review and update. J Am Acad Dermatol 55(6):929–942

Cockayne's Syndrome

Autosomal-recessive disorder caused by a defect in the DNA repair genes ERCC6 and ERCC8 that is characterized by cachectic dwarfism, bird-like facies, photodistributed erythema and telangiectasia, sensorineural deafness, "salt and pepper" retinitis pigmentosum, severe mental retardation, and intracranial calcifications

Differential Diagnosis

* <u>Ataxia–telangiectasia</u>
* <u>Bloom's syndrome</u>
* Kindler syndrome
* Hartnup syndrome
* Progeria
* <u>Rothmund–Thomson syndrome</u>
* Trichothiodystrophy
* Werner's syndrome
* Xeroderma pigmentosum

Further reading:
* Kraemer KH, Patronas NJ, Schiffmann R et al (2007) Xeroderma pigmentosum, trichothiodystrophy and Cockayne syndrome: a complex genotype–phenotype relationship. Neuroscience 145(4):1388–1396

Cold Panniculitis (Haxthausen Disease)

Physical type of panniculitis induced by cold exposure that predominantly affects children and is characterized by indistinct erythematous to violaceous, firm nodules on the exposed area, which is commonly the face in children and lateral thighs or arms in women

Differential Diagnosis

- Atopic dermatitis
- <u>Cellulitis</u>
- Chilblains
- Erythema infectiosum
- Morphea
- <u>Post-steroid panniculitis</u>
- Scleredema
- Sclerema neonatorum
- Sclerosing lipogranuloma
- Subcutaneous fat necrosis of the newborn

Further reading:

- Quesada-Cortés A, Campos-Muñoz L, Díaz-Díaz RM, Casado-Jiménez M (2008) Cold panniculitis. Dermatol Clin 26(4):485–489, vii

Collagenoma

Type of connective tissue nevus that is associated with an increased amount of collagen and that is characterized by solitary or multiple, flesh-colored plaques on the trunk, especially the lower back

Subtypes/Variants

- Eruptive collagenoma
- Familial cutaneous collagenoma
- Shagreen patch of tuberous sclerosis
- Solitary collagenoma

Differential Diagnosis

- Becker's nevus
- Cutis verticis gyrata

- Elastofibroma
- Elastoma
- Morphea
- Papular elastorrhexis
- Scar
- Smooth muscle hamartoma

Associations

- Down syndrome
- Ehlers–Danlos syndrome
- Tuberous sclerosis

Further reading:
- Ryder HF, Antaya RJ (2005) Nevus anelasticus, papular elastorrhexis, and eruptive collagenoma: clinically similar entities with focal absence of elastic fibers in childhood. Pediatr Dermatol 22(2):153–157

Colloid Milium (Wagner's Disease)

Deposition disease that is characterized by waxy papules and plaques on the sun-exposed areas that represent accumulations of colloid material as an acquired response in adults (most commonly to chronic sun exposure) or as an inherited phenomenon in children

Differential Diagnosis

- Erythropoietic protoporphyria
- Epidermal cyst
- Favre–Racouchot syndrome
- Lipoid proteinosis
- Nodular amyloidosis
- Papular mucinosis
- Porphyria cutanea tarda

- Sarcoidosis
- Sebaceous hyperplasia
- Trichoepithelioma
- Tuberous sclerosis
- Xanthoma

Associations

- Ligneous conjunctivitis (juvenile type)
- Ligneous periodontitis (juvenile type)
- Ultraviolet light

Further reading:
- Pourrabbani S, Marra DE, Iwasaki J et al (2007) Colloid milium: a review and update. J Drugs Dermatol 6(3):293–296

Coma Bullae

Uncommon, subepidermal bullous lesions of uncertain cause that are seen most often in the setting of drug-induced coma (but also coma unrelated to drugs) and are characterized by tense bullae located at sites of pressure

Differential Diagnosis

- Bullous impetigo
- Burn
- Contact dermatitis
- Epidermolysis bullosa acquisita
- Friction blisters
- Herpes simplex virus infection
- Insect bites
- Localized bullous pemphigoid
- Multiple fixed drug eruption
- Porphyria cutanea tarda

Further reading:

- Kakurai M, Umemoto N, Yokokura H et al (2006) Unusual clinical features of coma blister mimicking contact dermatitis in rhabdomyolysis: report of a case. J Eur Acad Dermatol Venereol 20(6):761–763

Common Variable Immunodeficiency

Type of acquired immunodeficiency that is characterized by a paucity of antibody-producing B lymphocytes and a decreased cellular immune response and that manifests as recurrent infections, autoimmunity, granulomatous skin lesions, and a tendency to develop lymphoproliferative malignancy

Differential Diagnosis

- Bruton's agammaglobulinemia
- Chronic mucocutaneous candidiasis
- <u>Chronic granulomatous disease</u>
- Hyper-IgM syndrome
- HIV infection
- Lymphoma
- Thymoma
- Sarcoidosis
- Severe combined immunodeficiency

Associations

- Alopecia areata
- Atopic dermatitis
- Polymorphous light eruption

Evaluation

- Immunoglobulin level
- T cell panel

- Antinuclear antibodies
- Complete blood count
- Skin tests to evaluate T cell function (candida, trichophyton, etc.)
- CT scan of chest, abdomen, and pelvis (if lymphoma is suspected)
- T and B cell marker studies

Further reading:
- Mitra A, Pollock B, Gooi J et al (2005) Cutaneous granulomas associated with primary immunodeficiency disorders. Br J Dermatol 153(1):194–199

Condylomata Acuminata (Genital Warts)

Sexually transmitted human papillomavirus infection characterized by verrucous papules occasionally coalescent into large cauliflower-like plaques on the penis, vulva, and perianal area

Differential Diagnosis

- Acantholytic dyskeratosis of the vulva
- Amyloid deposits
- Angiokeratoma
- Bowenoid papulosis
- Condylomata lata
- Epidermoid cysts
- Fordyce spots
- Granular cell tumor
- Granuloma annulare
- Lichen nitidus
- Lichen planus
- Lymphangioma
- Molluscum contagiosum
- Pearly penile papules
- Pseudoverrucous papules/nodules
- Raspberry-like papillomas (Goltz syndrome)
- Reiter syndrome

- Rhinosporidiosis
- Schistosomiasis
- Sebaceous hyperplasia
- <u>Seborrheic keratoses</u>
- Squamous cell carcinoma
- Syringomas
- Verruciform xanthoma
- <u>Verrucous carcinoma</u>

Evaluation

- HIV test

Treatment Options

- <u>Cryotherapy</u>
- <u>Imiquimod cream</u>
- <u>Topical sinecatechins ointment</u>
- <u>Podophyllin gel</u>
- Electrodessication and curettage
- Surgical excision
- CO_2 laser
- TCA chemical peels
- Cidofovir

Further reading:
- Brodell LA, Mercurio MG, Brodell RT (2007) The diagnosis and treatment of human papillomavirus-mediated genital lesions. Cutis 79(4 Suppl):5–10

Confluent and Reticulated Papillomatosis (of Gougerot and Carteaud)

Acquired keratinization disorder of uncertain cause that is possibility related to acanthosis nigricans and is characterized by hyperkeratotic and hyperpigmented, papillomatous skin changes in a reticulated pattern on the chest or back (Fig. 6.18)

Fig. 6.18 Confluent and reticulated papillomatosis (Courtesy of K. Guidry)

Differential Diagnosis

- <u>Acanthosis nigricans</u>
- Darier's disease
- Dermatopathia pigmentosa reticularis
- Dyschromatosis universalis
- Dyskeratosis congenita
- Epidermodysplasia verruciformis
- Eruptive syringomas
- Lichen amyloidosis
- Macular amyloidosis
- Naegeli–Franceschetti–Jadassohn syndrome
- Parapsoriasis
- Pityriasis rubra pilaris
- Prurigo pigmentosa
- Pseudoacanthosis nigricans
- Pseudoatrophoderma colli
- Seborrheic dermatitis
- <u>Terra firma–forme dermatosis</u>
- <u>Tinea versicolor</u>
- Verruca plana

Diagnostic Criteria

- Scaling brown macules and patches, at least part of which appear reticulated and papillomatous.
- Involvement of the upper trunk and neck.
- Fungal staining of scales is negative for fungus.
- No response to antifungal treatment.
- Excellent response to minocycline.

Treatment Options

- <u>Minocycline</u>
- Keratolytic moisturizers
- Tazarotene cream
- Topical vitamin D analogues
- Isotretinoin
- Selenium sulfide
- Oral ketoconazole
- Topical ketoconazole

Further reading:

- Davis MD, Weenig RH, Camilleri MJ (2006) Confluent and reticulate papillomatosis (Gougerot–Carteaud syndrome): a minocycline-responsive dermatosis without evidence for yeast in pathogenesis. A study of 39 patients and a proposal of diagnostic criteria. Br J Dermatol 154(2):287–293

Congenital Ichthyosiform Erythroderma, Bullous (Epidermolytic Hyperkeratosis)

Inherited (AD) disorder of keratinization that is caused by defects in the genes for keratin 1 or 10 and that is characterized by neonatal-onset erythroderma and bullae that improves during childhood; later in childhood, chronic, unremitting hyperkeratotic plaques with a ridged or cobblestone appearance develop, along with palmoplantar keratoderma in some patients (K1 deficient only)

Differential Diagnosis

- Bullous impetigo
- CHILD syndrome
- Congenital erosive and vesicular dermatosis
- Conradi–Hünermann–Happle syndrome
- <u>Epidermolysis bullosa</u>
- Erythrokeratodermia variabilis
- IBIDS (trichothiodystrophy)
- Ichthyosis bullosa of Siemens
- Ichthyosis hystrix, Curth–Macklin
- Incontinentia pigmenti
- KID syndrome
- Lamellar ichthyosis
- Omenn's syndrome
- Netherton syndrome
- Neutral lipid storage disease
- Peeling skin syndrome
- Sjögren–Larsson syndrome
- Staphylococcal scalded-skin syndrome
- Toxic epidermal necrolysis
- X-linked Ichthyosis

Further reading:

- Lacz NL, Schwartz RA, Kihiczak G (2005) Epidermolytic hyperkeratosis: a keratin 1 or 10 mutational event. Int J Dermatol 44(1):1–6

Congenital Ichthyosiform Erythroderma, Nonbullous

Inherited (AR) disorder of keratinization that is caused most commonly by a defect in the transglutaminase 1 gene and is characterized by a collodion baby presentation at birth, neonatal erythroderma, and chronic generalized scaling involving the face, with alopecia and ectropion common complications

Differential Diagnosis

- Atopic dermatitis
- Collodion baby
- IBIDS
- Ichthyosis vulgaris
- <u>Lamellar ichthyosis</u>
- Leiner's disease
- Omenn's syndrome
- Netherton syndrome
- Neutral lipid storage disease
- Seborrheic dermatitis
- Staphylococcal scalded-skin syndrome

Further reading:

- Akiyama M, Sawamura D, Shimizu H (2003) The clinical spectrum of nonbullous congenital ichthyosiform erythroderma and lamellar ichthyosis. Clin Exp Dermatol 28(3):235–240

Congenital Self-Healing Reticulohistiocytosis (Hashimoto–Pritzker Disease)

Self-limited type of Langerhans' cell histiocytosis that is present at birth, involutes in the first 6 months, and is characterized by solitary or multiple reddish-brown papules or nodules with occasional ulceration on any part of the body

Differential Diagnosis

- <u>Benign cephalic histiocytosis</u>
- Blueberry muffin baby
- Congenital candidiasis
- Congenital leukemia
- Congenital syphilis

- Diffuse neonatal hemangiomatosis
- Erythema toxicum neonatorum
- Herpes simplex virus infection
- Juvenile xanthogranuloma
- Langerhans cell histiocytosis (other types)
- Lymphoma
- Mastocytosis
- Neonatal listeriosis
- Neonatal varicella
- Transient neonatal pustular melanosis

Further reading:

- Kapur P, Erickson C, Rakheja D et al (2007) Congenital self-healing reticulohistiocytosis (Hashimoto–Pritzker disease): ten-year experience at Dallas Children's Medical Center. J Am Acad Dermatol 56(2):290–294

Connective Tissue Nevus

Abnormal collection of connective tissue occurring solitarily or as part of a syndrome that is characterized by localized collections of excessive collagen, elastic tissue, or ground substance that manifest as firm, flesh-colored dermal papules or nodules most often located on the lower back

Subtypes/Variants

- Dermatofibrosis lenticularis disseminata
- Eruptive collagenomas
- Familial cutaneous collagenoma
- Nevus elasticus
- Nevus mucinosis
- Papular elastorrhexis
- Plantar cerebriform collagenoma
- Shagreen patch

- Solitary collagenoma
- Solitary elastoma

Differential Diagnosis

- Dermatofibroma
- Dermatomyofibroma
- Elastofibroma
- Keloid
- Knuckle pads
- Morphea
- Papular mucinosis
- Scar
- Sclerotic fibroma

Associations

- Buschke–Ollendorf syndrome (dermatofibrosis lenticularis)
- Cardiac disease (familial collagenomas)
- Down syndrome
- Hunter syndrome (nevus mucinosis)
- Multiple endocrine neoplasia
- Tuberous sclerosis (shagreen patch)

Further reading:
- Foo CC, Kumarasinghe SP (2005) Juvenile elastoma: A forme fruste of the Buschke–OllendOrff syndrome? Australas J Dermatol 46(4):250–252

Contact Dermatitis

Type of dermatitis caused by exposure to one of countless environmental allergens or irritants and characterized by eczematous changes of varying degrees of severity that are localized to the areas to which the contactant was applied (Fig. 6.19)

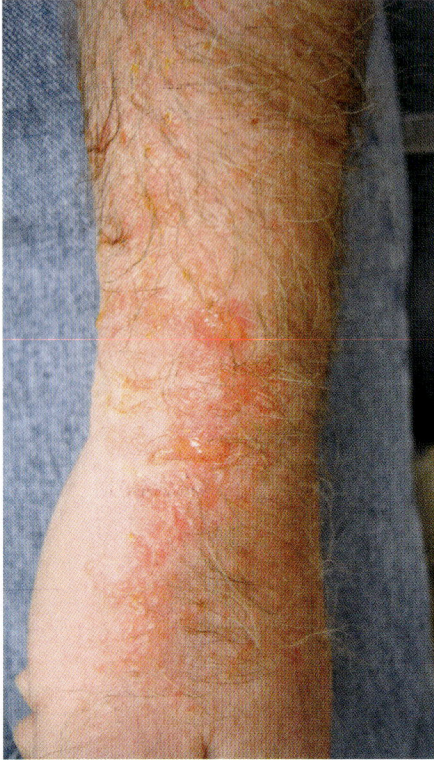

Fig. 6.19 Poison ivy dermatitis

Subtypes/Variants

- Airborne
- Allergic
- Dermal
- Erythema multiforme-like
- Follicular
- Granulomatous
- Ichthyosiform
- Irritant
- Leukodermic

- Lichenoid
- Lymphomatoid
- Photoallergic
- Phototoxic
- Phytophotodermatitis
- Protein
- Purpuric
- Pustular
- Systemic

Differential Diagnosis

Airborne
- Atopic dermatitis
- Chronic actinic dermatitis
- <u>Photoallergic contact dermatitis</u>
- Photoallergic drug eruption
- Seborrheic dermatitis

Allergic and Irritant
- <u>Asteatotic eczema</u>
- <u>Atopic dermatitis</u>
- Autoeczematization
- Autoimmune progesterone dermatitis
- Berloque dermatitis
- Contact urticaria
- Cutaneous T cell lymphoma
- Dermatomyositis
- Dermatophytosis
- Dyshidrotic eczema
- Erythema multiforme
- Folliculitis
- Grover's disease
- Id reaction

- Intertrigo
- Lichen nitidus
- Lichen simplex chronicus
- <u>Nummular eczema</u>
- Perioral dermatitis
- Phytophotodermatitis
- Pigmented purpuric dermatosis
- Prurigo nodularis
- Seborrheic dermatitis
- Stasis dermatitis
- Urticarial dermatitis

Phytophotodermatitis (Fig. 6.20)

- <u>Allergic contact dermatitis</u>
- Bleomycin pigmentation
- Burn
- Child abuse
- Jellyfish sting
- Mushroom dermatitis
- Porphyria cutanea tarda

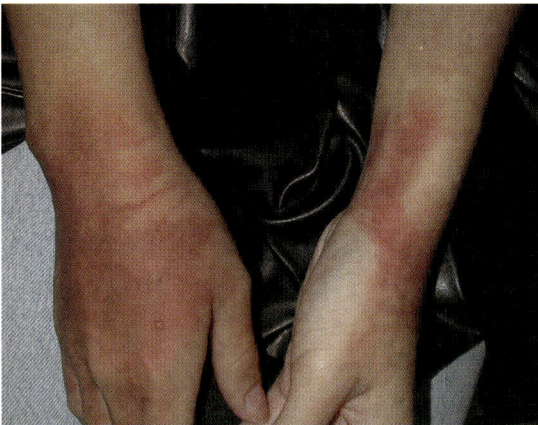

Fig. 6.20 Phytophotodermatitis (Courtesy of K. Guidry)

- Pseudoporphyria
- <u>Rhus dermatitis</u>
- Thrombophlebitis

Associations

Airborne

- Chromates
- Epoxy resin
- Sesquiterpene lactone
- Spray paint

Allergic Contact Dermatitis

Scalp, Face, and Eyelids

- Contact lens solution
- Cosmetics
- Dental products
- Elastic headbands
- Eyebrow pencils
- Eyedrops
- Eyeglass frames
- Eyelash curlers
- Fingernail polish
- Foods
- Fragrances
- Glaucoma medications
- Goggles
- Hair dye
- Hats
- Lipstick
- Makeup
- Masks
- Nasal sprays
- Permanent wave solutions

- Pillow material
- Rubber makeup applicators
- Shampoo
- Shaving products
- Spices
- Topical medications

Ears and Neck

- Cosmetics
- Ear drops
- Eyeglass frames
- Fragrance
- Hair care products
- Hearing aids
- Jewelry
- Nail polish
- Pillow material
- Shampoo
- Shaving products
- Telephone
- Topical medications

Trunk and Axilla

- Cobalt
- Clothing dyes
- Deodorants and antiperspirants
- Detergents
- Fabric softeners
- Formaldehyde and formaldehyde releasers
- Fragrances
- Perfumes
- Preservatives in lotion
- Nickel fasteners
- Resins
- Rubber accelerators

Hands

- Acrylic monomers
- Alcohol
- Antibacterials soap
- Bacitracin
- Balsam of Peru
- Benzalkonium chloride
- Benzocaine
- Chromates
- Colophony
- Copper
- Essential oils
- Formalin
- Fragrance
- Fruits
- Gloves
- Glutaraldehyde
- Gold
- Latex
- Local anesthetics
- Neomycin
- Nickel
- Paraphenylenediamine
- Plants and flowers
- Resins
- Rubber accelerators
- Vegetables

Extremities

- Adhesives
- Chromates
- Clothing dyes
- Neomycin
- Nickel

- Preservatives
- Rhus
- Rubber accelerators
- Topical medications

Feet

- Chromates
- Diisocyanates
- Dyes
- Formaldehyde
- Paraphenylenediamine
- P-tert-butylphenol formaldehyde resin
- Rubber accelerators
- Shoe padding
- Tar
- Topical medications

Generalized

- Balsam of Peru
- Quaternium-15
- Formaldehyde
- Fragrance mix
- Methyldibromoglutaronitrile
- Propylene glycol
- Diazolidinyl urea
- Imidazolidinyl urea
- Bronopol
- Tixocortol pivalate
- DMDM hydantoin
- Cocamidopropyl betaine
- Ethylene urea melamine formaldehyde
- Amidoamine
- Budesonide

Lichenoid

- Amalgam
- Aminoglycoside antibiotics
- Gold
- Musk ambrette
- Nickel
- Paraphenylenediamine

Lymphomatoid

- Cobalt
- Ethylenediamine
- Gold
- Nickel
- Paraphenylenediamine
- Phosphorus

Photoallergic

- 6-Methylcoumarin
- Benzophenones
- Chlorhexidine
- Cinnamates
- Dibenzoylmethanes
- Musk ambrette
- Oil of sandalwood
- Para-amino benzoic acid
- Sunscreen
- Triclosan

Phytophotodermatitis

- Agrimony
- Angelica
- Buttercup

- Celery
- Common rice
- Cowslip
- Dill
- Fennel
- Fig
- Grapefruit
- Lichens
- Lime/lemon
- Mango
- Meadow grass
- Mokihana berry
- Mustard
- Oak moss
- Oil of bergamot
- Orange
- Parsley
- Parsnips
- St. John's wort
- Wild carrot

Purpuric

- Benzoyl peroxide
- Cobalt
- Disperse dyes
- Eutectic mixture of lidocaine and prilocaine
- Methylmethacrylate
- Paraphenylenediamine
- Rubber

Systemic

- Nickel
- Cobalt
- Chromate
- Sesquiterpene lactones

- Thimerosal
- Aminophylline
- Preservatives

Treatment Options

- Avoidance of causative allergen
- Topical corticosteroids
- Systemic corticosteroids
- Tacrolimus ointment
- Cyclosporine
- Azathioprine
- Mycophenolate mofetil
- Methotrexate

Further reading:

- Rietschel RL (2004) Clues to an accurate diagnosis of contact dermatitis. Dermatol Ther 17(3):224–230
- [No authors listed] (2009) Adults with generalized dermatitis: what are the common causes? J Drugs Dermatol 8(1):80–81

Cowden Disease (Multiple Hamartoma Syndrome)

Autosomal-dominant syndrome of variable age of onset that is caused by a mutation in the *PTEN* tumor suppressor gene and that is characterized by trichilemmomas, oral papules with a cobblestone appearance, hyperkeratotic papules in the acral areas, and benign and malignant neoplasms arising in the thyroid, breast, and gastrointestinal tract

Differential Diagnosis

- Acanthosis nigricans, malignancy associated
- Angiofibromas
- <u>Bannayan–Riley–Ruvalcaba syndrome</u>
- Basaloid follicular hamartoma syndrome

- <u>Birt–Hogg–Dube syndrome</u>
- Darier's disease
- Epidermodysplasia verruciformis
- Fibrofolliculoma
- Fibrous papule
- Focal epithelial hyperplasia
- Goltz syndrome
- Lipoid proteinosis
- Multiple endocrine neoplasia (especially type IIB)
- Muir–Torre syndrome
- Multiple trichoepitheliomas
- Neurofibromatosis
- Nevoid basal cell carcinoma syndrome
- Oral florid papillomatosis
- Proteus syndrome
- Seborrheic keratoses
- Steatocystoma multiplex
- Syringomas
- Tuberous sclerosis
- Verruca

Diagnostic Criteria (Simplified; Need Two Major with One Out of Macrocephaly or LDD or One Major and Three Minor Criteria or Four Minor Criteria)

- Major criteria
  - Breast cancer
  - Thyroid cancer (follicular type)
  - Macrocephaly
  - Lhermitte–Duclos disease
  - Endometrial carcinoma
- Minor criteria
  - Thyroid goiter or adenoma
  - Mental retardation
  - Gastrointestinal hamartomas

- Fibrocystic disease of the breast
- Lipomas
- Sclerotic fibromas
- Uterine fibroids, renal cell carcinoma, or urinary tract malformation
- ≥6 facial papules (≥3 must be trichilemmomas) *or* cutaneous facial papules and mucosal papillomatosis *or* mucosal papillomatosis and acral keratoses *or* ≥6 palmoplantar keratoses

Evaluation

- Thyroid ultrasound
- Mammography
- CT/MRI scan of the brain
- Pelvic exam
- Endometrial biopsy

Further reading:
- Kovich O, Cohen D (2004) Cowden's syndrome. Dermatol Online J 10(3):3
- Eng C (2000) Will the real Cowden syndrome please stand up: revised diagnostic criteria. J Med Genet 37(11):828–830

CREST Syndrome (Limited Systemic Sclerosis, Thibierge–Weissenbach Syndrome)

Limited form of systemic sclerosis associated with anticentromere antibodies, calcinosis cutis, Raynaud's phenomenon, esophageal dysmotility, sclerodactyly, mat-like telangiectasias, and pulmonary hypertension

Differential Diagnosis

- Carcinoid syndrome
- Dermatomyositis
- Diabetic cheiroarthropathy

- <u>Diffuse systemic sclerosis</u>
- Eosinophilia–myalgia syndrome
- Eosinophilic fasciitis
- Generalized essential telangiectasia
- Hereditary hemorrhagic telangiectasia
- <u>Mixed connective tissue disease</u>
- Raynaud's disease
- Spider angiomas
- Thromboangiitis obliterans
- Unilateral nevoid telangiectasia
- Werner syndrome

Associations

- Primary biliary cirrhosis (Reynolds syndrome)

Evaluation

- Anticentromere antibodies
- Antimitochondrial antibodies
- Antinuclear antibodies
- Anti-Scl 70 antibodies
- Barium swallow
- Echocardiography
- Liver function test
- Pulmonary function test
- Renal function test

Treatment Options

- <u>Nifedipine</u>
- Diltiazem
- <u>ACE inhibitors</u>

- Alprostadil
- Bosentan
- Systemic corticosteroids
- Methotrexate
- Penicillamine
- Fluoxetine
- Sildenafil
- Cilostazol
- Proton pump inhibitors
- H2 blockers
- Topical nitroglycerine
- Pulsed dye laser

Further reading:

- Chung L, Lin J, Furst DE, Fiorentino D (2006) Systemic and localized scleroderma. Clin Dermatol 24(5):374–392

Crohn's Disease, Cutaneous

Cutaneous involvement in Crohn's disease that most often occurs as a result of direct extension of inflammation to the skin or mucous membranes but can occur distally (metastatic Crohn's disease) and is characterized by a variable clinical presentation, including genital swelling, erythematous papules, nodules, or plaques with or without ulceration, cobblestone appearance of the oral cavity, and pyostomatitis vegetans

Differential Diagnosis

- Actinomycosis
- Behçet's disease
- Cheilitis granulomatosis
- Deep fungal infections
- Panniculitis

- Foreign body reactions
- Granuloma inguinale
- <u>Hidradenitis suppurativa</u>
- Lupus vulgaris
- Lymphogranuloma venereum
- <u>Mycobacterial infections</u>
- Pyoderma gangrenosum
- <u>Sarcoidosis</u>
- Tuberculosis
- Wegener's granulomatosis

Evaluation

- Colonoscopy
- Barium swallow with small bowel follow-through
- Anti-*Saccharomyces cerevisiae* antibodies

Treatment Options

- <u>Metronidazole</u>
- Topical corticosteroids
- Intralesional corticosteroids
- <u>Infliximab</u>
- Adalimumab
- Systemic corticosteroids
- Methotrexate
- Tacrolimus ointment
- Sulfasalazine
- 6MP
- Azathioprine

Further reading:

- Eames T, Landthaler M, Karrer S (2009) Crohn's disease: an important differential diagnosis of granulomatous skin diseases. Eur J Dermatol 19(4):360–364

Cronkhite–Canada Syndrome

Acquired disorder of unknown cause that affects older patients and is characterized by gastrointestinal polyposis, diffuse hyperpigmentation of the skin and mucous membranes, generalized alopecia, nail dystrophy, and weight loss and nutritional deficiency as a consequence of chronic diarrhea

Differential Diagnosis

- Bandler syndrome
- Celiac disease and Addison's disease
- Dermatopathia pigmentosa reticularis
- Familial polyposis
- Gardner's syndrome
- Intestinal parasitic disease
- Laugier–Hunziker disease
- Peutz–Jeghers syndrome
- Protein-losing enteropathy
- Whipple disease

Evaluation

- Antinuclear antibodies
- B12 and folate levels
- Colonoscopy and gastroscopy
- Complete blood count
- CT scan of chest, abdomen, and pelvis
- Iron studies
- Serum albumin and protein levels
- Serum electrolyte studies including calcium and magnesium level
- Stool for occult blood
- Thyroid function tests

Further reading:
- Bruce A, Ng CS, Wolfsen HC et al (1999) Cutaneous clues to Cronkhite–Canada syndrome: a case report. Arch Dermatol 135(2):212

Cryoglobulinemia/Cryofibrinogenemia

Disorder caused by cold precipitation of circulating immunoglobulins or fibrinogens that is characterized by livedo reticularis, acral retiform purpura (type I), inflammatory purpura (types II or III), and acral necrosis

Subtypes/Variants

- Type I (monoclonal immunoglobulins)
- Type II (monoclonal rheumatoid factor and polyclonal IgG)
- Type III (polyclonal rheumatoid factor and polyclonal IgG)

Differential Diagnosis

- Acrocyanosis
- Antiphospholipid antibody syndrome
- Atrial myxoma
- Calciphylaxis
- Churg–Strauss syndrome
- Cholesterol emboli syndrome
- Cocaine-associated vasculopathy
- Disseminated intravascular coagulation
- Microscopic polyangiitis
- Oxalosis
- Polyarteritis nodosa
- Raynaud's phenomenon
- Sarcoidosis
- Septic vasculitis
- Serum sickness
- Systemic lupus erythematosus
- Wegener's granulomatosis

Associations

Cryofibrinogens
- Diabetes
- Chronic lung disease
- <u>Connective tissue disease</u>
- Hypothyroidism
- Internal malignancy
- Pregnancy
- Oral contraceptive drugs
- Thromboembolic disease

Cryoglobulins
- Chronic lymphocytic leukemia
- <u>Hepatis C infection (types II/III)</u>
- HIV infection
- Inflammatory bowel disease
- Lymphoma (type II/III)
- <u>Multiple myeloma (type I)</u>
- Rheumatoid arthritis
- Sjögren's syndrome
- Subacute bacterial endocarditis
- <u>Systemic lupus erythematosus</u>
- Waldenstrom's macroglobulinemia (type I)

Evaluation

- Antinuclear antibodies
- Complement levels
- Complete blood count
- CT scan of chest, abdomen, and pelvis (if lymphoma is suspected)
- Renal function test
- Rheumatoid factor
- Serum/urinary protein electrophoresis

- Test for cryoglobulins and cryofibrinogens
- Urinalysis
- Viral hepatitis panel

Treatment Options

- <u>Treatment of underlying cause</u>
- <u>Systemic corticosteroids</u>
- <u>Plasmapheresis</u>
- Cyclophosphamide
- Azathioprine
- Mycophenolate mofetil
- <u>Rituximab</u>

Further reading:

- Carlson JA, Chen KR (2006) Cutaneous vasculitis update: small vessel neutrophilic vasculitis syndromes. Am J Dermatopathol 28(6):486–506

Cryptococcosis (European Blastomycosis, Busse–Buschke Disease)

Infection with the opportunistic encapsulated yeast, *Cryptococcus neoformans*, that is characterized most commonly by cutaneous lesions in the setting of disseminated disease including molluscum-like lesions, cellulitis, erythematous papules, nodules, and ulcers

Differential Diagnosis

- Acanthamebiasis
- Acne
- Aspergillosis
- Bacillary angiomatosis
- Bacterial cellulitis
- Blastomycosis
- Coccidioidomycosis

- Granuloma annulare
- <u>Histoplasmosis</u>
- Lymphoma (especially CNS)
- <u>Molluscum contagiosum</u>
- Nocardiosis
- Syphilis
- Toxoplasmosis
- Tuberculosis

Evaluation

- CT/MRI scan of brain
- HIV test
- Lumbar puncture
- Serum latex agglutination test for cryptococcal antigen

Further reading:
- Lafleur L, Beaty S, Colome-Grimmer MI et al (2004) Cryptococcal cellulitis in a patient on prednisone monotherapy for myasthenia gravis. Cutis 74(3):165–170

Cutis Laxa

Inherited (AD, AR, XLR) or acquired disorder of elastic tissue with a variety of associated conditions that is caused by inadequate/faulty production of or a loss of elastic tissue and is characterized by focal or widespread loose, saggy, redundant, aged-appearing skin in a generalized or localized distribution (Fig. 6.21)

Differential Diagnosis

- Anetoderma
- Atrophoderma of Pasini and Pierini
- Costello syndrome
- <u>Cutis pleonasmus</u>

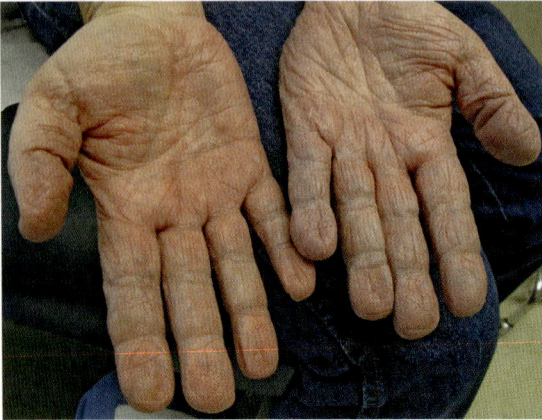

Fig. 6.21 Digital cutis laxa

- De Barsy syndrome
- Ehlers–Danlos syndrome
- <u>Granulomatous slack skin</u>
- Marfan syndrome
- Michelin tire baby syndrome
- Middermal elastolysis
- Pseudoatrophoderma colli
- <u>Pseudoxanthoma elasticum</u>
- SCARF syndrome
- Striae distensae

Associations

Hereditary

- Aneurysms
- Emphysema
- Gastrointestinal diverticula
- Hernias
- Valve disease
- Vocal cord abnormalities

Acquired

- Amyloidosis
- Angioedema
- *Borrelia burgdorferi* infection
- Celiac disease
- Hemolytic anemia
- Dermatitis herpetiformis
- Erythema multiforme
- <u>Myeloma</u>
- Nephrotic syndrome
- Penicillamine
- Rheumatoid arthritis
- Sarcoidosis
- Sweet's syndrome
- Systemic lupus erythematosus
- Urticaria

Evaluation

- Serum/urinary protein electrophoresis (acquired generalized)
- Chest radiography (inherited)
- Antinuclear antibodies (acquired generalized)
- Echocardiography

Further reading:
- Ringpfeil F (2005) Selected disorders of connective tissue: pseudoxanthoma elasticum, cutis laxa, and lipoid proteinosis. Clin Dermatol 23(1):41–46

Cutis Marmorata Telangiectatica Congenita (van Lohuizen Syndrome)

Congenital vascular anomaly of unknown cause that is associated with a variety of disorders and characterized by persistent, reticulated vascular mottling on the lower extremities that does not resolve with warming

Differential Diagnosis

- <u>Benign cutis marmorata</u>
- Bockenheimer syndrome
- Diffuse cutaneous mastocytosis
- <u>Focal dermal hypoplasia</u>
- Homocystinuria
- <u>Klippel–Trenaunay syndrome</u>
- Livedo reticularis
- <u>Neonatal lupus erythematosus</u>
- Reticular infantile hemangioma
- <u>Reticular port-wine stain</u>

Associations

- Adams–Oliver syndrome
- Capillary malformations
- Craniofacial abnormalities
- Glaucoma
- Hypospadias
- Klippel–Trenaunay syndrome
- Mental retardation
- Phakomatosis pigmentovascularis, type V
- Rothmund–Thomson syndrome
- Sturge–Weber syndrome
- Syndactyly

Further reading:
- Heughan CE, Kanigsberg N (2007) Cutis marmorata telangiectatica congenita and neonatal lupus. Pediatr Dermatol 24(3):320

Cutis Verticis Gyrata

Scalp condition that can be a primary disorder or secondary to a variety of causes and is characterized by deep, linear, and convoluted folds on the scalp

Differential Diagnosis

- AL amyloidosis
- Cerebriform melanocytic nevus
- Connective tissue nevus
- Cutis laxa
- Lipedematous alopecia
- Multiple cylindromas
- Nevus lipomatosus
- Sarcoidosis

Associations

- Acanthosis nigricans
- Acromegaly
- Amyloidosis
- Beare–Stevenson syndrome
- Darier's disease
- Ehlers–Danlos syndrome
- Epilepsy
- Fragile X syndrome
- Hyperinsulinism
- Leukemia
- Myxedema
- Noonan syndrome
- Pachydermoperiostosis
- Schizophrenia
- Syphilis
- Tuberous sclerosis
- Turner syndrome

Evaluation

- Endocrine evaluation (if suspect pituitary abnormality)
- EEG and MRI of brain (if neurologic abnormality is suspected)

Further reading:
- Larsen F, Birchall N (2007) Cutis verticis gyrata: three cases with different aetiologies that demonstrate the classification system. Australas J Dermatol 48(2):91–94

Cylindroma

Benign adnexal neoplasm of questionable apocrine or eccrine origin which, when multiple and familial, is associated with a defect in the CYLD gene and is characterized by flesh-colored to erythematous to red "tomato-like" tumors most commonly located on the scalp

Differential Diagnosis

- Angiolymphoid hyperplasia with eosinophilia
- Cutis verticis gyrata
- Eccrine spiradenoma
- Lymphoma
- Metastatic disease
- Pilar cyst
- Proliferating pilar tumor
- Sebaceous adenoma

Associations

- Brooke–Spiegler syndrome

Further reading:
- Retamar RA, Stengel F, Saadi ME et al (2007) Brooke–Spiegler syndrome – report of four families: treatment with CO_2 laser. Int J Dermatol 46(6):583–586

Cysticercosis

Infestation with the pork tapeworm *Taenia solium* that is characterized most commonly by CNS disease and less commonly by subcutaneous nodules

Differential Diagnosis

- Brain abscess
- Brain tumor
- Cerebrovascular accident
- Coccidioidomycosis
- Cryptococcosis
- Encephalitis
- Nocardiosis
- Sarcoidosis
- Toxoplasmosis
- Tuberculosis

Further reading:

- Uthida-Tanaka AM, Sampaio MC, Velho PE et al (2004) Subcutaneous and cerebral cysticercosis. J Am Acad Dermatol 50(2 Suppl):S14–S17

Cytophagic Histiocytic Panniculitis

Type of panniculitis that lies on spectrum of disease with subcutaneous T cell lymphoma and is characterized by erythematous, painful nodules on the extremities and trunk, fever, and a hemophagocytic syndrome, with cytopenias, hepatosplenomegaly, and liver failure

Differential Diagnosis

- Antitrypsin deficiency panniculitis
- Erythema nodosum
- Factitial disease
- Lupus panniculitis
- Nodular vasculitis
- Polyarteritis nodosa
- Pancreatic panniculitis
- Subcutaneous panniculitis-like T cell lymphoma

- Sweet's syndrome
- Traumatic panniculitis

Evaluation

- Antinuclear antibodies
- Bone marrow biopsy
- Complete blood count
- CT scan of chest, abdomen, and pelvis
- Immunophenotyping and T cell gene rearrangement of tissue
- Lactate dehydrogenase level
- Liver function test
- Renal function test

Further reading:
- Secmeer G, Sakalli H, Gok F et al (2004) Fatal cytophagic histiocytic panniculitis. Pediatr Dermatol 21(3):246–249

Dabska Tumor (Endovascular Papillary Angioendothelioma)

Rare, low-grade angiosarcoma that affects predominantly children, is likely lymphatic in origin, and is characterized by a slow-growing, violaceous, or blue subcutaneous mass on the head and neck, trunk, or extremities

Differential Diagnosis

- Angiolymphoid hyperplasia with eosinophilia
- Angiosarcoma
- Benign intravascular endothelial hyperplasia
- Glomeruloid hemangioma
- Hobnail hemangioma
- Infantile hemangioma, deep type
- Kaposi's sarcoma

- Reactive angioendotheliomatosis
- Retiform hemangioendothelioma
- <u>Venous malformation</u>
- <u>Tufted angioma</u>

Further reading:
- Schwartz RA, Dabski C, Dabska M (2000) The Dabska tumor: a thirty-year retrospect. Dermatology 201(1):1–5

Darier's Disease (Keratosis Follicularis)

Keratinization disorder that is caused by an autosomal-dominantly inherited defect in the ATP2A2 gene which encodes the SERCA2 calcium pump and is characterized by childhood or adolescent onset of keratotic papules that become coalescent into greasy, markedly hyperkeratotic and vegetating plaques on the central chest, upper back, neck, scalp, and intertriginous areas, as well as verrucous papules on the dorsal hands and nail changes (Fig. 6.22)

Differential Diagnosis

- Acrokeratosis verruciformis of Hopf
- Blastomycosis-like pyoderma
- Familial dyskeratotic comedones
- Folliculitis
- Grover's disease
- <u>Langerhans cell histiocytosis</u>
- Hailey–Hailey disease
- Pemphigus foliaceus
- Pemphigus vegetans
- Pityriasis lichenoides chronica
- Pityriasis rubra pilaris
- Seborrheic dermatitis

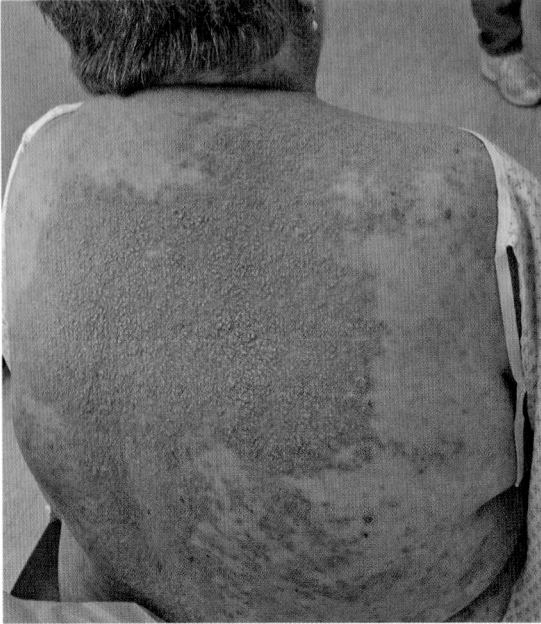

Fig. 6.22 Darier's disease (Courtesy of K. Guidry)

Associations

- Bipolar personality disorder
- Epilepsy

Treatment Options

- Topical retinoids
- <u>Systemic retinoids</u>
- Systemic steroids
- Oral antibiotics

Further reading:

- Sehgal VN, Srivastava G (2005) Darier's (Darier–White) disease/keratosis follicularis. Int J Dermatol 44(3):184–192

Decubitus Ulcer

Type of ulcer that is caused by ischemia related to prolonged pressure and is characterized by a superficial or deep punched-out ulcer most commonly located on the sacral area or lower extremities

Differential Diagnosis

- Bullous pemphigoid
- Burn
- Cellulitis
- Coma bullae
- Contact dermatitis, irritant
- Factitial ulcer
- Pyoderma gangrenosum
- Squamous cell carcinoma
- Spider bite
- Stasis ulcer
- Vasculitis

Staging

- Stage I – blanchable erythema
- Stage II – partial thickness (into dermis)
- Stage III – intermediate thickness (into subcutaneous layer)
- Stage IV – full thickness (into muscle, fascia, tendons, bone)

Treatment Options

- Relief of pressure
- Debridement and wound care
- Topical antibiotics
- Hydrocolloid dressings
- Becaplermin gel

Further reading:
- Parish LC, Lowthian P, Witkowski JA (2007) The decubitus ulcer: many questions but few definitive answers. Clin Dermatol 25(1):101–108

Delusions of Parasitosis (Ekbom's Disease)

Type of monosymptomatic hypochondriasis that is caused by a fixed, incontrovertible delusion held by the patient that he or she is infested with insects, worms, or other ectoparasites and is characterized by excoriations, prurigo nodularis, ulcers, and presentation to the physician evidence of infestation, usually in the form of a bag containing various debris (matchbox sign)

Differential Diagnosis

- B12 deficiency
- Bird mites
- Canine scabies
- Cheyletiella
- Cocaine abuse
- Dermatitis herpetiformis
- Formication
- Lymphoma
- Multiple sclerosis
- Papular urticaria
- Pediculosis
- Scabies
- Substance abuse
- Thyroid storm

Evaluation

- Microscopic examination of patient specimens
- Thyroid function test

- Serum B12 and folate levels
- Urine drug screen
- Liver function test
- Renal function test

Treatment Options

- Pimozide
- <u>Risperidone</u>
- Olanzapine

Further reading:
- Koo J, Lee CS (2001) Delusions of parasitosis. A dermatologist's guide to diagnosis and treatment. Am J Clin Dermatol 2(5):285–290

Demodicosis

Cutaneous infestation with the hair follicle mite *Demodex folliculorum* that manifests as a papulopustular rosacea-like eruption (often unilateral), a follicular-based papular eruption with fine scale (pityriasis folliculorum), blepharitis, or hyperpigmentation

Differential Diagnosis

- Acne vulgaris
- Contact dermatitis
- Cutaneous lymphoma
- Eosinophilic folliculitis
- Favus
- Perioral dermatitis
- <u>Rosacea</u>
- Seborrheic dermatitis
- Tinea faciei

Treatment Options

- <u>Permethrin 5% cream</u>
- Ivermectin

Further reading:
- Hsu CK, Hsu MM, Lee JY (2009) Demodicosis: a clinicopathological study. J Am Acad Dermatol 60(3):453–462

Dengue Fever

Flaviviral infection that is caused by the dengue virus, a virus that is endemic in various tropical and subtropical regions, is transmitted by the *Aedes* mosquito, and is characterized by fever, a centrifugal exanthem with islands of sparing, and hemorrhage

Differential Diagnosis

- Ebola virus
- Endemic typhus
- Epidemic typhus
- <u>Influenza</u>
- Leptospirosis
- <u>Malaria</u>
- <u>Meningococcemia</u>
- Pityriasis rubra pilaris
- Rocky Mountain spotted fever
- Scarlet fever
- Viral hepatitis
- <u>Yellow fever</u>

Evaluation

- Chest radiograph
- Complete blood count

- Liver function tests
- Prothrombin and partial thromboplastin time
- Serum chemistry
- Serum ELISA for dengue virus

Further reading:
- Pincus LB, Grossman ME, Fox LP (2008) The exanthem of dengue fever: clinical features of two US tourists traveling abroad. J Am Acad Dermatol 58(2):308–316

Dental Sinus

Sinus tract that originates from a dental abscess and is characterized by a fistulous opening or erythematous nodule most commonly on the jaw line (Fig. 6.23)

Differential Diagnosis

- Actinomycosis
- Basal cell carcinoma
- Chronic factitial ulcer of the chin

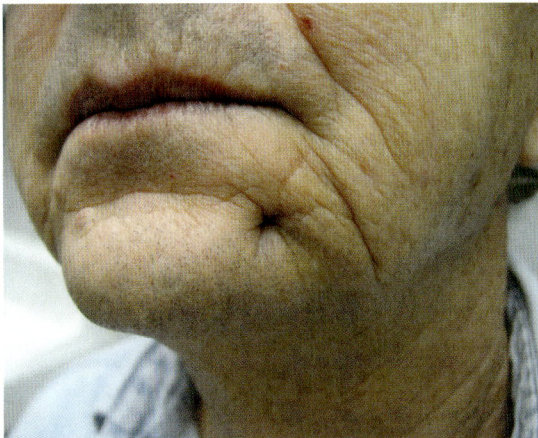

Fig. 6.23 Dental sinus

- Dermoid sinus
- <u>Epidermal inclusion cyst</u>
- Granuloma faciale
- Lupus erythematosus
- Melanoma
- Nocardiosis
- Orificial tuberculosis
- Osteomyelitis
- Paracoccidioidomycosis
- Pyogenic granuloma
- Scrofuloderma
- Squamous cell carcinoma
- Sporotrichosis
- Tinea barbae

Evaluation

- Panoramic radiograph of the jaw

Further reading:

- Cantatore JL, Klein PA, Lieblich LM (2002) Cutaneous dental sinus tract, a common misdiagnosis: a case report and review of the literature. Cutis 70(5):264–267

Dercum's Disease (Adiposis Dolorosa)

Disorder predominantly affecting postmenopausal women with psychiatric illness that is characterized by multiple, symmetric, painful lipomas on the trunk and extremities

Differential Diagnosis

- <u>Familial multiple lipomatosis</u>
- Fibromyalgia
- Multiple symmetrical lipomatosis (Madelung's disease)

- Neurofibromatosis
- Lipodystrophy, acquired progressive
- Proteus syndrome

Diagnostic Criteria

- Multiple, painful, fatty masses
- Generalized obesity, usually in menopausal age
- Asthenia, weakness, and fatigability
- Mental disturbances, including emotional instability, depression, epilepsy, confusion, and dementia

Further reading:
- Brodovsky S, Westreich M, Leibowitz A, Schwartz Y (1994) Adiposis dolorosa (Dercum's disease): 10-year follow-up. Ann Plast Surg 33(6):664–668
- Wortham NC, Tomlinson IP (2005) Dercum's disease. Skinmed 4(3):157–162

Dermatitis Artefacta

Self-inflicted skin disease associated with stress, psychological illness, or secondary gain that is characterized by skin lesions with bizarre morphology or distribution, angulated or linear borders, erosions, ulcers, or necrosis in areas that are accessible to the patient (Fig. 6.24)

Differential Diagnosis

- Arthropod-bite reaction
- Atopic dermatitis
- Bacterial pyoderma
- Herpes simplex virus infection
- Herpes zoster
- Nodular vasculitis
- Polyarteritis nodosa
- Pyoderma gangrenosum

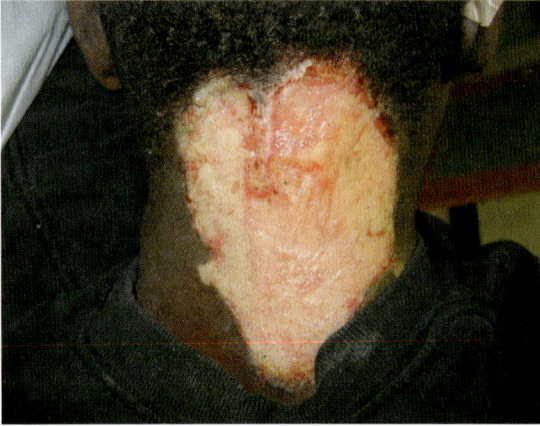

Fig. 6.24 Dermatitis artefacta

- Scabies
- Septic vasculitis
- Subcutaneous lymphoma
- Wegener's granulomatosis

Treatment Options

- Cognitive therapy
- SSRIs

Further reading:
- Kwon EJ, Dans M, Koblenzer CS et al (2006) Dermatitis artefacta. J Cutan Med Surg 10(2):108–113

Dermatitis Herpetiformis

Subepidermal autoimmune blistering disease with onset in early to mid-adulthood that is associated with granular IgA deposition at the basement membrane zone and is characterized by pruritic, grouped vesicles and excoriations located most commonly on the buttocks, knees, and elbows

Differential Diagnosis

- Allergic contact dermatitis
- Atopic dermatitis
- Autosensitization eczema
- Brachioradial pruritus
- Bullous erythema multiforme
- Bullous lupus erythematosus
- Bullous pemphigoid
- Epidermolysis bullosa acquisita
- Grover's disease
- Herpes simplex virus infection
- Id reaction
- Insect bites
- Linear IgA bullous dermatosis
- Neurotic excoriations
- Nummular eczema
- Papular eczema
- Pemphigus foliaceus
- Pemphigus herpetiformis
- Scabies
- Zoster

Associations

- Achlorhydria/atrophic gastritis
- Gluten-sensitive enteropathy
- Iron or folate deficiency
- Lupus erythematosus
- Pernicious anemia
- Potassium iodide
- Sjögren's syndrome
- Small bowel lymphoma
- Thyroid disease
- Vitiligo

Evaluation

- Antinuclear antibodies
- Complete blood count
- Direct immunofluorescence of perilesional skin
- Evaluation for gluten-sensitive enteropathy
- Liver function test
- Renal function test
- Small bowel study (if lymphoma is suspected)
- Thyroid function test
- Tissue transglutaminase antibodies

Treatment Options

- <u>Gluten-free diet</u>
- <u>Dapsone</u>
- Sulfasalazine
- Systemic steroids
- Colchicine
- Nicotinamide and tetracycline

Further reading:
- Alonso-Llamazares J, Gibson LE, Rogers RS III (2007) Clinical, pathologic, and immunopathologic features of dermatitis herpetiformis: review of the Mayo Clinic experience. Int J Dermatol 46(9):910–919

Dermatofibroma (Fibrous Histiocytoma)

Benign neoplasm possibly derived from the dermal dendrocyte that is characterized by a firm, solitary, circular, fibrous nodule most commonly on trauma-prone areas such as the lower extremity

Differential Diagnosis

- Angioma
- Blue nevus
- Calcification
- Chondroma
- Clear cell acanthoma
- <u>Dermatofibrosarcoma protuberans</u>
- Desmoplastic trichoepithelioma
- Epidermal cyst
- Foreign body granuloma
- Granular cell tumor
- Histioid leprosy
- Insect-bite reaction
- Juvenile xanthogranuloma
- Keloid
- Leiomyoma
- Leprosy
- Mastocytoma
- <u>Melanocytic nevus</u>
- <u>Melanoma</u>
- Metastasis
- Nodular scabies
- Papular sarcoidosis
- Perforating disorder
- Pilomatrixoma
- Prurigo nodule
- <u>Scar</u>
- Sclerosing sweat duct tumor
- Spindle cell xanthogranuloma
- Spitz nevus
- Wart

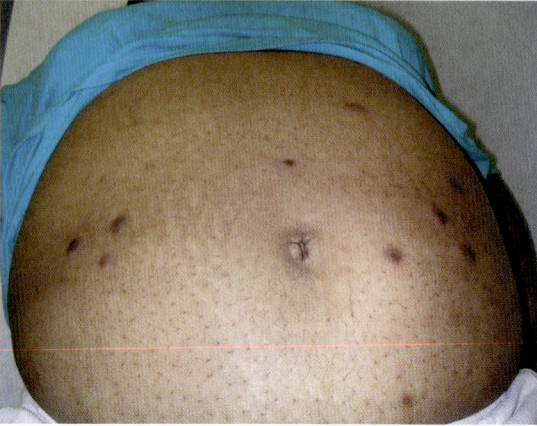

Fig. 6.25 Multiple dermatofibromas

Associations (Multiple; *Fig. 6.25*)

- Chronic myelogenous Leukemia
- HAART therapy
- HIV infection
- Immunosuppression
- Systemic lupus erythematosus

Further reading:
- Chan I, Robson A, Mellerio JE (2005) Multiple dermatofibromas associated with lupus profundus. Clin Exp Dermatol 30(2):128–130

Dermatofibrosarcoma Protuberans

Low-grade malignant neoplasm that is locally aggressive, frequently recurrent, but rarely metastatic and is characterized by a firm, multinodular mass or plaque with a sclerotic base most commonly located on the trunk (Fig. 6.26)

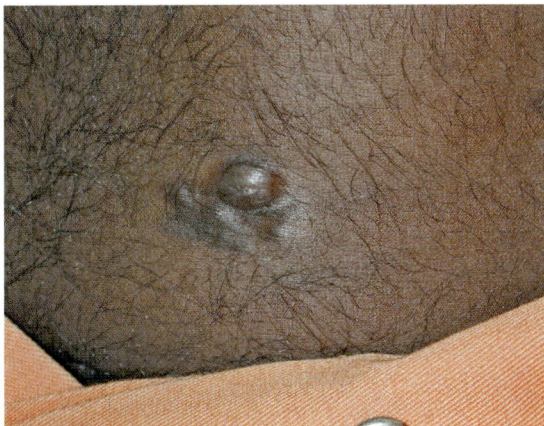

Fig. 6.26 Dermatofi-
brosarcoma
protuberans
(Courtesy of
K. Guidry)

Subtypes/Variants

- Bednar tumor (pigmented variant)
- Giant cell fibroblastoma (juvenile variant)

Differential Diagnosis

- Breast cancer
- Cellular blue nevus
- Dermatofibroma
- Dermatomyofibroma
- Desmoid tumor
- Epidermoid cyst
- Fibrosarcoma
- Fibrous hamartoma of infancy
- Keloid
- Leiomyosarcoma
- Lobomycosis
- Lipoma

- Lymphoma
- <u>Malignant fibrous histiocytoma</u>
- Melanoma
- Metastases
- Morphea
- Neurofibroma (including plexiform)
- Nodular fasciitis
- Sarcoidosis
- Sclerosing hemangioma
- Sweat gland carcinoma
- Syphilitic gumma

Treatment Options

- Excisional surgery
- <u>Mohs micrographic surgery</u>
- Imatinib

Further reading:
- Monnier D, Vidal C, Martin L et al (2006) Dermatofibrosarcoma protuberans: a population-based cancer registry descriptive study of 66 consecutive cases diagnosed between 1982 and 2002. J Eur Acad Dermatol Venereol 20(10):1237–1242

Dermatographism

Type of physical urticaria that develops within minutes of stroking the skin and is characterized by linear, pruritic wheals

Differential Diagnosis

- Cold urticaria
- Contact urticaria
- <u>Darier's sign of mastocytosis</u>
- Delayed pressure urticaria

- White dermatographism
- Trauma

Associations

- Hypereosinophilic syndrome
- Mastocytosis
- Scabies

Treatment Options

- <u>Oral antihistamines</u>
- Montelukast
- Dapsone
- Colchicine
- Cyclosporine
- Mycophenolate mofetil

Further reading:
- Taskapan O, Harmanyeri Y (2006) Evaluation of patients with symptomatic dermographism. J Eur Acad Dermatol Venereol 20(1):58–62

Dermatomyofibroma

Benign proliferation of myofibroblasts that arises predominantly in young women and is characterized by an erythematous to brown, firm, circumscribed plaque on the upper trunk or neck

Differential Diagnosis

- <u>Connective tissue nevus</u>
- Cutaneous lymphoid hyperplasia
- Dermatofibroma

- <u>Dermatofibrosarcoma protuberans</u>
- Desmoid tumor
- Elastofibroma
- Fibrous hamartoma of infancy
- Granuloma annulare
- Keloid
- Kaposi's sarcoma
- Leiomyoma
- Neurofibroma

Further reading:

- Gilaberte Y, Coscojuela C, Doste D et al (2005) Dermatomyofibroma in a male child. J Eur Acad Dermatol Venereol 19(2):257–259

Dermatomyositis (Wagner–Unverricht Syndrome)

Autoimmune disease with variable clinical features that is characterized by myositis, potential internal malignancy, and numerous skin findings, including Gottron's papules and sign, heliotrope erythema, calcinosis cutis, photodistributed poikiloderma, a pityriasis-rubra-pilaris-like eruption, flagellate erythema, Raynaud's phenomenon, a seborrheic-dermatitis-like eruption, panniculitis, and nail-fold telangiectasias

Differential Diagnosis

Skin and Systemic

- Acrokeratosis paraneoplastica
- Aldosteronism
- Atopic dermatitis
- Cutaneous T cell lymphoma
- CREST syndrome
- Cyclophosphamide side effect
- Dermatophytosis
- Dermatomyositis–meningoencephalitis syndrome

- Erythema dyschromicum perstans
- Graft-vs-host disease
- Hepatitis-B-related dermatomyositis-like syndrome
- Leishmaniasis
- Lichen myxedematosus
- Lichen planus
- <u>Mixed connective tissue disease</u>
- Multicentric reticulohistiocytosis
- Mycosis fungoides
- Parapsoriasis
- Parvovirus B19 infection
- Pemphigus foliaceus
- Photosensitive drug eruption
- Pityriasis lichenoides chronica
- Pityriasis rubra pilaris
- Polymorphous light eruption
- Poikiloderma of Civatte
- Psoriasis
- Rosacea
- Sarcoidosis
- Scleroderma
- Seborrheic dermatitis
- <u>Systemic lupus erythematosus</u>
- Thyroid disease
- Toxoplasmosis
- Trichinosis

Myositis

- Amyotrophic laterosclerosis
- Antimalarials
- Colchicine
- Cushing's disease
- Diabetic neuropathy
- Guillain–Barre syndrome

- Hyperthyroidism
- Hypokalemia
- Hypothyroidism
- Inclusion body myositis
- Isotretinoin
- Metabolic myopathies
- Muscular dystrophy
- Myasthenia gravis
- Rheumatic disease
- Statin myopathy
- Steroid myopathy
- Viral myositis
- Zidovudine

Diagnostic Criteria (Must Have First; Four Is Definite; Three Is Probable)

- Compatible cutaneous disease
- Progressive proximal symmetrical weakness
- Elevated muscle enzyme levels
- Abnormal findings on electromyograms
- Abnormal findings from muscle biopsy

Associated Medications

- Etoposide
- Hydroxyurea
- NSAIDS
- Phenytoin
- Statins

Evaluation

- Aldolase level
- Chest radiograph

- Complete blood count
- Creatine kinase level
- CT/MRI scan of chest, abdomen, and pelvis
- Electromyography
- Electrocardiogram
- Esophageal studies
- Jo-1, PM, Ku, Mi-2 antibodies
- Muscle biopsy (with or without prebiopsy MRI scan)
- Pelvic and breast examination
- Pulmonary function tests
- Thyroid function
- Urinalysis
- Urinary creatine level

Treatment Options

- <u>Sun avoidance</u>
- Topical corticosteroids
- Topical calcineurin inhibitors
- <u>Systemic corticosteroids (muscle)</u>
- <u>Hydroxychloroquine (skin)</u>
- Methotrexate
- <u>Mycophenolate mofetil (skin)</u>
- Azathioprine
- Dapsone
- Diltiazem
- <u>Intravenous immunoglobulin (muscle)</u>
- <u>Rituximab (muscle)</u>
- Etanercept
- Infliximab
- Plasmapheresis

Further reading:

- Bohan A, Peter JB (1975) Polymyositis and dermatomyositis. N Engl J Med 292(Part l):344–347

Dermatosis Papulosa Nigra (Castellani Dermatosis)

Benign, often familial dermatosis affecting predominantly patients of African descent that is characterized by small hyperpigmented seborrheic-keratosis-like papules on the face, neck, and, occasionally, the chest

Differential Diagnosis

- Acrochordons
- Adenoma sebaceum
- Centrofacial lentiginosis
- Melanocytic nevi
- Seborrheic keratosis
- Solar lentigines
- Syringomas
- Trichilemmomas
- Trichoepitheliomas
- Verrucae

Further reading:
- Schwartzberg JB, Ricotti CA Jr, Ballard CJ, Nouri K (2007) Eruptive dermatosis papulosa nigra as a possible sign of internal malignancy. Int J Dermatol 46(2):186–187

Dermoid Cyst

Developmental anomaly typically identified at birth or early in life that is caused by failure of normal distribution of several different ectodermal structures as embryonic fusion lines close and characterized by a subcutaneous mass usually in a periocular or midline distribution of the head and neck

Differential Diagnosis

- Ectopic meningeal tissue
- Encephalocele

- <u>Epidermal inclusion cyst</u>
- Fibrosarcoma
- <u>Hemangioma</u>
- Metastatic disease
- <u>Nasal glioma</u>
- Pilar cyst
- Rhabdomyosarcoma
- Steatocystoma

Further reading:

- Golden BA, Zide MF (2005) Cutaneous cysts of the head and neck. J Oral Maxillofac Surg 63(11):1613–1619

Desmoid Tumor

A deeply infiltrating benign tumor derived from the myofibroblast and often associated with a history of abdominal surgery that is characterized by a firm, deep-seated adherent mass with normal overlying skin most commonly located on the anterior abdominal wall

Subtypes/Variants

- Intra-abdominal
- Abdominal
- Extra-abdominal

Differential Diagnosis

- <u>Dermatofibrosarcoma protuberans</u>
- Dermatomyofibroma
- Fibrosarcoma
- <u>Keloid</u>
- Leiomyosarcoma
- Metastasis
- Nodular fasciitis

Associations

- Gardner syndrome
- Previous abdominal surgery

Further reading:
- Owens CL, Sharma R, Ali SZ (2007) Deep fibromatosis (desmoid tumor): cytopathologic characteristics, clinicoradiologic features, and immunohistochemical findings on fine-needle aspiration. Cancer 111(3):166–172

Diabetic Dermopathy

Cutaneous manifestation of diabetes mellitus that is characterized by erythematous to brown atrophic macules and patches most commonly located on the anterior lower extremity

Differential Diagnosis

- Lupus erythematosus
- Lichen sclerosus
- Lichen planus
- Morphea
- Necrobiosis lipoidica
- Pigmented purpuric dermatosis
- Scars

Treatment Options

- Control of diabetes
- Observation and reassurance

Further reading:
- Ahmed I, Goldstein B (2006) Diabetes mellitus. Clin Dermatol 24(4):237–246

Digital Mucous Cyst

Mucin-containing pseudocyst that is likely derived from the synovium of underlying arthritic joints and is characterized by a periungual, translucent papule or nodule with or without associated nail dystrophy

Differential Diagnosis

- Acquired digital fibrokeratoma
- Acral persistent papular mucinosis
- <u>Epidermoid cyst</u>
- Giant cell tumor of the tendon sheath
- Gouty tophus
- <u>Heberden node</u>
- Myxoid liposarcoma
- Myxoma
- Rheumatoid nodule
- Subcutaneous granuloma annulare
- Xanthoma

Associations

- Connective tissue disease (multiple)
- <u>Osteoarthritis</u>

Further reading:
- Connolly M, de Berker DA (2006) Multiple myxoid cysts secondary to occupation. Clin Exp Dermatol 31(3):404–406

Digitate Hyperkeratosis, Multiple Minute

Rare skin eruption characterized by nonfollicular digitate hyperkeratosis affecting the trunk and extremities

Differential Diagnosis

- Arsenical keratosis
- Darier's disease
- Hyperkeratotic spicules of myeloma
- Multiple filiform verrucae
- Multiple minute digitate hyperkeratosis
- Lichen spinulosus
- Phrynoderma
- Spiny keratoderma
- Postirradiation digitate keratosis
- Trichodysplasia spinulosa

Further reading:

- Caccetta TP, Dessauvagie B, McCallum D et al (2010) Multiple minute digitate hyperkeratosis: a proposed algorithm for the digitate keratoses. J Am Acad Dermatol

Dilated Pore of Winer

Follicular dilatation of unknown cause that is characterized by a keratin-filled pore most commonly on the head, neck, or back of men

Differential Diagnosis

- <u>Epidermoid cyst</u>
- Favre–Racouchot syndrome
- <u>Pilar sheath acanthoma</u>
- <u>Pore-like basal cell carcinoma</u>
- Trichoepithelioma
- Trichofolliculoma

Further reading:

- Mittal RR, Sethi PS, Jha A (2002) Dilated pore of Winer. Indian J Dermatol Venereol Leprol 68(4):239–240

Diphtheria, Cutaneous

Tropical bacterial infection of the skin caused by *Corynebacterium diphtheriae* that is characterized by a punched-out ulcer or ulcers most commonly located on the extremities

Differential Diagnosis

- Aspergillosis
- Atypical mycobacterial infection
- Chancroid
- Ecthyma
- Erythema multiforme
- Granuloma inguinale
- Majocchi's granuloma
- Nocardiosis
- Bacterial pyoderma
- Pyoderma gangrenosum
- Syphilis
- Tropical ulcer

Further reading:
- Wagner J, Ignatius R, Voss S et al (2001) Infection of the skin caused by *Corynebacterium ulcerans* and mimicking classical cutaneous diphtheria. Clin Infect Dis 33(9):1598–1600

Dissecting Cellulitis of the Scalp (Perifolliculitis Capitis Abscedens et Suffodiens, Hoffman's Disease)

Chronic inflammatory dermatosis involving the hair follicles of the scalp that is characterized by pustules, interconnecting abscesses, sinus tracts, and scarring alopecia

Differential Diagnosis

- <u>Acne keloidalis nuchae</u>
- Alopecia neoplastica
- <u>Bacterial infection</u>
- <u>Folliculitis decalvans</u>
- Keratosis follicularis spinulosa decalvans
- Lichen planopilaris
- Lupus erythematosus
- Sarcoidosis
- <u>Tinea capitis (especially kerion)</u>

Associations

- Acne conglobata
- Acne keloidalis
- Hidradenitis suppurativa
- Pilonidal sinus
- Spondyloarthropathy

Evaluation

- Bacterial and fungal culture of purulent material

Treatment Options

- <u>Incision and drainage</u>
- <u>Systemic antibiotics</u>
- <u>Intralesional corticosteroids</u>
- Systemic corticosteroids
- Dapsone
- Sulfasalazine
- Adalimumab
- Infliximab
- Zinc sulfate

- <u>Isotretinoin</u>
- Excision and grafting

Further reading:
- Salim A, David J, Holder J (2003) Dissecting cellulitis of the scalp with associated spondylarthropathy: case report and review. J Eur Acad Dermatol Venereol 17(6):689–691

Disseminate and Recurrent Infundibulofolliculitis (of Hitch and Lund)

Idiopathic, pruritic eruption most commonly affecting patients of African descent that is characterized by a widespread, monomorphic, papular, keratosis-pilaris-like eruption on the trunk (Fig. 6.27)

Differential Diagnosis

- Acne vulgaris
- Darier's disease

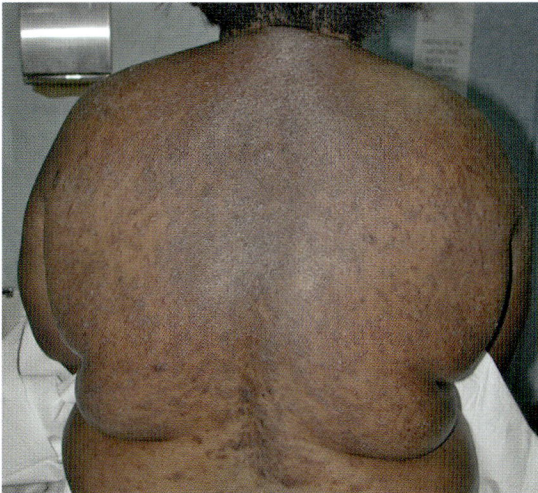

Fig. 6.27 Disseminate and recurrent infundibulofolliculitis (Courtesy of K. Guidry)

- Folliculitis
- Juxtaclavicular beaded lines
- <u>Keratosis pilaris</u>
- Lichen nitidus
- Lichen planopilaris
- Miliaria
- Papular eczema
- Phrynoderma
- Pityriasis rosea
- Pityriasis rubra pilaris
- <u>Pityrosporum folliculitis</u>
- <u>Trichostasis spinulosa</u>

Associations

- Atopic dermatitis

Treatment Options

- <u>Topical corticosteroids</u>
- Isotretinoin

Further reading:
- Aroni K, Grapsa A, Agapitos E (2004) Disseminate and recurrent infundibulofolliculitis: response to isotretinoin. J Drugs Dermatol 3(4):434–435

Dowling–Degos Disease

Familial disorder (AD) that is associated with keratin-5 gene mutations and that is characterized by reticulated hyperpigmentation of the neck, axilla, and inguinal regions, along with pitted scars and comedones around the mouth, neck, and trunk (Fig. 6.28)

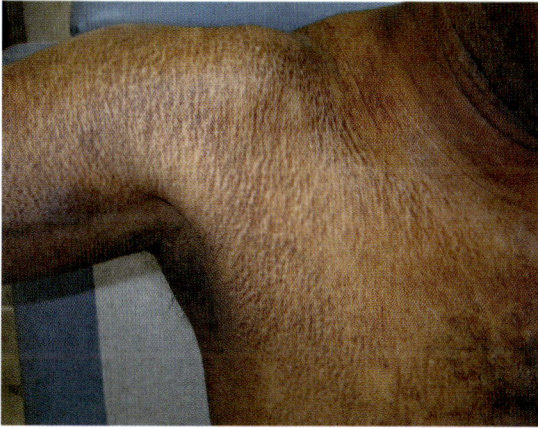

Fig. 6.28 Dowling–Degos disease

Differential Diagnosis

- Acanthosis nigricans
- Carney's complex
- Chloracne
- Confluent and reticulated papillomatosis
- Dermatosis neglecta
- Dyskeratosis congenita
- Galli–Galli disease
- Haber syndrome
- Naegeli–Franceschetti–Jadassohn syndrome
- Reticulate acropigmentation of Kitamura
- Scleroderma
- Terra firma–forme dermatosis

Associations

- Follicular occlusion triad
- Hidradenitis suppurativa

Treatment Options

- <u>Topical retinoids</u>
- <u>Hydroquinone</u>
- Erbium YAG laser
- Azelaic acid cream
- Isotretinoin

Further reading:
- Wu YH, Lin YC (2007) Generalized Dowling–Degos disease. J Am Acad Dermatol 57(2):327–334

Drug Eruption

Immunologic or nonimmunologic reaction of variable morphologies that is caused by numerous drugs and is most commonly characterized by a morbilliform, pruritic symmetric eruption involving the trunk and extremities

Subtypes/Variants

- Acneiform
- Acute generalized exanthematous pustulosis
- Autoimmune bullous disease
- Bullous
- Drug reaction with eosinophilia and systemic symptoms
- Erythrodermic
- Exanthematous (morbilliform)
- Fixed
- Lichenoid
- Photosensitive
- Pseudoporphyria
- Serum sickness-like
- Subacute cutaneous lupus erythematosus

- Toxic epidermal necrolysis
- Urticarial
- Vasculitis

Differential Diagnosis

- Autoimmune blistering disease
- Contact dermatitis
- Erythema multiforme
- Exfoliative erythroderma
- Folliculitis
- Graft-vs-host disease
- Kawasaki disease
- Lichen planus
- Lymphoma
- Pityriasis rosea
- Pustular psoriasis
- Scarlet fever
- Serum sickness
- Staphylococcal scalded-skin syndrome
- Still's disease
- Syphilis
- Urticaria
- Vasculitis
- Viral exanthem

Evaluation

- Liver function test
- Complete blood count
- Urinalysis
- Renal function test
- Antinuclear antibodies (including SS-A and SS-B)

Treatment Options

- <u>Discontinue offending medication</u>
- Topical corticosteroids
- Oral antihistamines
- Systemic corticosteroids

Further reading:
- Wolf R, Orion E, Marcos B (2005) Life-threatening acute adverse cutaneous drug reactions. Clin Dermatol 23(2):171–181

Drug Reaction with Eosinophilia and Systemic Symptoms (DRESS)

Potentially fatal type of drug-induced hypersensitivity syndrome that typically develops several weeks or months into therapy with the triggering medication and is characterized by facial edema, a morbilliform or bullous eruption, fever, eosinophilia, and hepatotoxicity

Differential Diagnosis

- Angioimmunoblastic lymphadenopathy with dysproteinemia
- Cutaneous lymphoid hyperplasia
- Simple drug eruption
- Hypereosinophilic syndrome
- Lymphoma
- Serum-sickness-like reactions
- <u>Viral illness</u>

Diagnostic Criteria (Japanese Consensus Group)

- HHV-6 reactivation
- Prolonged clinical symptoms 2 week after discontinuation of causative drug
- Maculopapular rash developing >3 week after starting with limited number of drugs

- Fever >38°C
- Lymphadenopathy
- Liver abnormalities
- Leukocytosis, atypical lymphocytosis, or eosinophilia

Associated Medications

- Abacavir
- Allopurinol
- Beta-lactam antibiotics
- Carbamazepine
- Dapsone
- Gold
- Lamotrigine
- Minocycline
- Nitrofurantoin
- Phenytoin
- Sulfonamides
- Terbinafine
- Valproic acid

Evaluation

- Complete blood count
- Liver function test
- Renal function test
- Thyroid function test (3 months after)
- Urinalysis

Treatment Options

- Discontinue offending medication
- Topical corticosteroids
- Oral antihistamines
- Systemic corticosteroids

Further reading:

- Ang CC, Wang YS, Yoosuff EL et al (2010) Retrospective analysis of drug-induced hypersensitivity syndrome: a study of 27 cases. J Am Acad Dermatol 63(2):219–27. Epub 2010 Jun 3
- Wolf R, Orion E, Marcos B, Matz H (2005) Life-threatening acute adverse cutaneous drug reactions. Clin Dermatol 23(2):171–181

Dupuytren's Contracture

Idiopathic fibromatosis with various associated diseases that affects the palm and is characterized by a cord-like, often bilateral thickening of the palm overlying the fourth metacarpal joint with flexion contracture of the fourth digit

Differential Diagnosis

- Calcifying aponeurotic fibroma
- Calluses
- Epithelioid sarcoma
- Ganglion cysts
- Giant cell tumor of the tendon sheath
- Soft tissue sarcoma
- Tenosynovitis
- Ulnar nerve injury

Associations

- Cirrhosis
- Diabetes
- Epilepsy
- Gardner syndrome
- Indinavir
- Knuckle pads
- Peyronie's disease
- Plantar fibromatosis
- Smoking

Treatment Options

- Needling
- Intralesional corticosteroids
- Collagenase clostridium hystolyticum injections
- Surgery

Further reading:
- Shaw RB Jr, Chong AK, Zhang A et al (2007) Dupuytren's disease: history, diagnosis, and treatment. Plast Reconstr Surg 120(3):44e–54e

Dyschromatosis Universalis Hereditaria

Inherited dyschromatosis (AD, AR) of unknown cause that is characterized by childhood onset of hyperpigmented and hypopigmented macules in a generalized distribution, including the face, palms, and soles, but not the mucous membranes

Differential Diagnosis

- Acropigmentation of Dohi
- Arsenical dyschromia
- Dowling–Degos disease
- Dyskeratosis congenita
- Epidermolysis bullosa with mottled pigmentation
- Pinta
- Primary cutaneous amyloidosis
- Syphilitic leukoderma
- Xeroderma pigmentosum
- Ziprkowski–Margolis syndrome

Further reading:
- Al Hawsawi K, Al Aboud K, Ramesh V, Al Aboud D (2002) Dyschromatosis universalis hereditaria: report of a case and review of the literature. Pediatr Dermatol 19(6):523–526

Dyshidrotic Eczema (Pompholyx, Chronic Vesiculobullous Hand Eczema)

Form of hand and foot eczema characterized by recurrent crops of pruritic, small tapioca-like deep-seated vesicles, pustules, and occasional bullae which are located primary on the sides of the palms, soles, and digits

Differential Diagnosis

- Blistering distal dactylitis
- Bullosis diabeticorum
- Bullous drug eruption
- Bullous pemphigoid
- Bullous tinea manuum
- Bullous tinea pedis
- Contact dermatitis
- Id reaction
- Juvenile plantar dermatitis
- Keratoderma climacterium
- Keratolysis exfoliativa
- Lichen nitidus
- Lichen planus
- Mycosis fungoides palmaris et plantaris
- Palmoplantar psoriasis
- Scabies
- Secondary syphilis

Associations

- Atopic diathesis
- Dermatophytosis
- Nickel allergy
- Intravenous immunoglobulin
- Stress

Treatment Options

- Topical corticosteroids
- Topical calcineurin inhibitors
- Systemic corticosteroids
- Acitretin
- Methotrexate
- Cyclosporine

Further reading:
- Wollina U (2010) Pompholyx: a review of clinical features, differential diagnosis, and management. Am J Clin Dermatol 11(5):305–314

Dyskeratosis Congenita (Zinsser–Engman–Cole Syndrome)

Inherited syndrome (XLR, AR, or AD) caused by defects in genes regulating telomerase function (especially dyskerin in the XLR form) that is characterized by reticulated pigmentation in the sun-exposed areas, atrophic nail changes, premalignant oral leukoplakia, pancytopenia, and tendency toward developing skin cancer and other malignancies later in life

Differential Diagnosis

- Acanthosis nigricans
- Acropigmentation of Dohi
- Ataxia–telangiectasia
- Bloom syndrome
- Dowling–Degos disease
- Graft-vs-host disease
- Fanconi anemia
- Naegeli–Franceschetti–Jadassohn syndrome
- Reticulate acropigmentation of Kitamura
- Rothmund–Thomson syndrome

Evaluation

- Appropriate cancer screening
- Bone marrow biopsy
- Chest radiograph
- Complete blood count

Further reading:
- Bessler M, Wilson DB, Mason PJ (2004) Dyskeratosis congenita and telomerase. Curr Opin Pediatr 16(1):23–28

Eccrine Acrospiroma

Broad term for a family of benign acrosyringeal neoplasms that vary based on depth of the proliferation and the clinical presentation and most commonly arise on the soles (poroma), the head and neck (nodular and clear cell hidradenoma), or anywhere on the body (dermal duct tumor)

Subtypes/Variants

- Clear cell hidradenoma
- Dermal duct tumor
- Hidroacanthoma simplex
- Nodular hidradenoma
- Poroma
- Solid–cystic hidradenoma

Differential Diagnosis

- Amelanotic melanoma
- Basal cell carcinoma
- Chondroid syringoma
- Cylindroma

- Dermatofibroma
- <u>Eccrine spiradenoma</u>
- Eccrine carcinoma
- Epidermal cyst
- Glomus tumor
- Hemangioma
- Lymphangioma
- Pyogenic granuloma
- Sebaceous adenoma
- Seborrheic keratosis
- Squamous cell carcinoma

Further reading:

- Gilaberte Y, Grasa MP, Carapeto FJ (2006) Clear cell hidradenoma. J Am Acad Dermatol 54(5 Suppl):248–249

Eccrine Angiomatous Hamartoma (Sudoriparous Angioma)

Hamartoma of both eccrine and endothelial derivation that usually arises in childhood and is characterized by a bluish or violaceous tender nodule on the distal extremities, with hypertrichosis and hyperhidrosis (upon stroking). The term sudoriparous angioma is considered by some to be a distinct entity.

Differential Diagnosis

- Blue rubber bleb nevus
- Eccrine nevus
- <u>Glomangioma</u>
- <u>Glomus tumor</u>
- Smooth muscle hamartoma
- Solitary mastocytoma
- Traumatic hemorrhage

- Tufted angioma
- Venous malformations

Further reading:
- Dadlani C, Orlow SJ (2006) Eccrine angiomatous hamartoma. Dermatol Online J 12(5):9

Eccrine Spiradenoma

Eccrine neoplasm that arises in young adults and is characterized by a solitary, tender, pink or blue, subcutaneous nodule typically located on the scalp, neck, or upper trunk

Differential Diagnosis

- Angiolipoma
- Blue rubber bleb nevus
- Cylindroma
- Dermatofibroma
- Cutaneous endometriosis
- Glomus tumor
- Leiomyoma
- Neuroma
- Poroma
- Schwannoma

Associations

- Brooke–Spiegler syndrome

Further reading:
- Ter Poorten MC, Barrett K, Cook J (2003) Familial eccrine spiradenoma: a case report and review of the literature. Dermatol Surg 29(4):411–414

Eccrine Syringosquamous Metaplasia

Rare eruption named for its histologic feature that is characterized by a micropapular, vesicular, pustular, or erosive eruption on the trunk more often than the extremities

Differential Diagnosis

- Bullous pyoderma gangrenosum
- Drug hypersensitivity
- Erythema multiforme
- Graft-vs-host disease
- Herpes simplex virus infection
- Leukemia cutis
- Neutrophilic eccrine hidradenitis
- Pressure necrosis
- Recall phenomenon
- Septic emboli
- Squamous cell carcinoma
- Sweet's syndrome
- Urticaria
- Vasculitis

Associations

- Burn scars
- Chemotherapy
- Lichen simplex chronicus
- Morphea
- Neutrophilic eccrine hidradenitis
- Pyoderma gangrenosum
- Radiation ports
- Thromboangiitis obliterans
- Ulcers

Further reading:

- El Darouti MA, Marzouk SA, El Hadidi HA, Sobhi RM (2001) Eccrine syringosquamous metaplasia. Int J Dermatol 40(12):777–781

Ecthyma

Streptococcal or staphylococcal infection that leads to ulceration of the entire thickness of the epidermis and part of the upper dermis and is characterized by well-circumscribed ulcers with a firm crust and surrounding erythema

Differential Diagnosis

- Anthrax
- Atypical mycobacterial infection
- Cutaneous diphtheria
- Excoriation
- Herpes simplex virus infection
- Insect-bite reaction
- Leishmaniasis
- Lymphoma
- Nocardia
- Pyoderma gangrenosum
- Spider bite
- Sporotrichosis
- Sweet's syndrome
- Tungiasis

Evaluation

- Gram stain and culture of exudate

Treatment Options

- Systemic antibiotics
- Topical antibiotics

Further reading:

- Matz H, Orion E, Wolf R (2005) Bacterial infections: uncommon presentations. Clin Dermatol 23(5):503–508

Ecthyma Gangrenosum

Cutaneous manifestation of blood-borne infection with several different vessel-invasive bacterial and fungal pathogens (classically *Pseudomonas*) and characterized by an erythematous plaque that develops hemorrhagic bullous changes and subsequently "gun-metal gray" gangrenous ulceration most commonly on the buttocks and perineum

Differential Diagnosis

- Antiphospholipid antibody syndrome
- Chemotherapy reaction
- Cholesterol emboli syndrome
- Cocaine-associated vasculopathy
- Cryoglobulinemia
- Ecthyma
- Herpes simplex virus infection
- HUS/TTP
- Meningococcemia
- Paroxysmal nocturnal hemoglobinuria
- Purpura fulminans (disseminated intravascular coagulation)
- Pyoderma gangrenosum
- Vasculitis
- Warfarin necrosis

Associations

- *Aeromonas*
- *Aspergillus fumigatus*
- *Candida*

- *Escherichia coli*
- *Fusarium*
- *Klebsiella*
- *Mucor*
- *Pseudomonas*
- *Serratia*
- *Staphylococcus aureus*

Evaluation

- Blood cultures
- Complete blood count

Treatment Options

- Systemic antibiotics

Further reading:
- Duman M, Ozdemir D, Yis U et al (2006) Multiple erythematous nodules and ecthyma gangrenosum as a manifestation of *Pseudomonas aeruginosa* sepsis in a previously healthy infant. Pediatr Dermatol 23(3):243–246

Ectodermal Dysplasias

A group of inherited disorders (XLR, AD, or AR) characterized by various combinations of defects in ectodermal structures, including hair, nails, sweat glands, and teeth

Subtypes/Variants

- ADULT syndrome
- APECED syndrome
- Cleft lip/palate–ectodermal dysplasia (Margarita Island type)
- Ectodermal dysplasia with absent dermatoglyphics (Basan syndrome)

- Ectodermal dysplasia with skin fragility (McGrath syndrome)
- EEC syndrome (Rudiger syndrome)
- Ellis–van Creveld syndrome
- Hay–Wells syndrome (AEC syndrome)
- Hidrotic ectodermal dysplasia (Clouston)
- Hypohidrotic ectodermal dysplasia
- Hypohidrotic ectodermal dysplasia with immunodeficiency (Zonana)
- Lelis syndrome
- Limb–Mammary syndrome
- Rapp–Hodgkin syndrome

Differential Diagnosis

- Adams–Oliver syndrome
- Aplasia cutis congenita
- Congenital ichthyosis
- Congenital syphilis
- CHANDS syndrome
- Dyskeratosis congenita
- Epidermolysis bullosa
- Goltz syndrome
- KID syndrome
- Incontinentia pigmenti
- Naegeli–Franceschetti–Jadassohn syndrome
- Netherton syndrome
- Odontotrichomelic syndrome
- Pachyonychia congenita
- Papular atrichia
- Tooth-and-nail syndrome (Witkop)

Further reading:
- Lamartine J (2003) Towards a new classification of ectodermal dysplasias. Clin Exp Dermatol 28(4):351–355

Ectodermal Dysplasia, Anhidrotic (Christ–Siemens–Touraine Syndrome)

X-linked recessive type of ectodermal dysplasia caused by a defect in the ectodysplasin A gene that is characterized by early childhood onset of hypohidrosis, hyperthermia, sparse hair, midface hypoplasia with frontal bossing, partial or total anodontia, nail dystrophy, and sinusitis

Differential Diagnosis

- APECED syndrome
- Bazex–Dupre–Christol syndrome
- Congenital syphilis
- EEC syndrome
- Hidrotic ectodermal dysplasia
- Naegeli–Franceschetti–Jadassohn syndrome
- Netherton syndrome
- Rapp–Hodgkin syndrome
- Tooth-and-nail syndrome

Further reading:
- Palit A, Inamadar AC (2006) What syndrome is this? Christ–Siemens–Touraine syndrome (anhidrotic/hypohidrotic ectodermal dysplasia). Pediatr Dermatol 23(4):396–398

Ectodermal Dysplasia, Hidrotic (Clouston Syndrome)

Autosomal-dominant disorder caused by defective GJB6 gene (encoding connexin 30) that has normal sweat gland function and normal facial features and that is characterized by alopecia, nail dystrophy, palmoplantar keratoderma, and cataracts

Differential Diagnosis

- Chronic mucocutaneous candidiasis
- Dyskeratosis congenita
- Anhidrotic ectodermal dysplasia
- Pachyonychia congenita
- Hereditary palmoplantar keratodermas
- Naegeli–Franceschetti–Jadassohn syndrome
- Netherton syndrome
- Tooth-and-nail syndrome

Further reading:

- van Steensel MA, Jonkman MF, van Geel M et al (2003) Clouston syndrome can mimic pachyonychia congenita. J Invest Dermatol 121(5):1035–1038

Eczema Herpeticum

A serious complication of atopic dermatitis involving superinfection with herpes simplex virus that is characterized by grouped, umbilicated vesicles in areas of eczema

Differential Diagnosis

- Bacterial superinfection
- Bullous pemphigoid
- Contact dermatitis
- Dermatitis herpetiformis
- Erythema multiforme
- Herpes gladiatorum
- Hydroa vacciniforme
- Impetigo

- Molluscum contagiosum
- Pemphigus
- Varicella

Evaluation

- Bacterial and viral culture of vesicles
- Direct fluorescent antibody for herpes simplex virus

Treatment Options

- Systemic antivirals
- Treatment of eczema

Further reading:
- Wollenberg A, Zoch C, Wetzel S et al (2003) Predisposing factors and clinical features of Eczema herpeticum: a retrospective analysis of 100 cases. J Am Acad Dermatol 49(2):198–205

Ehlers–Danlos Syndrome

Inherited disorder (AD or AR) of connective tissue of which there are at least six major subtypes that is caused by a variety of defects in collagen synthesis and is characterized by joint hypermobility, increased stretchability of skin, molluscum pseudotumors, easy bruising, broad "fishmouth" scarring, and blood vessel fragility

Subtypes/Variants

- Classic (types I and II)
- Hypermobility (type III)
- Vascular (type IV)
- Kyphoscoliosis (type VI)
- Arthrochalasis (types VIIA and VIIB)

- Dermatosparaxis (type VIIC)
- Others (types V, VIII, X, XI)

Differential Diagnosis

- Cartilage–hair syndrome
- Cutis laxa
- Marfan syndrome
- Menkes syndrome
- Pseudoxanthoma elasticum
- Turner syndrome

Further reading:
- Uitto J (2005) The Ehlers–Danlos syndrome: phenotypic spectrum and molecular genetics. Eur J Dermatol 15(5):311–312

Ehrlichiosis/Anaplasmosis

Identical illnesses caused by related tick-borne bacteria that infect granulocytes (human granulocytic anaplasmosis by *Anaplasma phagocytophilum* or human granulocytic ehrlichiosis by *Ehrlichia equi*) or monocytes (human monocytic ehrlichiosis by *Ehrlichia chaffeensis*) and are characterized by fever, headache, and rarely, a morbilliform exanthem

Differential Diagnosis

- Exanthematous drug eruption
- Infectious mononucleosis
- Leptospirosis
- Meningococcemia
- Q fever
- Rocky Mountain spotted fever
- Thrombotic thrombocytopenic purpura
- Tularemia
- Typhus
- Viral hepatitis

Evaluation

- Complete blood count with smear
- Serum immunofluorescent antibody (IgG)
- Liver function test

Further reading:
- Wormser GP, Dattwyler RJ, Shapiro ED et al (2006) The clinical assessment, treatment, and prevention of Lyme disease, human granulocytic anaplasmosis, and babesiosis: clinical practice guidelines by the Infectious Diseases Society of America. Clin Infect Dis 43(9):1089–1134

Elastofibroma Dorsi

Uncommon, reactive, elastic tissue pseudotumor possibly induced by repeated, strenuous, mechanical labor and characterized by a large subcutaneous, fibrous mass on the scapular area of the back

Differential Diagnosis

- Connective tissue nevus
- Desmoid tumor
- Dermatofibrosarcoma protuberans
- Hemangiomas
- Lipoma
- Liposarcoma
- Malignant fibrous histiocytoma
- Metastatic disease
- Morphea (especially deep type)
- Neurofibroma (especially plexiform)

Further reading:
- Parodi PC, Nadalig B, Rampino Cordaro E et al (2007) Non-traumatic elastofibroma dorsi. Eur J Dermatol 17(2):169–170

Elastosis Perforans Serpiginosa (Lutz–Miescher Syndrome)

Rare, perforating dermatosis of elastic tissue with onset in the first or second decade of life that is characterized by keratotic papules arrayed in circinate or serpiginous patterns, most commonly on the face or neck (Fig. 6.29)

Differential Diagnosis

- Acne keloidalis nuchae
- Actinic granuloma
- Cutaneous larva migrans
- Folliculitis

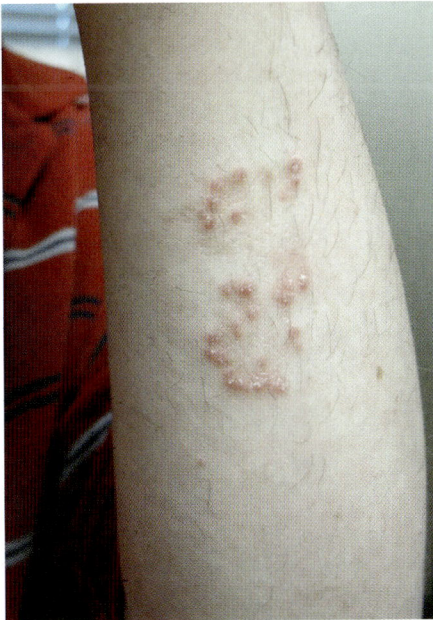

Fig. 6.29 Elastosis perforans serpiginosa

- Kyrle's disease
- Lupus erythematosus
- <u>Perforating folliculitis</u>
- <u>Perforating granuloma annulare</u>
- Perforating pseudoxanthoma elasticum
- Porokeratosis of Mibelli
- Prurigo nodularis
- Reactive perforating collagenosis
- Sarcoidosis
- Tinea corporis

Associations

- Acrogeria
- <u>Down syndrome</u>
- Ehlers–Danlos syndrome
- Marfan syndrome
- Osteogenesis imperfecta
- Penicillamine therapy
- Pseudoxanthoma elasticum
- Rothmund–Thomson syndrome
- Scleroderma
- XYY syndrome

Treatment Options

- Tazarotene cream
- <u>Cryosurgery</u>
- Isotretinoin

Further reading:
- Vearrier D, Buka RL, Roberts B et al (2006) What is standard of care in the evaluation of elastosis perforans serpiginosa? A survey of pediatric dermatologists. Pediatr Dermatol 23(3):219–224

Elastotic Nodule of the Ear

Nodule comprised of degenerated elastic tissue that arises on the ear of patients with a history of chronic sun exposure and is characterized by a flesh-colored nodule most commonly located on the antihelix

Differential Diagnosis

- Actinic keratosis
- Basal cell carcinoma
- Calcinosis cutis
- Chondrodermatitis nodularis helicis
- Colloid milium
- Gout
- Granuloma annulare
- Milia
- Nodular amyloidosis
- Rheumatoid nodule
- Sarcoidosis
- Squamous cell carcinoma
- Weathering nodule
- Xanthoma

Further reading:
- Seite S, Zucchi H, Septier D et al (2006) Elastin changes during chronological and photo-ageing: the important role of lysozyme. J Eur Acad Dermatol Venereol 20(8):980–987

Elephantiasis Nostras Verrucosa

Term for secondary changes occurring in the skin as a result of chronic lymphedema that are characterized by hyperkeratosis, verrucous or cobblestone appearance, massive thickening, and fibrosis of the affected area, most commonly the lower extremity

Differential Diagnosis

- Chromoblastomycosis
- Lobomycosis
- Podoconiosis
- <u>Pretibial myxedema, elephantiasic type</u>
- Tuberculosis verrucosa cutis

Associations

- Congenital lymphedema
- Klippel–Trenaunay syndrome
- Lymphatic filariasis
- <u>Morbid obesity</u>
- Venous insufficiency
- Recurrent cellulitis

Treatment Options

- Systemic antibiotics
- Bleach baths
- Acitretin
- Compression
- Weight loss/weight loss surgery

Further reading:
- Vaccaro M, Borgia F, Guarneri F, Cannavo SP (2000) Elephantiasis nostras verrucosa. Int J Dermatol 39(10):764–766

Encephalocele

Developmental anomaly caused by a neural tube defect that contains heterotopic CNS tissue and a persistent connection to the subarachnoid space and is characterized by a soft, compressible, transilluminating mass on the midline, which increases in size with crying

Differential Diagnosis

- Aplasia cutis congenita
- Arteriovenous malformation
- <u>Dermoid cyst</u>
- <u>Infantile hemangioma</u>
- Lipoma
- Meningioma
- <u>Nasal glioma</u>
- Sinus pericranii
- Venous malformation

Evaluation

- CT/MRI scan of the skull or spine

Further reading:
- Petrick MG, Kwong PC (2004) Anterior encephalocele with subcutaneous right facial nodule. J Am Acad Dermatol 51(2 Suppl):S77–S79

Endometriosis, Cutaneous (Villar Tumor)

Ectopic endometrial tissue in the skin that is characterized by tender, brown, occasionally hemorrhagic nodules on the abdominal wall, especially around the umbilicus (Fig. 6.30), and typically after pelvic surgical procedures

Differential Diagnosis

- Cutaneous ciliated cyst
- Eccrine spiradenoma
- <u>Epidermal cyst</u>
- Glomangioma

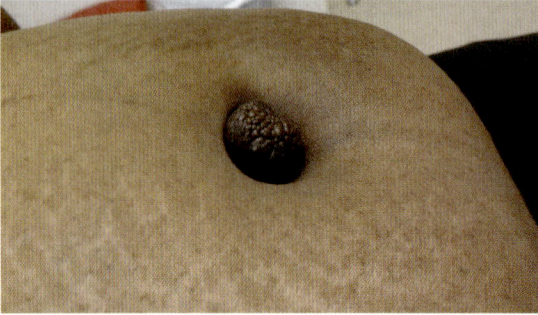

Fig. 6.30 Cutaneous endometriosis (Courtesy of E. Bardin)

- Hidradenoma papilliferum
- Lipoma
- <u>Metastatic lesion</u>
- <u>Pyogenic granuloma</u>
- Sister Mary Joseph nodule
- Suture granuloma

Further reading:
- Friedman PM, Rico MJ (2000) Cutaneous endometriosis. Dermatol Online J 6(1):8

Eosinophilic Cellulitis (Wells Syndrome)

Acquired, recurrent inflammatory skin condition of uncertain etiology but with a variety of associated triggers that is characterized by a pruritic, erythematous, indurated plaque most commonly on the trunk or extremities (Fig. 6.31)

Subtypes

- Annular granuloma-like
- Bullous
- Fixed drug eruption-like

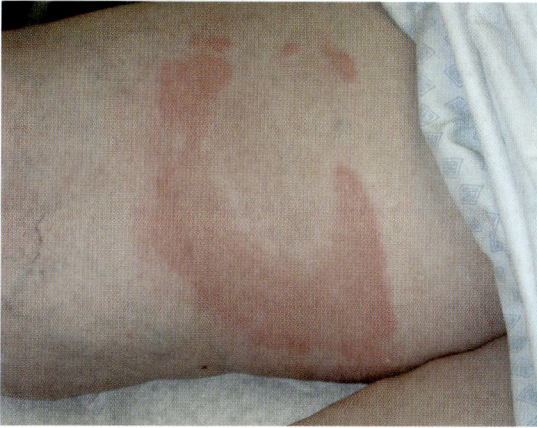

Fig. 6.31 Wells syndrome (Courtesy of K. Guidry)

- Papulovesicular
- Plaque type
- Urticaria-like

Differential Diagnosis

- <u>Allergic contact dermatitis</u>
- <u>Bacterial cellulitis</u>
- Bullous pemphigoid
- Churg–Strauss syndrome
- Erysipelas
- Erythema migrans
- Erythema multiforme
- <u>Fixed drug eruption</u>
- Granuloma annulare
- Hypereosinophilic syndrome
- Inflammatory metastases
- <u>Insect-bite reaction</u>
- Morphea
- Panniculitis

- *Toxocara canis* infection
- Urticaria
- Urticarial dermatitis

Associations

- Arthropod bites
- Atopic dermatitis
- Churg–Strauss syndrome
- Dermatophytosis
- HIV infection
- Hypereosinophilic syndrome
- Immunization
- Intestinal parasites
- Internal malignancy
- Mumps
- Myeloproliferative disease
- Onchocerciasis
- Tetanus vaccine
- Varicella

Evaluation

- Complete blood count
- Direct immunofluorescence (if bullous)

Treatment Options

- Systemic corticosteroids
- Topical corticosteroids
- Dapsone

Further reading:

- Caputo R, Marzano AV, Vezzoli P, Lunardon L (2006) Wells syndrome in adults and children: a report of 19 cases. Arch Dermatol 142(9):1157–1161
- Chung CL, Cusack CA (2000) Wells syndrome: an enigmatic and therapeutically challenging disease. J Drugs Dermatol 5(9):908–911

Eosinophilia–Myalgia Syndrome

Acquired scleroderma-like syndrome associated with the consumption of L-tryptophan that is characterized by sclerodermoid skin lesions sparing the digits, absence of Raynaud's phenomenon, peripheral eosinophilia, severe proximal muscle weakness and myalgias, and arthralgias, among other systemic features

Differential Diagnosis

- CREST syndrome
- Dermatomyositis
- Eosinophilic fasciitis
- Hypereosinophilic syndrome
- Mixed connective tissue disease
- Systemic sclerosis
- Toxic oil syndrome
- Trichinosis

Diagnostic Criteria

- Blood eosinophil count greater than 1,000 cells/ml
- Incapacitating myalgias
- No evidence of infectious (e.g., trichinosis), allergic, or neoplastic conditions that would account for these findings

Evaluation

- Antinuclear antibodies
- Chest radiograph
- Complete blood count
- Creatine kinase and aldolase
- CT scan of chest, abdomen, and pelvis
- Electromyography
- Liver function test
- MRI scan of affected area
- MRI scan of the brain
- Pulmonary function test
- Serum protein electrophoresis

Treatment Options

- Avoidance of L-tryptophan
- Systemic corticosteroids

Further reading:

- Hertzman PA, Clauw DJ, Duffy J et al (2001) Rigorous new approach to constructing a gold standard for validating new diagnostic criteria, as exemplified by the eosinophilia–myalgia syndrome. Arch Intern Med 161(19):2301–2306

Eosinophilic Fasciitis (Shulman's Syndrome)

Acquired scleroderma-like syndrome of unknown cause and associated with strenuous physical exertion that is characterized by rapid-onset skin tightening and induration (most commonly involving the forearms) and possible evolution to flexion contractures

Differential Diagnosis

- *Borrelia burgdorferi* infection
- Eosinophilia–myalgia syndrome

- Morphea
- Nephrogenic fibrosing dermopathy
- <u>Scleroderma</u>
- Scleromyxedema
- Toxic oil syndrome

Associations

- Aplastic anemia
- Carpal tunnel syndrome
- Hemolytic anemia
- Leukemia/lymphoma
- Monoclonal gammopathy
- Multiple myeloma
- Myelodysplasia
- Statin therapy
- Systemic lupus erythematosus
- Thrombocytopenia
- Thyroiditis

Evaluation

- Antinuclear antibodies
- Chest radiograph
- Complete blood count
- Creatine kinase and aldolase
- Electromyography
- Gamma globulin level
- Liver function test
- MRI scan of affected area
- Pulmonary function tests
- Serum protein electrophoresis

Treatment Options

- <u>Systemic corticosteroids</u>
- Hydroxychloroquine
- Cyclosporine
- Methotrexate
- Cimetidine
- Azathioprine
- Sulfasalazine

Further reading:
- Antic M, Lautenschlager S, Itin PH (2006) Eosinophilic fasciitis 30 years after: what do we really know? Report of 11 patients and review of the literature. Dermatology 213(2):93–101

Eosinophilic Pustular Folliculitis, Adult

Idiopathic type of folliculitis that is characterized by pruritic papules and pustules sometimes in an annular configuration on the head, neck, and upper chest and occasionally the palms and soles

Subtypes/Variants

- Classic eosinophilic folliculitis of Ofuji
- HIV-associated eosinophilic folliculitis

Differential Diagnosis

- Acne vulgaris
- *Demodex* folliculitis
- Dermatitis herpetiformis
- Dermatophyte folliculitis
- Drug-induced folliculitis
- Erosive pustular dermatosis

- Follicular mucinosis
- Folliculitis decalvans
- Herpes simplex virus infection
- Infectious folliculitis
- Langerhans cell histiocytosis
- Papular urticaria
- Pemphigus foliaceus
- Pemphigus erythematosus
- Pemphigus herpetiformis
- <u>Pityrosporum folliculitis</u>
- Pseudofolliculitis barbae
- Pustular psoriasis
- Rosacea
- Scabies
- Seborrheic dermatitis
- <u>Staphylococcal folliculitis</u>
- Subcorneal pustular dermatosis

Associations

- <u>HIV infection</u>
- Kimura disease

Evaluation

- HIV test
- CD4 count
- Complete blood count
- Direct immunofluorescence

Treatment Options

- <u>Indomethacin</u>
- <u>Topical corticosteroids</u>

- Systemic corticosteroids
- Dapsone
- Permethrin cream
- Tetracycline antibiotics
- Ivermectin
- Cetirizine
- Antiretroviral therapy
- Metronidazole
- Ultraviolet B phototherapy

Further reading:
- Nervi SJ, Schwartz RA, Dmochowski M (2006) Eosinophilic pustular folliculitis: a 40-year retrospect. J Am Acad Dermatol 55(2):285–289

Eosinophilic Pustular Folliculitis, Infantile

Uncommon dermatosis affecting infants and characterized by repeated crops of pruritic tiny pustules most often located on the scalp and distal extremities

Differential Diagnosis

- Acropustulosis of infancy
- Bacterial folliculitis
- Benign cephalic histiocytosis
- Candidiasis
- Erythema toxicum neonatorum
- Impetigo
- Infantile acne
- Langerhans cell histiocytosis
- Miliaria pustulosa
- Scabies
- Seborrheic dermatitis
- Transient neonatal pustular melanosis

Evaluation

- Wright stain of pustule
- Culture for bacteria and fungus

Treatment Options

- <u>Topical corticosteroids</u>
- <u>Ketoconazole cream</u>
- Selenium sulfide
- Tacrolimus ointment
- Cetirizine
- Permethrin

Further reading:
- Buckley DA, Munn SE, Higgins EM (2001) Neonatal eosinophilic pustular folliculitis. Clin Exp Dermatol 26(3):251–255

Eosinophilic Ulcer of the Tongue

Trauma-induced oral ulcer with an eosinophilic infiltrate that is characterized by a solitary, asymptomatic or painful ulcer with an indurated border which lasts weeks to months and is most commonly located on the dorsal tongue

Differential Diagnosis

- Allergic stomatitis
- <u>Aphthous ulcer</u>
- <u>Fixed drug eruption</u>
- Lymphoma (especially CD30+ types)
- Pyogenic granuloma
- <u>Pyostomatitis vegetans</u>
- <u>Riga–Fede disease</u>

- <u>Squamous cell carcinoma</u>
- Syphilis
- <u>Traumatic ulcer</u>
- Tuberculosis

Treatment Options

- Magic mouthwash
- Topical corticosteroids
- Topical anesthetics
- <u>Intralesional corticosteroids</u>
- NSAIDs
- <u>Systemic corticosteroids</u>

Further reading:

- Segura S, Romero D, Mascaro JM Jr et al (2006) Eosinophilic ulcer of the oral mucosa: another histological simulator of CD30+ lymphoproliferative disorders. Br J Dermatol 155(2):460–463

Ephelides (Freckles)

Hyperpigmented macules affecting patients with fair skin that are composed of melanocytes that have undergone increased melanin production as a response to sun exposure and that are accentuated and more numerous in the summer months

Differential Diagnosis

- Café-au-lait macules
- Junctional nevi
- Seborrheic keratosis
- <u>Multiple lentigines</u>
- Solar lentigines
- Tinea versicolor

Associations

- Neurofibromatosis (Crowe's sign)
- Xeroderma pigmentosum

Epidermal Growth Factor Receptor Inhibitor Acneiform Eruption

Acneiform rash triggered by cetuximab, erlotinib, and gefitinib that is characterized by erythematous papules and pustules without comedones on the face, chest, shoulders, and back and associated with an increased response of the cancer to the medication

Differential Diagnosis

- Acne vulgaris
- Demodicosis
- Exfoliative erythroderma
- Folliculitis
- Halogenoderma
- Neutrophilic eccrine hidradenitis
- Toxic epidermal necrolysis

Grading

- I – asymptomatic macular or papular eruption
- II – symptomatic macular or papular eruption or desquamation affecting <50% BSA
- III – symptomatic macular, papular, or vesicular eruption affecting =50% BSA
- IV – generalized exfoliative, ulcerative, or bullous dermatitis

Treatment Options

- Benzoyl peroxide
- Topical clindamycin

- Topical erythromycin
- Tetracycline antibiotics
- Isotretinoin

Further reading:
- Hu JC, Sadeghi P, Pinter-Brown LC et al (2007) Cutaneous side effects of epidermal growth factor receptor inhibitors: clinical presentation, pathogenesis, and management. J Am Acad Dermatol 56(2):317–326

Epidermal Nevus

Congenital hamartoma of ectodermal tissue that is often linear in shape, follows Blaschko's lines, and is comprised of either epidermal, sebaceous, follicular, apocrine, or eccrine structures or any of these in combination

Subtypes/Variants

- Acantholytic dyskeratotic epidermal nevus
- Apocrine nevus
- Becker's nevus
- Cowden nevus
- Eccrine nevus
- Ichthyosis hystrix
- Inflammatory linear verrucous epidermal nevus
- Nevus comedonicus
- Nevus sebaceus
- Nevus unius lateris
- Porokeratotic eccrine ostial and dermal duct nevus
- Systematized epidermal nevus
- Verrucous epidermal nevus
- White sponge nevus

Differential Diagnosis

Linear Verrucous Type

- Acanthosis nigricans
- Darier's disease
- <u>Incontinentia pigmenti, verrucous stage</u>
- Juvenile xanthogranuloma
- Lichen striatus
- Linear porokeratosis
- Linear psoriasis
- <u>Nevus sebaceus</u>
- Seborrheic keratoses
- Wart
- Xanthoma

Ichthyosis Hystrix

- <u>Bullous congenital ichthyosiform erythroderma</u>
- <u>Hystrix-like ichthyosis with deafness (HID) syndrome</u>
- <u>Ichthyosis hystrix Curth–Macklin</u>
- Keratitis–ichthyosis–deafness (KID) syndrome
- Widespread porokeratotic eccrine ostial and dermal duct nevus

Associations

- <u>Epidermal nevus syndrome</u>
- Gardner's syndrome
- KID syndrome
- Phakomatosis pigmentovascularis
- Proteus syndrome
- Rubinstein–Taybi syndrome
- <u>Vitamin-D-resistant rickets</u>
- Various anomalies

Treatment Options

- Shave excision
- Cryotherapy
- <u>Surgical excision</u>
- Dermabrasion
- Ablative laser
- Systemic retinoids

Further reading:

- Kriner J, Montes LF (1997) Gigantic ichthyosis hystrix. J Am Acad Dermatol 36(4):646–647
- Sarifakioglu E, Yenidunya S (2007) Linear epidermolytic verrucous epidermal nevus of the male genitalia. Pediatr Dermatol 24(4):447–448

Epidermal Nevus Syndrome

Autosomal-dominant group of disorders caused by a lethal mutation that is rescued by mosaicism and characterized by an epidermal nevus in association with several systemic defects, including skeletal abnormalities, CNS disturbance (seizures), and ocular disease (cataracts), among many other reported defects

Subtypes/Variants

- CHILD syndrome
- Nevus comedonicus syndrome
- Phakomatosis pigmentokeratotica
- Becker nevus syndrome
- Proteus syndrome
- Schimmelpenning syndrome

Differential Diagnosis

- Bullous congenital ichthyosiform erythroderma
- Cowden's disease

- <u>Encephalocraniocutaneous lipomatosis</u>
- Darier's disease
- Neurofibromatosis
- Oculocerebrocutaneous syndrome
- Phakomatosis pigmentovascularis
- <u>Tuberous sclerosis</u>

Evaluation

- CT/MRI scan of the brain
- Ophthalmologic exam
- Electroencephalogram
- Skeletal radiographs

Further reading:
- Chatproedprai S, Wananukul S, Prasarnnaem T, Noppakun N (2007) Epidermal nevus syndrome. Int J Dermatol 46(8):858–860

Epidermodysplasia Verruciformis

Inherited disorder caused by depressed cell-mediated immunity against several different types of human papillomavirus that is characterized by numerous flat warts on the face, upper trunk, and arms that have a potential to become squamous cell carcinoma, especially in those with a history of chronic, cumulative sun exposure

Differential Diagnosis

- Acrokeratosis verruciformis of Hopf
- Actinic keratosis
- Basal cell carcinoma
- <u>Darier's disease</u>
- Papular mucinosis
- Seborrheic keratoses
- Squamous cell carcinoma

- Solar elastosis
- Tinea versicolor
- Trichoepithelioma
- Verruca plana

Treatment Options

- Sunscreen
- Cryotherapy
- 5-FU cream
- Topical retinoids
- Systemic retinoids
- Interferon
- Imiquimod cream
- Photodynamic therapy

Further reading:
- Yanagi T, Shibaki A, Tsuji-Abe Y et al (2006) Epidermodysplasia verruciformis and generalized verrucosis: The same disease? Clin Exp Dermatol 31(3):390–393

Epidermoid Cyst (Epidermal Inclusion Cyst)

Very common keratinous cyst caused by proliferation of the infundibular portion of the hair follicle within the dermis that is characterized by a circumscribed dermal nodule with a central punctum and a malodorous, cheese-like keratinous substance

Differential Diagnosis

- Branchial cleft cyst
- Calcinosis cutis
- Dermoid cyst

- Dilated pore of Winer
- Foreign body granuloma
- Granuloma annulare
- Hybrid cyst
- Insect-bite reactions
- Keloid
- <u>Lipoma</u>
- Lymphocytic infiltrate
- Metastasis
- Nodular fasciitis
- Phaeohyphomycotic cyst
- Proliferating epidermoid cyst
- Rheumatoid nodule
- Sarcoidosis
- Steatocystoma multiplex
- Subcutaneous dirofilariasis
- Traumatic arteriovenous fistula
- <u>Trichilemmal cyst</u>
- Verrucous cyst

Associations

- Acne vulgaris
- <u>Gardner syndrome</u>
- Leukonychia and renal calculi
- Imiquimod use
- Nevoid basal cell syndrome
- Pachyonychia congenita
- Squamous cell carcinoma

Further reading:

- Garcia-Zuazaga J, Ke MS, Willen M (2009) Epidermoid cyst mimicry: report of seven cases and review of the literature. J Clin Aesthet Dermatol 2(10):28–33

Epidermolysis Bullosa Acquisita

Subepidermal autoimmune blistering disease that is caused by deposition of antibodies against type VII collagen and is characterized by either noninflammatory mechanobullous features (skin fragility, blisters in trauma-prone areas, etc.) or a less common generalized inflammatory bullous eruption

Differential Diagnosis

- Bullosis diabeticorum
- Bullous drug eruption
- Bullous lupus erythematosus
- <u>Bullous pemphigoid</u>
- Cicatricial pemphigoid
- Dermatitis herpetiformis
- Dystrophic epidermolysis bullosa
- Erythema multiforme
- <u>Porphyria cutanea tarda</u>
- <u>Pseudoporphyria</u>
- Pyridoxine excess

Diagnostic Criteria

- Adult onset
- Blister formation beneath basal lamina
- Clinical lesions of dystrophic EB with increased skin fragility, trauma-induced blistering, milia over extensor surfaces, and nail dystrophy
- Deposition of IgG below basal lamina
- Direct immunofluorescence positive for IgG at the dermoepidermal junction
- Exclusion of bullous pemphigoid, bullous drug eruption, porphyria cutanea tarda, and dermatitis herpetiformis
- Lack of a family history of epidermolysis bullosa

Associations

- Amyloidosis
- Chronic lymphocytic leukemia
- Dermatitis herpetiformis
- Diabetes
- Inflammatory bowel disease
- Lung cancer
- Lymphoma
- Monoclonal cryoglobulinemia
- Myeloma
- Psoriasis
- Rheumatoid arthritis
- Thyroiditis

Evaluation

- 24-h urine porphyrins
- Antinuclear antibodies
- Appropriate cancer screening
- Colonoscopy
- Direct immunofluorescence
- Fasting blood glucose
- Indirect immunofluorescence (with salt-split skin)
- Rheumatoid factor
- Serum/urinary protein electrophoresis

Treatment Options

- Systemic corticosteroids
- Dapsone
- Azathioprine
- Colchicine
- Intravenous immunoglobulin

- Mycophenolate mofetil
- Cyclophosphamide
- Cyclosporine
- Rituximab
- Plasmapheresis

Further reading:
- Hallel–Halevy D, Nadelman C, Chen M, Woodley DT (2001) Epidermolysis bullosa acquisita: update and review. Clin Dermatol 19(6):712–718

Epidermolysis Bullosa, Junctional and Dystrophic

Inherited group of mechanobullous disorders (AD, AR) that are caused by several different defects in structural proteins or basement membrane zone and are characterized by skin fragility, blisters in trauma-prone areas, variable mucosal involvement, and scarring and potential for severe deformity

Subtypes

Recessive Dystrophic
- Generalized
- Severe (Hallopeau–Siemens)
- Mitis
- Inversa
- Centripetalis

Dominant Dystrophic
- Cockayne–Touraine type
- Pasini type
- Transient bullous dermolysis of the newborn

Junctional
- Generalisata mitis
- Generalized atrophic benign epidermolysis bullosa

- Herlitz type
- Inversa
- Localisata
- Progressiva
- With pyloric atresia (Carmi syndrome)

Differential Diagnosis

- <u>Bullous impetigo</u>
- Bullous pemphigoid
- Burns
- <u>Bullous congenital ichthyosiform erythroderma</u>
- Congenital erosive and vesicular dermatosis
- <u>Ectodermal dysplasia with skin fragility</u>
- Epidermolysis bullosa acquisita
- Friction blisters
- Herpes simplex virus infection
- <u>Linear IgA bullous dermatosis</u>
- Peeling skin syndrome
- Pemphigus vulgaris
- Porphyria cutanea tarda
- Shabbir syndrome
- <u>Weary–Kindler disease</u>

Treatment Options

- <u>Specialized wound care</u>
- Infection control
- Skin cancer monitoring
- Pain control
- Oral hygiene
- Ophthalmologic care
- Tetracycline
- Phenytoin
- Thalidomide

Further reading:

- Pasmooij AM, Pas HH, Jansen GH et al (2007) Localized and generalized forms of blistering in junctional epidermolysis bullosa due to COL17A1 mutations in the Netherlands. Br J Dermatol 156(5):861–870

Epidermolysis Bullosa Simplex

Inherited group of intraepidermal mechanobullous diseases (AD, AR) most commonly caused by defects in keratins 5 and 14 that are characterized by either localized vesicles, bullae, and milia on the hands, elbows, knees, and/or feet or a more generalized presentation

Subtypes

- Dowling–Meara type
- Koebner type
- Ogna type
- Superficialis type
- Weber–Cockayne type
- With mottled pigmentation
- With muscular dystrophy

Differential Diagnosis

- Acrodermatitis enteropathica
- Autoimmune blistering diseases
- Bart syndrome
- Bullous congenital ichthyosiform erythroderma
- Bullous impetigo
- Bullous mastocytosis
- Congenital erosive and vesicular dermatosis
- Ectodermal dysplasia with skin fragility
- Erythrokeratodermia variabilis

- <u>Friction blisters</u>
- Gunther disease
- Herpes simplex virus infection
- Ichthyosis bullosa of Siemens
- Kindler syndrome
- <u>Peeling skin syndrome (especially superficialis)</u>
- Staphylococcal scalded-skin syndrome
- Sucking blisters

Treatment Options

- Wound care

Further reading:
- Okulicz JF, Kihiczak NI, Janniger CK (2002) Epidermolysis bullosa simplex. Cutis 70(1):19–21

Episodic Angioedema with Eosinophilia (Gleich's Syndrome)

Cytokine-mediated syndrome with a benign course that is characterized by recurrent episodes of angioedema of the face and extremities, urticaria, fever, elevated IgM, and marked eosinophilia

Differential Diagnosis

- <u>Drug-induced angioedema</u>
- <u>Hereditary angioedema</u>
- Hypereosinophilic syndrome
- Muckle–Wells syndrome
- Nonepisodic angioedema with eosinophilia
- Schnitzler's syndrome
- Secretan's syndrome

Evaluation

- Complete blood count
- Immunoglobulin levels
- Complement levels

Treatment Options

- <u>Antihistamines</u>
- <u>Systemic corticosteroids</u>
- Cyclosporine

Further reading:
- Banerji A, Weller PF, Sheikh J (2006) Cytokine-associated angioedema syndromes including episodic angioedema with eosinophilia (Gleich's syndrome). Immunol Allergy Clin North Am 26(4):769–781

Epithelioid Sarcoma

Malignant fibrous neoplasm with a poor prognosis that arises predominantly in young adult men and is characterized by a subcutaneous nodule on the hand or wrist or, less commonly, the genitals, with eventual ulceration (Fig. 6.32)

Differential Diagnosis

- Angiosarcoma
- Calcifying aponeurotic fibroma
- Dupuytren's contracture
- Epithelioid angiosarcoma
- Epithelioid hemangioendothelioma
- Fibroma of tendon sheath
- Ganglion cyst
- Giant cell tumor of the tendon sheath

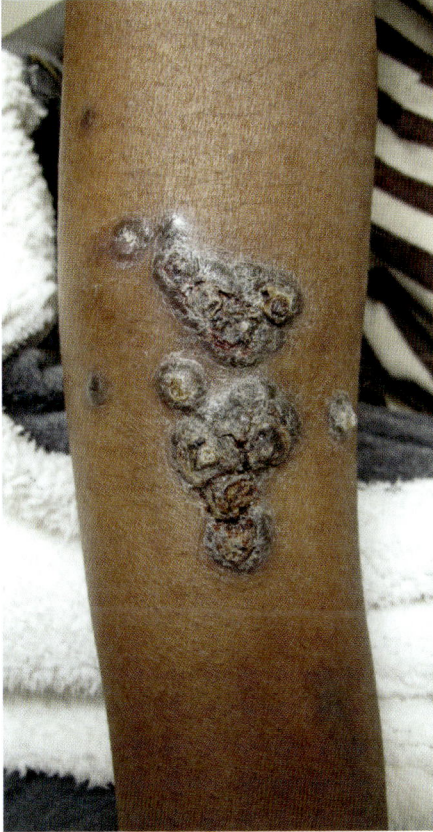

Fig. 6.32 Epithelioid sarcoma

- <u>Granuloma annulare (especially subcutaneous type)</u>
- Metastatic carcinoma
- Myxoid cyst
- Nodular fasciitis
- Rheumatoid nodule

Further reading:

- Pai KK, Pai SB, Sripathi H, Pranab, Rao P (2006) Epithelioid sarcoma: a diagnostic challenge. Indian J Dermatol Venereol Leprol 72(6):446–448

Erosive Adenomatosis of the Nipple (Papillary Adenoma of the Nipple)

Benign neoplasm of the lactiferous duct that is characterized by a unilateral, erythematous, eroded, crusted nodule on the nipple

Differential Diagnosis

- Apocrine gland tumors
- Basal cell carcinoma
- Breast cancer
- Contact dermatitis
- Eczema
- Hidradenoma papilliferum
- Nevoid hyperkeratosis of the nipple
- Paget's disease of breast
- Syringocystadenoma papilliferum

Further reading:
- Lee HJ, Chung KY (2002) Erosive adenomatosis of the nipple: conservation of nipple by Mohs micrographic surgery. J Am Acad Dermatol 47(4):578–580

Erosive Pustular Dermatosis

Erosive disorder affecting the scalp that predominantly affects the elderly; that is associated with trauma, actinic damage, and atrophy; and that is characterized by superficial crusted plaques that are unroofed to reveal moist, erythematous, nonhealing erosions with pustules, surrounding atrophy, and cicatricial alopecia

Differential Diagnosis

- Amicrobial pustulosis with autoimmunity
- Bacterial folliculitis

- Blastomycosis-like pyoderma
- Brunsting–Perry cicatricial pemphigoid
- Erosive candidiasis
- Folliculitis decalvans
- Hypertrophic actinic keratoses
- Kerion
- Pemphigus
- Pyoderma gangrenosum
- Squamous cell carcinoma
- Temporal arteritis

Evaluation

- Bacterial and fungal cultures
- Direct immunofluorescence

Treatment Options

- Topical corticosteroids
- Tacrolimus ointment
- Tetracycline antibiotics
- Topical vitamin D analogues
- Acitretin

Further reading:
- Patton D, Lynch PJ, Fung MA, Fazel N (2007) Chronic atrophic erosive dermatosis of the scalp and extremities: a recharacterization of erosive pustular dermatosis. J Am Acad Dermatol 57(3):421–427

Eruptive Lingual Papillitis

Type of acute stomatitis of possible viral etiology that affects infants and is characterized by hypertrophy of the fungiform papillae, burning sensation, hypersalivation, and difficulty feeding

Differential Diagnosis

- <u>Candidiasis</u>
- Food allergy
- Geographic tongue
- <u>Herpes stomatitis</u>
- Hand–foot–mouth disease
- Nutritional deficiency
- Teething

Treatment Options

- Observation and reassurance

Further reading:

- Roux O, Lacour JP (2004) Paediatricians of the region var-Cote d'azur. Eruptive lingual papillitis with household transmission: a prospective clinical study. Br J Dermatol 150(2):299–303

Eruptive Pseudoangiomatosis

Uncommon, benign, asymptomatic eruption with probable viral etiology that arises in childhood and is characterized by an acute eruption of erythematous, angioma-like papules on the face and trunk, with resolution typically in a few days

Differential Diagnosis

- Bacillary angiomatosis
- Carcinoma telangiectaticum
- Cholinergic urticaria
- Chronic meningococcemia
- Cherry angiomas

- Gianotti–Crosti syndrome
- Insect bites
- Papular pityriasis rosea
- Papular urticaria
- Secondary syphilis
- Spider telangiectasias
- Verruga peruana

Treatment Options

- Observation and reassurance

Further reading:

- Pitarch G, Torrijos A, Garciaescriva D, Martinezmenchon T (2007) Eruptive pseudoangiomatosis associated to cytomegalovirus infection. Eur J Dermatol 17(5):455–456

Eruptive Vellus Hair Cysts

Tiny vellus hair-containing cysts arising as a result of abnormal development of vellus hair follicles that are characterized by small, acneiform papules on the chest and extremities

Differential Diagnosis

- Acne vulgaris
- Eruptive syringoma
- Folliculitis
- Keratosis pilaris
- Milia
- Nevus of Ota
- Steatocystoma multiplex
- Trichostasis spinulosa

Associations

- Ectodermal dysplasias
- Pachyonychia congenita
- Steatocystoma multiplex

Further reading:
- Chan KH, Tang WY, Lam WY, Lo KK (2007) Eruptive vellus hair cysts presenting as bluish-grey facial discoloration masquering as naevus of Ota. Br J Dermatol 157(1):188–189

Erysipeloid of Rosenbach

Trauma-related bacterial infection caused by *Erysipelothrix rhusiopathiae* that is characterized by a well-demarcated, tender, erythematous to violaceous, erysipelas-like eruption most commonly affecting the dorsal hand, digits, and web spaces

Differential Diagnosis

- Cellulitis
- Cutaneous larva migrans
- Erysipelas
- Fixed drug eruption
- Herpetic whitlow
- Leishmaniasis
- Milker's nodule
- *Mycobacterium marinum* infection
- Orf
- Seal finger
- Spider bites
- Sporotrichosis
- *Streptococcus iniae* infection

- Sweet's syndrome
- *Vibrio vulnificus* infection

Evaluation

- Complete blood count
- Gram stain and bacterial culture (special media) of tissue and blood
- Echocardiography

Further reading:
- Varella TC, Nico MM (2005) Erysipeloid. Int J Dermatol 44(6):497–498

Erythema Ab Igne

Refers to changes that occur in the skin after localized, chronic exposure to a heat source, such as a heating pad, that are characterized by reticulate hyperpigmentation, telangiectasias, poikiloderma, and the potential to develop squamous cell carcinoma (Fig. 6.33)

Differential Diagnosis

- Carcinoma telangiectaticum
- Cutaneous T cell lymphoma
- Cutis marmorata
- Dermatomyositis
- Dyschromia
- Livedo reticularis/racemosa
- Livedoid vasculopathy
- Morphea
- Poikiloderma atrophicans vasculare
- Radiation dermatitis
- Unilateral nevoid telangiectasia

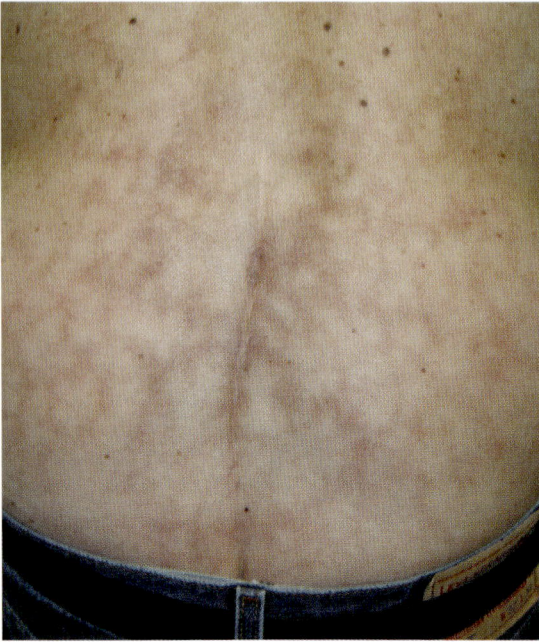

Fig. 6.33 Erythema ab igne

Associations

- Low back pain
- Pain from underlying malignancy

Treatment Options

- Observation and reassurance
- Topical retinoids
- 5-FU cream

Further reading:
- Mohr MR, Scott KA, Pariser RM, Hood AF (2007) Laptop computer-induced erythema ab igne: a case report. Cutis 79(1):59–60

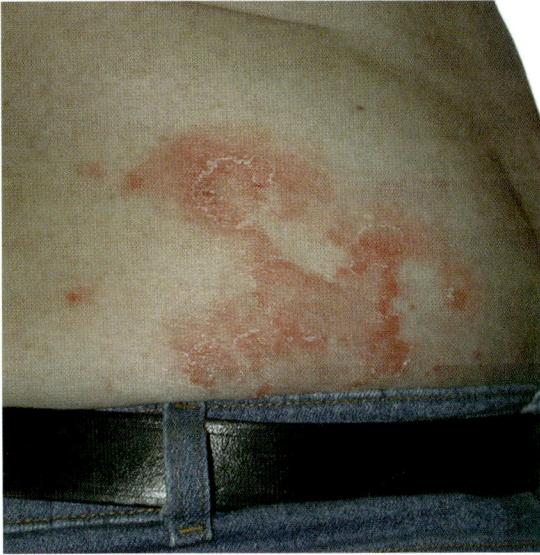

Fig. 6.34 Erythema annulare centrifugum (Courtesy of K. Guidry)

Erythema Annulare Centrifugum

Type of gyrate erythema that is probably caused by hypersensitivity to various pathogens, drugs, or foods and is characterized by slowly enlarging, annular or figurate erythematous plaques with a trailing scale which are most commonly located on the thigh (Fig. 6.34)

Differential Diagnosis

- <u>Annular psoriasis</u>
- Annular syphilis
- Autoimmune progesterone dermatitis
- Benign lymphocytic infiltrate
- <u>Erythema gyratum repens</u>
- Erythema marginatum
- Erythema migrans
- Granuloma annulare

- Jessner's lymphocytic infiltrate
- Leprosy
- Lupus erythematosus tumidus
- Lymphoma cutis
- Metastatic carcinoma
- Mycosis fungoides
- Sarcoidosis
- Seborrheic dermatitis
- Sjögren syndrome
- Subacute cutaneous lupus erythematosus
- Tinea corporis
- Urticaria
- Urticarial dermatitis

Associations

- Blue cheese consumption
- Candidiasis
- Dermatophytosis
- Graves disease
- Insect bites
- Internal malignancy
- Medications
- Parasitic infestation
- Sarcoidosis
- Tomato consumption
- Tuberculosis
- Urinary tract infection

Associated Medications

- Amitriptyline
- Antimalarials
- Cimetidine
- Diuretics

- Gold
- Piroxicam
- Salicylates

Evaluation

- Antinuclear antibodies
- Appropriate cancer screening
- Complete blood count
- Examination for dermatophytosis
- Liver function tests
- Potassium hydroxide evaluation of scale
- Stool examination for parasites
- Tuberculin skin test
- Urinalysis

Treatment Options

- Topical corticosteroids
- Systemic corticosteroids
- Systemic antibiotics
- Topical calcipotriene
- Systemic antifungals

Further reading:

- Weyers W, Diaz-Cascajo C, Weyers I (2003) Erythema annulare centrifugum: results of a clinicopathologic study of 73 patients. Am J Dermatopathol 25(6):451–462

Erythema Dyschromicum Perstans (Ashy Dermatosis, Ramirez Syndrome)

Idiopathic disorder affecting predominantly Latin American patients that is possibly related to lichen planus and is characterized by gray macules and patches with an elusive, thin erythematous border which are typically located on the face, trunk, and upper extremities

Differential Diagnosis

- Contact dermatitis
- Erythema multiforme
- Hemochromatosis
- <u>Idiopathic eruptive macular hyperpigmentation</u>
- Leprosy
- Lichen planus
- <u>Lichen planus pigmentosus</u>
- Lichenoid drug eruption
- Maculae cerulea
- Macular amyloidosis
- Macular urticaria pigmentosum
- Multiple fixed drug eruption
- Parapsoriasis
- Pinta
- Pityriasis rosea
- <u>Postinflammatory hyperpigmentation</u>
- <u>Tinea versicolor</u>
- Urticaria pigmentosum

Treatment Options

- <u>Observation and reassurance</u>
- Clofazimine
- Dapsone
- Systemic corticosteroids

Further reading:
- Muñoz C, Chang AL (2011) A case of Cinderella: erythema dyschromicum perstans (ashy dermatosis or dermatosis cinecienta). Skinmed 9(1):63–64

Erythema Elevatum Diutinum (Bury Disease)

Uncommon, chronic fibrosing type of cutaneous leukocytoclastic vasculitis with various associated diseases that is characterized by yellow-red firm nodules located over the joints, on the dorsal hands, and buttocks

Differential Diagnosis

- Dermatofibroma
- Dermatomyositis
- Erythema multiforme
- Gout
- Granuloma annulare
- Insect-bite reaction
- Keloid
- Multicentric reticulohistiocytosis
- Neutrophilic dermatosis of the dorsal hands
- Rheumatoid nodules
- Sarcoidosis
- Sweet's syndrome
- Xanthomas

Associations

- Celiac disease
- Dermatitis herpetiformis
- HIV infection
- Hyper-IgD syndrome
- Erythropoietin therapy
- IgA monoclonal gammopathy
- IgA antineutrophil cytoplasmic antibodies

- Inflammatory bowel disease
- Myelodysplastic syndrome
- Ocular abnormalities
- Pyoderma gangrenosum
- Relapsing polychondritis
- Rheumatoid arthritis
- Streptococcal infection
- Tuberculosis

Evaluation

- Antineutrophilic cytoplasmic antibodies (especially IgA type)
- Antinuclear antibodies
- Antistreptolysin O antibodies
- Complete blood count
- HIV test
- Immunoglobulin levels
- Rheumatoid factor
- Serum/urinary protein electrophoresis

Treatment Options

- Dapsone
- Systemic corticosteroids
- Colchicine
- Antimalarials
- Cyclophosphamide

Further reading:

- Wahl CE, Bouldin MB, Gibson LE (2005) Erythema elevatum diutinum: clinical, histopathologic, and immunohistochemical characteristics of six patients. Am J Dermatopathol 27(5):397–400

Erythema Gyratum Repens (Gammel Syndrome)

Type of gyrate erythema associated with internal malignancy (most commonly lung cancer) that is characterized by extensive, bizarre configurations of pruritic, rapidly migrating, wood grain-like erythematous annular and figurate plaques on the trunk and extremities

Differential Diagnosis

- Bullous pemphigoid
- Erythema annulare centrifugum
- Erythema marginatum
- Erythrokeratodermia variabilis
- Figurate psoriasis
- Granuloma annulare
- Necrolytic migratory erythema
- Pityriasis rubra pilaris
- Sarcoidosis
- Sjögren's syndrome
- Subacute cutaneous lupus erythematosus
- Tinea corporis
- Tinea imbricata
- Urticaria

Associations

- Internal malignancy
- Tuberculosis

Evaluation

- Appropriate cancer screening (especially CT scan of chest)

Treatment Options

• Treat the underlying cause

Further reading:
• Stone SP, Buescher LS (2005) Life-threatening paraneoplastic cutaneous syndromes. Clin Dermatol 23(3):301–306

Erythema Induratum of Bazin

Term for tuberculid form of nodular vasculitis affecting patients with pulmonary tuberculosis that is characterized by recurrent crops of erythematous, tender, subcutaneous nodules with or without ulceration that are most commonly located on the posterior calf

Differential Diagnosis

• Antitrypsin deficiency panniculitis
• Chilblains
• Cold panniculitis
• Cytophagic histiocytic panniculitis
• Erythema induratum of Whitfield (nodular vasculitis)
• Erythema nodosum
• Erythema nodosum leprosum
• Factitial panniculitis
• Infectious panniculitis
• Lupus panniculitis
• Lymphoma
• Pancreatic panniculitis
• Perniosis
• Polyarteritis nodosa
• Subcutaneous panniculitis-like lymphoma
• Thrombophlebitis
• Venous stasis

Evaluation

- Bacterial, mycobacterial, and fungal cultures of blood and lesional tissue
- Chest radiograph
- Complete blood count
- PCR of lesional skin
- Sedimentation rate
- Tuberculin skin test

Treatment Options

- Treat the underlying cause

Further reading:

- Jacinto SS, Nograles KB (2003) Erythema induratum of Bazin: role of polymerase chain reaction in diagnosis. Int J Dermatol 42(5):380–381

Erythema Infectiosum (Fifth Disease)

Self-limited childhood illness caused by parvovirus B19 that is characterized by a bright-red macular eruption of the cheeks, followed by a morbilliform exanthem on the trunk and extremities, and then a lacy, reticulated, heat-exacerbated, erythematous rash on the extremities

Differential Diagnosis

- Acute hemorrhagic edema of infancy
- Allergic hypersensitivity reaction
- Cutis marmorata
- Drug reaction
- Enteroviral infection
- Erythema marginatum
- Juvenile rheumatoid arthritis
- Livedo reticularis

- Lupus erythematosus
- Lyme disease
- Measles
- Roseola infantum
- Rubella
- Scarlet fever

Treatment Options

- Observation and reassurance

Further reading:
- Vafaie J, Schwartz RA (2005) Erythema infectiosum. J Cutan Med Surg 9(4):159–161

Erythema Marginatum

Cutaneous eruption associated with early rheumatic fever that is characterized by evanescent, polycyclic, erythematous patches on the trunk and proximal extremities

Differential Diagnosis

- Erythema annulare centrifugum
- Erythema infectiosum
- Erythema migrans
- Erythema multiforme
- Juvenile rheumatoid arthritis
- NOMID syndrome
- Urticaria
- Viral exanthem

Evaluation

- Antistreptolysin O antibody titers
- Cardiac enzymes

- Echocardiography
- Electrocardiogram
- Joint-fluid aspiration
- Neurologic examination
- Throat culture

Treatment Options

- Antistreptococcal antibiotics

Further reading:
- Ravisha MS, Tullu MS, Kamat JR (2003) Rheumatic fever and rheumatic heart disease: clinical profile of 550 cases in India. Arch Med Res 34(5):382–387

Erythema Migrans

The earliest cutaneous manifestation of Lyme disease that is characterized by a centrifugally expanding, erythematous annular patch around the site of the original tick bite with or without smaller satellite lesions

Differential Diagnosis

- Arthropod-bite reaction
- Cellulitis
- Contact dermatitis
- Dermatophytosis
- Drug reactions
- Erysipelas
- Erythema annulare centrifugum
- Erythema marginatum
- Erythema multiforme
- Fixed drug reaction
- Granuloma annulare
- Jessner's lymphocytic infiltrate

- Lymphocytoma cutis
- Sarcoidosis
- Spider bite
- Tularemia
- Urticaria
- <u>Wells syndrome</u>

Evaluation

- Lyme disease ELISA and Western blot

Further reading:
- Tibbles CD, Edlow JA (2007) Does this patient have erythema migrans? J Am Med Assoc 297(23):2617–2627

Erythema Multiforme

Acute, potentially recurrent skin eruption possibly resulting from a cellular immune reaction against pathogen-derived (most commonly HSV) or medication-derived antigens that is characterized by target lesions (containing central dusky necrosis, a middle ring of pink edema, and peripheral erythema) which are located most consistently on the dorsal hands, palms, extremities, and mucosal surfaces (Fig. 6.35)

Differential Diagnosis

- Acute hemorrhagic edema of infancy
- Aphthous stomatitis
- Autosensitization dermatitis
- Behçet's disease
- Bullous arthropod-bite reaction
- <u>Bullous pemphigoid</u>
- <u>Contact dermatitis, erythema multiforme-like</u>
- Erythema annulare centrifugum

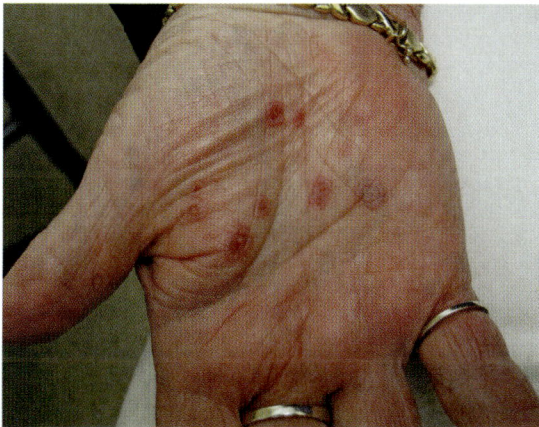

Fig. 6.35 Erythema multiforme

- Erythema-multiforme-like pityriasis rosea
- Fixed drug eruptions
- Granuloma annulare
- Hand foot and mouth disease
- Henoch–Schonlein purpura
- Herpes gestationis
- Herpes gingivostomatitis
- Id reaction
- Kawasaki disease
- Linear IgA bullous dermatosis
- Lupus erythematosus
- Mycosis fungoides
- Paraneoplastic pemphigus
- Pernio
- Polymorphous light eruption
- Rowell syndrome
- Secondary syphilis
- Staphylococcal scalded-skin syndrome
- Stevens–Johnson syndrome
- Subacute cutaneous lupus erythematosus

- Sweet's syndrome
- Urticaria
- Urticarial vasculitis
- Vasculitis
- Viral exanthem

Associations

- Erythema multiforme
- BCG immunization
- Deep fungal infections
- Herpes simplex virus infection
- Inflammatory bowel disease
- Medications (especially sulfonamides)
- Mononucleosis
- *Mycoplasma* infection
- Orf
- Phenytoin
- Pregnancy
- Radiation (especially cranial while on anticonvulsant therapy)
- Sarcoidosis
- Sulfonamides
- Systemic lupus erythematosus
- Tuberculosis
- Viral infection
- Yersinia infections

Contact Erythema Multiforme

- Bermuda fire sponge
- Disperse blue dyes
- DNCB
- Nickel
- Nitrogen mustard
- Oxybenzone

- <u>Paraphenylenediamine</u>
- Primula
- Rhus dermatitis
- Rosewood
- Topical steroids

Evaluation

- Direct immunofluorescence
- Herpes simplex virus serologic tests
- Viral culture

Treatment Options

- <u>Systemic antivirals</u>
- <u>Systemic corticosteroids</u>
- Topical corticosteroids
- Dapsone
- Antimalarials
- Cyclosporine
- Azathioprine

Further reading:

- Aurelian L, Ono F, Burnett J (2003) Herpes simplex virus (HSV)-associated erythema multiforme (HAEM): a viral disease with an autoimmune component. Dermatol Online J 9(1):1

Erythema Nodosum

Immune-mediated panniculitis associated with numerous diseases that is characterized by acute, self-resolving (or less commonly, chronic) erythematous, tender nodules most commonly on the anterior lower extremities that heal to bruise-like lesions

Differential Diagnosis

- Arthropod bites
- B cell lymphoma of the leg
- Behçet's disease erythema-nodosum-like nodules
- Bowel-associated dermatosis–arthritis syndrome
- Cellulitis
- Cytophagic histiocytic panniculitis
- Erysipelas
- Erythema induratum
- Familial Mediterranean fever
- Halogenoderma
- Infective panniculitis
- Intravascular lymphoma
- Lipodermatosclerosis (especially early)
- Lymphomatoid granulomatosis
- Polyarteritis nodosa
- Pancreatic panniculitis
- Rheumatoid nodules
- Subcutaneous sarcoidosis
- Subcutaneous T cell lymphoma
- Superficial thrombophlebitis
- Traumatic panniculitis

Associations

- Amebiasis
- Behçet's disease
- Blastomycosis
- *Brucellosis*
- *Campylobacter*
- *Chlamydia*
- CMV infection
- Coccidioidomycosis
- Dermatophyte infection
- EBV infection

- Giardiasis
- Hepatitis B
- Histoplasmosis
- <u>Inflammatory bowel disease</u>
- Lymphomas
- Medications
- Pregnancy
- Reiter syndrome
- *Salmonella*
- <u>Sarcoidosis</u>
- Sjögren syndrome
- <u>Streptococcal infection</u>
- Systemic lupus erythematosus
- Toxoplasmosis
- Tuberculosis
- *Yersinia*

Associated Medications

- Bromides
- Echinacea
- Gold salts
- Hepatitis B vaccine
- Iodides
- Isotretinoin
- Minocycline
- <u>Oral contraception</u>
- Penicillins
- Sulfonamides
- Thalidomide

Evaluation

- ACE level
- Antistreptolysin O titer
- Appropriate cancer screening

- Chest radiograph
- Evaluation for inflammatory bowel disease
- Pregnancy test
- Throat culture
- Tuberculin skin test

Treatment Options

- Rest
- Indomethacin
- Systemic corticosteroids
- Potassium iodide
- Colchicine
- Hydroxychloroquine
- Dapsone
- Mycophenolate mofetil

Further reading:

- Mana J, Marcoval J (2007) Erythema nodosum. Clin Dermatol 25(3):288–294

Erythema Nodosum Leprosum (Type II Lepra Reaction)

A serious complication of Hansen's disease that is mediated by immune complex deposition and characterized by widespread painful, erythematous dermal nodules and a variety of systemic symptoms, including peripheral neuropathy and ocular inflammation

Differential Diagnosis

- Behçet's disease
- Erythema elevatum diutinum
- Erythema nodosum
- Leprosy
- Polyarteritis nodosa

- Subcutaneous panniculitis-like lymphoma
- Vasculitis

Treatment Options

- <u>Aspirin</u>
- Pentoxifylline
- <u>Systemic corticosteroids</u>
- <u>Thalidomide</u>
- Clofazimine

Further reading:

- Cuevas J, Rodriguez-Peralto JL, Carrillo R et al (2007) Erythema nodosum leprosum: reactional leprosy. Semin Cutan Med Surg 26(2):126–130

Erythema Toxicum Neonatorum

Benign eruption affecting healthy newborns that starts around day 2 of life and resolves by day 10 and is characterized by erythematous macules, papules, and pustules predominantly affecting the face, trunk, and extremities, but not the palms and soles

Differential Diagnosis

- Benign cephalic histiocytosis
- Bullous impetigo
- <u>Congenital candidiasis</u>
- Dermatophytosis
- Eosinophilic pustular folliculitis
- Folliculitis
- Herpes simplex virus infection
- Incontinentia pigmenti
- Infantile acropustulosis
- Insect-bite reactions

- Miliaria rubra
- Neonatal acne
- Scabies
- Transient neonatal pustular melanosis
- Urticaria

Evaluation

- Wright stain of pustule
- Viral, bacterial, and fungal cultures

Treatment Options

- Observation and reassurance

Further reading:
- Akoglu G, Ersoy Evans S, Akca T, Sahin S (2006) A unusual presentation of erythema toxicum neonatorum: delayed onset in a preterm infant. Pediatr Dermatol 23(3):301–302

Erythrasma

Superficial bacterial infection caused by the porphyrin-producing diphtheroid *Corynebacterium minutissimum* and characterized by a well-demarcated red-brown plaque in the axilla, groin, or toe-web spaces

Differential Diagnosis

- Acanthosis nigricans
- Candidiasis
- Contact dermatitis
- Intertrigo
- Inverse psoriasis
- Lichen simplex chronicus

- <u>Seborrheic dermatitis</u>
- Tinea corporis
- <u>Tinea cruris</u>
- <u>Tinea versicolor</u>

Associations

- Diabetes mellitus
- Obesity

Treatment Options

- <u>Topical clindamycin</u>
- Topical erythromycin
- Benzoyl peroxide
- Oral macrolide antibiotics

Further reading:
- Lee PL, Lemos B, O'Brien SH et al (2007) Cutaneous diphtheroid infection and review of other cutaneous Gram-positive *Bacillus* infections. Cutis 79(5):371–377

Erythrokeratodermia, Progressive Symmetric (Gottron Syndrome)

Rare autosomal-dominant type of erythrokeratodermia with onset in childhood that is characterized by fixed, symmetric, sharply marginated hyperkeratotic plaques with an erythematous base that are most commonly located on face, buttocks, and extremities, but not the trunk

Differential Diagnosis

- Atopic dermatitis
- <u>Erythrokeratodermia variabilis</u>
- <u>Erythrokeratodermia with ataxia</u>
- Erythrokeratolysis hiemalis

- Ichthyosis linearis circumflexa
- Lamellar ichthyosis
- Mycosis fungoides
- <u>Pityriasis rubra pilaris</u>
- <u>Psoriasis</u>
- <u>Vohwinkel syndrome</u>

Further reading:

- Gray LC, Davis LS, Guill MA (1996) Progressive symmetric erythrokeratodermia. J Am Acad Dermatol 34(5 Pt 1):858–859

Erythrokeratodermia Variabilis (Mendes de Costa Syndrome)

Inherited disorder (AD) of keratinization that is caused by a defect in the gene encoding connexin 31 or 30.3 and is characterized by neonatal onset of transient, variable erythematous patches which eventually become less common and childhood-onset fixed, hyperkeratotic thick plaques on the extremities (including the palms and soles) and trunk, with sparing of the face (Fig. 6.36)

Differential Diagnosis

- Atopic dermatitis
- <u>Erythrokeratodermia with ataxia</u>
- Erythrokeratolysis hiemalis
- Gyrate erythema
- Ichthyosis linearis circumflexa
- Lamellar ichthyosis
- Mycosis fungoides
- Pityriasis rubra pilaris
- <u>Progressive symmetric erythrokeratodermia</u>
- <u>Psoriasis</u>
- Vohwinkel syndrome

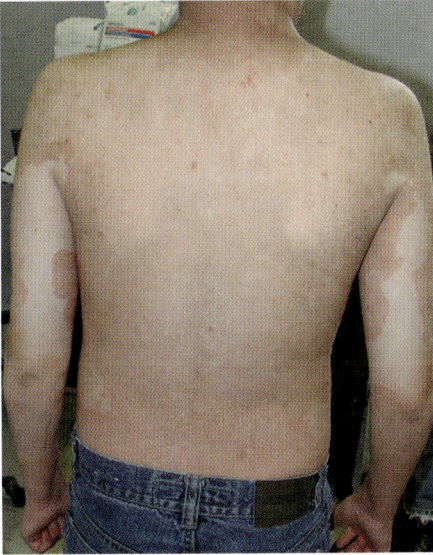

Fig. 6.36 Erythrokeratodermia variabilis (Courtesy of K. Guidry)

Treatment Options

- Keratolytic moisturizers
- Topical retinoids
- Acitretin
- Isotretinoin

Further reading:
- Strober BE (2003) Erythrokeratodermia variabilis. Dermatol Online J 9(4):5

Erythromelalgia (Mitchell Syndrome)

Disorder of peripheral vasodilation with a variety of possible mechanisms that is characterized by heat-induced episodic swelling, pain, erythema, and warmth of the feet, and, less commonly, the hands

Differential Diagnosis

- Acrodynia
- Carpal tunnel syndrome
- Chemotherapy-associated acral erythema
- Cellulitis
- Diabetic autonomic neuropathy
- Diabetic stiff skin (diabetic cheiroarthropathy)
- Fabry's disease
- Frostbite
- Immersion foot syndrome
- Peripheral vascular disease
- Mushroom poisoning
- Myeloproliferative disease
- Peripheral neuropathy
- Raynaud phenomenon
- Reflex sympathetic dystrophy

Associations

- Calcium channel blockers
- Cyclosporine
- Diabetes mellitus
- Essential thrombocytosis
- Fabry's disease
- Hypercholesterolemia
- Multiple sclerosis
- Mushroom poisoning
- Polycythemia vera
- Systemic lupus erythematosus
- Isopropyl alcohol
- Thrombotic thrombocytopenic purpura

Evaluation

- Antinuclear antibodies
- Complete blood count
- Fasting blood glucose
- HIV test
- Nerve conduction study
- Rheumatoid factor

Treatment Options

- Aspirin
- <u>Gabapentin</u>
- Pregabalin
- Sertraline
- Venlafaxine

Further reading:

- Brill TJ, Funk B, Thaçi D, Kaufmann R (2009) Red ear syndrome and auricular erythromelalgia: the same condition? Clin Exp Dermatol 34(8):e626–e628
- Ljubojevic S, Lipozenic J, Pustisek N (2005) Erythromelalgia. Skinmed 4(1):55–57

Erythromelanosis Follicularis Faciei et Colli

Uncommon, idiopathic skin disorder that predominantly affects young men and that is characterized by well-demarcated erythema, hyperpigmentation, and follicular papules with an irregular border and a symmetric distribution over the bilateral cheeks, jaws, and sides of neck. A variant involving the medial aspect of the face is more common in women and is called erythrosis pigmentosa peribuccalis

Differential Diagnosis

- Berloque dermatitis
- <u>Keratosis pilaris rubra</u>
- Keratosis pilaris atrophicans faciei
- Lichen spinulosus
- <u>Melasma</u>
- Poikiloderma of Civatte
- Riehl melanosis
- Rosacea

Treatment Options

- <u>Topical retinoids</u>
- Hydroquinone
- Azelaic acid
- Ammonium lactate lotion

Further reading:
- Karakatsanis G et al (2007) Erythromelanosis follicularis faciei et colli. Cutis 79:459–461

Erythroplasia of Queyrat

Squamous cell carcinoma in situ of the glans or prepuce that affects uncircumcised men and is characterized by a chronic, nonhealing solitary or multiple erythematous plaques with or without overlying scale, crusts, or verrucous changes

Differential Diagnosis

- Balanitis xerotica obliterans
- <u>Bowen's disease</u>

- Candidiasis
- Condyloma acuminatum
- Contact dermatitis
- Erosive lichen planus
- Fixed drug eruption
- Lichen planus
- Paget's disease
- Psoriasis
- Squamous cell carcinoma
- Trauma
- Zoon balanitis

Treatment Options

- <u>5-FU cream</u>
- <u>Imiquimod cream</u>
- <u>Surgical excision</u>
- Mohs micrographic surgery
- Radiation
- Photodynamic therapy
- Cryotherapy

Further reading:
- Porter WM, Francis N, Hawkins D et al (2002) Penile intraepithelial neoplasia: clinical spectrum and treatment of 35 cases. Br J Dermatol 147(6):1159–1165

Erythropoietic Protoporphyria

Autosomal-dominantly inherited type of porphyria caused by a defect in the ferrochelatase gene that is characterized by a sunlight-induced burning and pruritic reaction, scarring, waxy papules and plaques, gallstones, hepatotoxicity, and end-stage liver disease (if untreated)

Differential Diagnosis

- Actinic prurigo
- Congenital erythropoietic porphyria
- Hereditary coproporphyria
- Hydroa vacciniforme
- Juvenile colloid milium
- Lipoid proteinosis
- Porphyria cutanea tarda
- Phototoxic drug reactions
- Polymorphous light eruption
- Solar urticaria
- Xeroderma pigmentosum

Associations

- Myelodysplasia (late onset)

Evaluation

- Erythrocyte and plasma protoporphyrin levels
- Liver function tests
- Complete blood count
- Abdominal ultrasound
- 24-h urine porphyrins
- Liver biopsy
- Antinuclear antibodies
- Iron studies

Treatment Options

- Sunscreen
- Beta-carotene
- UVB phototherapy

- Vitamin C
- Vitamin E
- Liver transplant

Further reading:
- Murphy GM (2003) Diagnosis and management of the erythropoietic porphyrias. Dermatol Ther 16(1):57–64

Essential Fatty Acid Deficiency

Type of nutritional deficiency with prominent cutaneous effects that is characterized by infections, impaired wound healing, alopecia, xerosis, and moist, erythematous, erosions predominantly in the intertriginous areas

Differential Diagnosis

- Acquired zinc deficiency
- Acrodermatitis enteropathica
- Biotin deficiency
- Contact dermatitis
- Glucagonoma syndrome
- Pellagra
- Pyridoxine deficiency
- Riboflavin deficiency

Associations

- Cystic fibrosis
- Inflammatory bowel disease
- Malabsorption
- Total parenteral nutrition

Further reading:
- Darmstadt GL, McGuire J, Ziboh VA (2000) Malnutrition-associated rash of cystic fibrosis. Pediatr Dermatol 17(5):337–347

Extramammary Paget's Disease

Intraepidermal adenocarcinoma with or without an underlying adnexal, genitourinary tract, or gastrointestinal tract carcinoma that is characterized by a chronic, pruritic, erythematous, eczematous plaque in the groin or, less commonly, the axilla

Differential Diagnosis

- Basal cell carcinoma
- Bowen's disease
- Bowenoid papulosis
- Candidiasis
- Contact dermatitis
- Erythrasma
- Eyelid dermatitis
- Hailey–Hailey disease
- Intertrigo
- Lichen planus
- Lichen sclerosus
- Melanoma
- Otitis externa
- Pagetoid dyskeratosis
- Psoriasis
- Seborrheic dermatitis
- Superficial spreading melanoma
- Tinea cruris

Treatment Options

- Excisional surgery
- Mohs micrographic surgery
- Photodynamic therapy
- Radiation

- Systemic 5-FU
- Topical 5-FU
- Imiquimod cream
- CO_2 laser

Further reading:
- Kanitakis J (2007) Mammary and extramammary Paget's disease. J Eur Acad Dermatol Venereol 21(5):581–590

Fabry Disease

X-linked recessive disease with onset in childhood or adolescence that is caused by a deficiency in the lysosomal enzyme alpha-galactosidase A and is characterized by angiokeratoma corporis diffusum, acral paresthesias, corneal opacities, hypohidrosis, recurrent abdominal pain, and other renal, cardiac, and CNS changes

Differential Diagnosis

- Aspartylglycosaminuria
- Erythromelalgia
- Fucosidosis
- Galactosialidosis
- GM1 gangliosidosis
- Kanzaki disease
- Mercury poisoning
- Rheumatic fever
- Sialidosis
- ß-mannosidase

Evaluation

- Urinalysis (maltese cross-lipid globules)
- Renal function test

- MRI of the brain
- Echocardiogram
- Ophthalmologic exam for cornea verticillata
- Serum alpha-galactosidase level (if negative, consider other causes)

Further reading:
- Larralde M, Boggio P, Amartino H, Chamoles N (2004) Fabry disease: a study of 6 hemizygous men and 5 heterozygous women with emphasis on dermatologic manifestations. Arch Dermatol 140(12):1440–1446

Familial Dyskeratotic Comedones

Rare, inherited dermatosis (AD) of unknown pathogenesis that develops in childhood and is characterized by numerous noninflammatory, comedone-like keratotic papules on the trunk and extremities

Differential Diagnosis

- Acantholytic dyskeratosis of the vulva
- Acne vulgaris
- Darier's disease
- Flegel's disease
- Grover's disease
- Keratosis pilaris
- Kyrle's disease
- Lichen spinulosus
- Nevus comedonicus
- Perforating folliculitis
- Reactive perforating collagenosis

Further reading:
- Van Geel NA, Kockaert M, Neumann HA (1999) Familial dyskeratotic comedones. Br J Dermatol 140(5):956–959

Familial Mediterranean Fever

Autosomal-recessive disorder caused by mutation of the pyrin gene that is characterized by periodic fever, erysipelas-like erythema on the legs, pleuritis and abdominal serositis, arthritis, orchitis, and renal AA amyloidosis

Differential Diagnosis

- Appendicitis
- CINCA/NOMID syndrome
- Cyclic neutropenia
- Drug-induced lupus erythematosus
- Erysipelas
- Henoch–Schonlein purpura
- Hereditary angioedema
- Hyperimmunoglobulin D syndrome
- Juvenile rheumatoid arthritis
- Muckle–Wells syndrome
- Pancreatitis
- Pelvic inflammatory disease
- PFAPA syndrome
- Pleurisy
- Pneumonia
- Polyarteritis nodosa
- Porphyria
- Pretibial fever
- Septic arthritis
- Systemic lupus erythematosus
- Tumor necrosis factor alpha receptor periodic fever syndrome (TRAPS)

Diagnostic Criteria (Two Major or One major and Two minor)

- Major criteria
  - Recurrent febrile episodes of peritonitis, synovitis, or pleuritis
  - AA amyloidosis with no predisposing disease
  - Favorable response to continuous colchicine treatment
- Minor criteria
  - Recurrent febrile episodes
  - Erysipelas-like erythema
  - FMF in a first-degree relative

Evaluation

- Serum/urinary protein electrophoresis
- Kidney or rectal biopsy
- Urinalysis
- Renal function test
- Sedimentation rate
- Complete blood count
- Blood cultures
- Antinuclear antibodies
- 24-h urine protein
- Chest radiography
- Echocardiography
- Abdominal CT scan

Treatment Options

- Colchicine
- TNF inhibitors
- Anakinra
- Interferon

Further reading:
- Livneh A, Langevitz P, Zemer D et al (1997) Criteria for the diagnosis of familial Mediterranean fever. Arthritis Rheum 40(10):1879–1885

- Samuels J, Ozen S (2006) Familial Mediterranean fever and the other autoinflammatory syndromes: evaluation of the patient with recurrent fever. Curr Opin Rheumatol 18(1):108–117

Favre–Racouchot Syndrome

Cutaneous disorder affecting photoaged men that is characterized by symmetric, multiple comedones and solar elastosis on the temples, periocular area, and, occasionally, the neck

Differential Diagnosis

- <u>Acne vulgaris</u>
- Actinic granuloma
- Chloracne
- Colloid milia
- <u>Milia en plaque</u>
- Nevus comedonicus
- Sebaceous hyperplasia
- Syringoma
- Trichoepitheliomas
- Xanthoma

Associations

- Smoking

Treatment Options

- Topical retinoids

Further reading:
- Patterson WM, Fox MD, Schwartz RA (2004) Favre–Racouchot disease. Int J Dermatol 43(3):167–169

Favus

Chronic type of tinea capitis caused by *Trichophyton schoenleinii* and characterized by yellowish, cup-shaped crusts called scutula

Differential Diagnosis

- Chronic mucocutaneous candidiasis
- Discoid lupus erythematosus
- Dissecting cellulitis
- Folliculitis decalvans
- Langerhans cell histiocytosis
- Pediculosis capitis
- Pemphigus foliaceus
- Pityriasis amiantacea
- Psoriasis
- Scalp demodicosis
- Scalp impetigo
- Seborrheic dermatitis

Treatment Options

- Terbinafine
- Griseofulvin
- Fluconazole
- Itraconazole

Further reading:
- Cecchi R, Paoli S, Giomi A, Rossetti R (2003) Favus due to *Trichophyton schoenleinii* in a patient with metastatic bronchial carcinoma. Br J Dermatol 148(5):1057

Fibroelastolytic Papulosis of the Neck
(White Fibrous Papulosis, PXE-Like Papillary Dermal Elastolysis)

Acquired disorder of elastic tissue that affects middle-aged to elderly patients that is characterized by asymptomatic white-yellow papules in cobblestone-like plaques on the neck

Differential Diagnosis

- Colloid milium
- Papular elastorrhexis
- Pseudoxanthoma elasticum
- Eruptive xanthomas
- Solar elastosis

Further reading:
- Song YC, Oh BH, Ko JH et al (2011) A case of fibroelastolytic papulosis on the neck of a young man. Ann Dermatol 23(2):193–197

Fibroepithelioma of Pinkus

Uncommon variant of basal cell carcinoma that is characterized by a pedunculated, flesh-colored, fibrous nodule on the lower back, groin, or thigh

Differential Diagnosis

- <u>Acrochordon</u>
- Amelanotic melanoma
- Melanocytic nevus
- Neurofibroma
- Nevus sebaceus

- Seborrheic keratosis (especially reticulated)
- Tumor of follicular infundibulum

Further reading:
- Su MW, Fromer E, Fung MA (2006) Fibroepithelioma of Pinkus. Dermatol Online J 12(5):2

Fibrofolliculoma

Benign neoplasm of follicular derivation that is associated with Birt–Hogg–Dube syndrome (when multiple) and that is characterized by a small flesh-colored papule on the head and neck, often on the face

Differential Diagnosis

- Acrochordon
- Angiofibroma
- Basal cell carcinoma
- Fibrous papule
- Perifollicular fibroma
- Syringoma
- Trichodiscoma
- Trichoepithelioma
- Trichofolliculoma

Further reading:
- Vincent A, Farley M, Chan E, James WD (2003) Birt–Hogg–Dube syndrome: a review of the literature and the differential diagnosis of firm facial papules. J Am Acad Dermatol 49(4):698–705

Fibrokeratoma, Acquired Digital

Benign fibrous neoplasm possibly induced by trauma that is found on acral skin, has a dome-shaped or protuberant shape, is located on the palms or periungual area, and has a peripheral collarette (Fig. 6.37)

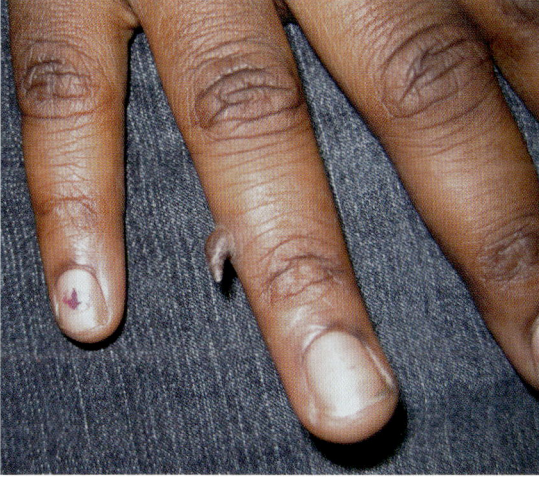

Fig. 6.37 Acquired digital fibrokeratoma

Differential Diagnosis

- Acral fibromyxoma
- Cutaneous horn
- Dermatofibroma
- Eccrine poroma
- Infantile digital fibromatosis
- Periungual fibroma (Koenen tumor)
- Pyogenic granuloma
- Supernumerary digit
- Traumatic neuroma
- Verruca

Further reading:
- Baykal C, Buyukbabani N, Yazganoglu KD, Saglik E (2007) Acquired digital fibrokeratoma. Cutis 79(2):129–132

Fibrous Hamartoma of Infancy

Type of benign fibrous proliferation that is present at birth or that arises in the first year of life that is characterized by a firm nodule or plaque in the axilla, upper trunk, or proximal extremities which continues to grow with the child

Differential Diagnosis

- Connective tissue nevus
- Dermatofibroma
- Dermatomyofibroma
- Infantile digital fibromatosis
- Neuroblastoma
- Leukemia cutis
- Lipoblastoma
- Lipoma
- Mucinosis of infancy
- Leiomyosarcoma
- Epidermal inclusion cyst
- Rhabdomyosarcoma
- Subcutaneous fat necrosis

Further reading:
- Scott DM, Pena JR, Omura EF (1999) Fibrous hamartoma of infancy. J Am Acad Dermatol 41(5 Pt 2):857–859

Fibrous Papule

Type of angiofibroma that develops in early adulthood that is characterized by a flesh-colored or red-brown dome-shaped papule on the central face

Differential Diagnosis

- Angioma
- Appendageal tumor
- <u>Basal cell carcinoma</u>
- <u>Intradermal melanocytic nevus</u>
- Milium
- Perifollicular fibroma
- Pyogenic granuloma
- Rhinophyma
- Seborrheic keratosis
- Syringoma
- Trichoblastoma
- Trichodiscoma
- Trichoepithelioma

Further reading:
- Lee AN, Stein SL, Cohen LM (2005) Clear cell fibrous papule with NKI/C3 expression: clinical and histologic features in six cases. Am J Dermatopathol 27(4):296–300

Fibroxanthoma, Atypical

Rapidly growing, malignant neoplasm possibly derived from the dermal dendrocyte that is seen in the elderly and characterized by an erythematous nodule with ulceration on the head and neck or other sun-exposed areas

Differential Diagnosis

- <u>Amelanotic melanoma</u>
- Basal cell carcinoma
- Cutaneous metastasis
- Dermatofibrosarcoma protuberans

- Leiomyosarcoma
- Merkel cell carcinoma
- Malignant fibrous histiocytoma
- Pyogenic granuloma
- Spindle cell neoplasm
- Squamous cell carcinoma

Further reading:
- Farley R, Ratner D (2006) Diagnosis and management of atypical fibroxanthoma. Skinmed 5(2):83–86

Filariasis, Lymphatic

Parasitic infestation of the lymphatic system with several filarial worms (most commonly *Wuchereria bancrofti*, *Brugia malayi*, and *Brugia timori*) that is characterized by chronic lymphedema, elephantiasis, and verrucous or papillomatosis skin changes

Differential Diagnosis

- Bacterial or fungal lymphadenitis
- Hydrocele
- Klippel–Trenaunay syndrome
- Leprosy
- Lymphogranuloma venereum
- Lymphedema-related elephantiasis
- Lymphoma
- Milroy disease
- Podoconiosis
- Traumatic lymphedema

Further reading:
- Melrose WD (2002) Lymphatic filariasis: new insights into an old disease. Int J Parasitol 32(8):947–960

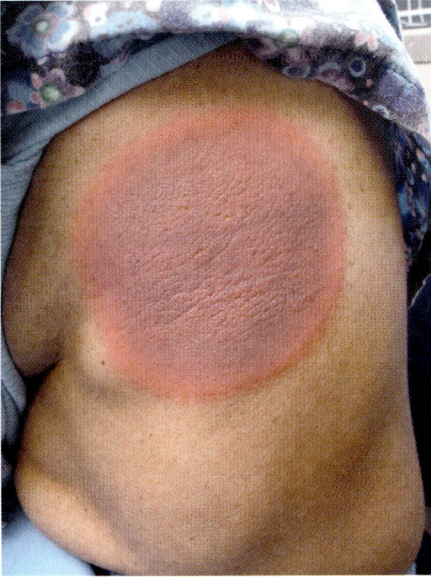

Fig. 6.38 Fixed drug eruption

Fixed Drug Eruption

Type of drug eruption that recurs in the same location upon re-exposure
to the causative agent and that is characterized by a solitary (or multiple)
erythematous patch, often on the genital or oral mucosa, that eventually
blisters, erodes, and, with withdrawal of the triggering medication, heals
with hyperpigmentation (Fig. 6.38)

Differential Diagnosis

- Arthropod-bite reaction
- Bullosis diabeticorum
- Bullous pemphigoid
- Cellulitis
- Chemical burn

- Contact dermatitis
- Eosinophilic ulcer of the tongue
- Erosive lichen planus
- Erythema dyschromicum perstans
- Erythema migrans
- Erythema multiforme
- Erythroplasia of Queyrat
- Factitial disease
- Herpes simplex virus infection
- Large plaque parapsoriasis
- Lichenoid drug eruption
- Lupus erythematosus
- Pityriasis rotunda
- Postinflammatory hyperpigmentation
- Psoriasis
- Pyoderma gangrenosum (superficial type)
- Spider bite
- Stevens–Johnson syndrome
- Zoon's balanitis

Associated Medications

- Acetaminophen
- Allopurinol
- Aspirin
- Barbiturates
- Ciprofloxacin
- Fluconazole
- Griseofulvin
- Hydrochlorothiazide
- Ketoconazole
- Metronidazole
- Naproxen/NSAIDs
- Phenolphthalein

- Pseudoephedrine
- <u>Sulfonamides</u>
- Terbinafine
- Tetracycline
- Trimethoprim

Treatment Options

- <u>Discontinuation of offending medication</u>
- Topical corticosteroids
- Systemic corticosteroids

Further reading:
- Sehgal VN, Srivastava G (2006) Fixed drug eruption (FDE): changing scenario of incriminating drugs. Int J Dermatol 45(8):897–908

Focal Dermal Hypoplasia (Goltz Syndrome)

X-linked dominant disorder of unknown cause that affects females and presents at birth with linear, reticulate, or whorled areas of dermal atrophy, telangiectasia and fat herniation, hypodontia, lobster-claw deformity, coloboma, raspberry-like papillomas in the periorificial areas, and osteopathia striata and other musculoskeletal deformities

Differential Diagnosis

- <u>Adams–Oliver syndrome</u>
- <u>Aplasia cutis congenita</u>
- Bart syndrome
- CHILD syndrome
- Congenital erosive and vesicular dermatosis
- Conradi–Hünermann–Happle syndrome
- EEC syndrome
- Goldenhar syndrome

- <u>Incontinentia pigmenti</u>
- <u>MIDAS syndrome</u>
- Nevus lipomatosus superficialis
- Oculocerebrocutaneous syndrome
- Proteus syndrome

Evaluation

- Ophthalmologic examination
- Skeletal survey
- CT/MRI scan of the brain

Further reading:
- Mianda SB, Delmaestro D, Bertoli R et al (2005) Focal dermal hypoplasia with exuberant fat herniations and skeletal deformities. Pediatr Dermatol 22(5):420–423

Fogo Selvagem (Endemic Pemphigus)

Endemic form of pemphigus foliaceus affecting young patients in Brazil that is possibly related to exposure to the *Simulium* black fly and is characterized by superficial vesicles, bullae, and crusts in a seborrheic distribution or occasionally a generalized distribution

Differential Diagnosis

- Atopic dermatitis
- Epidermolysis bullosa
- Erythema multiforme
- <u>Impetigo</u>
- Lupus erythematosus
- Necrolytic migratory erythema
- <u>Pemphigus vulgaris</u>
- <u>Seborrheic dermatitis</u>
- Subcorneal pustular dermatosis

Evaluation

- Direct immunofluorescence
- Antidesmoglein 1 and antidesmoglein 3 antibody titers

Treatment Options

- See Treatment Options of "Pemphigus"

Further reading:
- Rocha-Alvarez R, Ortega-Loayza AG, Friedman H et al (2007) Endemic pemphigus vulgaris. Arch Dermatol 143(7):895–899

Folliculitis

Inflammation of the hair follicle due to a variety of infectious and noninfectious causes that is characterized follicular erythematous papules and pustules

Subtypes/Variants

- Bacterial
- Candida
- Demodex
- Drug induced
- Eosinophilic
- Fungal
- Gram-negative
- Herpes simplex virus
- Hot tub
- Occlusion
- Perforating
- Pityrosporum
- Pseudolymphomatous folliculitis

- Staphylococcal folliculitis
- Steroid related

Differential Diagnosis

- <u>Acne vulgaris</u>
- Acquired perforating disease
- Acute graft-vs-host disease
- Darier's disease
- Disseminate and recurrent infundibulofolliculitis
- <u>Drug eruption (including acneiform eruptions)</u>
- Eruptive syringomas
- Eruptive vellus hair cysts
- <u>Follicular eczema</u>
- Follicular lichen planus
- Follicular mucinosis
- Folliculotropic mycosis fungoides
- <u>Grover's disease</u>
- Hailey–Hailey disease
- Halogenoderma
- Insect-bite reaction
- <u>Keratosis pilaris</u>
- Miliaria
- Pemphigus foliaceus
- Perioral dermatitis
- Pityriasis rubra pilaris
- Pseudofolliculitis barbae
- Rosacea
- Scabies

Further reading:
- Luelmo-Aguilar J, Santandreu MS (2004) Folliculitis: recognition and management. Am J Clin Dermatol 5(5):301–310

Folliculitis Decalvans (Quinquaud Disease)

Type of scarring alopecia possibly caused by staphylococcal infection of the scalp that is characterized by tender inflammatory plaques of hyperkeratosis, pustules, crusts, erosions, and tufting

Differential Diagnosis

- <u>Central centrifugal cicatricial alopecia</u>
- Cicatricial pemphigoid, Brunsting–Perry type
- <u>Dissecting cellulitis</u>
- Erosive pustular dermatosis of the scalp
- Favus
- <u>Keratosis follicularis spinulosa decalvans</u>
- Lichen planopilaris
- Lupus erythematosus
- Pemphigus foliaceus
- Pemphigus vulgaris
- <u>Tinea capitis, especially kerion</u>

Evaluation

- Bacterial and fungal culture of lesional tissue

Treatment Options

- <u>Systemic antibiotics</u>
- Topical antibiotics
- <u>Intralesional corticosteroids</u>
- Zinc sulfate
- Dapsone
- <u>Isotretinoin</u>
- Excision

Further reading:
- Brooke RC, Griffiths CE (2001) Folliculitis decalvans. Clin Exp Dermatol 26(1):120–122

Folliculitis, Hot Tub

Self-limited type of folliculitis caused most commonly by *Pseudomonas* spp. and characterized by discrete erythematous papules and pustules on the trunk and proximal extremities

Differential Diagnosis

- Acne vulgaris
- Contact dermatitis
- Eosinophilic folliculitis
- Grover's disease
- Insect bites, including bed bugs
- Majocchi granuloma
- Miliaria
- Papular urticaria
- Pityriasis lichenoides et varioliformis acuta
- Scabies
- Seabather's eruption
- Staphylococcal folliculitis
- Swimmer's itch

Treatment Options

- Observation and reassurance
- Fluoroquinolone antibiotics

Further reading:
- Yu Y, Cheng AS, Wang L et al (2007) Hot tub folliculitis or hot hand–foot syndrome caused by *Pseudomonas aeruginosa*. J Am Acad Dermatol 57(4):596–600

Foreign Body Granuloma

Persistent foreign body reaction to a variety of environmental substances that is characterized by a firm, erythematous to brown papule or nodule anywhere on the body

Differential Diagnosis

- <u>Dermatofibroma</u>
- <u>Epidermal inclusion cyst</u>
- Granuloma annulare
- Granuloma faciale
- Kerion
- Leprosy
- Lymphoma
- Phaeohyphomycosis cyst
- Ruptured cyst
- <u>Sarcoidosis</u>
- Sporotrichosis
- Tuberculosis

Associations

- Aluminum (vaccinations)
- Beryllium
- Cactus spines
- Calcinosis
- Coral fragments
- Corticosteroid injection
- Dermal filler substances
- Foreign collagen
- Gout
- Ingrown hair
- Jellyfish stings

- Keratin
- Paraffin
- Ruptured epidermoid cyst
- Ruptured follicle
- Sea urchin spines
- Silica
- Silicone
- Starch
- Suture material
- Suture
- Talc
- Tattoo pigment
- Thorns
- Tick mouth parts
- Wood splinter
- Zirconium

Further reading:

- Ghislanzoni M, Bianchi F, Barbareschi M, Alessi E (2006) Cutaneous granulomatous reaction to injectable hyaluronic acid gel. Br J Dermatol 154(4):755–758

Fox–Fordyce Disease (Apocrine Miliaria)

Chronic dermatosis related to obstruction of apocrine sweat ducts that affects the axillary and inguinal areas of young women and is characterized by pruritic monomorphous flesh-colored to erythematous papules

Differential Diagnosis

- Candidiasis
- Contact dermatitis
- Follicular hamartoma
- Folliculitis
- Granular parakeratosis

- Hidradenitis suppurativa
- Intertriginous xanthomas
- Lichen nitidus
- Lichen planus
- Milia
- Miliaria
- Pseudofolliculitis
- Pseudoxanthoma elasticum
- Syringomas

Treatment Options

- Topical steroids
- Oral contraceptive pills
- Topical clindamycin
- Topical retinoids
- Isotretinoin

Further reading:
- Ozcan A, Senol M, Aydin NE, Karaca S, Sener S (2003) Fox–Fordyce disease. J Eur Acad Dermatol Venereol 17(2):244–245

Friction Blisters

Intraepidermal blister caused by repeated frictional trauma to the skin

Differential Diagnosis

- Bullous amyloidosis
- Bullosis diabeticorum
- Callus
- Coma blister
- Contact dermatitis
- Dyshidrotic eczema

- Epidermolysis bullosa acquisita
- Epidermolysis bullosa simplex (especially Weber–Cockayne type)
- Pemphigus foliaceus
- Suction blister

Further reading:
- Mailler EA, Adams BB (2004) The wear and tear of 26.2: dermatological injuries reported on marathon day. Br J Sports Med 38(4):498–501

Frictional Lichenoid Dermatitis

Dermatosis affecting young boys that is probably caused by friction and characterized by scaly, grouped, flesh-colored papules most commonly located on the extensor extremities, especially around the elbows and knees

Differential Diagnosis

- Atopic dermatitis
- Gianotti–Crosti syndrome
- Lichen nitidus
- Lichen spinulosus
- Molluscum
- Pityriasis rubra pilaris (circumscribed type)
- Psoriasis
- Verruca plana

Treatment Options

- Topical corticosteroids
- Ammonium lactate
- Salicylic acid
- Glycolic acid
- Urea

Further reading:

- Serna MJ, Espana A, Idoate MA, Quintanilla E (1994) Lichenoid papular eruption in a child. Frictional lichenoid dermatitis of childhood (FLDC). Arch Dermatol 130(1):106–107, 109–110

Frontal Fibrosing Alopecia

Distinct clinical subtype of scarring alopecia that predominantly affects postmenopausal women, has the histologic features of lichen planopilaris, and is characterized by a band of alopecia with perifollicular erythema and eventual loss of follicles on the frontotemporal scalp, often with eyebrow involvement (Fig. 6.39)

Differential Diagnosis

- Actinic granuloma/annular elastolytic giant cell granuloma
- Alopecia areata (especially ophiasis type)
- Alopecia neoplastica
- Androgenetic alopecia
- Lupus erythematosus
- Sarcoidosis
- Traction alopecia

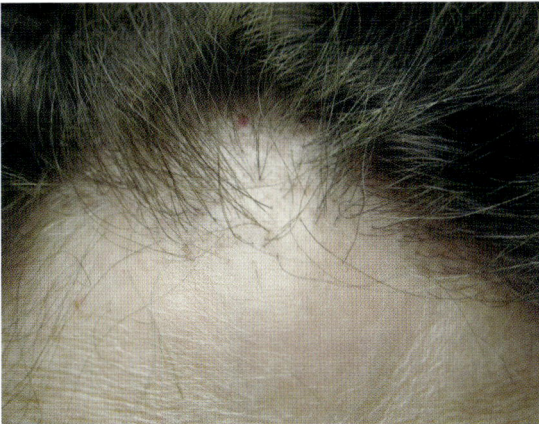

Fig. 6.39 Frontal fibrosing alopecia

Treatment Options

- See "Lichen Planopilaris"

Further reading:
- Conde Fernandes I, Selores M, Machado S (2011) Frontal fibrosing alopecia: a review of eleven patients. Eur J Dermatol 21(5):750–752

Frostbite

Most severe form of cold injury that is characterized by cold, firm and edematous, initially painless and later painful, cyanotic, or gangrenous skin changes with or without bullae

Differential Diagnosis

- Acrocyanosis
- Chilblains (pernio)
- Cold panniculitis
- Cryoglobulinemia
- Immersion foot syndromes
- Raynaud phenomenon
- Subcutaneous fat necrosis

Treatment Options

- Rapid rewarming
- Debridement of devitalized tissue

Further reading:
- Meffert JJ (1999) Environmental skin diseases and the impact of common dermatoses on medical readiness. Dermatol Clin 17(1):1–17

Furuncle/Carbuncle

Common type of cutaneous infection centered around a hair follicle that is most commonly caused by *Staphylococcus* and is characterized by a solitary (furuncle) or multiloculated (carbuncle) tender erythematous cutaneous abscess

Differential Diagnosis

- Atypical mycobacterium
- Bites
- Cystic acne
- Deep fungal infection
- Dental abscess
- Erythema nodosum
- Factitial disease
- Folliculitis
- Foreign body reaction
- Furuncular myiasis
- Hidradenitis suppurativa
- Inflamed epidermal inclusion cyst
- Kerion
- Leishmaniasis
- Metastatic disease
- Nocardiosis
- Panniculitis
- Phaeohyphomycosis cyst
- Ruptured pilar cyst
- Spider bite
- Syphilis
- Tuberculosis
- Tularemia
- Yaws

Associations

- Diabetes mellitus
- Immunodeficiency

Treatment Options

- <u>Incision and drainage</u>
- Antibiotics guided by sensitivity

Further reading:
- Sidwell RU, Ibrahim MA, Bunker CB (2002) A case of common variable immunodeficiency presenting with furunculosis. Br J Dermatol 147(2):364–367

Ganglion Cyst

Benign tumor arising from the periarticular soft tissue of the hand that is characterized by a firm, compressible, asymptomatic subcutaneous mass most commonly located on the dorsal wrist

Differential Diagnosis

- Aneurysm
- Arteriovenous malformations
- Arthritis
- Digital mucous cyst
- <u>Epidermoid inclusion cyst</u>
- Extensor digitorum brevis manus muscle
- Fibroma of the tendon sheath
- Foreign body granuloma
- <u>Giant cell tumor of the tendon sheath</u>
- Gouty tophus
- Lipoma
- Neurilemmoma

- Neuroma
- Nodular fasciitis
- <u>Rheumatoid nodule</u>
- Sarcoma

Further reading:
- Nahra ME, Bucchieri JS (2004) Ganglion cysts and other tumor related conditions of the hand and wrist. Hand Clin 20(3):249–260

Gardner Syndrome

Inherited syndrome (AD) caused by mutation of the APC tumor suppressor gene that is characterized by colonic polyposis with potential for colon carcinoma, desmoid tumors, epidermoid cysts, pilomatrixomas, osteomas of the jaw, and congenital hypertrophy of the pigmented retinal epithelium

Differential Diagnosis

- Cowden's disease
- <u>Familial adenomatous polyposis</u>
- Juvenile polyposis
- Muir–Torre syndrome
- Multiple epidermoid cysts
- Peutz–Jeghers syndrome
- Turcot syndrome

Evaluation

- Colonoscopy
- Ophthalmologic examination
- Radiography of the mandible and long bones
- Thyroid function test and ultrasound
- Appropriate cancer screening

Further reading:

- Herrmann SM, Adler YD, Schmidt-Petersen K et al (2003) The concomitant occurrence of multiple epidermal cysts, osteomas and thyroid gland nodules is not diagnostic for Gardner syndrome in the absence of intestinal polyposis: a clinical and genetic report. Br J Dermatol 149(4):877–883

Gardner–Diamond Syndrome (Autoerythrocyte Sensitization, Psychogenic Purpura)

Poorly understood, possibly factitial syndrome affecting women with psychiatric illness that is characterized by recurrent, spontaneous bruises on the extremities with preceding and concomitant pain and a variety of associated symptoms, including headache, gastrointestinal disturbance, and arthralgias

Differential Diagnosis

- Amyloidosis
- Bleeding disorder
- Child abuse
- Ehlers–Danlos syndrome
- Factitial disorder
- Henoch–Schonlein purpura
- Leukemia
- Solar purpura

Evaluation

- Antinuclear antibodies
- Bleeding time
- Complete blood count
- Prothrombin time and partial thromboplastin time
- Psychiatric evaluation

Further reading:

- Siddi GM, Montesu MA (2006) Gardner–Diamond syndrome. J Eur Acad Dermatol Venereol 20(6):736–737

Gaucher's Disease

Autosomal-recessive lysosomal storage disease with onset at any age that is caused by deficiency of acid beta-glucosidase and is characterized by a collodion membrane presentation (infantile type), bronze melasma-like pigmentation on the face and hands (adult type), symmetric hyperpigmentation on the lower legs, Erlenmeyer flask deformity of the femur and bone pain, pancytopenia, pinguecula, and progressive neurologic deterioration (infantile type)

Subtypes/Variants

- Type I – adult type
- Type II – infantile type
- Type III – juvenile type

Differential Diagnosis

- Addison's disease
- Adrenoleukodystrophy (Schilder's disease)
- Farber's disease
- Hemochromatosis
- Krabbe disease
- Niemann–Pick disease
- Neutral lipid storage disease
- Sjögren–Larsson disease
- Tay–Sachs disease

Evaluation

- Glucocerebrosidase activity study
- Complete blood count
- Liver function test
- Abdominal MRI
- Skeletal survey
- Bone marrow biopsy

Further reading:
- Holleran WM, Ziegler SG, Goker-Alpan O et al (2006) Skin abnormalities as an early predictor of neurologic outcome in Gaucher disease. Clin Genet 69(4):355–357

Geographic Tongue (Benign Migratory Glossitis)

Benign inflammatory disorder of the dorsal tongue possibly related to psoriasis that is characterized by serpiginous erythematous plaques devoid of filiform papillae with a yellow hyperkeratotic border

Differential Diagnosis

- Burns
- Candidiasis
- Contact stomatitis
- Eruptive lingual papillitis
- Herpetic geometric glossitis
- Lichen planus
- Lingua plicata
- Median rhomboid glossitis
- Syphilis

Associations

- AIDS
- Atopic dermatitis

- Fissured tongue
- Lithium therapy
- Psoriasis

Treatment Options

- Soothing mouthwashes
- Topical corticosteroids
- Fluconazole
- Topical retinoids
- Topical calcineurin inhibitors

Further reading:

- Zargari O (2006) The prevalence and significance of fissured tongue and geographical tongue in psoriatic patients. Clin Exp Dermatol 31(2):192–195

Gianotti–Crosti Syndrome (Papular Acrodermatitis of Childhood)

Self-limited childhood eruption caused by a variety of viruses, including EBV and hepatitis B, that is characterized by erythematous papules and papulovesicles on the face, buttocks, and extremities, but not the trunk (Fig. 6.40)

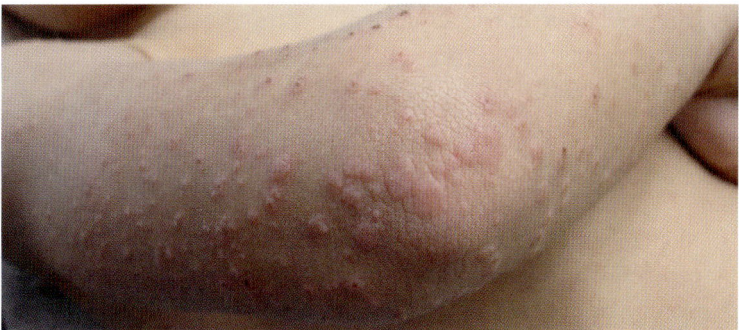

Fig. 6.40 Gianotti–Crosti syndrome

Differential Diagnosis

- Arthropod bites
- Atopic dermatitis
- Contact dermatitis
- Dermatophytosis
- Drug eruption
- Eruptive pseudoangiomatosis
- Erythema multiforme
- Frictional lichenoid dermatitis
- Granuloma annulare
- Henoch–Schonlein purpura
- Langerhans cell histiocytosis
- Lichen nitidus
- Lichen planus
- Lichen striatus
- Molluscum contagiosum
- Papular and purpuric gloves and socks syndrome
- Papular urticaria
- Pityriasis lichenoides
- Pityriasis rosea
- Polymorphous light eruption
- Sarcoidosis
- Scabies
- Unilateral laterothoracic exanthem
- Verruca plana
- Viral exanthem

Diagnostic Criteria

- Monomorphous, flat-topped, pink to red-brown papular or papulovesicular lesions 1–10 mm in diameter
- Symmetric distribution favoring cheeks, extensor surfaces of the extremities, and buttocks

- Lesions remain for at least 10 days
- Spares trunk and not scaly

Treatment Options

- Systemic corticosteroids
- Topical corticosteroids
- Oral antihistamines

Further reading:

- Brandt O, Abeck D, Gianotti R, Burgdorf W (2006) Gianotti–Crosti syndrome. J Am Acad Dermatol 54(1):136–145

Giant Cell Tumor of the Tendon Sheath

Benign tumor arising from the tendons of young adults that is characterized by a firm subcutaneous nodule most commonly located on the flexor tendons of the hand and wrist

Differential Diagnosis

- Calcifying aponeurotic fibroma
- Clear cell sarcoma
- Epithelioid sarcoma
- Fibroma of the tendon sheath
- Ganglion cyst
- Morton's neuroma
- Myxoid cyst
- Rheumatoid nodule
- Subcutaneous granuloma annulare

Further reading:

- Walsh EF, Mechrefe A, Akelman E, Schiller AL (2005) Giant cell tumor of tendon sheath. Am J Orthop 34(3):116–121

Glanders (Farcy)

Rare, potentially fatal, zoonotic infection affecting horse and donkey handlers or laboratory personnel that is caused by *Burkholderia mallei* and is characterized by multiple erythematous nodules along the lymphatics that ulcerate and drain a purulent exudate

Differential Diagnosis

- Anthrax
- Atypical mycobacteriosis
- Blastomycosis
- Brucellosis
- Coccidioidomycosis
- Melioidosis
- Nocardiosis
- Plague
- Sporotrichosis
- Tuberculosis
- Tularemia

Evaluation

- Gram stain and culture of blood and tissue
- Complement fixation test

Further reading:
- Lupi O, Madkan V, Tyring SK (2006) Tropical dermatology: bacterial tropical diseases. J Am Acad Dermatol 54(4):559–578

Glomangioma (Glomuvenous Malformation)

Type of vascular malformation associated with glomulin gene mutation that is present at birth, resembles a venous malformation, and is characterized by multiple, bluish, and hyperkeratotic, noncompressible, painful nodules predominantly located on the extremities (Fig. 6.41)

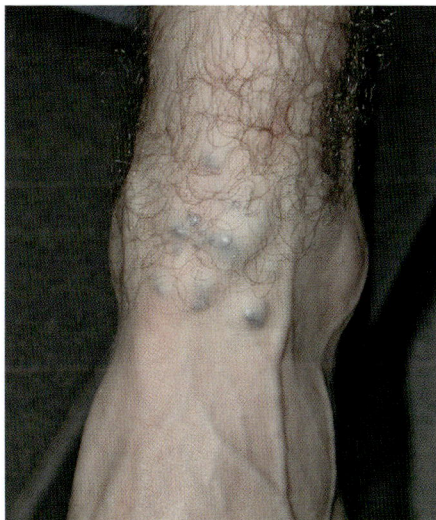

Fig. 6.41 Glomangiomas (Courtesy of K. Guidry)

Differential Diagnosis

- <u>Blue rubber bleb nevus</u>
- Glomus tumor
- Infantile hemangioma
- Maffucci syndrome
- Venous malformation

Further reading:
- Lu R, Krathen RA, Sanchez RL et al (2005) Multiple glomangiomas: potential for confusion with blue rubber bleb nevus syndrome. J Am Acad Dermatol 52(4):731–732

Glomus Tumor (Barre–Masson Syndrome)

Benign proliferation of glomus cells that is characterized by a small blue papule on the acral areas, typically the nail bed, and associated with cold-induced pain

Differential Diagnosis

- Angioleiomyoma
- Angiolipoma
- Arteriovenous malformation
- Blue nevus
- Blue rubber bleb nevus
- Hemangioma
- Kaposi's sarcoma
- Leiomyoma
- Maffucci syndrome
- Melanoma
- Neurilemmoma
- Spiradenoma
- Tufted angioma

Associations (Multiple)

- Neurofibromatosis I

Further reading:
- D'Acri AM, Ramos-e-Silva M, Basilio-de-Oliveira C et al (2002) Multiple glomus tumors: recognition and diagnosis. Skinmed 1(2):94–98

Glomeruloid Hemangioma

Benign, reactive vascular proliferation associated with POEMS syndrome and Castleman's disease that is characterized by multiple red angioma-like papules on the trunk or proximal extremities

Differential Diagnosis

- Cherry angiomas
- Dabska's tumor

- Intravascular papillary endothelial hyperplasia
- Intravascular pyogenic granuloma
- <u>Microvenular hemangioma</u>
- Multinucleate cell angiohistiocytoma
- Tufted angioma

Evaluation (for POEMS)

- Serum/urinary protein electrophoresis
- Endocrine evaluation
- Complete blood count
- Cerebrospinal fluid examination
- Skeletal survey
- Bone marrow biopsy (if myeloma is suspected)
- Lymph node biopsy (if Castleman's disease is suspected)
- Nerve conduction studies

Further reading:

- Phillips JA, Dixon JE, Richardson JB et al (2006) Glomeruloid hemangioma leading to a diagnosis of POEMS syndrome. J Am Acad Dermatol 55(1):149–152

Gonococcemia

Bacteremia with *Neisseria gonorrhea* that predominantly affects women and is characterized by fever, arthralgias, acral hemorrhagic pustules, and, if untreated, septic arthritis and other systemic complications

Differential Diagnosis

- Bowel bypass dermatitis–arthritis syndrome
- Candidemia
- Cryoglobulinemia
- <u>Infective endocarditis</u>
- Lupus erythematosus

- Lyme disease
- Meningococcemia
- Polyarteritis nodosa
- Rat-bite fever
- Reactive arthritis
- Rheumatic fever
- Rheumatoid arthritis
- <u>Rickettsial diseases</u>
- <u>Septic vasculitis</u>
- Syphilis
- Typhoid fever

Associations

- Pregnancy
- Menstruation
- HIV infection
- Systemic lupus erythematosus

Evaluation

- Gram stain and culture (with antibiotic sensitivity) of urethra, cervix, joint fluid, and blood
- Joint-fluid studies

Further reading:
- Mehrany K, Kist JM, O'Connor WJ, Dicaudo DJ (2003) Disseminated gonococcemia. Int J Dermatol 42(3):208–209

Gout, Chronic Tophaceous

Chronic form of gout characterized by the deposition of urate crystals in the joints and skin, which appears to have firm, erythematous to yellow nodules most commonly of the helix of the ear but also the hands, feet, and elbows

Differential Diagnosis

- <u>Calcinosis cutis</u>
- Chondrodermatitis nodularis helicis
- Erythema elevatum diutinum
- Foreign body granuloma
- Granuloma annulare
- Heberden's nodes
- Multicentric reticulohistiocytosis
- Pilomatrixoma
- <u>Rheumatoid nodule</u>
- Sarcoidosis
- Weathering nodule
- <u>Xanthoma</u>

Associations

- Acidosis
- Alcohol ingestion
- Dehydration
- Diuretics
- Drugs
- Hemodialysis
- <u>High-purine diet</u>
- Hypothyroidism
- Idiopathic
- Lead poisoning
- Lesch–Nyhan syndrome
- Leukemia
- Lymphoma
- Obesity
- Psoriasis
- Renal failure
- Tumor lysis syndrome

Evaluation

- Serum uric acid level
- Renal function test
- Urinalysis
- Joint-fluid examination
- Radiography of affected joints

Further reading:
- Falasca GF (2006) Metabolic diseases: gout. Clin Dermatol 24(6):498–508

Graft-vs-Host Disease

Common complication of bone marrow transplant that is caused by his-toincompatible donor lymphocytes reacting against epithelial tissues and characterized by an early acute phase (first 100 days), which manifests cutaneously as a follicular-based erythematous eruption that begins acrally and a later chronic phase, which is characterized by lichen-planus-like lesions or sclerodermoid skin changes

Differential Diagnosis

Acute
- Acute radiation dermatitis
- Chemotherapy-induced acral erythema
- Chemotherapy-related reaction
- Contact dermatitis
- Eruption of lymphocytic recovery
- Erythema multiforme (especially radiation related)
- Lupus erythematosus
- Morbilliform drug eruption
- Necrolytic acral erythema
- Paraneoplastic pemphigus
- Staphylococcal scalded-skin syndrome

- Thymoma
- Toxic epidermal necrolysis
- <u>Viral exanthem</u>

Chronic Lichenoid

- Lichenoid drug eruption
- <u>Lichen planus</u>
- Lichen sclerosus et atrophicus
- Lupus erythematosus
- Paraneoplastic pemphigus
- Pityriasis lichenoides chronica
- <u>Pseudoporphyria (esp. voriconazole)</u>

Chronic Sclerodermoid

- <u>Lichen sclerosus et atrophicus</u>
- <u>Morphea</u>
- Porphyria cutanea tarda
- Progressive systemic sclerosis
- <u>Pseudoporphyria (esp. voriconazole)</u>
- Sclerodermatous drug reaction (e.g., bleomycin)

Evaluation

- Liver function tests
- Serum chemistry
- Complete blood count

Treatment Options

- Acute
  - <u>Systemic corticosteroids</u>
  - Cyclosporine
  - <u>Tacrolimus</u>
  - Mycophenolate mofetil

- — <u>Sirolimus</u>
- — Antithymocyte globulin
- — Extracorporeal photochemotherapy
- — Infliximab
- Chronic
  - — <u>Tacrolimus</u>
  - — Mycophenolate mofetil
  - — Thalidomide
  - — Acitretin
  - — Hydroxychloroquine
  - — Infliximab
  - — Extracorporeal photochemotherapy
  - — UVB phototherapy
  - — <u>UVA1 phototherapy</u>

Further reading:

- Schaffer JV (2006) The changing face of graft-versus-host disease. Semin Cutan Med Surg 25(4):190–200

Graham–Little–Piccardi–Lasseur Syndrome

Uncommon idiopathic lichenoid dermatosis characterized by lichen planopilaris of the scalp, nonscarring alopecia of the axilla and groin, and follicular lichen planus of the trunk, with or without a history of classic lichen planus

Differential Diagnosis

- Cutaneous T cell lymphoma
- Discoid lupus erythematosus
- Folliculitis decalvans
- <u>Lichenoid drug reaction</u>
- Lichen planus
- Keratosis follicularis spinulosa decalvans

- Pityriasis rubra pilaris
- Sarcoidosis

Treatment Options

- See "Lichen Planus"

Further reading:
- Srivastava M, Mikkilineni R, Konstadt J (2007) Lasseur–Graham–Little–Piccardi syndrome. Dermatol Online J 13(1):12

Gram-Negative Toe-Web Infection

Gram-negative bacterial infection of the toe-web spaces that is character-ized by inflammation (can be quite severe), desquamation, pustules, ero-sions, and maceration affecting the toe-web spaces and neighboring areas

Differential Diagnosis

- <u>Allergic contact dermatitis</u>
- Bullosis diabeticorum
- Bullous drug eruption
- Candidiasis
- Epidermolysis bullosa (especially Weber–Cockayne type)
- Erythrasma
- Juvenile plantar dermatosis
- Immersion foot
- <u>Interdigital tinea pedis (especially bullous type)</u>
- Intertrigo
- Necrolytic acral erythema
- Pitted keratolysis
- <u>Pompholyx</u>

Evaluation

- Potassium hydroxide preparation and fungal culture
- Gram stain and culture of tissue

Treatment Options

- <u>Systemic antibiotics</u>
- <u>Systemic corticosteroids</u>
- Topical antibiotics
- Topical antifungals
- Systemic antifungals
- Vinegar and water soaks

Further reading:
- Aste N, Atzori L, Zucca M et al (2001) Gram-negative bacterial toe web infection: a survey of 123 cases from the district of Cagliari, Italy. J Am Acad Dermatol 45(4):537–541

Granular Cell Tumor (Abrikossoff Tumor)

Benign neural tumor (with a malignant counterpart) arising predominantly in adults, especially adults of African descent, that is characterized by a solitary, smooth, or verrucous papule or nodule on the head and neck, especially the tongue, or, less commonly, other areas of the body

Differential Diagnosis

Cutaneous

- Adnexal tumor
- Compound nevi
- Condyloma acuminatum

- Dermatofibroma
- Epidermal inclusion cyst
- Fibroma
- Neurofibroma
- Squamous cell carcinoma
- Verruca
- Verrucous carcinoma

Oral
- Ameloblastoma
- Congenital epulis
- Fibroma
- Foreign body granuloma
- Odontogenic cyst
- Neurofibroma
- Warty dyskeratoma
- Verruciform xanthoma

Associations (Multiple)

- Phacomatosis pigmentovascularis, type III

Further reading:
- Tomson N, Abdullah A, Tan CY (2006) Multiple granular cell tumors in a child with growth retardation. Report of a case and review of the literature. Int J Dermatol 45(11):1358–1361

Granular Parakeratosis

Idiopathic dermatosis that affects the axilla and less commonly the inguinal folds and that is characterized by hyperkeratotic, hyperpigmented papules and plaques (Fig. 6.42)

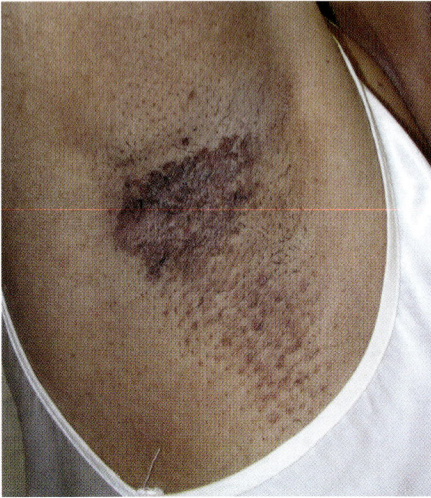

Fig. 6.42 Granular parakeratosis
(Courtesy of A. Record)

Differential Diagnosis

- Acanthosis nigricans
- Contact dermatitis
- Confluent and reticulated papillomatosis
- Darier's disease
- Dermatophytosis
- Erythrasma
- Fox–Fordyce disease
- Hailey–Hailey disease
- Intertrigo
- Pemphigus vegetans
- Psoriasis inversa
- Seborrheic keratosis

Treatment Options

- Topical corticosteroids
- Topical vitamin D analogues

- Topical retinoids
- Ammonium lactate
- Tacrolimus ointment
- Cryotherapy
- Curettage

Further reading:
- Scheinfeld N et al (2005) Granular parakeratosis: pathologic and clinical correlation of 18 cases of granular parakeratosis. J Am Acad Dermatol 52:863–867

Granulocytic Sarcoma (Chloroma)

Tumor of immature granulocytes that is associated with myelogenous leukemia and is characterized by solitary or multiple violaceous (and less commonly, green) nodules or plaques on the head and neck or trunk

Differential Diagnosis

- Extramedullary hematopoiesis
- Lymphoma
- Neuroblastoma
- Mastocytoma
- Melanoma
- Merkel cell carcinoma
- Metastatic carcinoma
- Rhabdomyosarcoma
- Sweet's syndrome

Evaluation

- Bone marrow biopsy
- Complete blood count

Further reading:

- Beswick SJ, Jones EL, Mahendra P, Marsden JR (2002) Chloroma (aleukaemic leukaemia cutis) initially diagnosed as cutaneous lymphoma. Clin Exp Dermatol 27(4):272–274

Granuloma Annulare

Idiopathic dermatosis with a variable clinical presentation in both children and adults that is characterized by annular arrangements of erythematous dermal papules (or less commonly, subcutaneous nodules) that are localized to the extensor surfaces of the extremities or in a more generalized distribution (Fig. 6.43)

Subtypes

- Plaque
- Patch
- Subcutaneous

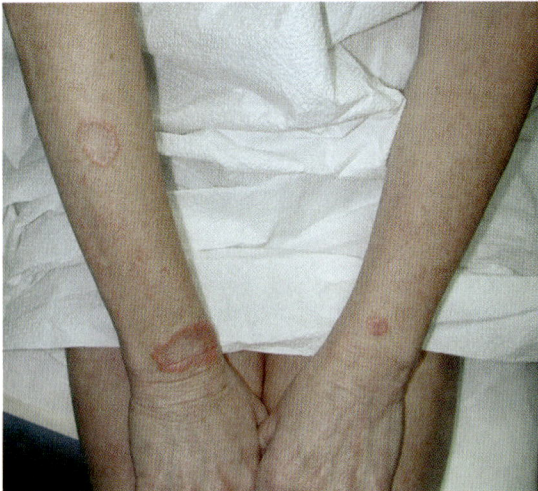

Fig. 6.43 Granuloma annulare (Courtesy of K. Guidry)

- Acute-onset painful acral
- Disseminated papular
- Perforating

Differential Diagnosis

- Acquired perforating dermatosis
- <u>Actinic granuloma</u>
- Annular lichen planus
- Arthropod bites
- Deep morphea
- Dermatofibroma
- Drug eruption
- Elastosis perforans serpiginosa
- <u>Epithelioid sarcoma</u>
- <u>Erythema annulare centrifugum, deep type</u>
- Erythema elevatum diutinum
- Erythema migrans
- Frictional lichenoid dermatitis
- Granuloma multiforme
- Granulomatous mycosis fungoides
- Granulomatous skin lesions associated with systemic lymphoma
- Immunodeficiency-related noninfectious granuloma
- Insect-bite reactions
- <u>Interstitial granulomatous dermatitis with arthritis</u>
- <u>Interstitial granulomatous drug reaction</u>
- Kaposi's sarcoma
- Keratoacanthoma
- Knuckle pads
- Lennert's lymphoma
- Leprosy
- Lichen myxedematosus
- Lichen planus
- Lichenoid drug reaction

- Lipoma
- Lupus erythematosus
- Lyme disease
- Metastatic disease
- Molluscum contagiosum
- Multinucleate cell angiohistiocytoma
- *Mycobacterium marinum* infection
- Necrobiosis lipoidica
- Nodular amyloidosis
- Nodular fasciitis
- Nodular syphilis
- Non-X-type histiocytoses
- Palisaded neutrophilic and granulomatous dermatitis
- Papular sarcoidosis
- Reactive perforating collagenosis
- Rheumatic fever nodules
- Rheumatoid neutrophilic dermatosis
- Rheumatoid nodules
- Sarcoidosis
- Secondary syphilis
- Subcutaneous sarcoidosis
- Tertiary syphilis
- Tinea
- Tuberculosis
- Xanthomas

Associations

- Allopurinol
- Amlodipine
- Autoimmune thyroiditis
- Diabetes mellitus
- Hepatitis B vaccine
- Herpes zoster scars

- HIV
- Hodgkin's disease
- <u>Hyperlipidemia</u>
- Necrobiosis lipoidica
- Non-Hodgkin's lymphoma
- Tetanus vaccination
- Thyroid disease

Treatment Options

- Topical corticosteroids
- <u>Intralesional corticosteroids</u>
- Topical calcineurin inhibitors
- Dapsone
- Isotretinoin
- Cyclosporine
- <u>Hydroxychloroquine</u>
- <u>Pentoxifylline</u>
- <u>Nicotinamide</u>
- Infliximab
- Etanercept
- Adalimumab

Further reading:
- Kovich O, Burgin S (2005) Generalized granuloma annulare. Dermatol Online J 11(4):23

Granuloma Faciale

Uncommon idiopathic dermatosis affecting predominantly the face of middle-aged patients that is characterized by solitary or multiple erythematous to brown papules, nodules, or plaques with patulous follicles (Fig. 6.44)

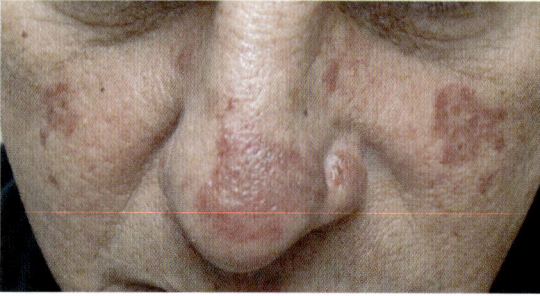

Fig. 6.44 Granuloma faciale

Differential Diagnosis

- Angiolymphoid hyperplasia with eosinophilia
- Basal cell carcinoma
- Cutaneous lymphoid hyperplasia
- Cutaneous Rosai–Dorfman disease
- Discoid lupus erythematosus
- Erythema elevatum diutinum
- Fixed drug eruption
- Follicular mucinosis
- Foreign body granuloma
- Granulomatous rosacea
- Jessner's lymphocytic infiltrate
- Leprosy
- Lupus vulgaris
- Lymphoma
- Rhinophyma
- Sarcoidosis
- Syphilis
- Sweet's syndrome
- Tumid lupus

Association

- Angiocentric eosinophilic fibrosis

Treatment Options

- Topical corticosteroids
- Intralesional corticosteroids
- Topical tacrolimus
- Dapsone
- Pulsed dye laser

Further reading:
- Ortonne N et al (2005) Granuloma faciale: a clinicopathologic study of 66 patients. J Am Acad Dermatol 53:1002–1009

Granuloma Gluteale Infantum

Uncommon, multifactorial dermatosis affecting infants with concomitant diaper dermatitis that is characterized by erythematous or violaceous papules and nodules in the skin folds of the groin and perineum and, occasionally, the neck

Differential Diagnosis

- Candidiasis
- Cold abscesses
- Contact dermatitis
- Folliculitis
- Foreign body granuloma
- Furunculosis
- Halogenoderma
- Jacquet's erosive diaper dermatitis
- Juvenile xanthogranuloma
- Langerhans cell histiocytosis
- Lymphoma
- Mastocytosis
- Molluscum contagiosum
- Nodular scabies

- Pseudoverrucous papules and nodules
- Pyogenic granuloma
- Sarcoma
- Syphilis
- Tuberculosis

Associations

- Candidiasis
- Fluorinated steroids
- Irritation and maceration

Treatment Options

- Observation and reassurance
- Discontinuation of topical steroids
- Anticandidal therapy

Further reading:

- Robson KJ, Maugham JA, Purcell SD (2006) Erosive papulonodular dermatosis associated with topical benzocaine: a report of two cases and evidence that granuloma gluteale, pseudoverrucous papules, and Jacquet's erosive dermatitis are a disease spectrum. J Am Acad Dermatol 55(5 Suppl):S74–S80

Granuloma Inguinale (Donovanosis)

Tropical bacterial infection that is possibly transmitted sexually, caused by *Klebsiella granulomatis*, and characterized by painful genital ulcers with beefy-red granulation tissue and lymphedema that have the potential to evolve to squamous cell carcinoma in long-standing cases

Differential Diagnosis

- Amebiasis
- Chancriform pyoderma
- Chancroid

- <u>Chronic herpes simplex virus infection</u>
- Condylomata lata
- Crohn's disease
- Leishmaniasis
- Lymphogranuloma venereum
- Lichen sclerosus
- Pyoderma gangrenosum
- Scrofuloderma
- <u>Squamous cell carcinoma</u>
- Syphilis
- Tuberculosis

Evaluation

- Tissue crush examination with Wright stain (Donovan bodies)

Further reading:

- Lupi O, Madkan V, Tyring SK (2006) Tropical dermatology: bacterial tropical diseases. J Am Acad Dermatol 54(4):559–578

Granuloma Multiforme (of Leiker)

Idiopathic granulomatous disease predominantly diagnosed in Africa that is characterized by indurated papules that evolve to large annular plaques with central hypopigmentation on the arms and upper trunk

Differential Diagnosis

- Actinic granuloma
- Annular elastolytic giant cell granuloma
- Annular lichenoid dermatitis of youth
- Annular syphilis
- <u>Granuloma annulare</u>
- <u>Leprosy (especially tuberculoid type)</u>
- Lupus vulgaris

- Necrobiosis lipoidica
- Pinta
- <u>Sarcoidosis</u>
- Yaws

Further reading:

- Sandhu K, Saraswat A, Gupta S, Shukla R, Handa S (2004) Granuloma multiforme. Int J Dermatol 43(6):441–443

Granulomatous Drug Reaction, Interstitial

Type of drug reaction characterized by granuloma-annulare-like skin lesions with a predilection for the flexural areas, trunk, and extremities, but not the face

Differential Diagnosis

- Cutaneous T cell lymphoma
- Dermatomyositis
- Eczema
- Erythema annulare centrifugum
- <u>Granuloma annulare</u>
- Granulomatous mycosis fungoides
- <u>Interstitial granulomatous dermatitis with arthritis</u>
- Lichen planus
- Pigmented purpura
- Pityriasis rosea
- <u>Sarcoidosis</u>
- Subacute cutaneous lupus erythematosus

Associated Medications

- ACE inhibitors
- Allopurinol

- Anticonvulsants
- Antidepressants
- Antihistamines
- Calcium channel blockers
- Diuretics
- Gold
- Lipid-lowering agents
- NSAIDs
- Sennoside
- Soy

Treatment Options

- Discontinuation of offending medication

Further reading:
- Magro CM, Crowson AN, Schapiro BL (1998) The interstitial granulomatous drug reaction: a distinctive clinical and pathological entity. J Cutan Pathol 25(2):72–78

Granulomatous Periorificial Dermatitis (Facial Afro-Caribbean Childhood Eruption (FACE), Facial Idiopathic Granulomas with Regressive Evolution)

Idiopathic eruption affecting children, especially children of African descent, that is characterized by tiny erythematous papules around the mouth, nose, and eyes

Differential Diagnosis

- Benign cephalic histiocytosis
- Eruptive milia
- Granulomatous rosacea
- Lupus miliaris disseminata faciei
- Perioral dermatitis

- Sarcoidosis
- Syringomas
- Tinea incognito

Treatment Options

- Topical metronidazole
- <u>Tacrolimus ointment</u>
- Topical erythromycin
- Oral erythromycin
- Tetracycline antibiotics

Further reading:
- Kroshinsky D, Glick SA (2006) Pediatric rosacea. Dermatol Ther 19(4):196–201

Granulomatous Slack Skin

Clinical variant of cutaneous T cell lymphoma that is characterized by atrophic, redundant, pendulous plaques in the axilla and groin

Differential Diagnosis

- Anetoderma
- <u>Cutis laxa</u>
- <u>Granulomatous mycosis fungoides</u>
- Pseudoxanthoma elasticum
- Steroid atrophy
- Striae atrophicans

Treatment Options

- See "Lymphoma, Cutaneous T Cell"

Further reading:
- Teixeira M, Alves R, Lima M et al (2007) Granulomatous slack skin. Eur J Dermatol 17(5):435–438

Granulosis Rubra Nasi

Rare familial dermatosis affecting children that resolves by puberty and is characterized by hyperhidrosis, miliaria, and erythema of the central face, especially the tip of the nose

Differential Diagnosis

- Acne
- Erythrosis pigmentosa peribuccalis
- Keratosis pilaris rubra
- Lupus erythematosus
- Lupus pernio
- Miliaria
- Perioral dermatitis
- Perniosis
- Photosensitivity
- Rosacea

Associations

- Pheochromocytoma

Treatment Options

- Observation and reassurance

Further reading:
- Akhdari N (2007) Granulosis rubra nasi. Int J Dermatol 46(4):396

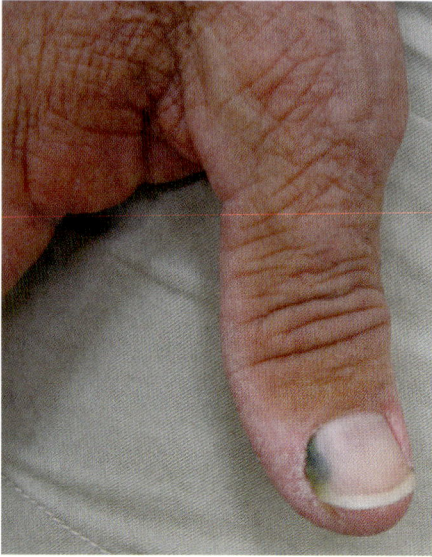

Fig. 6.45 *Pseudomonas* green-nail syndrome

Green-Nail Syndrome

Nail disorder caused by bacterial overgrowth of the nail unit with *Pseudomonas aeruginosa* that is characterized by onycholysis and greenish discoloration of the nail (Fig. 6.45)

Differential Diagnosis

- *Aspergillus* infection
- Dermatosis neglecta
- Foreign body
- Melanocytic nevus
- Melanoma
- Onychomycosis
- Subungual hematoma
- Subungual wart

Treatment Options

- <u>Topical gentamicin</u>
- Identify and treat underlying nail bed disease, such as wart
- Systemic fluoroquinolones
- <u>Vinegar and water soaks</u>
- Nail avulsion

Further reading:
- Sakata S, Howard A (2007) *Pseudomonas chloronychia* in a patient with nail psoriasis. Med J Aust 186(8):424

Griscelli Syndrome

Autosomal-recessive disorder caused by defects in the gene encoding the melanosomal transport proteins myosin Va (also known as Elejalde syndrome) or RAB27A that is characterized by partial albinism with silvery hair and either immunodeficiency with hemophagocytic syndrome (RAB27A) or severe neurologic and psychomotor symptoms (myosin Va)

Differential Diagnosis

- <u>Chediak–Higashi syndrome</u>
- Chronic granulomatous disease
- Familial hematophagocytic lymphohistiocytosis
- Hermansky–Pudlak syndrome
- <u>Oculocutaneous albinism</u>
- Phenylketonuria
- Wiskott–Aldrich syndrome
- X-linked lymphoproliferative syndrome (Duncan's disease)

Further reading:
- Emanuel PO, Sternberg LJ, Phelps RG (2007) Griscelli syndrome. Skinmed 6(3):147–149

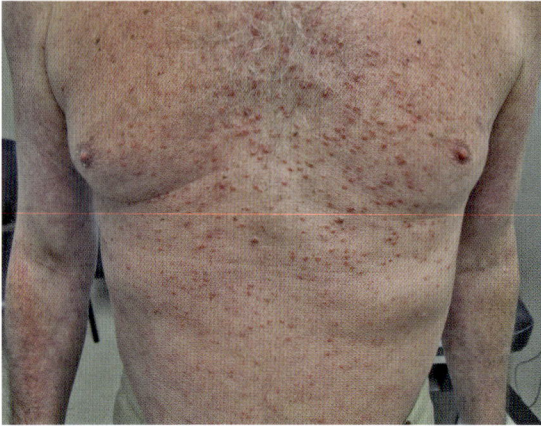

Fig. 6.46 Grover's disease

Grover's Disease (Transient Acantholytic Dermatosis)

Idiopathic acantholytic disease that predominantly affects older men and is characterized by a chronic, heat-exacerbated eruption of pruritic papulovesicles on the upper chest and shoulder area (Fig. 6.46)

Subtypes (Histologic)

- Benign familial pemphigus type
- Darier's disease type
- Pemphigus foliaceus type
- Pemphigus vulgaris type
- Spongiotic type

Differential Diagnosis

- Allergic contact dermatitis
- Asteatotic eczema
- Bullous pemphigoid

- Darier's disease
- Disseminate and recurrent infundibulofolliculitis
- Dermatitis herpetiformis
- Drug eruption
- Eczema herpeticum
- Familial dyskeratotic comedones
- <u>Folliculitis</u>
- <u>Galli–Galli disease</u>
- Hailey–Hailey disease
- Herpes simplex virus infection
- Insect bites
- <u>Miliaria rubra</u>
- Nummular eczema
- <u>Papular eczema</u>
- Papular urticaria
- Parapsoriasis
- Pemphigus foliaceus
- Pityriasis lichenoides et varioliformis acuta
- Pityriasis rosea
- Pityrosporum folliculitis
- Psoriasis
- Retiform parapsoriasis
- Scabies
- Secondary syphilis
- Subacute prurigo
- Tinea corporis
- Urticaria

Associations

- Asteatotic eczema
- Atopic dermatitis
- Chemotherapeutic agents

Treatment Options

- <u>Topical corticosteroids</u>
- <u>Systemic corticosteroids</u>
- <u>Tetracycline antibiotics</u>
- Antihistamines
- Isotretinoin
- Acitretin
- Methotrexate

Further reading:
- Davis MD, Dinneen AM, Landa N, Gibson LE (1999) Grover's disease: clinicopathologic review of 72 cases. Mayo Clin Proc 74(3):229–234

Hailey–Hailey Disease (Familial Benign Pemphigus)

Inherited disorder (AD) that is caused by a mutation in the gene (ATP2C1) encoding the epidermal calcium pump (hSPCA1) and is characterized by chronic, recurrent vesicles and erosions predominantly affecting the flexures that are made worse or triggered by bacterial and candidal super-infection, maceration, occlusion, moisture, and heat (Fig. 6.47)

Differential Diagnosis

- Acantholytic dyskeratosis of the vulva
- Atopic dermatitis
- <u>Candidiasis</u>
- Darier's disease
- Extramammary Paget's disease
- Granular parakeratosis
- Herpes simplex virus infection
- Impetigo
- <u>Intertrigo</u>
- Inverse psoriasis
- <u>Irritant dermatitis</u>

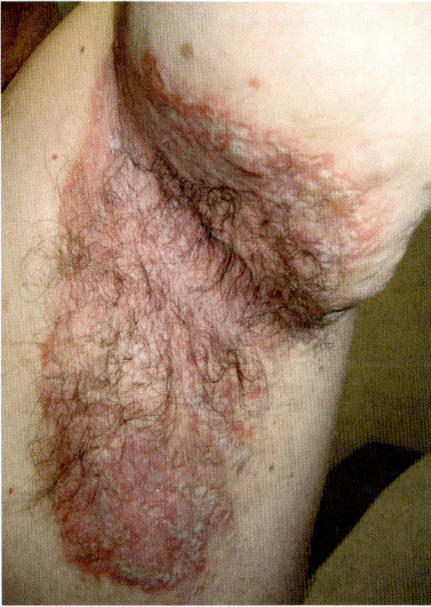

Fig. 6.47 Hailey–Hailey disease

- Lichen simplex chronicus
- Necrolytic migratory erythema
- Pemphigus foliaceus
- Pemphigus vegetans
- Pemphigus vulgaris
- Seborrheic dermatitis
- Tinea cruris

Evaluation

- Viral, bacterial, and fungal cultures of lesional tissue

Treatment Options

- Oral antibiotics
- Oral anticandidal therapy

- Topical corticosteroids
- Topical calcineurin inhibitors
- Dapsone
- Systemic corticosteroids
- Systemic retinoids
- Cyclosporine
- CO_2 laser

Further reading:
- Mckibben J, Smalling C (2006) Hailey–Hailey. Skinmed 5(5):250–252

Halo Nevus (Sutton's Nevus, Leukoderma Acquisitum Centrifugum)

Benign melanocytic nevus that develops an antimelanocyte lymphocytic infiltrate and is characterized by a typical nevus with or without signs of regression and a peripheral halo of hypopigmentation or depigmentation (Fig. 6.48)

Differential Diagnosis

- Atypical melanocytic nevi
- Cutaneous T cell lymphoma
- Dermatofibromas
- Lichen planus
- Melanoma
- Molluscum contagiosum
- Meyerson's nevus
- Nevus en cocarde
- Psoriasis
- Sarcoidosis
- Seborrheic keratoses
- Spitz nevi

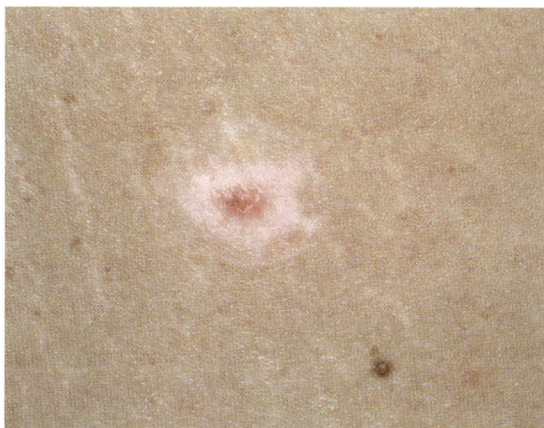

Fig. 6.48 Halo nevus (Courtesy of K. Guidry)

Associations

- Melanoma
- Turner syndrome
- <u>Vitiligo</u>

Evaluation

- Total body skin examination (for melanoma)

Further reading:

- Brazzelli V, Larizza D, Martinetti M et al (2004) Halo nevus, rather than vitiligo, is a typical dermatologic finding of Turner's syndrome: clinical, genetic, and immunogenetic study in 72 patients. J Am Acad Dermatol 51(3):354–358

Halogenoderma (Iododerma, Bromoderma)

Cutaneous eruption associated with the ingestion or administration of iodide-, bromide-, or fluoride-containing products that is characterized by vesiculopustular, vegetating, and ulcerative lesions on the face, trunk, or extremities

Differential Diagnosis

- Blastomycosis
- Chronic mucocutaneous candidiasis
- <u>Drug-induced acne</u>
- Erythema nodosum
- Folliculitis
- Multiple granular cell tumors
- Multiple keratoacanthoma
- Mycosis fungoides (tumoral or verrucous type)
- <u>Neutrophilic eccrine hidradenitis</u>
- <u>Pemphigus vegetans</u>
- Pyoderma gangrenosum, vegetative type
- Rosacea
- Sarcoidosis
- <u>Sweet's syndrome</u>
- Syphilitic gumma
- Tuberculosis

Evaluation

- Serum iodine and bromine levels

Further reading:
- Anzai S, Fujiwara S, Inuzuka M (2003) Bromoderma. Int J Dermatol 42(5):370–371

Hand–Foot–Mouth Disease

Common, benign enteroviral infection affecting children and characterized by vesicles that first arise on the palate, gingiva, buccal mucosa, and tongue and then later involve the edges of the palms and soles

Differential Diagnosis

- Acropustulosis of infancy
- Aphthous ulcers
- Dyshidrotic eczema
- Erythema multiforme
- Gonococcemia
- Herpangina
- Herpes stomatitis
- Reiter's syndrome
- Varicella
- Secondary syphilis

Further reading:
- Scott LA, Stone MS (2003) Viral exanthems. Dermatol Online J 9(3):4

Harlequin Ichthyosis (Riecke Syndrome)

Inherited (AR) ichthyosis that is associated with an ABCA12 gene defect and is characterized by severe, armor-plate-like hyperkeratosis, markedly distorted facial features with ectropion and eclabium, low birth weight, and early death or stillbirth

Differential Diagnosis

- Collodion baby (see Chap. 3)
- Neu–Laxova syndrome
- Restrictive dermopathy

Further reading:
- Akiyama M (2006) Pathomechanisms of harlequin ichthyosis and ABCA transporters in human diseases. Arch Dermatol 142(7):914–918

Hartnup Disease

Inherited metabolic disorder (AR) caused by a mutation in the SLC6A19 gene encoding a tryptophan transporter that results in decreased amounts of available tryptophan and episodes of photodistributed dermatitis, diarrhea, ataxia, and nystagmus

Differential Diagnosis

- <u>Actinic prurigo</u>
- Ataxia–telangiectasia
- Atopic dermatitis
- Carcinoid syndrome
- Cockayne syndrome
- Hydroa vacciniforme
- <u>Lupus erythematosus</u>
- <u>Pellagra</u>
- Phenylketonuria
- <u>Porphyria</u>
- Seborrheic dermatitis
- Xeroderma pigmentosum

Evaluation

- Urinary amino acid analysis

Further reading:
- Seyhan ME, Selimoglu MA, Ertekin V et al (2006) Acrodermatitis enteropathica-like eruptions in a child with Hartnup disease. Pediatr Dermatol 23(3):262–265

Hemangioendothelioma, Epithelioid

Low-grade angiosarcoma that arises in adolescents and young adults and is characterized by a slow-growing deep nodule or mass on the distal extremities

Differential Diagnosis

- Angiolymphoid hyperplasia with eosinophilia
- Arteriovenous malformation
- Epithelioid angiosarcoma
- Epithelioid sarcoma
- Melanoma
- Metastatic carcinoma
- Nodular fasciitis
- Pyogenic granuloma
- Reactive angioendotheliomatosis
- Retiform hemangioendothelioma
- Spindle cell hemangioendothelioma

Further reading:
- Requena L, Sangueza OP (1998) Cutaneous vascular proliferations. Part III. Malignant neoplasms, other cutaneous neoplasms with significant vascular component, and disorders erroneously considered as vascular neoplasms. J Am Acad Dermatol 38(2 Pt 1):143–175

Hemangioendothelioma, Kaposiform

Vascular proliferation presenting in the first 2 years of life that is associated with Kasabach–Merritt syndrome and is characterized by a large, rapidly growing, red, multinodular plaque on the trunk, extremities, or retroperitoneum

Differential Diagnosis

- Dabska tumor
- Infantile hemangioma
- Infantile hemangiopericytoma
- Infantile myofibromatosis
- Kaposi's sarcoma

- Spindle cell hemangioendothelioma
- <u>Tufted angioma</u>

Evaluation

- Complete blood count

Further reading:
- Gruman A, Liang MG, Mulliken JB et al (2005) Kaposiform hemangioendothelioma without Kasabach–Merritt phenomenon. J Am Acad Dermatol 52(4):616–622

Hemangioendothelioma, Retiform

Low-grade angiosarcoma arising that arises in young adults and is characterized by slowly growing exophytic mass or subcutaneous nodule most commonly on lower extremities

Differential Diagnosis

- Angiosarcoma
- Dabska tumor
- <u>Dermatofibrosarcoma protuberans</u>
- Hobnail hemangioma
- Lymphoma
- <u>Pyogenic granuloma</u>

Further reading:
- Ioannidou D, Panayiotides J, Krasagakis K et al (2006) Retiform hemangio-endothelioma presenting as bruise-like plaque in an adult woman. Int J Dermatol 45(1):53–55

Hemangioendothelioma, Spindle Cell

Benign vascular proliferation arising in children or young adults that is characterized by multiple blue nodules on the distal extremities

Differential Diagnosis

- Angiosarcoma
- <u>Glomangioma</u>
- Intravascular papillary endothelial hyperplasia
- Kaposi's sarcoma
- Pyogenic granuloma
- Tufted angioma
- <u>Venous malformation</u>

Associations

- Congenital lymphedema
- Klippel–Trenaunay syndrome
- <u>Maffucci syndrome</u>
- Varicose veins

Further reading:
- Dhawan SS, Raza M (2007) Spindle cell hemangioendothelioma. Cutis 79(2):125–128

Hemangioma, Infantile

Benign proliferation of endothelial cells that develops in the first few months of life (or, less commonly, is present at birth) that is characterized by a superficial, deep, or mixed vascular mass affecting any portion of the body which rapidly proliferates (and potentially ulcerates), reaches a peak size, then slowly and spontaneously involutes over the first 10 years

Differential Diagnosis

- Angiosarcoma
- <u>Arteriovenous malformation</u>
- <u>Capillary malformation</u>
- Eccrine angiomatous hamartoma
- Congenital fibrosarcoma

- Congenital hemangiopericytoma
- Gorham syndrome
- Infantile myofibromatosis
- Kaposiform hemangioendothelioma
- Lipoblastoma
- Maffucci syndrome
- Nasal glioma
- Neuroblastoma
- Noninvoluting congenital hemangioma (NICH)
- Primitive neuroectodermal tumor
- Pyogenic granuloma
- Rapidly involuting congenital hemangioma (RICH)
- Rhabdomyosarcoma
- Spindle cell hemangioendothelioma
- Telangiectasia
- Teratoma
- Tufted angioma
- Venous, lymphatic, or combined malformation

Associations

- Benign neonatal hemangiomatosis
- Cobb syndrome
- Diffuse neonatal hemangiomatosis
- Hypothyroidism
- PELVIS syndrome
- PHACES syndrome
- Spinal dysraphism

Evaluation (if PHACES Is Suspected)

- Doppler ultrasound (if deep component is suspected)
- MRI of brain
- Echocardiography and aortography
- Ophthalmologic examination
- Radiograph of the sternum

Treatment Options

- Topical corticosteroids
- Intralesional corticosteroids
- Systemic corticosteroids
- Propanolol
- Pulsed dye laser
- Surgical excision
- Vincristine

Further reading:
- Bruckner AL, Frieden IJ (2003) Hemangiomas of infancy. J Am Acad Dermatol 48(4):477–493
- Metry D, Heyet G, Hess C et al (2009) Consensus statement on diagnostic criteria for PHACE syndrome. Pediatrics 124(5):1447–1456. Epub 2009 Oct 26

Hemangiopericytoma, Infantile

Benign vascular neoplasm of periendothelial cell derivation (possibly myofibroblast cell) that appears in the first year of life and is characterized by solitary or multiple blue or red subcutaneous nodules most commonly located on the head and neck (but can occur anywhere)

Differential Diagnosis

- Angioleiomyoma
- Fibrous histiocytoma
- Glomangioma
- Infantile fibrosarcoma
- Infantile hemangioma
- Infantile myofibromatosis
- Malignant fibrous histiocytoma
- Mesenchymal chondrosarcoma
- Myxoid lipoma
- Myxoid liposarcoma
- Rapidly involuting congenital hemangioma
- Subcutaneous pyogenic granuloma
- Venous malformation

Further reading:
- Requena L, Sangueza OP (1997) Cutaneous vascular proliferation. Part II. Hyperplasias and benign neoplasms. J Am Acad Dermatol 37(6):887–919

Hemochromatosis, Hereditary (Hanot–Chauffard Syndrome)

Inherited disorder (AR) of iron metabolism that is caused by one of several different mutations in the HFE gene (which leads to excessive amounts of iron in tissues) and is characterized by diffuse hyperpigmentation accentuated in the sun-exposed areas, porphyria cutanea tarda, cirrhosis, diabetes, arthritis, and an increased incidence of hepatocellular carcinoma

Differential Diagnosis

- Addison's disease
- Alcoholic liver disease
- Argyria

- Chrysiasis
- <u>Drug-induced pigmentation</u>
- Gaucher disease
- Hepatitis C infection
- Niemann–Pick disease
- Polymorphous light eruption
- Postinflammatory pigmentation
- Rheumatoid arthritis
- Riehl melanosis
- Wilson's disease

Evaluation

- Iron studies
- Echocardiography
- HFE gene studies
- Fasting blood glucose
- Liver function test
- Liver biopsy
- Electrocardiography

Further reading:

- Franchini M (2006) Hereditary iron overload: update on pathophysiology, diagnosis, and treatment. Am J Hematol 81(3):202–209

Henoch–Schonlein Purpura (Anaphylactoid Purpura)

IgA-mediated systemic vasculitis syndrome that affects children more commonly than adults, is caused by IgA immune complex deposition in the skin and viscera, and is characterized by palpable purpura usually on the legs and buttocks, arthralgias, gastrointestinal bleeding and abdominal pain, and nephritis, with the potential to result in chronic renal failure

Differential Diagnosis

- Acute appendicitis
- <u>Acute hemorrhagic edema of childhood</u>
- Child abuse
- Churg–Strauss syndrome
- Cryoglobulinemia
- Endocarditis
- Erythema multiforme
- Hemolytic uremic syndrome
- Juvenile rheumatoid arthritis
- Lupus erythematosus
- <u>Meningococcemia</u>
- Polyarteritis nodosa
- Pigmented purpuric dermatosis
- Rheumatoid arthritis
- Rocky Mountain spotted fever
- <u>Urticaria</u>
- Urticarial vasculitis

Diagnostic Criteria (2/4)

- Age =20 years at presentation
- Bowel angina
- Palpable purpura
- Vessel wall neutrophils on biopsy

Associations

- Drugs
- IgA nephropathy
- Malignancy
- <u>Viral or bacterial upper respiratory infection</u>

Evaluation

- Abdominal ultrasound
- Antinuclear antibodies
- Antistreptolysin O titer
- Chest radiograph
- Complement levels
- Direct immunofluorescence of affected tissue
- Renal function tests
- Rheumatoid factor
- Stool for occult blood
- Upper or lower endoscopy
- Urinalysis

Treatment Options

- Observation and reassurance
- Topical corticosteroids
- Systemic corticosteroids
- NSAIDS
- Azathioprine
- Plasmapheresis
- Intravenous immunoglobulin
- Cyclophosphamide

Further reading:

- Mills JA, Michel BA, Bloeh DA et al (1990) The American College of Rheumatology criteria for the classification of Henoch–Schonlein purpura. Arthritis Rheum 33:1114–1121
- Roberts PF, Waller TA, Brinker TM et al (2007) Henoch–Schonlein purpura: a review article. South Med J 100(8):821–824

Heparin Necrosis

Drug-induced necrosis caused by heparin-dependent antiplatelet antibodies that can be localized to the injection site or more widespread and is characterized by erythematous, painful plaques that become purpuric and necrotic as well as excessive platelet aggregation leading to thrombosis and thrombocytopenia

Differential Diagnosis

- Antiphospholipid antibody syndrome
- Calciphylaxis
- Cholesterol emboli syndrome
- Cocaine-associated vasculopathy
- Coumadin necrosis
- Factitial disease
- Fixed drug eruption
- Herpes simplex virus infection
- Polyarteritis nodosa
- Purpura fulminans
- Spider-bite reaction
- Thrombotic thrombocytopenic purpura

Diagnostic Criteria

- Heparin exposure >5 days
- Relative thrombocytopenia: decrease in platelet count by 50% from baseline OR absolute thrombocytopenia: decrease in platelet count to less than $100–150\times10^9$/l
- Absence of other causes of thrombocytopenia
- Development of new thrombosis or extension of preexisting thrombosis while receiving heparin therapy
- Confirmation by laboratory testing
- Return to normal platelet count when heparin is discontinued

Evaluation

- Protein-C and protein-S level
- Factor V Leiden mutation study

- Complete blood count
- Prothrombin time and partial thromboplastin time
- Antithrombin III level
- Heparin-platelet factor IV antibody assay (with the heparin-induced platelet aggregation test or the serotonin release assay)

Treatment Options

- Warfarin
- Argatroban
- Lepirudin

Further reading:

- Harenberg J, Hoffmann U, Huhle G et al (2001) Cutaneous reactions to anticoagulants. Recognition and management. Am J Clin Dermatol 2(2):69–75
- Warkentin TE, Cook DJ (2005) Heparin, low molecular weight heparin, and heparin-induced thrombocytopenia in the ICU. Crit Care Clin 21(3):513–529

Hermansky–Pudlak Syndrome

Rare inherited syndrome (AR) caused by one of seven different defects in the genes (HSP1–HSP7) encoding proteins responsible for the formation of specialized lysosomes (melanosomes, dense bodies, etc.) that is characterized by bleeding tendency, oculocutaneous albinism, and ceroid lipofuscin deposition in the lungs (leading to pulmonary fibrosis) and other organs

Differential Diagnosis

- Chediak–Higashi syndrome
- Elejalde syndrome
- Griscelli syndrome
- Oculocutaneous albinism

Associations

- Inflammatory bowel disease
- Systemic lupus erythematosus

Evaluation

- Genetic testing
- Platelet function studies
- Chest CT scan and pulmonary function test
- Ophthalmologic examination

Further reading:
- Dimson O, Drolet BA, Esterly NB (1999) Hermansky–Pudlak syndrome. Pediatr Dermatol 16(6):475–477

Herpangina

Self-limited, acute viral disease caused by coxsackievirus A that mainly affects children and is characterized by fever, headache, sore throat, and small vesicles on the soft palate and pharynx with peripheral erythema

Differential Diagnosis

- <u>Aphthous stomatitis</u>
- Behçet's disease
- Drug eruption
- Erythema multiforme
- <u>Forschheimer's spots</u>
- <u>Hand, foot, and mouth disease</u>
- Koplik spots
- Lupus erythematosus
- <u>Primary herpetic gingivostomatitis</u>

Further reading:
- Scott LA, Stone MS (2003) Viral exanthems. Dermatol Online J 9(3):4

Herpes, Genital

Sexually transmitted HSV infection of the genital area with a predilection for recurrent disease and characterized by painful, grouped vesicles on an erythematous base

Differential Diagnosis

- Behçet's disease
- Chancriform pyoderma
- Chancroid
- CMV infection
- Erosive candidiasis
- Erythema multiforme
- Fixed drug eruption
- Granuloma inguinale
- Lipschutz ulcer
- Syphilis
- Trauma

Evaluation

- HSV serology
- Tzanck prep
- Direct fluorescent antibody test
- Viral culture

Treatment Options

- Systemic antivirals

Further reading:
- Yeung-Yue KA, Brentjens MH, Lee PC, Tyring SK (2002) Herpes simplex viruses 1 and 2. Dermatol Clin 20(2):249–266

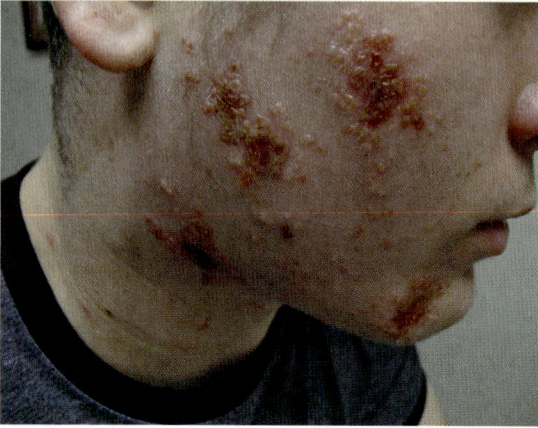

Fig. 6.49 Herpes gladiatorum

Herpes Gladiatorum

Herpes simplex virus infection that is spread among wrestlers and other athletes and that is characterized by randomly distributed umbilicated vesicles, bullae, and crusts, some of which are in herpetiform arrangements (Fig. 6.49)

Differential Diagnosis

- Bullous impetigo
- Contact dermatitis
- Eczema herpeticum
- Tinea gladiatorum

Evaluation

- Viral culture
- Bacterial culture
- Fungal culture

Treatment Options

- Oral antiviral therapy
- Suspension from wrestling for 7–10 days

Further reading:
- Johnson R (2004) Herpes gladiatorum and other skin diseases. Clin Sports Med 23(3):473–484

Herpes Labialis

HSV infection of the perioral area with a predilection for recurrent disease and characterized by painful, grouped vesicles on an erythematous base

Differential Diagnosis

- Aphthous stomatitis
- Behçet's disease
- Bullous pemphigoid
- Candidiasis
- Contact dermatitis
- Erythema multiforme
- Fixed drug eruption
- Herpangina
- Impetigo
- Lupus erythematosus
- Orificial tuberculosis
- Pemphigus vulgaris
- Stevens–Johnson syndrome
- Syphilis
- Varicella
- Zoster

Associations

- Emotional stress
- Erythema multiforme
- Febrile illness
- Sun exposure
- Trauma

Evaluation

- HSV serology
- Tzanck prep
- Direct fluorescent antibody test
- Viral culture

Treatment Options

- <u>Systemic antivirals</u>
- Topical docosanol
- Topical acyclovir
- Topical penciclovir
- L-lysine

Further reading:
- Yeung-Yue KA, Brentjens MH, Lee PC, Tyring SK (2002) Herpes simplex viruses 1 and 2. Dermatol Clin 20(2):249–266

Herpes, Neonatal

Infection with HSV2 that is transmitted through an infected birth canal, is characterized by grouped vesicles and erosions on a erythematous base with a predilection for the head and neck, and is associated with severe, life-threatening, disseminated disease

Differential Diagnosis

- Benign cephalic histiocytosis
- Bullous impetigo
- <u>Congenital candidiasis</u>
- Congenital syphilis
- <u>Congenital varicella</u>
- <u>Epidermolysis bullosa</u>
- <u>Erythema toxicum neonatorum</u>
- Langerhans cell histiocytosis
- Miliaria
- Neonatal acne
- Transient bullous dermolysis
- Transient neonatal pustular melanosis

Treatment Options

- Systemic antivirals

Further reading:
- Kimberlin DW, Whitley RJ (2005) Neonatal herpes: What have we learned? Semin Pediatr Infect Dis 16(1):7–16

Herpes Zoster

Acute eruption that is caused by reactivation of latent varicella-zoster virus and is characterized by painful grouped vesicles and erosions usually confined to a single dermatome

Subtypes/Variants

- Disseminated
- Nodular

- Ophthalmic
- Ramsay Hunt syndrome

Differential Diagnosis

- Appendicitis
- Bell's palsy
- Brachioradial pruritus
- Bullous impetigo
- Bullous pemphigoid
- Candidiasis
- Caterpillar dermatitis
- Cellulitis
- Cholecystitis
- Contact dermatitis
- Erysipelas
- Folliculitis
- Incontinentia pigmenti
- Intervertebral disc disease
- Jellyfish sting
- Lichen striatus
- Myocardial infarction
- Pemphigus
- Photoallergic reaction
- Phytophotodermatitis
- Pleurisy
- Renal stone
- Rhus dermatitis
- Trigeminal neuralgia
- Urticaria
- Zosteriform herpes simplex virus infection
- Zosteriform metastasis

Associations (Skin Disease in Zoster Scars)

- Chronic lymphocytic leukemia
- Cutaneous lymphoid hyperplasia
- Granuloma annulare
- Granulomatous vasculitis
- <u>Lichen planus</u>
- Lichen sclerosus
- Prurigo nodularis
- Reactive perforating collagenosis
- Rosai–Dorfman disease

Evaluation

- Direct fluorescent antibody test
- Viral culture
- Tzanck prep

Treatment Options

- <u>Systemic antivirals</u>
- <u>Systemic corticosteroids</u>
- <u>Gabapentin</u>
- Pregabalin
- Amitriptyline
- Topical anesthetics
- Capsaicin cream

Further reading:
- Chen TM, George S, Woodruff CA, Hsu S (2002) Clinical manifestations of varicella-zoster virus infection. Dermatol Clin 20(2):267–282

Herpetic Whitlow

Infection of the distal aspect of a finger with HSV1 or HSV2 character-ized by painful, grouped vesicles on an erythematous base

Differential Diagnosis

- Acrodermatitis continua
- Acute paronychia
- Bacterial paronychia
- Blistering distal dactylitis
- Bullous impetigo
- Contact dermatitis
- Dyshidrotic eczema
- Hand, foot, and mouth disease
- Orf

Treatment Options

- Systemic antivirals

Further reading:
- Bowling JC, Saha M, Bunker CB (2005) Herpetic whitlow: a forgotten diagnosis. Clin Exp Dermatol 30(5):609–610

Hidradenitis, Idiopathic Palmoplantar

Idiopathic, inflammatory disorder of the eccrine sweat glands that most commonly affects children and is characterized by recurrent episodes of sudden-onset erythematous tender nodules on the palms and soles that resolve spontaneously within a few days

Differential Diagnosis

- Arthropod-bite reaction
- Atypical erythema nodosum

- Chilblains
- Contact dermatitis
- Contact urticaria
- Erythema multiforme
- Granuloma annulare
- Juvenile plantar dermatosis
- Pseudomonal hot-foot syndrome
- Neutrophilic eccrine hidradenitis

Treatment Options

- Observation and reassurance
- NSAIDs

Further reading:

- Rubinson R, Larralde M, Santos-Munoz A et al (2004) Palmoplantar eccrine hidradenitis: seven new cases. Pediatr Dermatol 21(4):466–468

Hidradenitis Suppurativa

Chronic, recurrent inflammatory disorder involving follicular occlusion in the intertriginous areas and characterized papules, pustules, abscesses, and draining sinuses that heal with hypertrophic scarring

Differential Diagnosis

- Actinomycosis
- Bartholin cyst
- Carbuncle
- Crohn's disease
- Fox–Fordyce disease
- Furunculosis
- Granuloma inguinale
- Inflamed epidermal cyst
- Lymphogranuloma venereum

- Lymphoma
- Mycetoma
- Scrofuloderma
- Tularemia

Associations

- Acne conglobata
- Arthritis
- Dissecting cellulitis
- Dowling–Degos disease
- Fox–Fordyce disease
- Hirsutism
- Inflammatory bowel disease
- Lithium
- Obesity
- Pilonidal sinus
- Pityriasis rubra pilaris, type VI
- Pyoderma gangrenosum
- SAPHO syndrome
- Smoking
- Steatocystoma multiplex

Evaluation

- Bacterial culture of exudate

Treatment Options

- Oral antibiotics
- Surgical excision
- Spironolactone
- Oral contraceptive pills

- <u>Isotretinoin</u>
- Adalimumab
- Infliximab
- Dapsone
- Pentoxifylline

Further reading:
- Wiseman MC (2004) Hidradenitis suppurativa: a review. Dermatol Ther 17(1):50–54

Hidradenoma Papilliferum (Papillary Hidradenoma)

Benign neoplasm of apocrine derivation (a type of apocrine adenoma) that is characterized by a firm dermal or subcutaneous nodule most commonly located on the vulva or perianal area

Differential Diagnosis

- <u>Bartholin cyst</u>
- <u>Ciliated cyst of the vulva</u>
- Cutaneous endometriosis
- <u>Epidermoid cyst</u>
- Hemangioma
- Leiomyoma
- Melanoma
- Metastatic adenocarcinoma
- Pyogenic granuloma
- Squamous cell carcinoma
- Sweat gland carcinoma

Further reading:
- Handa Y, Yamanaka N, Inagaki H, Tomita Y (2003) Large ulcerated perianal hidradenoma papilliferum in a young female. Dermatol Surg 29(7):790–792

Hidroacanthoma Simplex

Superficial type of acrospiroma (essentially, an intraepidermal poroma) that predominantly arises in the elderly and is characterized by a seborrheic-keratosis-like papule on the lower extremities or trunk

Differential Diagnosis

- Actinic keratosis
- Basal cell carcinoma
- Benign lichenoid keratosis
- Bowen's disease
- Clear cell acanthoma
- Dermatofibroma
- Large cell acanthoma
- Pyogenic granuloma
- Seborrheic keratosis, especially clonal type

Further reading:
- Kurokawa I, Nishijima S, Kusumoto K et al (2005) A case report of hidroacanthoma simplex with an immunohistochemical study of cytokeratins. Int J Dermatol 44(9):775–776

Hidrocystoma, Apocrine/Eccrine

Benign cystic tumor of apocrine or eccrine derivation that is characterized by solitary or multiple translucent, bluish, or pigmented papules on the face, especially in the periorbital area

Differential Diagnosis

- Basal cell carcinoma (especially cystic type)
- Blue nevus
- Colloid milium

- Epidermal inclusion cyst
- Malignant melanoma
- <u>Milia</u>
- Mucous cyst
- <u>Syringoma</u>

Associations

- Focal dermal hypoplasia
- Schopf–Schulz–Passarge syndrome

Further reading:

- Anzai S, Goto M, Fujiwara S, Da T (2005) Apocrine hidrocystoma: a case report and analysis of 167 Japanese cases. Int J Dermatol 44(8):702–703

Histiocytosis, Benign Cephalic

Benign type of non-X-type histiocytosis that presents in the first year of life, spontaneously resolves within a few months to years, and is characterized by small, erythematous papules on the head and neck without any associated systemic symptoms

Differential Diagnosis

- <u>Congenital self-healing histiocytosis (Hashimoto–Pritzker disease)</u>
- Erythema toxicum neonatorum
- Generalized eruptive histiocytoma
- Infantile acne
- Juvenile xanthogranuloma
- <u>Langerhans cell histiocytosis</u>
- Molluscum contagiosum
- Neonatal cephalic pustulosis
- Transient neonatal pustular melanosis

Associations

- Generalized eruptive histiocytoma
- Juvenile xanthogranuloma

Treatment Options

- Observation and reassurance

Further reading:

- Sidwell RU, Francis N, Slater DN, Mayou SC (2005) Is disseminated juvenile xanthogranulomatosis benign cephalic histiocytosis? Pediatr Dermatol 22(1):40–43

Histoplasmosis (Darling's Disease)

Respiratory mycotic infection caused by *Histoplasma capsulatum* that is usually asymptomatic in the immunocompetent patient or widely disseminated in the immunocompromised patient and is characterized by a variable clinical presentation with erythematous papules, pustules, nodules, or purpuric lesions as well as mucocutaneous ulcerations and granulomatous lesions, often in the oropharynx or nasopharynx (Fig. 6.50)

Differential Diagnosis

- Acanthamebiasis
- Aphthous stomatitis
- Blastomycosis
- Coccidioidomycosis
- Cryptococcosis
- Herpes simplex virus infection
- Lymphoma
- Malignancy
- Paracoccidioidomycosis
- Sarcoidosis
- Squamous cell carcinoma

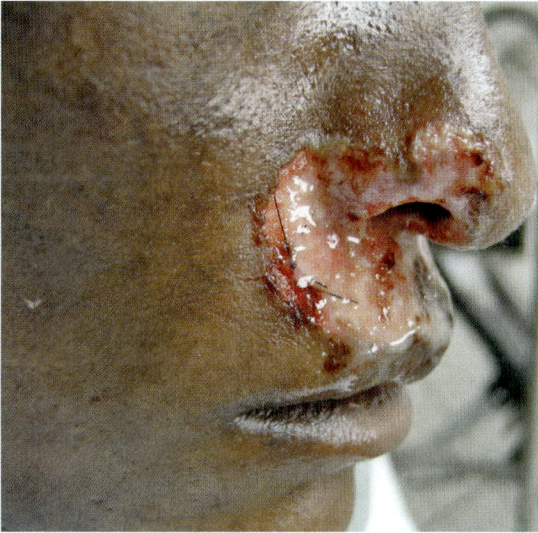

Fig. 6.50 Histoplasmosis

- Syphilis
- Tuberculosis (especially miliary or orificial types)

Evaluation

- Blood cultures
- Chest radiography
- Complete blood count
- CT/MRI scan of the brain
- HIV test
- Liver function test
- Lumbar puncture
- Renal function test
- Urinary histoplasmosis antigen test

Further reading:

- Verma SB (2006) Chronic disseminated cutaneous histoplasmosis in an immunocompetent individual – a case report. Int J Dermatol 45(5):573–576

Howel–Evans Syndrome

Autosomal-dominant disorder caused by mutation of the TOC gene that is characterized by childhood onset of focal nonepidermolytic palmoplantar keratoderma followed by esophageal carcinoma which develops in the fifth decade of life

Differential Diagnosis

- Acrokeratosis paraneoplastica of Bazex
- <u>Focal nonepidermolytic palmoplantar keratoderma with oral, genital, and follicular lesions</u>
- <u>Focal palmoplantar and gingival keratosis</u>
- <u>Hereditary painful callosities</u>
- Nummular epidermolytic palmoplantar keratoderma
- Pachyonychia congenita, type I
- Richner–Hanhart syndrome (tyrosinemia, type II)
- Tripe palms

Evaluation

- Esophageal gastroduodenoscopy

Further reading:
- Maillefer RH, Greydanus MP (1999) To B or not to B: Is tylosis B truly benign? Two North American genealogies. Am J Gastroenterol 94(3):829–834

Hunter Syndrome/Hurler Syndrome

Two mucopolysaccharidoses caused by deficiency of the enzymes, iduronate sulfatase (Hunter syndrome, X-linked) and alpha-L-iduronidase (Hurler syndrome, AR) that are characterized by coarse facial features, hypertrichosis, mental retardation, hepatosplenomegaly, gargoylism (Hurler syndrome), genital infantilism, corneal opacities (Hurler syndrome), flesh-colored papules on the scapular areas representing mucinous connective tissue nevi (nevus mucinosis, Hunter syndrome), extensive dermal melanocytosis, and early death

Differential Diagnosis

- Ambras syndrome
- Congenital syphilis
- Cornelia de Lange syndrome
- Donahue syndrome
- Ectodermal dysplasias
- Fetal alcohol syndrome
- Gaucher's disease
- Niemann–Pick disease
- Osteogenesis imperfecta
- Other mucopolysaccharidoses
- Phakomatosis pigmentovascularis
- Vitamin-D-resistant rickets
- Tuberous sclerosis

Further reading:
- Lonergan CL, Payne AR, Wilson WG et al (2004) What syndrome is this? Hunter syndrome. Pediatr Dermatol 21(6):679–681

Hydroa Vacciniforme

Childhood idiopathic photodermatosis that is characterized by photodistributed umbilicated vesicles that heal to smallpox-like scars

Differential Diagnosis

- Actinic prurigo
- EBV infection
- Erythema multiforme

- <u>Erythropoietic protoporphyria</u>
- Hartnup syndrome
- Herpes simplex virus infection
- <u>Hydroa-like cutaneous T cell lymphoma</u>
- Lupus erythematosus
- Lymphomatoid papulosis
- Pityriasis lichenoides et varioliformis acuta
- <u>Polymorphous light eruption</u>
- <u>Porphyria cutanea tarda</u>
- Pseudoporphyria
- Varicella infection

Evaluation

- Antinuclear antibodies
- Complete blood count
- EBV titers
- Erythrocyte, plasma, and urinary porphyrin studies
- Phototesting
- T cell gene rearrangement of lesional tissue (if lymphoma is suspected)

Treatment Options

- <u>Sunscreen</u>
- Phototherapy
- <u>Antimalarials</u>
- <u>Beta-carotene</u>
- Azathioprine
- Cyclosporine
- Thalidomide

Further reading:
- Gupta G, Man I, Kemmett D (2000) Hydroa vacciniforme: a clinical and follow-up study of 17 cases. J Am Acad Dermatol 42(2 Pt 1):208–213

Hypereosinophilic Syndrome

Acquired syndrome associated with idiopathic eosinophilia that is caused by excessive production of eosinophil-stimulating cytokines and characterized by pruritus, urticaria, erythroderma, and other eosinophil-rich cutaneous and visceral infiltrates

Subtypes/Variants

- Lymphoproliferative
- Myeloproliferative

Differential Diagnosis

- Angiolymphoid hyperplasia with eosinophilia
- Atopic dermatitis
- Bullous pemphigoid
- Churg–Strauss syndrome
- Drug reaction
- Eosinophilia–myalgia syndrome
- Eosinophilic fasciitis
- Eosinophilic leukemia
- Episodic angioedema with eosinophilia
- Leukemia
- Lupus erythematosus
- Lymphoma
- Parasitic infections
- Urticaria
- Urticarial dermatitis
- Wells syndrome

Diagnostic Criteria

- Eosinophils >1,500 for more than 6 months
- Evidence of parenchymal organ involvement

- No apparent underlying disease to explain eosinophilia
- No vasculitis

Associations

- Aquagenic pruritus
- Bullous pemphigoid
- Erythema annulare centrifugum
- Raynaud phenomenon
- Splinter hemorrhages
- Wells syndrome

Evaluation

- Bone marrow biopsy
- Chest radiograph
- Complete blood count
- Direct immunofluorescence
- Echocardiography
- Immunoglobulin levels
- Liver function test
- Renal function test
- Stool studies for parasites
- Urinalysis

Treatment Options

- Systemic corticosteroids
- Hydroxyurea
- Imatinib
- Chemotherapy
- Interferon
- Alemtuzumab

Further reading:

- Leiferman KM, Gleich GJ (2004) Hypereosinophilic syndrome: case presentation and update. J Allergy Clin Immunol 113(1):50–58

Hypergammaglobulinemic Purpura of Waldenstrom, Benign

Chronic, benign purpuric disorder association with elevated gamma globulins (especially IgG) and a variety of autoimmune diseases that is characterized by repeated episodes of noninflammatory petechiae and purpura all over the body, especially the lower extremities (Fig. 6.51)

Differential Diagnosis

- <u>Benign pigmented purpura</u>
- Chronic meningococcemia
- <u>Cutaneous small vessel vasculitis</u>
- Disseminated intravascular coagulation
- <u>Drug-induced purpura</u>

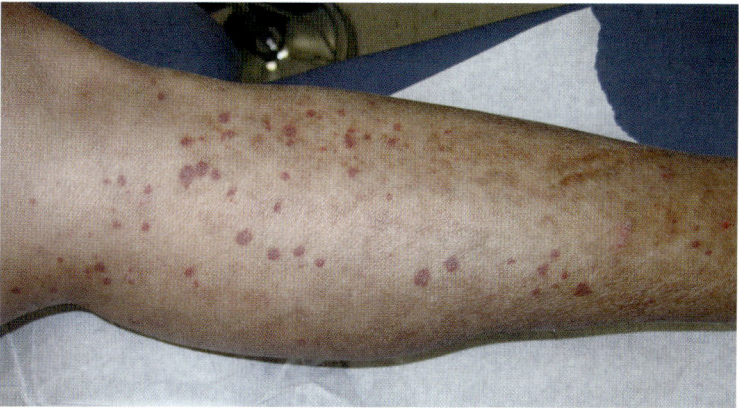

Fig. 6.51 Benign hypergammaglobulinemic purpura of Waldenstrom

- <u>Immune thrombocytopenic purpura</u>
- Platelet dysfunction
- Scurvy
- Thrombotic thrombocytopenic purpura

Associations

- Chronic lymphocytic leukemia
- Monoclonal gammopathy
- Hashimoto's thyroiditis
- Idiopathic
- <u>Rheumatoid arthritis</u>
- Sarcoidosis
- <u>Sjögren syndrome</u>
- Systemic lupus erythematosus

Evaluation

- Antinuclear antibodies (including SS-A and SS-B)
- Complement levels
- Complete blood count
- Immunoglobulin levels
- Prothrombin time and partial thromboplastin time
- Rheumatoid factor
- Serum/urinary protein electrophoresis
- Thyroid function test

Treatment Options

- <u>Treat underlying cause</u>
- Systemic corticosteroids
- Indomethacin
- Hydroxychloroquine

Further reading:

- Malaviya AN, Kaushik P, Budhiraja S et al (2000) Hypergammaglobulinemic purpura of Waldenstrom: report of 3 cases with a short review. Clin Exp Rheumatol 18(4):518–522

Hyperimmunoglobulin E Syndrome (Job Syndrome)

Inherited syndrome (AD) of uncertain cause characterized by coarse facies, potentially severe eczema, recurrent candidiasis and staphylococcal infections (presenting as cold abscesses), retention of primary teeth, bony fractures, various systemic infections (especially pulmonary), and high levels of IgE

Differential Diagnosis

- Atopic dermatitis
- Chronic granulomatous disease
- Chronic mucocutaneous candidiasis
- Common variable immunodeficiency
- DiGeorge syndrome
- Leukocyte adhesion deficiency
- Nezelof syndrome
- Omenn syndrome
- Recurrent furunculosis
- Wiskott–Aldrich syndrome
- X-linked hypogammaglobulinemia

Evaluation

- Bacterial and fungal cultures (of any infected sites)
- Chest radiograph or CT scan
- Complete blood count
- Immunoglobulin levels

- Panoramic radiograph of teeth
- Skeletal survey

Further reading:
- Dewitt CA, Bishop AB, Buescher LS et al (2006) Hyperimmunoglobulin E syndrome: two cases and a review of the literature. J Am Acad Dermatol 54(5):855–865

Hyperkeratosis Lenticularis Perstans (Flegel's Disease)

Uncommon, acquired dermatosis of unknown cause characterized by small, flat, brown, hyperkeratotic papules predominantly on the lower extremities

Differential Diagnosis

- Acquired perforating dermatosis
- Acrokeratosis verruciformis of Hopf
- Actinic keratoses
- Darier's disease
- Disseminated superficial actinic porokeratosis
- Epidermodysplasia verruciformis
- Guttate psoriasis
- Stucco keratoses
- Verruca plana

Treatment Options

- 5-FU cream
- Topical vitamin D analogues
- Topical retinoids
- Acitretin

Further reading:
- Vando K, Hattori H, Yamauchi Y (2006) Histopathological differences between early and old lesions of hyperkeratosis lenticularis perstans (Flegel's disease). Am J Dermatopathol 28(2):122–126

Hypertensive Ulcer (Martorell's Ulcer)

Type of ulcer associated with severe, uncontrolled hypertension that is characterized by an extremely painful ulcer on the lateral aspects on the lower extremity which is occasionally bilateral and symmetrical or surrounded by satellite lesions

Differential Diagnosis

- Antiphospholipid antibody syndrome
- Arterial insufficiency ulcer
- Arthropod-bite reaction
- Chancriform pyoderma
- Cholesterol emboli syndrome
- Dermatitis artefacta
- Livedoid vasculopathy
- Pyoderma gangrenosum
- Sickle cell ulcer
- Tropical ulcer
- Vasculitis

Treatment Options

- Wound care
- Control of hypertension

Further reading:
- Graves JW, Morris JC, Sheps SG (2001) Martorell's hypertensive leg ulcer: case report and concise review of the literature. J Hum Hypertens 15(4):279–283

Hypomelanosis of Ito (Incontinentia Pigmenti Achromians)

Pigmentary disturbance that may be associated with a variety of CNS defects and is characterized by linear and whorled hypomelanosis following Blaschko's lines that fails to have any preceding stage of vesicles and verrucous lesions that are classically seen in incontinentia pigmenti (Fig. 6.52)

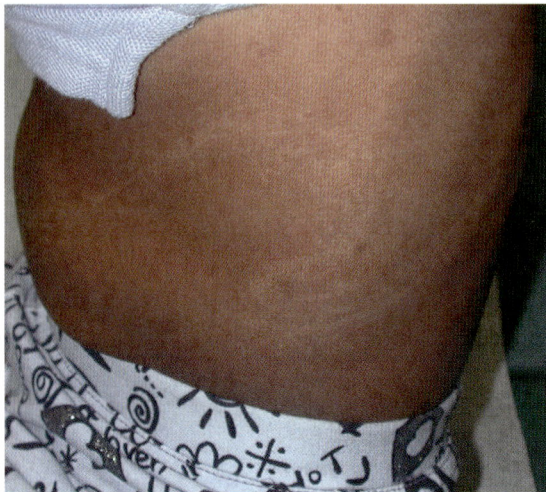

Fig. 6.52 Hypomel-
anosis of Ito
(Courtesy of
K. Guidry)

Differential Diagnosis

- <u>Incontinentia pigmenti, stage IV</u>
- Linear and whorled nevoid hypermelanosis
- <u>Nevus depigmentosus</u>
- Pallister–Killian syndrome
- Phylloid hypomelanosis
- <u>Postinflammatory hypopigmentation</u>
- Segmental vitiligo
- Tuberous sclerosis

Associations

- Deafness
- Developmental disturbance
- Mental retardation
- Seizures
- Skeletal abnormalities
- Visual disturbance

Evaluation

- CT/MRI scan of brain
- Electroencephalogram
- Hearing test
- Ophthalmologic exam
- Skeletal surgery
- Vision test

Further reading:

- Taibjee SM, Bennett DC, Moss C (2004) Abnormal pigmentation in hypomelanosis of Ito and pigmentary mosaicism: the role of pigmentary genes. Br J Dermatol 151(2):269–282

Ichthyosis Bullosa of Siemens

Autosomal-dominant ichthyosis caused by mutation of the keratin-2e gene that is characterized by mild trauma-induced blistering at birth that is replaced by mild flexural hyperkeratosis and superficial molting of the skin later in childhood

Differential Diagnosis

- <u>Bullous congenital ichthyosiform erythroderma</u>
- Collodion baby
- <u>Epidermolysis bullosa</u>
- <u>Lamellar ichthyosis</u>
- Omenn's syndrome
- <u>Peeling skin syndrome</u>
- Pemphigus foliaceus (including maternal disease)
- Staphylococcal scalded-skin syndrome
- Syphilitic pemphigus
- Transient bullous dermolysis
- Weary–Kindler syndrome

Further reading:
• Akiyama M, Tsuji-Abe Y, Yanagihara M et al (2005) Ichthyosis bullosa of Siemens: its correct diagnosis facilitated by molecular genetic testing. Br J Dermatol 152(6):1353–1356

Ichthyosis, Lamellar

Inherited disorder (AR) of keratinization that is caused by mutation of the gene encoding epidermal transglutaminase 1 and characterized by collodion baby presentation at birth, followed by chronic, generalized plate-like scaling, including the face and flexures

Differential Diagnosis

• Conradi–Hunermann–Happle disease
• CHIME syndrome
• IBIDS syndrome
• KID syndrome
• Leiner's disease
• Netherton syndrome
• Neutral lipid storage disorder
• Nonbullous congenital ichthyosiform erythroderma
• Psoriatic erythroderma
• Refsum disease
• Seborrheic dermatitis (generalized)
• Sjögren–Larsson syndrome
• X-linked ichthyosis

Further reading:
• Oji V, Traupe H (2006) Ichthyoses: differential diagnosis and molecular genetics. Eur J Dermatol 16(4):349–359

Ichthyosis Vulgaris

Inherited disorder (AD) of keratinization associated with decreased conversion of profilaggrin to filaggrin that is characterized by fine scaling predominantly affecting the extensor surfaces of the extremities with sparing of the flexures and tendency toward improvement in the summer months

Differential Diagnosis

- Acquired ichthyosis
- Asteatotic eczema
- Atopic dermatitis
- CHIME syndrome
- Dermatophytosis
- Dermatosis neglecta
- IBIDS syndrome
- KID syndrome
- Netherton syndrome
- Neutral lipid storage disease
- Refsum disease
- Sarcoidosis
- Sjögren–Larsson syndrome
- Xerosis
- X-linked ichthyosis

Associations

- Atopic dermatitis
- Keratosis pilaris

Further reading:

- Oji V, Traupe H (2006) Ichthyoses: differential diagnosis and molecular genetics. Eur J Dermatol 16(4):349–359

Ichthyosis, X-Linked

X-linked recessive disorder of keratinization caused by a defect in the gene encoding steroid sulfatase and characterized by large brown scales on the neck and extensor surfaces with sparing of the flexures, as well as cryptorchidism, a history of maternal failure of progression of labor, and comma-shaped corneal opacities

Differential Diagnosis

- Asteatotic eczema
- Atopic dermatitis
- CHIME syndrome
- Chondrodysplasia punctata
- Dermatosis neglecta
- Ichthyosis vulgaris
- Lamellar ichthyosis
- Multiple sulfatase deficiency
- Netherton syndrome
- Nonbullous congenital ichthyosiform erythroderma
- Peeling skin syndrome

Associations

- Androgenetic alopecia
- Kallmann syndrome
- Multiple sulfatase deficiency

Evaluation

- Testicular ultrasound
- Ophthalmologic exam

Further reading:
- Hazan C, Orlow SJ, Schaffer JV (2005) X-linked recessive ichthyosis. Dermatol Online J 11(4):12

Idiopathic Facial Aseptic Granuloma

Idiopathic granulomatous lesion that arises on the face of children and is characterized by a reddish-brown papule or nodule

Differential Diagnosis

- Dermoid cyst
- Epidermal inclusion cyst
- Foreign body granuloma
- Granulomatous infection
- Hemangioma
- Juvenile xanthogranuloma
- Molluscum contagiosum
- Nodulocystic acne
- Pilomatricoma
- Pyogenic granuloma
- Sarcoidosis
- Spitz nevus

Further reading:
- Boralevi F, Leaute-Labreze C, Lepreux S et al (2007) Idiopathic facial aseptic granuloma: a multicentre prospective study of 30 cases. Br J Dermatol 156(4):705–708

Idiopathic Guttate Hypomelanosis

Acquired idiopathic type of leukoderma that predominantly affects women and is characterized by small white macules on the anterior lower extremities and, less commonly, on the forearms

Differential Diagnosis

- Atrophie blanche
- Cryotherapy leukoderma
- Darier's disease leukodermic macules
- <u>Excoriation or arthropod-bite scars</u>
- Hypopigmented mycosis fungoides
- Leprosy
- Lichen sclerosus
- Malignant atrophic papulosis (Degos disease)
- Occupational leukoderma
- Pinta
- Pityriasis lichenoides chronica
- Postinflammatory hypopigmentation
- Secondary syphilis
- Tinea versicolor
- Verruca plana
- <u>Vitiligo, especially ponctue type</u>

Treatment Options

- Observation and reassurance

Further reading:
- Kaya TI, Yazici AC, Tursen U et al (2005) Idiopathic guttate hypomelanosis: Idiopathic or ultraviolet induced? Photodermatol Photoimmunol Photomed 21(5):270–271

Idiopathic Eruptive Macular Pigmentation

Rare, acquired pigmentary disorder with onset in the first two decades of life that is characterized by asymptomatic brown macules and patches on the face, trunk, and proximal extremities that spontaneously resolve within a few years

Differential Diagnosis

- Erythema dyschromicum perstans
- Lichenoid drug eruption
- Lichen planus pigmentosus
- Macula cerulea
- Multiple fixed drug eruption
- Postinflammatory hyperpigmentation, especially due to pityriasis rosea
- Tinea versicolor
- Urticaria pigmentosum

Treatment Options

- Observation and reassurance

Further reading:
- Jang KA, Choi JH, Sung KS et al (2001) Idiopathic eruptive macular pigmentation: report of 10 cases. J Am Acad Dermatol 44(2 Suppl):351–353

Id Reaction

Type of immune-mediated skin reaction caused by various infections or infestations that is characterized by symmetric erythematous papules, vesicles, or eczematous changes in areas distant to the site of initial triggering infection (Fig. 6.53)

Subtypes

- Eczematous
- Erythema annulare centrifugum
- Erythema multiforme-like
- Lichen trichophyticus
- Pompholyx-like

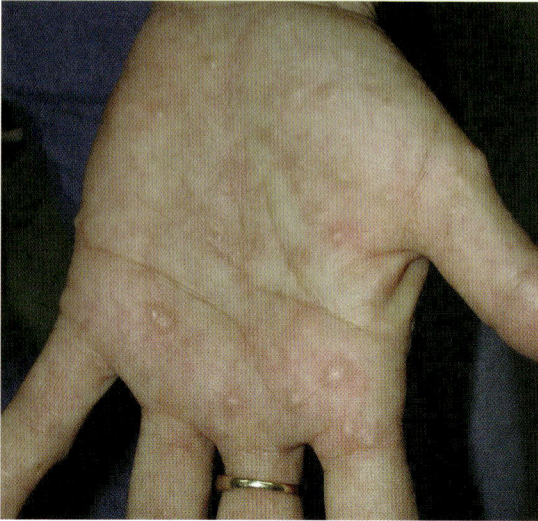

Fig. 6.53 Id reaction (Courtesy of K. Guidry)

- Psoriasiform
- Urticarial

Differential Diagnosis

- Atopic dermatitis
- Autosensitization dermatitis
- Contact dermatitis
- Dermatophytosis
- Drug eruption
- Dyshidrotic eczema
- Erysipelas
- Erythema multiforme
- Folliculitis
- Gianotti–Crosti syndrome
- Pityriasis lichenoides et varioliformis acuta
- Scabies

- Seborrheic dermatitis
- Stasis dermatitis

Associations

- Bacterial infection
- <u>Dermatophyte infection</u>
- Molluscum contagiosum
- Pediculosis capitis
- Scabies infestation
- Tick bite

Treatment Options

- <u>Treat underlying cause</u>
- <u>Systemic corticosteroids</u>
- Topical corticosteroids

Further reading:
- Atzori L, Pau M, Aste M (2003) Erythema multiforme ID reaction in atypical dermatophytosis: a case report. J Eur Acad Dermatol Venereol 17(6):699–701

IFAP Syndrome (Ichthyosis Follicularis, Alopecia, and Photophobia)

X-linked recessive disorder of unknown cause that is characterized by diffuse, congenital nonscarring alopecia, ichthyosis, spiny keratotic follicular papules, photophobia, facial dysmorphism, mental retardation, and a variety of other systemic features

Differential Diagnosis

- <u>Atrichia with papules</u>
- Cardiofaciocutaneous syndrome

- Down syndrome
- Graham–Little–Piccardi–Lasseur syndrome
- <u>Keratosis follicularis spinulosa decalvans</u>
- KID syndrome
- <u>Monilethrix</u>
- Noonan syndrome

Further reading:
- Alfadley A, Al Hawsawi K, Al Aboud K (2003) Ichthyosis follicularis: a case report and review of the literature. Pediatr Dermatol 20(1):48–51

Immersion Foot, Warm Water, and Tropical

Dermatosis predominantly affecting soldiers that results from immersion of the feet in warm water or mud (paddy foot) for several days and is characterized by wrinkling, maceration, pruritus, and burning of the soles of the feet (warm water) or swelling and pain of the dorsal feet (tropical) that persists for several days after the exposure

Differential Diagnosis

- <u>Aquagenic acrosyringeal keratoderma</u>
- Cellulitis
- Chilblains
- <u>Dermatophyte infection</u>
- Erosio interdigitalis blastomycetica
- Erythrasma
- <u>Erythromelalgia</u>
- Frostbite
- <u>Gram-negative toe-web infections</u>
- Pitted keratolysis
- Plantar hyperhidrosis
- Raynaud phenomenon

Further reading:

- Oumeish OY, Parish LC (2002) Marching in the army: common cutaneous disorders of the feet. Clin Dermatol 20(4):445–451

Impetigo Contagiosa

Superficial streptococcal or staphylococcal infection of the epidermis characterized by honey-crusted lesions (nonbullous) or flaccid vesiculobullous lesions and erosions (bullous) most commonly seen on the face but can occur anywhere the skin barrier is damaged

Differential Diagnosis

Bullous

- Acropustulosis of infancy
- Bullous arthropod-bite reaction
- Bullous dermatophyte infection
- Bullous erythema multiforme
- Bullous fixed drug eruption
- Bullous pemphigoid
- Bullous scabies
- Burn
- Candidiasis
- Contact dermatitis
- Dermatitis herpetiformis
- Herpes simplex infection
- Incontinentia pigmenti, stage I
- Pemphigus foliaceus
- Pemphigus vulgaris
- Staphylococcal scalded-skin syndrome
- Stevens–Johnson syndrome
- Subcorneal pustular dermatosis
- Thermal burns
- Varicella

Nonbullous

- Candidiasis
- Eczema
- Herpes simplex infection
- Insect-bite reaction
- Pediculosis
- Pemphigus foliaceus
- Rhus dermatitis
- Scabies
- Tinea corporis
- Varicella

Associations

- Glomerulonephritis

Treatment Options

- Topical antibiotics
- Systemic antibiotics

Further reading:
- Stanley JR, Amagai M (2006) Pemphigus, bullous impetigo, and the staphylococcal scalded-skin syndrome. N Engl J Med 355(17):1800–1810

Incontinentia Pigmenti (Bloch–Sulzberger Syndrome)

Inherited disorder (XLD) caused by a defect in the gene encoding the nuclear factor kappa beta essential modulator (NEMO) that is characterized by a neonatal-onset skin eruption along Blaschko's lines that progresses through stages, in addition to scarring alopecia at the vertex of the scalp, nail dystrophy, pegged-shaped teeth or partial anodontia, strabismus, and seizures

Stages

- Stage I – vesiculobullous
- Stage II – verrucous
- Stage III – hyperpigmented
- Stage IV – hypopigmented

Differential Diagnosis

Stage I

- <u>Bullous impetigo</u>
- Bullous mastocytosis
- Congenital erosive and vesicular dermatosis
- Congenital syphilis
- <u>Contact dermatitis</u>
- <u>Epidermolysis bullosa</u>
- Epidermolytic hyperkeratosis
- Erythema toxicum neonatorum
- Focal dermal hypoplasia (Goltz)
- Herpes simplex virus infection
- Infantile acropustulosis
- Langerhans cell histiocytosis
- Linear IgA bullous dermatosis
- Miliaria
- Scabies
- Transient neonatal pustular melanosis
- Varicella
- Zoster

Stage II

- Congenital ichthyosiform erythroderma
- Conradi–Hunermann syndrome
- Ichthyosis hystrix
- Ichthyosis hystrix, Curth–Macklin type
- <u>Inflammatory linear verrucous epidermal nevus</u>

- <u>Lichen striatus</u>
- Linear Darier's disease
- <u>Linear verrucous epidermal nevus</u>
- Linear porokeratosis
- Verruca vulgaris

Stage III

- Dermatopathia pigmentosa reticularis
- <u>Linear and whorled nevoid hypermelanosis</u>
- Naegeli–Franceschetti–Jadassohn syndrome
- Pallister–Killian syndrome
- Progressive cribriform and zosteriform hyperpigmentation
- XLD chondrodysplasia punctata
- X-linked reticulate pigmentary disorder

Stage IV

- Focal dermal hypoplasia
- <u>Hypomelanosis of Ito</u>
- <u>Nevus depigmentosus</u>
- Pallister–Killian syndrome
- Phylloid hypomelanosis
- Segmental vitiligo
- XLD chondrodysplasia punctata

Diagnostic Criteria

- Major criteria, no family history (one necessary)
  - Typical neonatal vesicular rash with eosinophilia
  - Typical blaschkoid hyperpigmentation on the trunk, fading in adolescence
  - Linear, atrophic hairless lesions
- Major criteria, positive family history (any suggests diagnosis)
  - Suggestive history or evidence of typical rash, hyperpigmentation, or atrophic hairless lesions
  - Vertex alopecia

- Dental anomalies
- Retinal disease
- Multiple male miscarriages
- Minor criteria (supports diagnosis)
  - Dental anomalies
  - Alopecia
  - Woolly hair
  - Abnormal nails

Evaluation

- Ophthalmologic exam
- CT/MRI scan of the brain
- Electroencephalogram
- Panoramic radiograph of the mandible

Treatment Options (Vesiculobullous Phase)

- <u>Topical corticosteroids</u>
- Tacrolimus ointment

Further reading:
- Lands SJ, Donnai D (1993) Incontinentia pigmenti (Bloch–Sulzberger syndrome). J Med Genet 30(1):53–59

Infantile Digital Fibromatosis (Reye Tumor)

Type of fibrous proliferation that is characterized by fibrous, flesh-colored nodules on the fingers and toes, with sparing of the thumb and great toe and a tendency to recur after excision

Differential Diagnosis

- Acral fibrokeratoma
- Angiofibroma

- Calcifying aponeurotic fibroma
- Dermatofibroma
- Fibrosarcoma
- Granuloma annulare
- <u>Juvenile hyaline fibromatosis</u>
- <u>Keloid</u>
- Knuckle pad
- Multicentric reticulohistiocytosis
- Neurilemmoma
- <u>Pachydermodactyly</u>
- Periungual fibromas
- Sarcoidosis
- Supernumerary digits
- Wart
- Xanthoma

Treatment Options

- <u>Observation and reassurance</u>
- Intralesional corticosteroids
- <u>Surgical excision</u>
- Mohs micrographic

Further reading:

- Niamba P, Leaute-Labreze C, Boralevi F et al (2007) Further documentation of spontaneous regression of infantile digital fibromatosis. Pediatr Dermatol 24(3):280–284

Infantile Myofibromatosis (Congenital Generalized Fibromatosis)

Type of infantile fibromatosis that is often present at birth and characterized by a solitary fibrous nodule or plaque on the head and neck or, less commonly, generalized dermal and subcutaneous nodules with skeletal and, uncommonly, visceral (particularly the lung) involvement (that can be associated with a poor prognosis, depending on the organs involved)

Differential Diagnosis

- Connective tissue nevus
- Cutaneous metastases
- <u>Fibrous hamartoma of infancy</u>
- Hemangioma
- Hemangiopericytoma
- Juvenile xanthogranuloma
- Leiomyoma
- Leukemia cutis
- Mastocytoma
- Neuroblastoma
- Neurofibroma
- Rhabdomyosarcoma
- Solitary histiocytoma
- Subcutaneous fat necrosis
- Urticaria pigmentosa

Evaluation

- CT/MRI scan of chest, abdomen, and pelvis
- Skeletal radiographs

Treatment Options

- Chemotherapy
- <u>Surgical excision</u>
- Radiation therapy

Further reading:
- Stanford D, Rogers M (2000) Dermatological presentations of infantile myofibromatosis: a review of 27 cases. Australas J Dermatol 41(3):156–161

Infectious Eczematoid Dermatitis (Engman's Disease)

Eczematous eruption and form of autosensitization that is localized around a draining focus of purulent infectious material

Differential Diagnosis

- <u>Allergic contact dermatitis (especially topical antibiotics or bandage)</u>
- Arthropod-bite reaction
- Id reaction
- Eczema herpeticum
- <u>Impetigo</u>
- Perioral dermatitis
- Seborrheic dermatitis

Associations

- Mastoiditis
- Nasal discharge
- Osteomyelitis
- Otitis externa
- Toe-web infection

Treatment Options

- Topical antibiotics
- <u>Topical corticosteroids</u>
- <u>Systemic antibiotics</u>

Infective Dermatitis

Childhood manifestation of HTLV-1 infection that is characterized by chronic, recalcitrant eczema with persistent staphylococcal or strep-tococcal infection, involvement of scalp and retroauricular area, dermatopathic lymphadenopathy, and predilection for the development of lymphoma and tropical paraparesis.

Differential Diagnosis

- <u>Atopic dermatitis</u>
- <u>Childhood mycosis fungoides</u>
- Impetigo
- Seborrheic dermatitis
- Psoriasis
- Tinea

Diagnostic Criteria (Four Major Required)

- Major criteria
  - Dermatitis involving two or more sites including the scalp, axillae, groin, external ear, retroauricular areas, eyelid margins, paranasal skin, and/or neck
  - Chronic rhinorrhea without other signs of rhinitis and/or crusting of the anterior nares
  - Chronic relapsing dermatitis with prompt response to antibiotics but prompt recurrence upon withdrawal
  - Onset in early childhood
  - Human T-lymphotropic virus type 1 seropositivity
- Minor criteria
  - Positive cultures for *Staphylococcus aureus* and/or ß-hemolytic streptococci from the skin or anterior nares
  - Generalized papular rash
  - Generalized lymphadenopathy with dermatopathic lymphadenitis
  - Anemia
  - Increased erythrocyte sedimentation rate
  - Elevated immunoglobulin levels (IgD and IgE)
  - Raised CD4 count, CD8 count, and CD4/CD8 ratio

Further reading:

- Lee R, Schwartz RA (2011) Human T-lymphotrophic virus type 1-associated infective dermatitis: a comprehensive review. J Am Acad Dermatol 64(1):152–160

Inflammatory Linear Verrucous Epidermal Nevus (ILVEN)

Type of verrucous epidermal nevus that appears in infancy or early childhood and that is characterized by chronic, pruritic and erythematous, verrucous, or psoriasiform plaques along Blaschko's lines (Fig. 6.54)

Differential Diagnosis

- Basaloid follicular hamartoma syndrome
- Ichthyosiform nevus of CHILD syndrome
- Incontinentia pigmenti, stage II
- Linear Darier's disease
- Linear lichen planus
- Linear lichen nitidus
- Linear lichen simplex chronicus

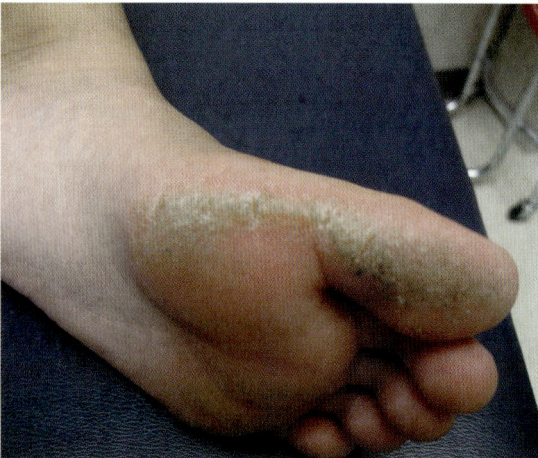

Fig. 6.54 Inflammatory linear verrucous epidermal nevus

- Linear porokeratosis
- <u>Linear verrucous epidermal nevus</u>
- Linear warts
- <u>Nevoid psoriasis</u>

Treatment Options

- <u>Topical corticosteroids</u>
- Topical vitamin D analogues
- <u>Topical retinoids</u>
- CO_2 laser
- <u>Surgical excision</u>

Further reading:
- Lee SH, Rogers M (2001) Inflammatory linear verrucous epidermal naevi: a review of 23 cases. Australas J Dermatol 42(4):252–256

Ingrown Toenail (Onychocryptosis, Unguis Incarnatus)

Common nail problem predominantly affecting the great toes that is caused by ingrowth of the nail under the lateral nail fold and is characterized by pain, erythema, swelling, and exuberant granulation tissue

Differential Diagnosis

- Amelanotic melanoma
- Metastatic lesion
- Paronychia
- <u>Pyogenic granuloma</u>

Association

- <u>Congenital malalignment of the great toenails</u>
- Isotretinoin

Treatment Options

- <u>Partial nail avulsion with or without chemical ablation</u>
- Topical antibiotics
- Systemic antibiotics

Further reading:
- Daniel CR III, Iorizzo M, Tosti A, Piraccini BM (2006) Ingrown toenails. Cutis 78(6):407–408

Interstitial Granulomatous Dermatitis with Arthritis

Idiopathic granulomatous disease that occurs predominantly in female patients with autoimmune disease, especially severe rheumatoid arthritis, and some infectious diseases (e.g., coccidioidomycosis) and is characterized by linear, erythematous subcutaneous cords (rope sign) distributed on the abdomen or flank as well as tender or burning, erythematous to violaceous indurated papules, nodules, and plaques

Differential Diagnosis

- Blau syndrome
- Churg–Strauss syndrome
- <u>Granuloma annulare</u>
- <u>Granulomatous drug reaction</u>
- Granulomatous mycosis fungoides
- Juvenile rheumatoid arthritis
- Leukemia cutis
- Lyme disease
- Lymphocytic infiltrate of Jessner
- Lymphoma
- Mondor's disease
- Morphea
- Necrobiosis lipoidica

- <u>Palisaded neutrophilic and granulomatous dermatitis</u>
- Rheumatoid nodule
- <u>Sarcoidosis</u>
- Superficial thrombophlebitis
- Tumid lupus erythematosus
- Urticarial vasculitis
- Wegener's granulomatosis

Associations

- Coccidioidomycosis
- Hemolytic anemia
- <u>Rheumatoid arthritis</u>
- Systemic lupus erythematosus
- Thyroiditis
- TNF inhibitor therapy

Evaluation

- Antinuclear antibodies
- Complete blood count
- Rheumatoid factor level
- Search for underlying infection

Treatment Options

- <u>Treat the underlying cause</u>
- Topical corticosteroids
- <u>Systemic corticosteroids</u>
- Infliximab

Further reading:

- Sayah A, English JC (2005) Rheumatoid arthritis: a review of the cutaneous manifestations. J Am Acad Dermatol 53(2):191–209

Intertrigo

Dermatosis affecting the intertriginous areas that is caused by a combination of occlusion, friction, heat, and moisture and is characterized by pruritus, erythema, scale, and maceration

Differential Diagnosis

- Acanthosis nigricans
- Acrodermatitis enteropathica
- Baboon syndrome
- Biotin deficiency
- Bowen's disease
- <u>Candidiasis</u>
- <u>Contact dermatitis</u>
- <u>Dermatophytosis</u>
- Erythrasma
- Extramammary Paget's disease
- <u>Hailey–Hailey disease</u>
- Granuloma gluteale infantum
- Langerhans cell histiocytosis
- Inverse psoriasis
- Necrolytic migratory erythema
- Pemphigus
- <u>Seborrheic dermatitis</u>
- Staphylococcal infection
- Streptococcal infection

Evaluation

- Gram stain and bacterial culture
- Potassium hydroxide examination and fungal culture

Treatment Options

- <u>Topical corticosteroids</u>
- Zinc oxide
- <u>Nystatin cream</u>
- Ketoconazole
- Protopic ointment
- Petrolatum
- Absorbent powders

Further reading:
- Farage MA, Miller KW, Berardesca E, Maibach HI (2007) Incontinence in the aged: contact dermatitis and other cutaneous consequences. Contact dermatitis 57(4):211–217

Inverted Follicular Keratosis (Helwig's Disease)

Benign neoplasm that affects older adults and is characterized by a hyper-keratotic, pink papule most commonly located on the face

Differential Diagnosis

- Actinic keratosis
- Basal cell carcinoma
- Bowen's disease
- Keratoacanthoma
- Melanoma
- Poroma
- <u>Squamous cell carcinoma</u>
- <u>Seborrheic keratosis</u>
- Trichilemmoma
- Verruca

Further reading:
- Ko CJ, Shintaku P, Binder SW (2005) Comparison of benign keratoses using p53, bcl-1, and bcl-2. J Cutan Pathol 32(5):356–359

IPEX Syndrome (Immune Dysregulation, Polyendocrinopathy, Enteropathy, and X-Linked Syndrome)

X-linked recessive syndrome that is caused by mutation of the gene-encoding FOXP3, which is required for the development of regulatory T cells, and is characterized by dermatitis, urticaria, alopecia universalis, pemphigoid, enteropathy, type I diabetes, thyroiditis, hemolytic anemia, and thrombocytopenia

Differential Diagnosis

- APECED syndrome
- Autoimmune polyendocrine syndrome, type II (Schmidt syndrome)
- Dermatitis herpetiformis
- Severe combined immune deficiency
- Systemic lupus erythematosus
- Wiskott–Aldrich syndrome

Further reading:
- Nieves DS, Phipps RP, Pollock SJ et al (2004) Dermatologic and immunologic findings in the immune dysregulation, polyendocrinopathy, enteropathy, X-linked syndrome. Arch Dermatol 140(4):466–472

Jellyfish Sting

Painful and pruritic eruption caused by aquatic contact with a variety of jellyfish and characterized by flagellate, streaky urticarial and vesicular plaques at the exposed site

Differential Diagnosis

- Herpes zoster
- Larva migrans
- Mushroom dermatitis

- <u>Phytophotodermatitis</u>
- Rhus dermatitis
- Zoster

Associations

- Allergic contact dermatitis
- Deep venous thrombosis
- Erythema nodosum
- Gangrene
- Granuloma annulare
- Keloids
- Mondor's disease
- Papular urticaria
- Postinflammatory hyperpigmentation
- Toxin-mediated eruption

Treatment Options

- <u>Vinegar rinse</u>
- Antivenom (box jellyfish)
- Removal of nematocysts
- Pain control

Further reading:

- Ulrich H, Landthaler M, Vogt T (2007) Granulomatous jellyfish dermatitis. J Dtsch Dermatol Ges 5(6):493–495

Jessner's Lymphocytic Infiltrate

Idiopathic disease caused by benign lymphocytic infiltration of the skin that is characterized by erythematous, nonscaly papules and plaques either solitary or grouped in circinate, annular, or semicircular arrays which are most commonly located on the face (especially the cheeks), neck, and back

Differential Diagnosis

- Arthropod-bite reaction
- Contact dermatitis, especially lymphomatoid type
- Cutaneous lymphoid hyperplasia
- Cutaneous lymphoma
- Erythema annulare centrifugum (especially deep variant)
- Fixed drug eruption
- Granuloma annulare
- Granuloma faciale
- Metastasis
- Polymorphous light eruption
- Reticular erythematous mucinosis
- Rosacea
- Sarcoidosis
- Sjögren syndrome
- Sweet's syndrome
- Tumid lupus erythematosus
- Urticarial dermatitis

Evaluation

- Antinuclear antibodies (including SS-A and SS-B)

Treatment Options

- Sunscreen
- Topical corticosteroids
- Hydroxychloroquine
- Systemic corticosteroids
- Methotrexate

Further reading:
- Lipsker D, Mitschler A, Grosshans E et al (2006) Could Jessner's lymphocytic infiltrate of the skin be a dermal variant of lupus erythematosus? An analysis of 210 cases. Dermatology 213(1):15–22

Juvenile Hyaline Fibromatosis

Autosomal-recessive disorder caused by mutation of the gene-encoding capillary morphogenesis protein 2 that is characterized by onset in early childhood of nodular skin lesions containing hyaline material on the hands, scalp, ears, and face, as well as gingival hypertrophy, and, later in childhood, joint contractures and osteopenia

Differential Diagnosis

- Farber lipogranulomatosis
- <u>Gingival fibromatosis</u>
- Infantile digital fibromatosis
- <u>Infantile myofibromatosis</u>
- <u>Lipoid proteinosis</u>
- Nodular amyloidosis
- <u>Winchester syndrome</u>

Evaluation

- Skeletal survey

Further reading:
- Thomas JE, Moossavi M, Mehregan DR et al (2004) Juvenile hyaline fibromatosis: a case report and review of the literature. Int J Dermatol 43(11):785–789

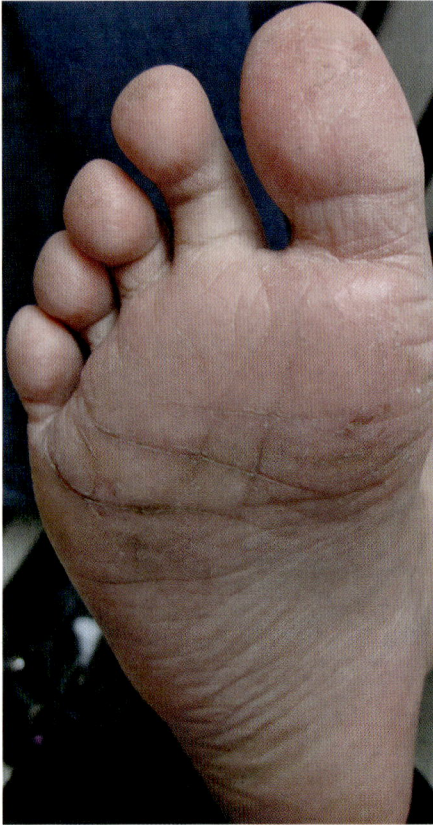

Fig. 6.55 Juvenile plantar dermatitis

Juvenile Plantar Dermatitis

Cutaneous eruption that affects children and is characterized by erythema, fissuring, and peeling on the anterior aspect of the sole, but not the toe-web spaces, and is exacerbated by sweating in occlusive footwear (Fig. 6.55)

Differential Diagnosis

- Dyshidrotic eczema
- Palmoplantar hyperhidrosis

- Palmoplantar psoriasis
- Pitted keratolysis
- Pityriasis rubra pilaris
- Pseudomonal hot-foot syndrome
- Shoe allergy
- Tinea pedis

Evaluation

- Potassium hydroxide examination of scale

Treatment Options

- Observation
- Emollients at night
- Drying measures during day
- Topical corticosteroids
- Topical calcineurin inhibitors

Further reading:
- Gibbs NF (2004) Juvenile plantar dermatosis. Can sweat cause foot rash and peeling? Postgrad Med 115(6):73–75

Juvenile Rheumatoid Arthritis (Still's Disease)

Arthritic disease with onset in childhood (and occasionally adulthood) that is associated with periodic episodes of spiking fever with a concomitant salmon-colored evanescent macular rash on the trunk and extremities

Differential Diagnosis

- Ankylosing spondylitis
- Blau syndrome
- Endocarditis
- Familial Mediterranean fever

- Farber lipogranulomatosis
- Hyper-IgD syndrome
- Kawasaki disease
- Leukemia
- Lyme disease
- Muckle–Wells syndrome
- Multicentric reticulohistiocytosis
- NOMID syndrome
- Reactive arthritis with urethritis and conjunctivitis
- Rheumatic fever
- Sarcoidosis
- Systemic lupus erythematosus
- Tumor necrosis factor receptor-associated periodic syndrome (TRAPS)
- Viral exanthem

Evaluation

- Antinuclear antibodies
- Complete blood count
- Echocardiography
- Immunoglobulin levels
- Joint-fluid examination
- Joint radiographs
- Liver function test
- Ophthalmologic exam
- Renal function test
- Rheumatoid factor
- Sedimentation rate
- Urinalysis

Further reading:

- Sayah A, English JC III (2005) Rheumatoid arthritis: a review of the cutaneous manifestations. J Am Acad Dermatol 53(2):191–209

Juvenile Spring Eruption

Variant of polymorphous light eruption affecting young boys in the spring that is characterized by erythematous, nonscarring papules and papulo-vesicles on the helices

Differential Diagnosis

- Actinic prurigo
- Herpes simplex virus infection
- Hydroa vacciniforme
- Impetigo
- Porphyria
- Pseudoporphyria
- Sunburn

Treatment Options

- Sunscreen
- Topical corticosteroids

Further reading:

- Stratigos AJ, Antoniou C, Papadakis P et al (2004) Juvenile spring eruption: clinicopathologic features and phototesting results in 4 cases. J Am Acad Dermatol 50(2 Suppl):S57–S60

Juvenile Xanthogranuloma

Histiocytic lesion of unknown cause that predominantly affects children and is characterized by a red-brown to yellow, solitary (less commonly, multiple) papule or nodule most commonly on the head or neck

Differential Diagnosis

- Benign cephalic histiocytosis
- Dermatofibroma
- Fibrous hamartoma of infancy
- Generalized eruptive histiocytoma
- Giant cell reticulohistiocytoma
- Idiopathic facial aseptic granuloma
- Indeterminate cell histiocytosis
- Infantile myofibromatosis
- Keloid
- Langerhans cell histiocytosis
- Melanocytic nevus
- Molluscum contagiosum
- Pyogenic granuloma
- Rhabdomyoma
- Self-healing reticulohistiocytosis
- Solitary mastocytoma
- Spitz nevus
- Xanthoma
- Xanthoma disseminatum

Associations

- Chronic myelogenous leukemia
- Neurofibromatosis
- Niemann–Pick disease
- Urticaria pigmentosa

Further reading:
- Redbord KP, Sheth AP (2007) Multiple juvenile xanthogranulomas in a 13-year-old. Pediatr Dermatol 24(3):238–240

Kaposi's Sarcoma

Mucocutaneous vascular malignancy affecting elderly patients of Mediterranean descent or profoundly immunocompromised AIDS patients that is caused by human herpes virus 8 (HHV-8) and is characterized by red to purple patches, plaques, and nodules that can occur anywhere, including the gastrointestinal tract and lungs, but most commonly occur on the distal lower extremities

Subtypes

- African endemic
- AIDS-related epidemic
- Classic
- Iatrogenic

Differential Diagnosis

- Acquired elastotic hemangioma
- Acquired progressive lymphangioma
- Acroangiodermatitis of Mali
- Aneurysmal fibrous histiocytoma
- Angiokeratoma
- Angiosarcoma
- Arteriovenous malformation
- Bacillary angiomatosis
- Blue nevus
- Blue rubber bleb nevus syndrome
- Dermatofibroma
- Ecchymosis
- Erythema elevatum diutinum
- Granuloma annulare

- Granuloma faciale
- Hemangiopericytoma
- Insect-bite reactions
- Kaposiform hemangioendothelioma
- Keloid
- Leiomyosarcoma
- Leishmaniasis (especially diffuse cutaneous)
- Lymphatic malformation
- Malignant fibrous histiocytoma
- Melanocytic nevus
- Melanoma
- Metastasis (especially renal cell carcinoma)
- Microvenular hemangioma
- Multinucleate cell angiohistiocytoma
- Myofibromatosis
- Nevus flammeus
- Polyarteritis nodosa
- Progressive lymphangioma
- Pyogenic granuloma
- Reactive angioendotheliomatosis
- Spindle cell hemangioendothelioma
- Stasis dermatitis
- Stewart–Bluefarb syndrome (pseudo-Kaposi's sarcoma)
- Targetoid hemosiderotic (hobnail) hemangioma
- Tufted angioma
- Varix
- Venous malformation

Evaluation

- Chest radiograph
- Stool for occult blood
- Complete blood count

Treatment Options

- HAART therapy
- Cryotherapy
- Intralesional vinblastine
- Radiation
- Systemic chemotherapy
- Intralesional interferon
- Systemic interferon
- Thalidomide
- Pulsed dye laser
- Surgical excision

Further reading:
- Jessop S (2006) HIV-associated Kaposi's sarcoma. Dermatol Clin 24(4):509–520

Kaposi's Varicelliform Eruption

Term given for viral (usually HSV) infection superimposed on one of several chronic or inflammatory skin conditions, most commonly eczema, that is characterized by umbilicated vesicles and erosions typically on the neck but also on any area affected with the underlying dermatosis

Differential Diagnosis

- Acute exacerbation of underlying disease
- Bullous impetigo
- Hydroa vacciniforme
- Varicella infection
- Zoster

Associations

- Allergic contact dermatitis
- Atopic dermatitis
- Burns
- Congenital ichthyosiform erythroderma
- Hailey–Hailey disease
- Ichthyosis vulgaris
- Darier's disease
- Mycosis fungoides
- Pemphigus
- Psoriasis
- Rosacea
- Seborrheic dermatitis
- Sézary's syndrome
- Wiskott–Aldrich syndrome

Treatment Options

- Systemic antivirals
- Treat underlying cause

Further reading:
- Santmyire-Rosenberger BR, Nigra TP (2005) Psoriasis herpeticum: three cases of Kaposi's varicelliform eruption in psoriasis. J Am Acad Dermatol 53(1):52–56

Kawasaki Disease (Mucocutaneous Lymph Node Syndrome)

Childhood vasculitis-like syndrome with a possible bacterial or viral etiology that is characterized by fever, a polymorphous skin eruption, desquamating rash on the acral areas, mucosal inflammation, lymphadenopathy, and the potential for coronary artery aneurysms

Differential Diagnosis

- <u>Drug eruption</u>
- Erythema multiforme
- <u>Juvenile rheumatoid arthritis</u>
- Kawasaki-like syndrome (HIV)
- Leptospirosis
- Lupus erythematosus
- Lyme disease
- Measles
- Mercury poisoning
- Parvovirus B19 infection
- Polyarteritis nodosa
- Rocky Mountain spotted fever
- <u>Scarlet fever</u>
- Serum sickness
- Staphylococcal scalded-skin syndrome
- <u>Stevens–Johnson syndrome</u>
- <u>Toxic shock syndrome</u>
- <u>Viral exanthem</u>

Diagnostic Criteria

- Fever for 5 or more days without other explanation *and*
- Four of the following five:
  - Bilateral nonexudative conjunctival injection
  - Injected or fissured lips, injected pharynx, or strawberry tongue
  - Erythema of the palms and soles, edema of hands and feet, or periungual desquamation
  - Polymorphous exanthem
  - Acute nonsuppurative cervical lymphadenopathy

Evaluation

- Complete blood count
- Echocardiography
- Electrocardiography
- Liver function test
- Renal function test
- Sedimentation rate
- Urinalysis

Treatment Options

- Aspirin
- Intravenous immunoglobulin
- Plasma exchange

Further reading:
- Mizuno Y, Suga Y, Muramatsu S et al (2006) Psoriasiform and palmoplanter pustular lesions induced after Kawasaki disease. Int J Dermatol 45(9):1080–1082

Keloid

Benign, exuberant proliferation of scar tissue that is characterized by nodules or plaques of fibrous tissue which extend beyond the boundary of the initial wound

Differential Diagnosis

- Carcinoma en cuirasse
- Connective tissue nevus
- Dermatofibroma
- Dermatofibrosarcoma protuberans
- Dermatomyofibroma
- Epidermal inclusion cyst

- Erythema elevatum diutinum
- <u>Hypertrophic scar</u>
- Keloidal basal cell carcinoma
- Keloidal Kaposi's sarcoma
- Kimura disease
- Lepromatous leprosy
- Lobomycosis (keloidal blastomycosis)
- Molluscum pseudotumors
- Morphea
- Neurofibroma
- Spitz nevus, keloid type
- Systemic sclerosis
- Xanthoma disseminatum

Associations

- Ehlers–Danlos syndrome
- Rubinstein–Taybi syndrome
- Turner syndrome

Treatment Options

- <u>Intralesional corticosteroids</u>
- Flurandrenolide tape
- Intralesional interferon
- Imiquimod cream
- Cryosurgery
- Radiation
- Verapamil
- <u>Surgical excision</u>

Further reading:
- Robles DT, Berg D (2007) Abnormal wound healing: keloids. Clin Dermatol 25(1):26–32

Keratitis–Ichthyosis–Deafness (KID) Syndrome (Senter Syndrome)

Sporadic genodermatosis associated with connexin 26 mutation that is characterized by vascularizing keratitis, ichthyosis, thick verrucous plaques on the face, perioral furrowing, palmoplantar keratoderma, and sensorineural deafness

Differential Diagnosis

- Bullous congenital ichthyosiform erythroderma
- Erythrokeratodermia variabilis
- HID syndrome
- Keratosis follicularis spinulosa decalvans
- Lamellar ichthyosis
- Netherton's syndrome
- Nonbullous congenital ichthyosiform erythroderma
- Progressive symmetric erythrokeratodermia
- Vohwinkel's syndrome with deafness

Further reading:

- Mazereeuw-Hautier J, Bitoun E, Chevrant-Breton J et al (2007) Keratitis–ichthyosis–deafness syndrome: disease expression and spectrum of connexin 26 (GJB2) mutations in 14 patients. Br J Dermatol 156(5):1015–1019

Keratoacanthoma

Low-grade type of squamous cell carcinoma with the potential to self-involute that is characterized by a circular dome-shaped erythematous papule or nodule with central ulceration most commonly on the sun-exposed areas

Subtypes/Variants

- Aggressive
- Eruptive keratoacanthomas of Grzybowski
- Giant type

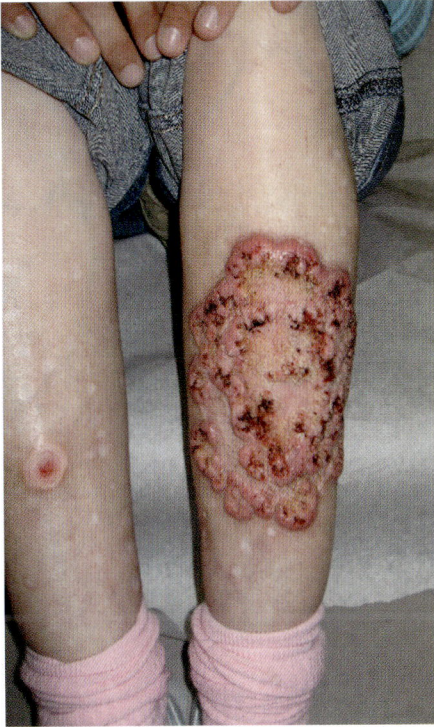

Fig. 6.56 Keratoacanthoma centrifugum marginatum (Courtesy of A. Zedlitz)

- Keratoacanthoma centrifugum marginatum (Fig. 6.56)
- Keratoacanthoma dyskeratoticum segregans
- Multinodular
- Multiple self-healing keratoacanthomas of Ferguson–Smith
- Solitary type
- Subungual type
- Witten and Zak syndrome

Differential Diagnosis

- Anaplastic large cell lymphoma
- Atypical fibroxanthoma

- Basal cell carcinoma
- Blastomycosis
- Coccidioidomycosis
- Halogenoderma
- <u>Hypertrophic actinic keratosis</u>
- Hypertrophic/verrucous cutaneous lupus erythematosus
- <u>Inverted follicular keratosis</u>
- Lupus vulgaris
- Merkel cell carcinoma
- Metastasis
- Molluscum contagiosum
- Orf/Milker's nodule
- Pilomatricoma
- <u>Prurigo nodularis</u>
- Sebaceous epithelioma
- Sporotrichosis
- Trichilemmoma
- Verruca

Associations

- Chronically inflamed area
- <u>Immunosuppression</u>
- Incontinentia pigmenti
- Muir–Torre syndrome
- Nevus sebaceus
- Stasis dermatitis
- Steel wool (periungual type)
- Trauma

Treatment Options

- <u>Surgical excision</u>
- Electrodessication and curettage
- Intralesional 5-FU

- Intralesional methotrexate
- Radiation
- Isotretinoin
- Acitretin

Further reading:
- Magalhães RF, Cruvinel GT, Cintra GF, Cintra ML, Ismael AP, de Moraes AM (2008) Diagnosis and follow-up of keratoacanthoma-like lesions: clinical-histologic study of 43 cases. J Cutan Med Surg 12(4):163–173

Keratoelastoidosis Marginalis (Degenerative Collagenous Plaques of the Hands)

Rare acquired disorder associated with both chronic trauma and chronic actinic damage that affects the hands and is characterized by asymptomatic, translucent, crateriform plaques on the margins of the hands, especially the radial aspect of the index finger and the opposing aspect of the thumb

Differential Diagnosis

- <u>Acrokeratoelastoidosis of Costa</u>
- Acrokeratosis verruciformis of Hopf
- Colloid milium
- Erythropoietic protoporphyria
- Focal acral hyperkeratosis

Further reading:
- Abulafia J, Vignale RA (2000) Degenerative collagenous plaques of the hands and acrokeratoelastoidosis: pathogenesis and relationship with knuckle pads. Int J Dermatol 39(6):424–432

Keratolysis Exfoliativa (Recurrent Focal Palmar Peeling, Lamellar Dyshidrosis)

Low-grade form of hand eczema characterized by small foci of dry peeling on the palms or soles

Differential Diagnosis

- Contact dermatitis
- Dyshidrotic eczema
- Kawasaki disease
- Psoriasis
- Secondary syphilis
- Tinea manuum or pedis
- Xerosis

Treatment Options

- Keratolytic moisturizers
- Topical corticosteroids

Further reading:
- Lee HJ, Ha SJ, Ahn WK et al (2001) Clinical evaluation of atopic hand–foot dermatitis. Pediatr Dermatol 18(2):102–106

Keratosis Follicularis Spinulosa Decalvans

X-linked recessive or dominant disorder characterized by generalized keratosis pilaris atrophicans, scarring alopecia of the scalp and eyebrows, palmoplantar keratoderma, photophobia, and, less consistently, deafness and mental retardation

Differential Diagnosis

- Atopic dermatitis
- Atrichia with papular lesions
- Graham–Little syndrome
- IFAP syndrome
- KID syndrome
- Lichen planopilaris

Further reading:

• Goh MS, Magee J, Chong AH (2005) Keratosis follicularis spinulosa decalvans and acne keloidalis nuchae. Australas J Dermatol 46(4):257–260

Keratosis Lichenoides Chronica (Nekam's Disease)

Rare, idiopathic disorder with onset in childhood that is characterized by linear or reticulate plaques of coalescent, hyperkeratotic, violaceous papules and nodules on the extremities and buttocks along with an erythematous, scaly, seborrheic dermatitis-like, or rosacea-like eruption on the face, oral ulcers, and nail dystrophy

Differential Diagnosis

• Graham–Little–Piccardi–Lasseur syndrome
• Haber syndrome
• <u>Hypertrophic lichen planus</u>
• Lichenoid drug eruption
• Lichen striatus
• <u>Lupus erythematosus</u>
• Mycosis fungoides
• Pityriasis lichenoides
• Porokeratosis of Mibelli
• Seborrheic dermatitis
• Secondary syphilis (especially verrucous type)

Associations

• Chronic lymphocytic leukemia
• Cutaneous amyloidosis
• Glomerulonephritis
• Hepatitis
• Multiple sclerosis
• Seborrheic dermatitis
• Toxoplasmosis

Treatment Options

- Tazarotene cream
- Acitretin
- Narrowband UVB phototherapy
- Topical vitamin D analogues

Further reading:
- Boer A (2006) Keratosis lichenoides chronica: proposal of a concept. Am J Dermatopathol 28(3):260–275

Keratosis Pilaris

Disorder of follicular hyperkeratosis affecting children and adults and characterized by keratotic papules with or without surrounding erythema located predominantly on the upper outer arms, anterior thighs, and buttocks and occasionally the cheeks (keratosis pilaris rubra faciei)

Differential Diagnosis

- Acne vulgaris
- Atrichia with papular lesions
- Darier's disease
- Disseminate and recurrent infundibulofolliculitis
- Familial dyskeratotic comedones
- Follicular eczema
- Folliculitis
- Gianotti–Crosti syndrome
- Graham–Little–Piccardi–Lasseur syndrome
- Infantile acne
- Keratosis pilaris atrophicans
- KID syndrome

- Lichen nitidus
- Lichen planus
- Lichen spinulosus
- Milia
- Phrynoderma
- Pityriasis rubra pilaris
- Trichostasis spinulosa

Associations

- <u>Atopic dermatitis</u>
- Cardiofaciocutaneous syndrome
- Carvajal syndrome
- Down syndrome
- <u>Ichthyosis vulgaris</u>
- Monilethrix
- Noonan syndrome

Treatment Options

- <u>Ammonium lactate</u>
- <u>Urea</u>
- <u>Salicylic acid</u>
- <u>Glycolic acid</u>
- Topical corticosteroids
- Topical retinoids
- Isotretinoin
- Systemic antibiotics

Further reading:
- Lateef A, Schwartz RA (1999) Keratosis pilaris. Cutis 63(4):205–207

Keratosis Pilaris Atrophicans

Uncommon group of disorders of follicular keratinization that can occur as isolated findings or as part of a syndrome and that are characterized by inflammatory keratotic papules, most commonly on the face, that evolve to atrophic scars

Subtypes/Variants

- Atrophoderma vermiculatum
- Folliculitis spinulosa decalvans
- Keratosis follicularis spinulosa decalvans
- Ulerythema ophryogenes

Differential Diagnosis

- <u>Acne vulgaris</u>
- <u>Atrophia maculosa varioliformis cutis</u>
- Folliculitis
- <u>Keratosis pilaris</u>
- Milia
- Pityriasis rubra pilaris

Associations

- Cardiofaciocutaneous syndrome
- Cornelia de Lange syndrome
- Noonan's syndrome
- Rubinstein–Taybi syndrome
- Woolly hair

Further reading:
- Callaway SR, Lesher JL Jr (2004) Keratosis pilaris atrophicans: case series and review. Pediatr Dermatol 21(1):14–17

Keratosis Punctata (Palmaris et Plantaris/of the Palmar Creases)

Two types of punctate keratoderma that are autosomal-dominantly inherited, that have onset in adulthood, that predominantly affect patients of African descent, and that are characterized by pruritic, keratotic papules or comedo-like pits diffusely over the palms and soles or confined to the creases

Differential Diagnosis

- Acrokeratoelastoidosis of Costa
- Arsenical keratoses
- Clavi
- Cowden's disease
- Darier's disease
- Focal acral hyperkeratosis
- Porokeratosis punctata
- Spiny keratoderma
- Verruca vulgaris

Treatment Options

- Paring, filing, and curettage
- Urea cream
- Salicylic acid
- Acitretin

Further reading:
- Kong MS, Harford R, O'Neill JT (2004) Keratosis punctata palmoplantaris controlled with topical retinoids: a case report and review of the literature. Cutis 74(3):173–179

Kikuchi–Fujimoto Disease (Histiocytic Necrotizing Lymphadenitis)

Acquired, uncommon, self-limited disorder that is possibly viral in etiology, predominantly affects women, and is characterized by cervical lymphadenopathy, fever, and, occasionally, a generalized, polymorphic skin eruption

Differential Diagnosis

- <u>Angioimmunoblastic dysproteinemia with lymphadenopathy</u>
- Cat-scratch disease
- <u>DRESS syndrome</u>
- <u>Hodgkin's disease</u>
- Lymphoma
- <u>Mononucleosis</u>
- Polyarteritis nodosa
- <u>Rosai–Dorfman disease</u>
- Secondary syphilis
- Still's disease
- Systemic lupus erythematosus
- Toxoplasmosis
- Tuberculosis

Evaluation

- Antinuclear antibodies
- Complete blood count
- EBV serologic tests
- Lymph node biopsy
- Sedimentation rate

Further reading:
- Lee HW, Yun WJ, Chang SE et al (2006) Generalized maculopapules with fever and cervical lymphadenopathy. Arch Dermatol 142(5):641–646

Kimura's Disease

Idiopathic inflammatory disorder that is possibly allergic in etiology and is characterized by an asymptomatic subcutaneous swelling or enlarged lymph node in the cervical area

Differential Diagnosis

- <u>Angiolymphoid hyperplasia with eosinophilia</u>
- <u>Benign lymphadenopathy</u>
- Cutaneous lymphoid hyperplasia
- Cylindroma
- Dermatofibrosarcoma protuberans
- Eosinophilic granuloma
- Kaposi's sarcoma
- <u>Keloid</u>
- Kikuchi's disease
- Langerhans cell histiocytosis
- <u>Lymphoma</u>
- Metastatic disease
- Mikulicz syndrome
- Parotid tumor
- Pyogenic granuloma
- <u>Rosai–Dorfman disease</u>
- Salivary gland tumor
- Sarcoidosis

Further reading:
- Chong WS, Thomas A, Goh CL (2006) Kimura's disease and angiolymphoid hyperplasia with eosinophilia: two disease entities in the same patient: case report and review of the literature. Int J Dermatol 45(2):139–145

Klippel–Trenaunay (Parkes Weber) Syndrome

Vascular malformation syndrome characterized by port-wine stain, varicose veins, bone and soft tissue hypertrophy, and, occasionally, an arteriovenous malformation (Parkes Weber syndrome)

Differential Diagnosis

- Bockenheimer syndrome
- Cutis marmorata telangiectatica congenita
- Extensive venous malformation
- Gorham syndrome
- Kaposiform hemangioendothelioma
- Maffucci syndrome
- Neurofibromatosis
- Proteus syndrome

Associations

- Sturge–Weber syndrome

Evaluation

- Venography
- Ultrasound
- Arteriography
- MRI studies

Treatment Options

- Pain control
- Compressive wraps
- Surgical excision
- Endovenous laser ablation

Further reading:

- Redondo P, Aguado L, Martínez-Cuesta A (2011) Diagnosis and management of extensive vascular malformations of the lower limb: part I. Clinical diagnosis. J Am Acad Dermatol 65(5):893–906; quiz 907–908

Knuckle Pads

Benign, acquired or familial, asymptomatic, fibrous nodules occurring on the knuckles

Differential Diagnosis

- Acanthosis nigricans, acral type
- Callus
- Diabetic finger pebbles
- Erythema elevatum diutinum
- Foreign body reaction
- Gottron's papules
- Gouty tophus
- Granuloma annulare
- Heberden nodules
- Infantile digital fibromatosis
- Lichen simplex chronicus
- Pachydermodactyly
- Psoriasis
- Rheumatoid nodules
- Russell's sign of bulimia
- Wart
- Xanthomas

Associations

- Bart–Pumphrey syndrome
- Dupuytren's contracture

- Esophageal carcinoma
- Plantar fibromatosis
- Pseudoxanthoma elasticum

Further reading:
- Dickens R, Adams BB, Mutasim DF (2002) Sports-related pads. Int J Dermatol 41(5):291–293

Langerhans Cell Histiocytosis

Collective term for a group of disorders caused by the proliferation of Langerhans cells that is characterized by either an adult-onset type with localized bony or pulmonary infiltrates (chronic focal); a childhood-onset type with bony infiltrates, exophthalmos, and diabetes insipidus (chronic multifocal); or an infancy-onset type with a diffuse, seborrheic-dermatitis-like eruption in the intertriginous areas, hepatosplenomegaly, lymphadenopathy, and bone marrow involvement (acute disseminated)

Subtypes/Variants

- Acute disseminated (Letterer–Siwe disease)
- Chronic multifocal (Hand–Schuller–Christian disease)
- Chronic focal (eosinophilic granuloma)
- Congenital self-healing (Hashimoto–Pritzker disease)

Differential Diagnosis

- Acrodermatitis enteropathica
- Benign cephalic histiocytosis
- Candidiasis
- Darier's disease
- Dermatomyositis
- Eosinophilic pustular folliculitis
- Generalized eruptive histiocytosis

- Granuloma gluteale infantum
- Herpes simplex virus infection
- Incontinentia pigmenti
- Indeterminate cell histiocytosis
- Infantile acropustulosis
- Leukemia
- Lichen nitidus
- Listeriosis
- Lymphoma
- Mastocytosis
- Miliaria
- Multiple myeloma
- Mycosis fungoides
- Neonatal lupus
- Pseudoverrucous papules
- Rosai–Dorfman disease
- Scabies
- <u>Seborrheic dermatitis</u>
- Transient neonatal pustular melanosis
- Urticaria pigmentosa
- Varicella
- Wiskott–Aldrich syndrome
- Xanthoma disseminatum

Associations

- Smoking (eosinophilic granuloma)
- Leukemia

Evaluation

- Bone marrow biopsy
- Chest radiograph
- Complete blood count

- Liver function test
- MRI scan of the brain/pituitary
- Neurologic examination
- Panoramic radiograph of teeth
- Serum chemistry
- Skeletal survey
- Urinalysis and urine electrolytes
- Urine osmolality

Treatment Options

- Topical nitrogen mustard
- PUVA phototherapy
- Systemic chemotherapy
- Systemic corticosteroids
- Azathioprine
- Methotrexate

Further reading:
- Querings K, Starz H, Balda BR (2006) Clinical spectrum of cutaneous Langerhans' cell histiocytosis mimicking various diseases. Acta Derm Venereol 86(1):39–43

Large Cell Acanthoma

Benign epidermal neoplasm that is possibly related to the solar lentigo and is characterized by a sharply demarcated, tan, slightly scaly, plaque most commonly located on the sun-exposed areas

Differential Diagnosis

- Actinic keratosis
- Bowen's disease
- Clear cell acanthoma
- Lichen-planus-like keratosis

- Melanoma
- <u>Seborrheic keratosis</u>
- Solar lentigo

Further reading:

- Mehregan DR, Hamzavi F, Brown K (2003) Large cell acanthoma. Int J Dermatol 42(1):36–39

Larva Migrans/Larva Currens, Cutaneous (Creeping Eruption)

Cutaneous infestation with the larvae of the hookworms *Ancylostoma braziliensis* or *Necator americanus* (migrans) or the roundworm *Strongyloides stercoralis* (currens) characterized by a migratory, erythematous, serpiginous eruption on the feet, buttocks, arms, hands, and back

Differential Diagnosis

- Allergic contact dermatitis
- Arthropod-bite reaction
- Chemical burn
- <u>Cutaneous pili migrans</u>
- Dermatographism
- <u>Dermatophytosis</u>
- Dirofilariasis
- <u>Erythema annulare centrifugum</u>
- Erythema gyratum repens
- Erythema marginatum
- Erythema migrans
- <u>Granuloma annulare</u>
- Jellyfish sting
- Lichen striatus
- Lymphangitis
- Mondor disease
- Myiasis

- Paragonimiasis
- Photoallergic dermatitis
- Phytophotodermatitis
- Scabies
- Sparganosis
- Thrombophlebitis

Treatment Options

- Cryotherapy
- <u>Topical thiabendazole</u>
- Mebendazole
- Albendazole
- Ivermectin

Further reading:
- Brenner MA, Patel MB (2003) Cutaneous larva migrans: the creeping eruption. Cutis 72(2):111–115

Laugier–Hunziker Syndrome

Rare mucocutaneous pigmentary disorder of unknown cause that is characterized by hypermelanotic macules on the oral mucosa (especially lips and buccal mucosa) and longitudinal pigmented streaks of the nails

Differential Diagnosis

- Addison's disease
- Amalgam tattoo
- Chemotherapy-related hyperpigmentation
- Cronkhite–Canada syndrome
- Hemochromatosis
- Racial pigmentation
- Periungual melanoma

- <u>Peutz–Jeghers syndrome</u>
- Smoker
- Traumatic melanonychia

Further reading:
- Fisher D, Field EA, Welsh S (2004) Laugier–Hunziker syndrome. Clin Exp Dermatol 29(3):312–313

Leiomyoma

Benign neoplasm derived from smooth muscle around blood vessels, the arrector pili muscle, or genital smooth muscle that is characterized by solitary or multiple, firm, occasionally painful, flesh-colored to red-brown papules or nodules

Subtypes/Variants

- Angioleiomyoma
- Genital leiomyoma
- Piloleiomyoma

Differential Diagnosis

- Adnexal tumors
- Angiofibroma
- <u>Collagenoma</u>
- Dermatofibroma
- <u>Eccrine spiradenoma</u>
- <u>Glomus tumor</u>
- Keloid
- Leiomyosarcoma
- Mastocytoma
- Metastases
- Neurofibroma

- Plasmacytoma
- Schwannoma

Associations (Multiple)

- Alport's syndrome (genital)
- Chronic lymphocytic leukemia
- HIV infection (angioleiomyomas)
- Renal cell carcinoma
- Uterine leiomyomas (Reed syndrome)

Evaluation

- Fumarate hydratase gene study
- Renal ultrasound or abdominal CT scan
- Pelvic examination

Further reading:
- Holst VA, Junkins-Hopkins JM, Elenitsas R (2002) Cutaneous smooth muscle neoplasms: clinical features, histologic findings, and treatment options. J Am Acad Dermatol 46(4):477–479

Leiomyosarcoma, Superficial

Malignant neoplasm of smooth muscle that can arise from the dermis (arrector pili muscles) or subcutaneous layer (blood vessels) and is characterized by a solitary nodule most commonly located on the head and neck (dermal) or hair-bearing area of the lower extremity (subcutaneous)

Differential Diagnosis

- Amelanotic melanoma
- Appendageal tumors
- Atypical fibroxanthoma

- Basal cell carcinoma
- Cyst
- Dermatofibromas
- <u>Dermatofibrosarcoma protuberans</u>
- Leiomyoma
- Merkel cell carcinoma
- Metastatic sarcoma
- <u>Squamous cell carcinoma</u>

Further reading:
- Annest NM, Grekin SJ, Stone MS, Messingham MJ (2007) Cutaneous leiomyosarcoma: a tumor of the head and neck. Dermatol Surg 33(5):628–633

Leishmaniasis

Infection of the skin or viscera caused by several species of the protozoa *Leishmania* that is transmitted by bite of the sandfly and characterized by an erythematous papule that evolves to a ulcerated nodule or plaque with a predilection for the exposed areas, especially the face, nose, ears, and extremities (Fig. 6.57)

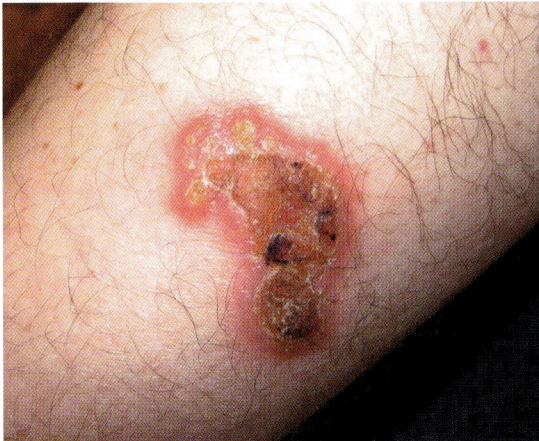

Fig. 6.57 Cutaneous leishmaniasis

Subtypes/Variants

- American mucocutaneous (espundia)
- Disseminated
- Leishmaniasis recidivans
- New World cutaneous (chiclero ulcer, uta, pian bois)
- Old World cutaneous (rural (moist) or urban (dry) types)
- Post–Kala-Azar dermal leishmaniasis
- Visceral leishmaniasis

Differential Diagnosis

- Angiocentric NK/T cell lymphomas
- Basal cell carcinoma
- Blastomycosis
- Chromoblastomycosis
- Granuloma inguinale
- Histoplasmosis
- Lepromatous leprosy
- Paracoccidioidomycosis
- Pyoderma gangrenosum
- Rhinoscleroma
- Sarcoidosis
- Squamous cell carcinoma
- Syphilis
- Tropical ulcer
- Tuberculosis
- Tularemia
- Wegener's granulomatosis

Differential Diagnosis (Disseminated Cutaneous)

- Histoplasmosis
- Lepromatous leprosy

- Lobomycosis
- Lymphoma
- Neurofibromatosis
- Paracoccidioidomycosis
- Verruga peruana
- Xanthoma tuberosum

Evaluation

- Culture on Novy–MacNeal–Nicolle medium
- ELISA for leishmanial antibodies
- PCR of lesional tissue
- Tissue examination with Giemsa stain

Treatment Options

- Cryotherapy
- Heat therapy
- Sodium stibogluconate
- Topical paromomycin
- Pentamidine
- Ketoconazole
- Surgical excision

Further reading:
- Bailey MS, Lockwood DN (2007) Cutaneous leishmaniasis. Clin Dermatol 25(2):203–211

Lentiginosis, Centrofacial

Localized type of lentiginosis with onset in the first few years of life that is characterized by lentigines on the nose and cheeks

Differential Diagnosis

- Carney's complex
- <u>Inherited patterned lentiginosis</u>
- LEOPARD syndrome
- Peutz–Jeghers syndrome

Associations

- Epilepsy
- Hypothyroidism
- Mental retardation
- Skeletal abnormalities

Further reading:
- Kaur TD, Kanwar AJ (2004) Giant nevus spilus and centrofacial lentiginosis. Pediatr Dermatol 21(4):516–517

Lentigo Maligna (Hutchinson Freckle)

Slowly evolving type of melanoma in situ affecting patients with a long history of sun exposure that is characterized by an unevenly pigmented, irregularly bordered macule or patch on the face and other sun-exposed areas

Differential Diagnosis

- Large cell acanthoma
- Lentigo simplex
- Pigmented actinic keratosis
- Seborrheic keratosis
- <u>Solar lentigo</u>

Treatment Options

- Excisional surgery
- Mohs micrographic surgery
- Imiquimod cream
- Radiation therapy
- Cryotherapy

Further reading:

- Mckenna JK, Florell SR, Goldman GD et al (2006) Lentigo maligna/lentigo maligna melanoma: current state of diagnosis and treatment. Dermatol Surg 32(4):493–504

Lentigo Simplex

Benign proliferation of basal layer melanocytes that can be solitary and occur anywhere (lentigo simplex) or multiple as a part of a variety of syndromes

Differential Diagnosis

- Blue nevus
- Café-au-lait macule
- Ephelides
- Junctional melanocytic nevi
- Labial melanotic macule
- Large cell acanthoma
- Lentigo maligna
- Melanoma
- Pigmented actinic keratosis
- Seborrheic keratosis
- Traumatic tattoo

Associations (Multiple)

- Arterial dissection
- Bandler syndrome
- Café-au-lait macules
- Cantu syndrome
- Carney complex (NAME/LAMB syndrome)
- Centrofacial lentiginosis
- Cowden's disease
- Cronkhite–Canada syndrome
- Eruptive lentiginosis
- Gastrocutaneous syndrome
- Generalized lentigines
- Inherited patterned lentiginosis
- Laugier–Hunziker syndrome
- LEOPARD syndrome
- Partial unilateral lentiginosis
- Peutz–Jeghers syndrome
- Tay's syndrome
- Xeroderma pigmentosum

Further reading:
- Chong WS, Klanwarin W, Giam YC (2004) Generalized lentiginosis in two children lacking systemic associations: case report and review of the literature. Pediatr Dermatol 21(2):139–145

Lentigo, Solar (Senile Lentigo)

Benign marker of chronic sun exposure that is characterized by multiple tan or brown macules on the sun-exposed areas, especially the face and dorsal hands

Differential Diagnosis

- Actinic keratosis, pigmented type
- Exogenous ochronosis

- Large cell acanthoma
- Lentigo maligna
- Lentigo simplex
- Lichen-planus-like keratosis
- Seborrheic keratosis

Further reading:
- Moreno-Ramirez D, Ferrandiz L, Camacho FM (2005) Are the ABCD signs useful for the management of solar lentigo? Br J Dermatol 153(5):1083–1084

LEOPARD Syndrome (Moynahan Syndrome)

Familial (AD) or sporadic syndrome caused by a mutation in the PTPN11 gene and that is characterized by multiple lentigines, ECG abnormalities, ocular hypertelorism, pulmonary stenosis, genital abnormalities, growth retardation, and deafness

Differential Diagnosis

- Arterial dissections with lentiginosis
- Carney complex
- Inherited pattern lentiginosis
- McCune–Albright syndrome
- Neurofibromatosis
- Noonan syndrome
- Peutz–Jeghers syndrome

Evaluation

- Electrocardiogram
- Echocardiogram
- Hearing test

Further reading:
- Dgilio MC, Sarkozy A, de Zorzi A et al (2006) LEOPARD syndrome: clinical diagnosis in the first year of life. Am J Med Genet A 140(7):740–746

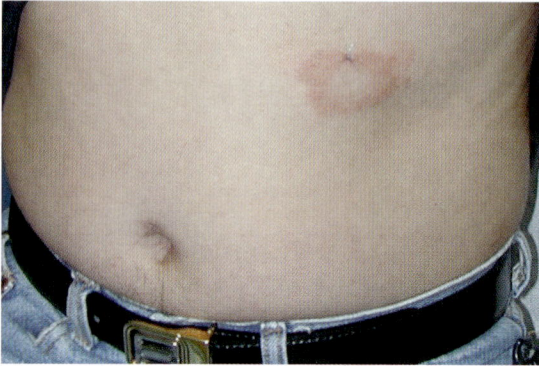

Leprosy (Hansen's Disease)

Chronic infection caused by the neurotropic *Mycobacterium leprae* and characterized by a spectrum of cutaneous lesions, determined by the patient's immunologic response, ranging from a few anesthetic and hypopigmented annular lesions (tuberculoid, good response) to many widespread infiltrated, nodular lesions (lepromatous, poor response)

Subtypes/Variants

- Borderline
- Borderline lepromatous
- Borderline tuberculoid
- Histioid
- Indeterminate
- Lepromatous
- Neural
- Tuberculoid (Fig. 6.58)

Differential Diagnosis

Lepromatous

- Chronic lichenified atopic dermatitis
- <u>Cutaneous tuberculosis</u>
- Granuloma annulare
- Granuloma multiforme
- Granulomatous mycosis fungoides
- Jessner's lymphocytic infiltrate
- Leishmaniasis
- Leonine facies
- Lobomycosis
- <u>Lymphoma</u>
- Melkersson–Rosenthal syndrome
- Midline nasal destructive lesion
- Multicentric reticulohistiocytosis
- Myxedema
- Neurofibromatosis
- <u>Sarcoidosis</u>
- Syphilis

Tuberculoid

- Annular lichenoid dermatitis of youth
- <u>Granuloma annulare</u>
- Lichen planus
- Lupus erythematosus
- <u>Mycosis fungoides</u>
- Pinta
- Pityriasis alba
- Pityriasis versicolor
- Postinflammatory pigmentary alteration
- Psoriasis
- <u>Sarcoidosis</u>
- Tinea corporis
- Vitiligo

Evaluation

- Liver and renal function test
- Neurologic examination
- Ophthalmologic examination
- PCR of lesional skin
- Complete blood count

Treatment Options

- <u>Dapsone</u>
- <u>Rifampin</u>
- <u>Clofazimine</u>
- Minocycline
- Ofloxacin
- Clarithromycin

Further reading:
- Ramos-E-Silva M, Oliveira ML, Munhoz-da-Fontoura GH (2005) Leprosy: uncommon presentations. Clin Dermatol 23(5):509–514

Leptospirosis (Weil's Disease, Pretibial Fever)

Spirochetal infection acquired from animal urine-contaminated drinking water that is caused by *Leptospira interrogans* spp. icterohemorrhagiae (Weil's disease) or autumnalis (pretibial fever) and is characterized by fever, jaundice, purpura, renal failure, and death (Weil's) or fever, headache, conjunctival hemorrhage, photophobia, and a erythematous patchy eruption most prominent on the shins (pretibial fever)

Differential Diagnosis

- Brucellosis
- Dengue fever

- Encephalitis
- Ehrlichiosis
- Hantavirus infection
- HIV infection
- Malaria
- Q fever
- <u>Rickettsial disease</u>
- Syphilis
- Tuberculosis
- Tularemia
- Typhoid fever
- Typhus
- <u>Viral hepatitis</u>
- Viral meningitis
- Yellow fever

Evaluation

- Complete blood count
- Liver function test
- Prothrombin time and partial thromboplastin time
- Renal function test
- Serologic test for *Leptospira* antibodies

Further reading:

- Mcbride AJ, Athanazio DA, Reis MG, Ko AI (2005) Leptospirosis. Curr Opin Infect Dis 18(5):376–386

Leukemia Cutis

Cutaneous infiltration with leukemic cells that can precede a diagnosis of leukemia or occur during the course of the disease and is characterized by erythematous or violaceous papules and nodules, hemorrhage, chloroma, or gingival infiltration

Differential Diagnosis

- Blueberry muffin baby
- Chilblains
- <u>Cutaneous lymphoid hyperplasia</u>
- Cutaneous small vessel vasculitis
- Erythema annulare centrifugum
- Erythema nodosum
- Extramedullary hematopoiesis
- Gingival hypertrophy
- Guttate psoriasis
- Hypereosinophilic syndrome
- Jessner's lymphocytic infiltrate
- Kaposi's sarcoma
- Langerhans cell histiocytosis
- Leonine facies
- <u>Lymphoma cutis</u>
- Mastocytoma
- <u>Metastatic disease</u>
- Neutrophilic eccrine hidradenitis
- Plasmacytoma
- <u>Pyoderma gangrenosum</u>
- Sarcoidosis
- Sister Mary Joseph's nodule
- Stasis dermatitis
- <u>Sweet's syndrome (including histiocytoid variant)</u>
- Urticaria pigmentosum

Associations

- Ataxia–telangiectasia
- Bloom syndrome
- Down syndrome

- Fanconi syndrome
- Wiskott–Aldrich syndrome

Evaluation

- Complete blood count
- Bone marrow biopsy

Further reading:
- Watson KM, Mufti G, Salisbury JR et al (2006) Spectrum of clinical presentation, treatment and prognosis in a series of eight patients with leukaemia Cutis. Clin Exp Dermatol 31(2):218–221

Leukocyte Adhesion Deficiency

Inherited (AR) immunodeficiency syndrome caused by a CD18 gene defect (type 1) or SLC35C1 (type 2) that leads to impaired neutrophil rolling and opsonization and that is characterized by recurrent bacterial and fungal infections, pyoderma-gangrenosum-like lesions, periodontitis, poor wound healing, and delayed separation of the umbilical cord

Differential Diagnosis

- Chediak–Higashi syndrome
- Chronic granulomatous disease
- Myelodysplastic syndrome
- Myeloperoxidase deficiency
- Pyoderma gangrenosum
- X-linked hypogammaglobulinemia

Further reading:
- Movahedi M, Entezari N, Pourpak Z et al (2007) Clinical and laboratory findings in Iranian patients with leukocyte adhesion deficiency (study of 15 cases). J Clin Immunol 27(3):302–307

Leukoderma, Chemical (Occupational Vitiligo)

Hypopigmented or depigmented patches resulting from contact exposure to a chemical that is either toxic to melanocytes or causes decreased production to melanin

Differential Diagnosis

- Burns
- Cutaneous lupus erythematosus
- Leprosy
- Mycosis fungoides
- Postinflammatory hypopigmentation
- Scars
- Vitiligo

Associations

- Catechols
- Hydroquinones
- Mercaptoamines
- Phenols
- Paraphenylenediamine

Further reading:
- Kumar A, Freeman S (1999) Leukoderma following occupational allergic contact dermatitis. Contact Dermatitis 41(2):94–98

Leukoplakia, Oral Hairy

Type of leukoplakia induced by EBV infection that occurs predominantly in patients with HIV and is characterized by white, verrucous plaques bilaterally on the sides of the tongue

Differential Diagnosis

- <u>Black hairy tongue</u>
- Geographic tongue
- Hypertrophic candidiasis
- Leukoedema
- <u>Lichen planus</u>
- <u>Premalignant leukoplakia</u>
- Smoker keratosis
- <u>Squamous cell carcinoma</u>
- Syphilis
- Traumatic leukoplakia
- Wart
- <u>White sponge nevus</u>

Treatment Options

- <u>HAART therapy</u>
- Acyclovir
- Valacyclovir
- Famciclovir
- Podophyllin
- Tretinoin gel

Further reading:
- Ikediobi NI, Tyring SK (2002) Cutaneous manifestations of Epstein–Barr virus infection. Dermatol Clin 20(2):283–289

Lichen Myxedematosus (Papular Mucinosis)

Idiopathic type of cutaneous mucinosis that can be associated with mono-clonal gammopathy and is characterized by discrete, often grouped, dome-shaped, flesh-colored papules in a generalized or localized distribution

Differential Diagnosis

- Colloid milium
- Darier disease
- Dermatomyositis
- Eruptive collagenoma
- Follicular mucinosis
- Granuloma annulare
- Leprosy
- Lichen amyloidosis
- Lichen planus
- Lipoid proteinosis
- Lymphoma
- Malignant atrophic papulosis
- Molluscum contagiosum
- Multiple trichoepithelioma
- Nevus mucinosis
- Nodular amyloidosis
- Sarcoidosis
- Scleredema
- Scleroderma
- Xanthomas (especially eruptive or papular types)

Evaluation

- Antinuclear antibodies
- HIV test
- Serum/urinary protein electrophoresis
- Thyroid function tests
- Viral hepatitis panel

Treatment Options

- Topical corticosteroids
- Intralesional corticosteroids

- Acitretin
- Isotretinoin
- Melphalan
- Plasmapheresis
- Intravenous immunoglobulin
- Methotrexate
- Cyclosporine
- Radiation
- Extracorporeal photopheresis
- Thalidomide
- Cyclophosphamide
- Chlorambucil
- Dermabrasion
- CO_2 laser

Further reading:
- Rongioletti F (2006) Lichen myxedematosus (papular mucinosis): new concepts and perspectives for an old disease. Semin Cutan Med Surg 25(2):100–104

Lichen Nitidus

Distinct eruption that most commonly affects children and is characterized by tiny, shiny, 1- to 2-mm flat-topped, occasionally pruritic papules associated with the Koebner phenomenon and clustered on the abdomen, extremities, and groin, including the penis (Fig. 6.59)

Subtypes/Variants

- Actinic (summertime actinic lichenoid eruption)
- Follicular
- Linear
- Hemorrhagic
- Keratodermic
- Mucous membrane
- Nail

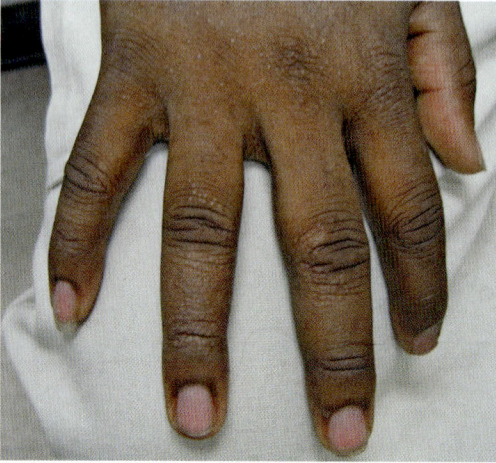

Fig. 6.59 Lichen nitidus

- Perforating
- Purpuric
- Vesicular

Differential Diagnosis

- Autoeczematization reaction
- Follicular prominence/lichen simplex
- Guttate lichen sclerosus
- Id reaction
- Keratosis pilaris
- Lichen planus
- Lichen scrofulosorum
- Lichen spinulosum
- Lichen striatus
- Lichenoid secondary syphilis
- Molluscum contagiosum
- Papular eczema
- Papular mucinosis

- Papular sarcoidosis
- Verruca plana

Associations

- Crohn's disease
- Lichen planus

Treatment Options

- <u>Topical corticosteroids</u>
- <u>Tacrolimus ointment</u>
- Cetirizine
- Systemic retinoids
- UVB phototherapy

Further reading:
- Tilly JJ, Drolet BA, Esterly NB (2004) Lichenoid eruptions in children. J Am Acad Dermatol 51(4):606–624

Lichen Planopilaris

Follicular variant of lichen planus that predominantly affects women and is characterized by follicular erythematous papules and scarring alopecia with or without classic lichen planus on the body or oral mucosa

Differential Diagnosis

- <u>Discoid lupus erythematosus</u>
- <u>Central centrifugal cicatricial alopecia</u>
- Folliculitis decalvans
- Frontal fibrosing alopecia
- Graham–Little–Piccardi–Lasseur syndrome
- Keratosis follicularis spinulosa decalvans
- Tinea capitis

Associations

- Dermatitis herpetiformis
- Lichen planus
- Gold
- Thyroiditis

Treatment Options

- Topical corticosteroids
- Systemic corticosteroids
- Intralesional corticosteroids
- Isotretinoin
- Acitretin
- Hydroxychloroquine
- Mycophenolate mofetil
- Griseofulvin
- Cyclosporine

Further reading:
- Cevasco NC, Bergfeld WF, Remzi BK et al (2007) A case-series of 29 patients with lichen planopilaris: the Cleveland Clinic Foundation experience on evaluation, diagnosis, and treatment. J Am Acad Dermatol 57(1):47–53

Lichen Planus

Immune-mediated cutaneous and mucosal eruption of uncertain cause that is characterized by localized or generalized grouped, pruritic, flat-topped violaceous papules with Koebner phenomenon and a white, reticulated surface (Wickham's striae) as well as streaky white changes with or without erosions on the oral mucosa

Subtypes/Variants

- Acral erosive (Fig. 6.60)
- Actinic

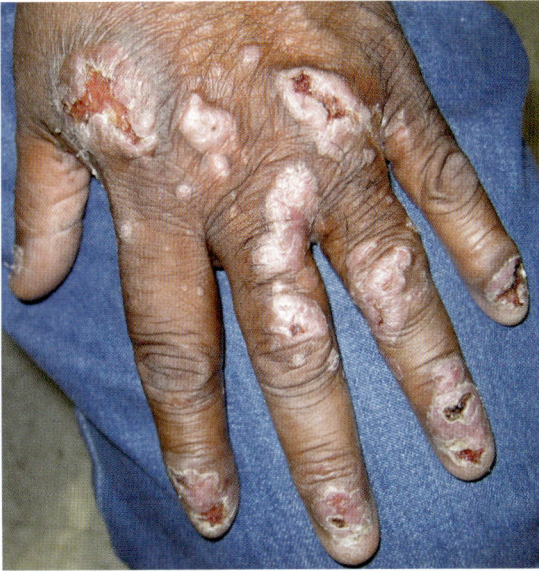

Fig. 6.60 Acral erosive lichen planus

- Annular
- Atrophic
- Bullous
- Classic
- Erosive
- Eruptive
- Follicular
- Genital
- Hypertrophic
- Lichen planus pigmentosus (pigmentosus–inversus)
- Linear (Fig. 6.61)
- Nail
- Oral
- Overlap with bullous pemphigoid (lichen planus pemphigoides)
- Overlap with lupus erythematosus
- Overlap with lichen sclerosus et atrophicus

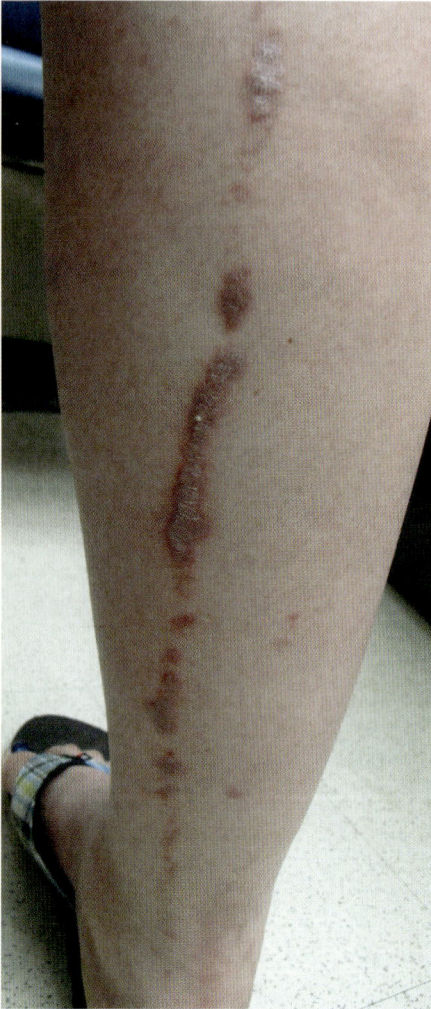

Fig. 6.61 Linear lichen planus

Differential Diagnosis

Actinic

- <u>Actinic lichen nitidus</u>
- <u>Melasma</u>

- Photoallergic contact dermatitis
- <u>Photolichenoid drug eruption</u>
- Photosensitive drug eruption
- Polymorphous light eruption

Annular

- Annular lichenoid dermatitis of youth
- Annular sarcoidosis
- Annular syphilis
- Erythema dyschromicum perstans
- <u>Granuloma annulare</u>
- Majocchi's granuloma
- Majocchi's pigmented purpuric dermatosis
- Morphea
- <u>Porokeratosis</u>
- Tinea

Classic

- Erythema dyschromicum perstans
- Graham–Little–Piccardi–Lasseur syndrome
- <u>Guttate psoriasis</u>
- Keratosis lichenoides chronica
- Lichen amyloidosis
- Lichen myxedematosus
- Lichen nitidus
- Lichen scrofulosorum
- Lichenoid contact dermatitis
- <u>Lichenoid drug eruption</u>
- Lichenoid graft-vs-host disease
- Lichenoid keratoses
- Lichenoid pigmented purpura of Gougerot and Blum
- Lupus erythematosus
- Paraneoplastic pemphigus
- Pityriasis lichenoides et varioliformis acuta
- <u>Pityriasis rosea</u>
- Scabies

- Secondary syphilis
- Syringomas

Eruptive

- <u>Guttate psoriasis</u>
- Lichen nitidus
- Lichen scrofulosorum
- <u>Lichenoid drug eruption</u>
- Lichenoid sarcoidosis
- Pityriasis rosea
- Secondary syphilis
- Syringomas
- Viral exanthem

Genital

- Behçet's disease
- Bowen's disease
- Cicatricial pemphigoid
- Condyloma acuminatum
- Extramammary Paget's disease
- Fixed drug eruption
- Lichen nitidus
- <u>Lichen sclerosus et atrophicus</u>
- <u>Lichen simplex chronicus</u>
- Vulvar eczema
- Zoon balanitis

Hypertrophic

- Bowen's disease
- Deep fungal infection
- Keratoacanthoma
- Keratosis lichenoides chronica
- <u>Hypertrophic lupus erythematosus</u>
- Lichen amyloidosis

- <u>Lichen simplex chronicus</u>
- Pagetoid reticulosis
- <u>Psoriasis</u>
- <u>Verrucous sarcoidosis</u>

Linear

- Inflammatory linear verrucous epidermal nevus
- <u>Lichen striatus</u>
- Linear Darier's disease
- Linear fixed drug eruption
- Linear graft-vs-host disease
- Linear porokeratosis
- <u>Linear psoriasis</u>

Nail

- <u>Alopecia areata</u>
- Digital ischemia
- Graft-vs-host disease
- Lichen striatus
- Onychomycosis
- <u>Psoriasis</u>
- Systemic amyloidosis
- Yellow nail syndrome

Oral

- Bite keratosis
- <u>Candidiasis</u>
- <u>Cicatricial pemphigoid</u>
- Gingivitis
- Graft-vs-host disease
- Leukoplakia
- Lichenoid contact stomatitis
- Linear IgA bullous dermatosis
- Lupus erythematosus

- Oral Crohn's disease
- Oral lichenoid drug reaction
- <u>Pemphigus</u>
- Squamous cell carcinoma
- Syphilis
- White sponge nevus

Associations

- Grinspan syndrome (oral)
- Hepatitis C infection (oral)
- Primary biliary cirrhosis
- Squamous cell carcinoma (oral, genital)

Evaluation

- Viral hepatitis panel (especially oral erosive type)

Treatment Options

- Topical corticosteroids
- Topical tacrolimus
- Intralesional corticosteroids
- <u>Systemic corticosteroids</u>
- Metronidazole
- Acitretin
- <u>UVB phototherapy</u>
- Griseofulvin
- Cyclosporine
- Azathioprine
- Mycophenolate mofetil
- Photodynamic therapy
- Low molecular weight heparin
- Methotrexate
- Thalidomide

Further reading:

- Reich HL, Nguyen JT, James WD (2004) Annular lichen planus: a case series of 20 patients. J Am Acad Dermatol 50(4):595–599

Lichen Sclerosus et Atrophicus

Immune-mediated cutaneous and mucosal eruption of uncertain cause that is characterized by pruritic, white, sclerotic, and atrophic plaques with occasional follicular plugging or erosive changes that are localized most commonly on the labia majora or prepuce of the penis with the potential to obliterate normal anatomic structures and lead to vulvar stenosis or phimosis

Differential Diagnosis

Extragenital
- Acrodermatitis chronica atrophicans
- Anetoderma
- Atrophic blanche
- Atrophoderma of Pasini and Pierini
- Bowen's disease
- Discoid lupus erythematosus
- Erythroplasia of Queyrat
- Excoriation scars
- Idiopathic guttate hypomelanosis
- Graft-vs-host disease
- Lichen planus
- Malignant atrophic papulosis
- Morphea
- Mycosis fungoides
- Postinflammatory hypopigmentation
- Sarcoidosis
- Scleroderma
- Tinea versicolor
- Vitiligo

Genital

- Bowen's disease
- Cicatricial pemphigoid
- <u>Contact dermatitis</u>
- Erythroplasia of Queyrat
- Extramammary Paget's disease
- <u>Lichen planus</u>
- <u>Lichen simplex</u>
- Morphea
- Phimosis
- Postinflammatory hypopigmentation
- <u>Sexual abuse</u>
- <u>Vitiligo</u>
- Vulvar eczema

Associations

- Alopecia areata
- Borreliosis
- <u>Morphea</u>
- Pernicious anemia
- Perianal pyramidal protrusion
- Scleroderma
- Thyroid disease
- Vitiligo

Evaluation

- Lyme disease ELISA and Western blot
- Complete blood count
- Thyroid function test and antithyroid antibodies

Treatment Options

- <u>Topical corticosteroids</u>
- Topical tacrolimus
- Topical retinoids
- Intralesional corticosteroids
- Acitretin
- Topical estrogen
- Topical vitamin D analogues
- CO_2 laser

Further reading:
- Funaro D (2004) Lichen sclerosus: a review and practical approach. Dermatol Ther 17(1):28–37

Lichen Scrofulosorum

Type of tuberculid most often affecting children with active tuberculosis and characterized by asymptomatic lichenoid papules on the trunk

Differential Diagnosis

- Atopic dermatitis
- Dermatophytid reactions
- Lichenoid drug eruption
- Lichen nitidus
- <u>Lichen planus</u>
- Lichen spinulosus
- Sarcoidosis
- <u>Secondary syphilis</u>

Treatment Options

- Antituberculous therapy

Further reading:
- Vashisht P, Sahoo B, Khurana N, Reddy BS (2007) Cutaneous tuberculosis in children and adolescents: a clinicohistological study. J Eur Acad Dermatol Venereol 21(1):40–47

Lichen Simplex Chronicus (Neurodermatitis Circumscripta)

Localized cutaneous changes which result from chronically rubbing and scratching the skin in response to pruritus and that are characterized by lichenified, thickened circumscribed plaques on the manipulated body surfaces, most commonly the lower legs, arms, neck, scalp, and genitalia

Differential Diagnosis

- Acanthosis nigricans
- Acne keloidalis nuchae
- Alopecia mucinosa
- Atopic dermatitis
- Berloque dermatitis
- Contact dermatitis
- Cutaneous T cell lymphoma
- Dermatitis herpetiformis
- Dermatophytosis
- Extramammary Paget's disease
- Hyperkeratosis of the nipple
- Insect-bite reaction
- Lichen amyloidosis
- Lichen nitidus
- Lichen planus

- Lichen striatus
- Lupus erythematosus
- Lupus vulgaris
- Macular amyloidosis
- Nummular eczema
- Phytophotodermatitis
- Pretibial myxedema
- <u>Psoriasis</u>
- Riehl melanosis
- Seborrheic dermatitis
- Stasis dermatitis

Associations

- Atopic dermatitis
- Dermatophytosis
- Contact dermatitis
- Insect bites
- Psoriasis
- Xerosis

Treatment Options

- <u>Topical corticosteroids with or without occlusion</u>
- Flurandrenolide tape
- <u>Intralesional corticosteroids</u>
- Doxepin cream
- Capsaicin cream
- Cryosurgery

Further reading:

- Lynch PJ (2004) Lichen simplex chronicus (atopic/neurodermatitis) of the anogenital region. Dermatol Ther 17(1):8–19

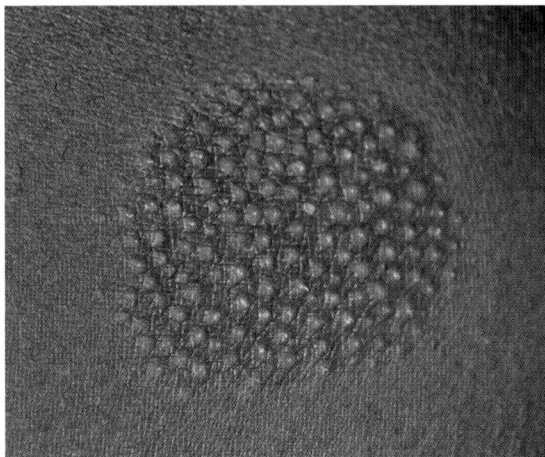

Fig. 6.62 Lichen spinulosus (Courtesy of K. Guidry)

Lichen Spinulosus

Keratotic dermatosis of uncertain cause that affects children and young adults and is characterized by solitary or multiple, discrete circular or oval clusters of keratotic papules on the trunk or extensor extremities (Fig. 6.62)

Differential Diagnosis

- Darier's disease
- Follicular mucinosis
- Frictional lichenoid dermatitis
- Hodgkin's disease
- Keratosis pilaris
- Keratotic spicules
- Lichen nitidus
- Lichen planopilaris
- Lichen scrofulosorum

- <u>Lichen simplex chronicus</u>
- Papular eczema
- Phrynoderma
- <u>Pityriasis rubra pilaris, circumscribed variant</u>
- Verruca plana

Associations

- <u>Atopic dermatitis</u>
- Crohn's disease
- Drug reaction
- HIV infection

Treatment Options

- <u>Ammonium lactate</u>
- <u>Salicylic acid</u>
- <u>Urea</u>
- Topical retinoids
- <u>Topical corticosteroids</u>
- Topical vitamin D analogues

Further reading:
- Tilly JJ, Drolet BA, Esterly NB (2004) Lichenoid eruptions in children. J Am Acad Dermatol 51(4):606–624

Lichen Striatus

Common childhood dermatosis that is probably viral in origin and is characterized by flesh-colored to hypopigmented lichenoid papules advancing in a linear pattern along Blaschko's lines that spontaneously resolve in about 1 year (Fig. 6.63)

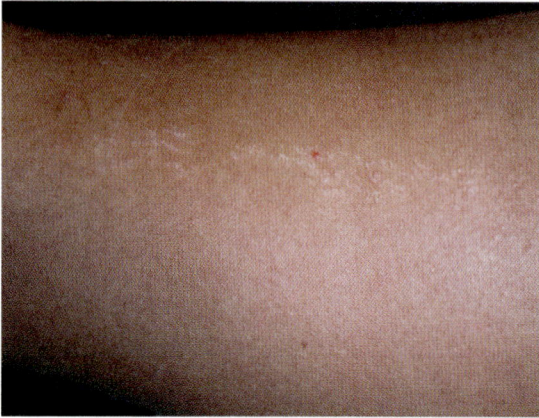

Fig. 6.63 Lichen striatus (Courtesy of K. Guidry)

Differential Diagnosis

- Atopic dermatitis
- Blaschkitis
- Inflammatory linear verrucous epidermal nevus
- Lichen simplex chronicus
- Linear Darier's disease
- Linear graft-vs-host disease
- Linear lichen planus
- Linear lupus erythematosus
- Linear psoriasis
- Porokeratosis
- Verruca

Treatment Options

- Observation and reassurance
- Topical corticosteroids
- Topical tacrolimus

Further reading:

- Tilly JJ, Drolet BA, Esterly NB (2004) Lichenoid eruptions in children. J Am Acad Dermatol 51(4):606–624

Lichenoid Drug Eruption

Drug eruption that resembles lichen planus and is characterized by either violaceous lichenoid papules and plaques, exfoliative dermatitis, a photo-distributed eruption or, least commonly, oral lesions

Subtypes/Variants

- Bullous
- Eczematous
- Lichen planus-like
- Photodistributed
- Psoriasiform
- Ulcerative

Differential Diagnosis

- Erythema dyschromicum perstans
- Guttate psoriasis
- Lichen planus, eruptive
- Lichen scrofulosorum
- Parapsoriasis
- Pityriasis lichenoides
- Pityriasis rosea
- Pityriasis-rosea-like drug eruption
- Secondary syphilis

Associated Medications

Lichen Planus-Like
- Allopurinol
- Antimalarials
- Beta-blockers
- Calcium channel blockers
- Captopril

- Carbamazepine
- Chlorpromazine
- Dapsone
- Furosemide
- Gold
- Hydrochlorothiazide
- Hepatitis B vaccination
- Metformin
- NSAIDS
- Penicillamine
- Spironolactone
- Sulfonylureas

Oral
- ACE inhibitors
- Allopurinol
- Dental amalgam
- Gold
- Ketoconazole
- Methyldopa
- NSAIDs
- Penicillamine
- Sulfonylureas

Photo
- 5-Fluorouracil
- Carbamazepine
- Chlorpromazine
- Ethambutol
- Furosemide
- Quinine
- Tetracyclines
- Thiazides

Treatment Options

- Discontinue offending medication
- Systemic corticosteroids

Further reading:
- Nigen S, Knowles SR, Shear NH (2003) Drug eruptions: approaching the diagnosis of drug-induced skin diseases. J Drugs Dermatol 2(3):278–299

Lichenoid Keratosis, Benign (Lichen-Planus-Like Keratosis)

Benign lesion that predominantly affects women, that evolves from a solar lentigo, is characterized by a keratotic erythematous or violaceous papule on the sun-exposed areas, and is histologically indistinguishable from lichen planus

Differential Diagnosis

- Actinic keratosis
- Basal cell carcinoma
- Bowen's disease
- Large cell acanthoma
- Solar lentigo
- Lichen planus
- Melanocytic nevus
- Melanoma
- Seborrheic keratosis
- Squamous cell carcinoma
- Wart

Further reading:
- Morgan MB, Stevens GL, Switlyk S (2005) Benign lichenoid keratosis: a clinical and pathologic reappraisal of 1040 cases. Am J Dermatopathol 27(5):387–392

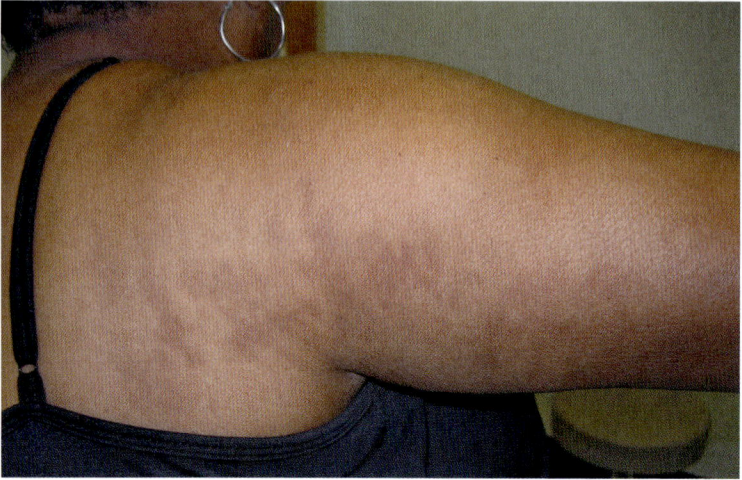

Fig. 6.64 Linear atrophoderma of Moulin

Linear Atrophoderma of Moulin

Acquired, idiopathic connective tissue disorder that may be related to linear morphea or atrophoderma of Pasini and Pierini and is characterized by a linear, hyperpigmented band of atrophoderma along Blaschko's lines (Fig. 6.64)

Differential Diagnosis

- Atrophoderma of Pasini and Pierini
- Blaschkitis
- Lichen sclerosus et atrophicus
- Lichen striatus
- Linear and whorled nevoid hypermelanosis
- Linear lichen planus
- Linear morphea
- Scar
- Striae atrophicans

Further reading:
- Miteva L, Nikolova K, Obreshkova E (2005) Linear atrophoderma of Moulin. Int J Dermatol 44(10):867–869

Linear and Whorled Nevoid Hypermelanosis

Sporadic disorder of epidermal hypermelanosis that develops in the first few weeks of life and is characterized by linear and whorled streaks of hyperpigmentation along Blaschko's lines without preceding inflammation and with occasional, variable extracutaneous abnormalities

Differential Diagnosis

- Becker's nevus
- Café-au-lait macule
- Hypomelanosis of Ito
- Incontinentia pigmenti, stage III
- Linear atrophoderma of Moulin
- Linear lichen planus
- Progressive cribriform and zosteriform hyperpigmentation
- X-linked chondrodysplasia punctata
- X-linked reticulate pigmentary disorder

Further reading:
- Di Lernia V (2007) Linear and whorled hypermelanosis. Pediatr Dermatol 24(3):205–210

Linear Focal Elastosis

Uncommon disorder of elastic tissue that predominantly affects older men and is characterized by linear, palpable, yellow bands on the middle to lower back (Fig. 6.65)

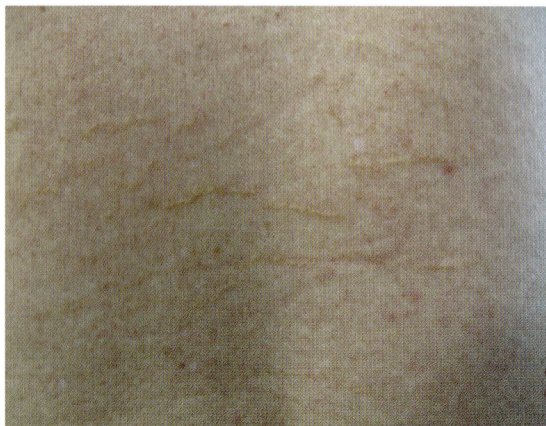

Fig. 6.65 Linear focal elastosis

Differential Diagnosis

- Cutaneous larva migrans
- Dermatofibrosis lenticularis disseminata
- Elastofibroma dorsi
- Interstitial granulomatous dermatitis (rope sign)
- Striae atrophicans

Further reading:
- Arroyo MP, Soter NA (2001) Linear focal elastosis. Dermatol Online J 7(2):18

Linear IgA Bullous Dermatosis

Autoimmune subepidermal blistering disorder affecting children and adults that is caused by IgA autoantibodies directed against a portion of BPAg2 and is characterized by discrete bullae and bullae in annular configurations that are located on the trunk, extremities, intertriginous areas, and occasionally the oral and ocular mucosa

Differential Diagnosis

- Bullous impetigo
- Bullous lupus erythematosus
- Bullous mastocytosis
- <u>Bullous pemphigoid</u>
- Bullous scabies
- <u>Dermatitis herpetiformis</u>
- Drug-induced pemphigus
- <u>Erythema multiforme</u>
- Epidermolysis bullosa acquisita
- Herpes simplex virus infection
- Pemphigus foliaceus
- Pemphigus vulgaris
- <u>Stevens–Johnson syndrome/toxic epidermal necrolysis</u>
- Zoster

Associations

- Internal malignancy
- Medications

Associated Medications

- Amiodarone
- Angiotensin receptor blockers
- Captopril
- Diclofenac
- Il-2
- Interferon gamma
- Furosemide
- Lithium
- Oxaprozin
- Penicillin
- Phenytoin

- PUVA
- Statins
- Tea tree oil
- <u>Vancomycin</u>

Evaluation

- Direct and indirect immunofluorescence
- Ophthalmologic examination

Treatment Options

- <u>Dapsone</u>
- Systemic corticosteroids
- Colchicine
- Tetracycline nicotinamide
- Sulfasalazine
- Methotrexate
- Mycophenolate mofetil
- Azathioprine
- Cyclosporine
- Intravenous immunoglobulins

Further reading:

- Guide SV, Marinkovich MP (2001) Linear IgA bullous dermatosis. Clin Dermatol 19(6):719–727

Lipodermatosclerosis (Sclerosing Panniculitis)

Type of panniculitis associated with chronic venous insufficiency that is characterized by woody induration of the bilateral lower extremities with an "inverted champagne bottle" appearance and with or without preceding cellulitis-like erythematous plaques

Differential Diagnosis

- Cellulitis
- Eosinophilic cellulitis
- Eosinophilic fasciitis
- Erythema induratum
- Erythema nodosum
- Lymphedema
- Morphea
- Nephrogenic fibrosing dermopathy
- Pretibial myxedema
- Sarcoidosis
- Scleromyxedema

Evaluation

- Venous ultrasound of the lower extremities

Treatment Options

- Compression
- Pentoxifylline
- Stanozolol
- Niacin
- Tetracycline antibiotics

Further reading:
- Huang TM, Lee JY (2009) Lipodermatosclerosis: a clinicopathologic study of 17 cases and differential diagnosis from erythema nodosum. J Cutan Pathol 36(4):453–460

Lipodystrophy, Acquired

Group of acquired disorders of fat distribution that are characterized by absence of fat in a localized or generalized distribution and that may be associated with insulin resistance, diabetes mellitus, hypertriglyceridemia, renal failure, and liver failure in some patients

Subtypes/Variants

- Acquired generalized (Lawrence syndrome)
- Acquired partial (Barraquer–Simons syndrome)
- HIV associated
- Injection related (insulin, corticosteroids)
- Lipoatrophia semicircularis
- Lipodystrophia centifugalis abdominalis infantilis

Differential Diagnosis

- Anorexia
- Atrophoderma of Pasini and Pierini
- Cachexia
- Congenital lipodystrophy
- Cushing syndrome
- Lupus panniculitis
- Malnutrition
- Parry–Romberg syndrome
- Subcutaneous T cell lymphoma

Associations

- Connective tissue disease (especially dermatomyositis)
- Febrile illness
- Glomerulonephritis
- Hypocomplementemia

Further reading:
- Pope E, Janson A, Khambalia A, Feldman B (2006) Childhood acquired lipodystrophy: a retrospective study. J Am Acad Dermatol 55(6):947–950

Lipodystrophy, Congenital

Group of congenital disorders of fat distribution that are characterized by localized or generalized absence of fat and that may be associated with insulin resistance, diabetes mellitus, hypertriglyceridemia, pancreatitis, cardiomyopathy, renal failure, and liver failure in some patients

Subtypes/Variants

- Congenital generalized (Berardinelli–Seip syndrome)
- Familial partial (Kobberling–Dunnigan syndrome)

Differential Diagnosis

- Acquired lipodystrophy
- Cushing syndrome
- Donahue syndrome
- Malnutrition
- SHORT syndrome

Further reading:
- Helm TN, Bisker E, Bergfeld WF (2001) Lipodystrophy. Cutis 67(2):163–164

Lipoid Proteinosis (Hyalinosis Cutis et Mucosae, Urbach–Wiethe Syndrome)

Rare AR disease that is caused by a mutation in the ECM1 gene encoding extracellular matrix protein 1 which causes the deposition of hyaline material in the skin and mucous membranes and is characterized by infiltrated waxy papules, nodules, and plaques on the vocal cords (hoarseness), tongue, lips (cobblestone appearance), face, eyelids (beaded appearance), and elbows and knees (verrucous appearance), as well as bilateral intracranial bean-shaped calcifications of the temporal lobe

Differential Diagnosis

- Acanthosis nigricans, oral
- Colloid milium, juvenile
- Cowden's disease
- Erythropoietic protoporphyria
- Infantile systemic hyalinosis
- Familial amyloidosis syndromes
- Leprosy
- Ligneous gingival hyperplasia
- Juvenile hyaline fibromatosis
- Myxedema
- Papular mucinosis
- Primary systemic amyloidosis
- Pseudoxanthoma elasticum
- Scleromyxedema
- Xanthoma disseminatum
- Xanthomas

Evaluation

- Otorhinolaryngologic examination
- CT or MRI scan of the brain

Further reading:
- Ringpfeil F (2005) Selected disorders of connective tissue: pseudoxanthoma elasticum, cutis laxa, and lipoid proteinosis. Clin Dermatol 23(1):41–46

Lipoma

Common benign tumor of adipose tissue with several histologic variants that is associated with numerous disorders or clinical presentations and is characterized by a large circumscribed soft subcutaneous mass most commonly located anywhere on the body

Subtypes/Variants

- Angiolipoleiomyoma
- Angiolipoma
- Chondroid lipoma
- Hibernoma
- Lipoblastoma
- Multiple
- Neural fibrolipoma
- Pleomorphic lipoma
- Segmental
- Spindle cell lipoma

Differential Diagnosis

Lipoma

- Desmoid tumor
- Elastofibroma dorsi
- Epidermoid cyst
- Glomus tumor
- Hibernoma
- Leiomyoma
- Liposarcoma
- Malignant fibrous histiocytoma
- Nevus lipomatosus superficialis

- Neurofibroma (especially plexiform)
- Nodular fasciitis
- Panniculitis
- Sarcoma
- Schwannoma
- Spiradenoma
- Traumatic arteriovenous fistula

Angiolipoma

- Dercum's disease
- Eccrine spiradenoma
- Glomus tumor
- Hibernoma
- Kaposiform hemangioendothelioma
- Leiomyoma
- Lipoma
- Liposarcoma
- Neuroma

Multiple

- Cysticercosis
- Epidermal cysts
- Hemangiomas
- Metastatic disease
- Neurofibromatosis
- Steatocystoma multiplex
- Subcutaneous granuloma annulare
- Subcutaneous sarcoidosis

Associations

Multiple

- Adiposis dolorosa (Dercum's disease)
- Bannayan–Riley–Ruvalcaba syndrome

- Diffuse lipomatosis
- Encephalocraniocutaneous lipomatosis
- Familial multiple lipomatosis
- Gardner's syndrome
- Madelung's disease (benign symmetric lipomatosis, Launois–Bensaude disease)
- Multiple endocrine neoplasia, type I
- Protease inhibitor therapy
- Proteus syndrome

Angiolipoma

- Antiretroviral therapy
- Diabetes mellitus

Further reading:

- Mentzel T (2001) Cutaneous lipomatous neoplasms. Semin Diagn Pathol 18(4):250–257

Lipomatosis, Benign Symmetric (Madelung's Disease, Launois–Bensaude Syndrome)

Type of lipomatosis predominantly affecting middle-aged men that is characterized by asymptomatic lipomas in a horse collar-like distribution around the neck

Differential Diagnosis

- Dercum's disease
- Goiter
- Lymphadenopathy
- Obesity
- Sialadenitis
- Soft tissue neoplasia

Associations

- Alcoholism
- Diabetes
- Gout

Further reading:
- Fernandez-Vozmediano J, Armario-Hita J (2005) Benign symmetric lipomatosis (Launois–Bensaude syndrome). Int J Dermatol 44(3):236–237

Liposarcoma

Uncommon malignant tumor of adipose tissue that affects older patients and is characterized by a circumscribed, often large, subcutaneous mass that grows slowly and is most commonly located on the thigh

Differential Diagnosis

- Dermatofibrosarcoma protuberans
- Leiomyosarcoma
- Lipoblastoma
- Lipoma
- Metastases
- Malignant fibrous histiocytoma
- Malignant schwannoma
- Neurofibroma (especially plexiform)
- Pleomorphic lipoma
- Plexiform neurofibroma
- Rhabdomyosarcoma
- Soft tissue sarcoma
- Spindle cell lipoma
- Tropical pyomyositis

Further reading:
- Dei Tos AP, Mentzel T, Fletcher CD (1998) Primary liposarcoma of the skin: a rare neoplasm with unusual high grade features. Am J Dermatopathol 20(4):332–338

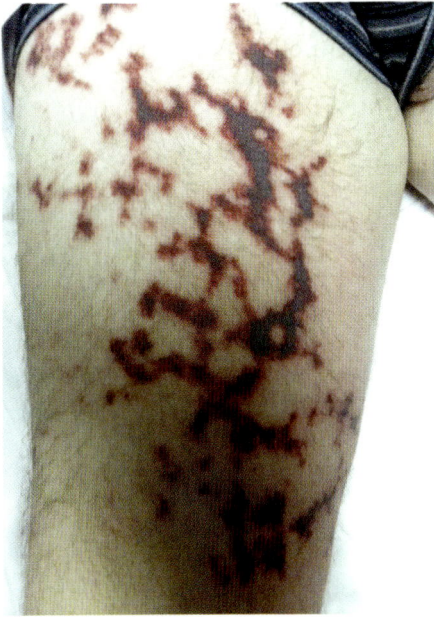

Fig. 6.66 Livedo racemosa

Livedo Reticularis/Racemosa

Vascular disorder that is caused by cutaneous hypoperfusion most often in the setting of hypercoagulability related to a variety of underlying diseases and is characterized by a net-like pattern of reddish to cyanotic discoloration of the extremities, especially the legs, that is accentuated with cold exposure and that may (reticularis) or may not (racemosa) improve with rewarming (Fig. 6.66)

Subtypes/Variants

- Without systemic associations
  - Congenital (physiologic cutis marmorata)
  - Idiopathic
  - Primary

- With systemic associations
  - Congenital (cutis marmorata telangiectatica congenita)
  - Hematologic/hypercoagulable
  - Autoimmune
  - Embolic
  - Medication induced
  - Infectious related
  - Neurologic

Differential Diagnosis

- Acrocyanosis
- Angioma serpiginosum
- Bier spots
- Cutis marmorata
- Cutis marmorata telangiectatica congenita
- Drug reactions
- Erythema ab igne
- Erythema infectiosum
- Livedo vasculopathy
- Poikilodermatous diseases
- Reticulated erythematous mucinosis
- Retiform purpura
- Viral exanthem

Associations

- Amantadine therapy
- Antiphospholipid antibody syndrome
- Antithrombin III deficiency
- Apoplexy
- Arteriosclerosis
- Calciphylaxis
- Carcinoid syndrome

- <u>Cholesterol emboli</u>
- Churg–Strauss syndrome
- CNS disease or injury
- <u>Cocaine-associated vasculopathy</u>
- Cold agglutinins
- Cryoglobulinemia/cryofibrinogenemia
- Cushing's syndrome
- Dermatomyositis
- Encephalitis
- Endocarditis
- Factor V Leiden mutation
- Fat emboli
- Felty syndrome
- Hemolytic uremic syndrome/thrombotic thrombocytopenic purpura
- Homocystinuria
- Hyperoxaluria
- Hypothyroidism
- Intravascular B cell lymphoma
- Leukemia
- Livedoid vasculopathy
- <u>Lupus erythematosus</u>
- Microscopic polyangiitis
- Moyamoya disease
- Multiple sclerosis
- Neurofibromatosis
- Pancreatitis
- Paraproteinemia
- Parkinson's disease
- Pellagra
- Pheochromocytoma
- Poliomyelitis
- Polyarteritis nodosa
- Polycythemia vera
- Protein-S, protein-C deficiency

- Quinine
- Rheumatoid arthritis
- Sepsis
- Septic vasculitis
- Sharp syndrome
- Sjögren syndrome
- Sneddon syndrome
- Still's disease
- Syphilis
- Systemic sclerosis
- Takayasu's disease
- Temporal arteritis
- Thromboangiitis obliterans
- Thrombocytosis
- Tuberculosis
- Wegener's granulomatosis

Evaluation

- Anticardiolipin antibodies
- Antineutrophilic cytoplasmic antibodies
- Antinuclear antibodies
- Antithrombin III level
- Factor V Leiden assay
- Homocysteine levels
- Lupus anticoagulant test
- Protein-C and protein-S level
- Renal function test
- Rheumatoid factor
- Serum/urinary protein electrophoresis
- Serum cryoglobulins and cryofibrinogens
- Viral hepatitis panel

Treatment Options

- <u>Treat underlying cause</u>
- Aspirin
- Pentoxifylline
- Dipyridamole

Further reading:
- Gibbs M et al (2005) Livedo reticularis: an update. J Am Acad Dermatol 52:1009–1019

Livedoid Vasculopathy

Distinct vascular disorder caused by thrombosis that is characterized by livedo reticularis and painful ulcerations around the ankles which heal to small atrophic white scars (atrophie blanche)

Differential Diagnosis

- <u>Antiphospholipid antibody syndrome</u>
- Arterial ulcer
- Cholesterol emboli
- Malignant atrophic papulosis
- Hydroxyurea-related ulceration
- Hypersensitivity vasculitis
- Hypertensive ulcer
- Lupus erythematosus
- Lichen sclerosus
- Lipodermatosclerosis
- Livedo reticularis
- <u>Polyarteritis nodosa</u>
- Scleroderma
- Septic emboli

- Sickle cell anemia
- Trauma
- Ulcerative necrobiosis lipoidica
- <u>Venous stasis ulcer</u>
- Vasculitis

Associations

- <u>Antiphospholipid antibody syndrome</u>
- Livedo reticularis
- Raynaud phenomenon
- Stasis dermatitis (can occur as a secondary phenomenon)

Evaluation

- Anticardiolipin antibodies
- Antineutrophilic cytoplasmic antibodies
- Antinuclear antibodies
- Antithrombin III level
- Beta-2 glycoprotein-1 antibodies
- Factor V Leiden assay
- Homocysteine levels
- Lupus anticoagulant test
- Protein-C and protein-S level
- Renal function test
- Rheumatoid factor
- Serum/urinary protein electrophoresis
- Serum cryoglobulins and cryofibrinogens
- Viral hepatitis panel

Treatment Options

- <u>Aspirin</u>
- <u>Dipyridamole</u>

- <u>Pentoxifylline</u>
- Danazol
- Heparin
- Warfarin
- Dapsone
- Niacin

Further reading:
- Hairston BR, Davis MD, Pittelkow MR et al (2006) Livedoid vasculopathy: further evidence for procoagulant pathogenesis. Arch Dermatol 142(11):1413–1418

Lobomycosis (Keloidal Blastomycosis)

Chronic fungal infection affecting patients in South and Central America that is caused by *Lacazia loboi* and is characterized by keloid-like papules, nodules, and plaques on the ears, trunk, and extremities

Differential Diagnosis

- Chromoblastomycosis
- Dermatofibrosarcoma protuberans
- Leishmaniasis
- Leprosy
- Kaposi's sarcoma
- <u>Keloid</u>
- Paracoccidioidomycosis
- Xanthoma

Further reading:
- Paniz-Mondolfi AE, Reyes Jaimes O, Davila Jones L (2007) Lobomycosis in Venezuela. Int J Dermatol 46(2):180–185

Loose Anagen Hair

Hair disorder possibly caused by defective keratinization of the inner root sheath that affects blonde-haired girls and is characterized by diffuse thinning or patchy alopecia with easily and painlessly plucked hairs that demonstrate a rumpled cuticle on hair mount

Differential Diagnosis

- <u>Alopecia areata</u>
- Anagen effluvium
- Iron deficiency
- Nutritional deficiency
- <u>Telogen effluvium</u>
- Thyroid disease
- Tinea capitis
- Traction alopecia
- Trichorrhexis invaginata
- Trichorrhexis nodosa
- Trichotillomania
- Uncombable hair syndrome

Associations

- Coloboma
- Hypohidrotic ectodermal dysplasia
- Noonan's syndrome

Treatment Options

- Observation and reassurance

Further reading:
- Tosti A, Piraccini BM (2002) Loose anagen hair syndrome and loose anagen hair. Arch Dermatol 138(4):521–522

Lupus Erythematosus, Cutaneous

Term encompassing a spectrum of autoimmune disease of the skin that may or may not be associated with systemic lupus and is characterized by a prominent erythema and photosensitivity (acute), papulosquamous, or annular lesions (subacute) or scarred, hypopigmented plaques (chronic), along with several other less common subtypes

Subtypes/Variants

- Acute
  - Exfoliative erythroderma-like
  - Malar erythema
  - Photodistributed
  - TEN-like eruption (ASAP syndrome)
- Chronic
  - Chilblains
  - Discoid
  - Hypertrophic
  - Lichen planus – lupus erythematosus overlap
  - Lupus panniculitis (Kaposi–Irgand syndrome)
  - Mucosal
  - Rowell's syndrome
  - Tumid
- Subacute
  - Annular
  - Exfoliative erythroderma-like
  - Papulosquamous
- Other Types of Lupus
  - Acute syndrome of apoptotic pan-epidermolysis
  - Bullous
  - Complement deficiency related
  - Neonatal
  - Systemic

Differential Diagnosis

Acute

- <u>Dermatomyositis</u>
- Eczema
- Erythema multiforme
- Pemphigus erythematosus
- Photoallergic contact dermatitis
- <u>Photosensitive drug eruption</u>
- Polymorphous light eruption
- Porphyria cutanea tarda
- Pseudoporphyria
- <u>Rosacea</u>
- Seborrheic dermatitis
- Solar urticaria
- Sunburn
- Tinea faciei
- Toxic epidermal necrolysis

Bullous

- Bullosis diabeticorum
- Bullous pemphigoid
- Dermatitis herpetiformis
- <u>Epidermolysis bullosa acquisita</u>
- Linear IgA bullous dermatosis
- Pemphigus
- <u>Toxic epidermal necrolysis</u>

Discoid

- Actinic keratosis
- Actinic prurigo
- Angiolymphoid hyperplasia with eosinophilia
- Bowen's disease
- Cicatricial pemphigoid
- Dermatomyositis

- Graham–Little–Piccardi–Lasseur syndrome
- Granuloma annulare
- <u>Granuloma faciale</u>
- Jessner's lymphocytic infiltrate
- Keratoacanthoma
- Leprosy
- Lichen planopilaris
- <u>Lichen planus (especially atrophic type)</u>
- Lichen sclerosus et atrophicus
- Lupus vulgaris
- Lymphocytoma cutis
- Lymphoma cutis
- Polymorphous light eruption
- Psoriasis
- Reticular erythematous mucinosis
- Rosacea
- <u>Sarcoidosis</u>
- Squamous cell carcinoma
- Sporotrichosis
- Tertiary syphilis
- Tinea faciei

Hypertrophic/Verrucous

- Deep fungal infection
- <u>Hypertrophic lichen planus</u>
- Keratoacanthomas
- Lichen simplex chronicus
- Prurigo nodularis
- Psoriasis
- Warts

Lupus Panniculitis

- Atrophoderma of Pasini and Pierini
- Carcinoma en cuirasse
- Erythema induratum

- <u>Erythema nodosum</u>
- Epidermal inclusion cyst
- Lipoatrophy
- <u>Morphea profunda</u>
- Pancreatic panniculitis
- Rheumatoid nodule
- Steroid lipoatrophy
- <u>Subcutaneous T cell lymphoma</u>
- Superficial thrombophlebitis
- Thrombophlebitis

Neonatal

- Acute hemorrhagic edema of infancy
- <u>Annular erythema of infancy</u>
- Bloom syndrome
- Congenital rubella
- Congenital syphilis
- Cutaneous lymphoid hyperplasia
- Cutis marmorata telangiectatica congenita
- Erythema toxicum neonatorum
- Langerhans cell histiocytosis
- Lymphangioma circumscriptum
- Rothmund–Thomson syndrome
- Serum-sickness-like reaction
- Urticaria

Subacute

- Actinic prurigo
- Dermatomyositis
- Disseminated superficial actinic porokeratosis
- <u>Erythema annulare centrifugum</u>
- Erythema gyratum repens
- Erythema multiforme
- Granuloma annulare
- Leprosy

- Lichen planus
- Lyme disease
- Mycosis fungoides
- <u>Nummular eczema</u>
- Pemphigus erythematosus
- <u>Photosensitive drug eruption</u>
- Photosensitive eczema
- Pityriasis rubra pilaris
- Polymorphous light eruption
- <u>Psoriasis</u>
- Rowell's syndrome
- Sarcoidosis
- Seborrheic dermatitis
- Sjögren's syndrome
- <u>Tinea corporis</u>

Tumid

- <u>Arthropod-bite reaction</u>
- Cutaneous lymphoid hyperplasia
- <u>Erythema annulare centrifugum (especially deep type)</u>
- Granuloma annulare
- Granuloma faciale
- <u>Jessner's lymphocytic infiltrate</u>
- Lupus panniculitis
- Lymphoma cutis
- Polymorphous light eruption
- <u>Reticular erythematous mucinosis</u>
- Sarcoidosis
- Wells syndrome

Diagnostic Criteria

Bullous (4/4)

- Fulfillment of the ARA criteria for SLE
- Vesicles and/or bullae

- Subepidermal blistering with leukocyte infiltrates in the dermis
- Linear or granular deposition of IgG (with or without IgA and/or IgM antibodies) at the dermal–epidermal junction of normal and/or affected skin sample

Rowell's Syndrome

- Major criteria (3/3)
  - Lupus erythematosus (LE): systemic LE, discoid LE, or subacute cutaneous LE
  - Erythema-multiforme-like lesions (with/without involvement of the mucous membranes)
  - Speckled pattern of antinuclear antibody
- Minor (1/3)
  - Chilblains
  - Anti-Ro antibody or anti-La antibody
  - Positive rheumatoid factor

Associated Medications (Subacute)

- ACE inhibitors
- Anticonvulsants
- Calcium channel blockers
- Glyburide
- Gold
- Griseofulvin
- Hydrochlorothiazide
- Penicillamine
- Piroxicam
- Procainamide
- PUVA
- Ranitidine
- Spironolactone
- Sulfonylureas
- Terbinafine

Evaluation

- Complete blood count
- Antinuclear antibodies (including SS-A and SS-B)
- Renal function test
- Lupus band test

Treatment Options

- Topical corticosteroids
- Intralesional corticosteroids
- Systemic corticosteroids
- Topical tacrolimus
- Sunscreen
- <u>Hydroxychloroquine</u>
- Chloroquine
- Quinacrine
- Dapsone
- <u>Mycophenolate mofetil</u>
- <u>Methotrexate</u>
- Acitretin
- Thalidomide
- Cyclophosphamide
- Sulfasalazine

Further reading:

- Crowson AN, Magro C (2001) The cutaneous pathology of lupus erythematosus: a review. J Cutaneous Pathol 28:1–23
- Yell JA, Allen J, Wojnarowska F, Kirtschig G et al (1995) Bullous systemic lupus erythematosus: revised criteria for diagnosis. Br J Dermatol 132(6):921–928
- Zeitouni NC, Funaro D, Cloutier RA et al (2000) Redefining Rowell's syndrome. Br J Dermatol 142(2):343–346

Lupus Erythematosus, Systemic

Autoimmune disorder with variable cutaneous and systemic features that is characterized by autoantibody production and immune complex deposition which affects a variety of organs including the kidneys, CNS, joints, serosal surfaces, and skin

Diagnostic Criteria (4/11)

- Anti-DNA antibodies, anti-Smith antibodies, or false-positive VDRL
- Antinuclear antibodies
- Discoid lesions
- Hemolytic anemia, leukopenia, lymphopenia, or thrombocytopenia
- Malar rash
- Neurologic disorder: seizures
- Nonerosive arthritis
- Oral ulcers (observed by a physician)
- Photosensitivity
- Proteinuria or cellular casts in the urine
- Serositis: pleuritis or pericarditis

Associations

- Acanthosis nigricans
- Benign hypergammaglobulinemic purpura of Waldenstrom
- Complement deficiency
- Dermatitis herpetiformis
- Eosinophilic fasciitis
- Pemphigus
- Porphyria cutanea tarda
- Rheumatoid arthritis
- Scleroderma
- Sjögren's syndrome
- Sweet's syndrome

- Ulcerative colitis
- Toxic-epidermal-necrolysis-like presentation

Associated Medications (Drug-Induced LE)

- Anticonvulsants
- Captopril
- Ciprofloxacin
- Etanercept
- Hydralazine
- Hydroxyurea
- Infliximab
- Isoniazid
- Minocycline
- Oral contraceptives
- Penicillin
- Penicillamine
- Procainamide
- Rifampin
- Spironolactone
- Sulfonamides

Evaluation

- Antinuclear antibodies and extractable nuclear antigen panel
- Antiphospholipid antibodies
- Chest radiograph
- Complete blood count
- Complement levels
- Direct immunofluorescence
- Echocardiography
- Electrocardiogram
- Renal function test
- Rheumatoid factor

- Serum protein electrophoresis
- Urinalysis

Further reading:
- Rothfield N, Sontheimer RD, Bernstein M (2006) Lupus erythematosus: systemic and cutaneous manifestations. Clin Dermatol 24(5):348–362

Lupus Miliaris Disseminata Faciei (Acne Agminata)

Chronic skin disorder of unknown cause that is characterized by multiple small, red-brown papules on the face, most commonly in a periocular distribution

Differential Diagnosis

- <u>Acne vulgaris</u>
- Cutaneous lymphoid hyperplasia
- <u>Demodicosis</u>
- Granuloma faciale
- Granulomatous periorificial dermatitis
- <u>Granulomatous rosacea</u>
- Histiocytoses
- Lupus vulgaris
- Multicentric reticulohistiocytosis
- Papular xanthoma
- Perioral dermatitis
- Sarcoidosis
- Syringoma
- Trichoepithelioma
- Verruca plana

Treatment Options

- <u>Tetracycline antibiotics</u>
- Dapsone

- Systemic corticosteroids
- Antimalarials

Further reading:

- Nino M, Barberio E, Delfino M (2003) Lupus miliaris disseminatus faciei and its debated link to tuberculosis. J Eur Acad Dermatol Venereol 17(1):97

Lyme Disease

Spirochetal disease that is caused by several subspecies of *Borrelia burg-dorferi*, is transmitted by *Ixodes* ticks, and is characterized by an initial stage associated with erythema migrans; a second stage associated with neuropathy, meningitis, cardiac inflammation, and cutaneous lymphoid hyperplasia; and a third-stage characterized by arthritis, CNS disturbance, and acrodermatitis chronica atrophicans

Differential Diagnosis

- Arbovirus encephalitis
- Ehrlichiosis
- Guillain–Barre syndrome
- HIV infection
- Juvenile rheumatoid arthritis
- Leptospirosis
- Lupus erythematosus
- Ramsay Hunt syndrome
- Rat-bite fever
- Rheumatoid arthritis
- Rocky Mountain spotted fever
- Southern tick-associated rash illness
- Syphilis
- Tick paralysis

Evaluation

- Complete blood count
- Electrocardiogram
- Joint-fluid analysis
- Liver function test
- Lumbar puncture
- Lyme disease ELISA and Western blot
- Polymerase chain reaction for borrelial antigen
- Renal function test

Treatment Options

- <u>Doxycycline</u>
- Amoxicillin
- Cefuroxime

Further reading:

- Wormser GP, Dattwyler RJ, Shapiro ED et al (2006) The clinical assessment, treatment, and prevention of Lyme disease, human granulocytic anaplasmosis, and babesiosis: clinical practice guidelines by the Infectious Diseases Society of America. Clin Infect Dis 43(9):1089–1134

Lymphadenoma, Cutaneous

Rare, benign neoplasm that contains both basaloid epithelial islands and a lymphocytic infiltrate and is characterized as a solitary, erythematous nodule on the head and neck, often in the preauricular area or cheek

Differential Diagnosis

- Accessory tragus
- Angiolymphoid hyperplasia with eosinophilia
- <u>Basal cell carcinoma</u>

- Clear cell syringoma
- <u>Cutaneous lymphoid hyperplasia</u>
- Follicular neoplasms
- Lymphoepithelioma-like carcinoma
- <u>Lymphoma cutis</u>
- Intradermal melanocytic nevus
- Sebaceous adenoma
- Trichoblastoma

Further reading:

- Alsadhan A, Taher M, Shokravi M (2003) Cutaneous lymphadenoma. J Am Acad Dermatol 49(6):1115–1116

Lymphangioma

Term referring to either a congenital lymphatic malformation or an acquired postsurgical or postinflammatory lymphatic lesion that is characterized by verrucous clusters of hyperkeratotic superficial vesicle-like papules (congenital microcystic or acquired) or deeper subcutaneous cystic dilatations that are most commonly located on the head and neck (congenital macrocystic)

Subtypes/Variants

- Congenital macrocystic (cavernous/cystic hygroma)
- Congenital microcystic (lymphangioma circumscriptum)
- Acquired

Differential Diagnosis

- Amyloidosis
- <u>Angiokeratoma circumscriptum</u>
- Branchiogenic cyst
- Condyloma acuminatum

- Deep hemangioma
- Epidermal inclusion cyst
- <u>Epidermal nevus</u>
- Hemangioma
- Herpes simplex virus infection
- Kaposi's sarcoma
- Lipoma
- Melanoma
- Mucocele
- Neurofibroma
- Ranula
- Soft tissue tumor
- Telangiectatic cutaneous metastasis
- Thyroglossal cyst
- <u>Warts</u>

Associations

Macrocystic/Cystic Hygroma

- Achondroplasia
- Down syndrome
- Klinefelter syndrome
- Multiple pterygium syndrome
- Noonan syndrome
- Turner syndrome

Acquired

- Esthiomene
- Hidradenitis suppurativa
- Lymph node dissection
- Radiation

Further reading:

- Gupta S, Radotra BD, Javaheri SM et al (2003) Lymphangioma circumscriptum of the penis mimicking venereal lesions. J Eur Acad Dermatol Venereol 17(5):598–600

Lymphogranuloma Venereum (Nicolas–Favre Disease)

Sexually transmitted disease caused by L serotypes of *Chlamydia trachomatis* that is characterized by an often unrecognized, asymptomatic genital ulcer, followed by painful inguinal lymphadenopathy that is bisected by Poupart's ligament (groove sign), and, if untreated, elephantiasis resulting from lymphatic obstruction with markedly enlarged and distorted genitalia (esthiomene)

Differential Diagnosis

- Brucellosis
- Bubonic plaque
- Cat-scratch disease
- Chancroid
- Crohn's disease
- Elephantiasis
- Filariasis
- Granuloma inguinale
- Hidradenitis suppurativa
- Hodgkin's disease
- Infectious mononucleosis
- Lymphoma
- Metastasis
- Scrofuloderma
- Syphilis
- Tuberculosis
- Tularemia

Evaluation

- Complement fixation serologic test
- HIV test
- Lymph node aspiration, Gram stain, and culture
- Syphilis serologic tests

Further reading:
- Lupi O, Madkan V, Tyring SK (2006) Tropical dermatology: bacterial tropical diseases. J Am Acad Dermatol 54(4):559–578

Lymphoid Hyperplasia, Cutaneous (Lymphocytoma Cutis, Pseudolymphoma, Spiegler–Fendt Sarcoid)

Term for several different types of benign lymphocytic infiltration (with a mix of T cells and B cells; Fig. 6.67) that clinically and histologically mimic cutaneous lymphoma occur in response to a variety of antigenic stimuli and are characterized most commonly by plum-colored papules or nodules on the head and neck (B cell lymphoma-like) or erythematous scaly patches and plaques (T cell lymphoma-like)

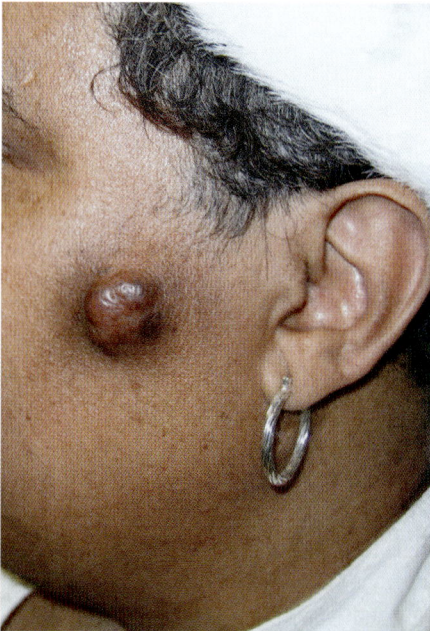

Fig. 6.67 Cutaneous lymphoid hyperplasia

Subtypes/Variants

- Acral pseudolymphomatous angiokeratoma of children (APACHE)
- Angioimmunoblastic lymphadenopathy
- Angiolymphoid hyperplasia with eosinophils
- Castleman's disease
- Kimura's disease
- Lymphocytic infiltrates
- Lymphomatoid contact dermatitis
- Lymphomatoid drug reaction
- Lymphomatoid keratosis
- Lymphomatoid papulosis
- Pseudolymphomatous folliculitis
- Pseudomycosis fungoides
- Syringolymphoid hyperplasia

Differential Diagnosis

- Adnexal tumor
- Basal cell carcinoma
- Cutaneous metastasis
- Cylindroma
- Foreign body granuloma
- Granuloma annulare
- Granuloma faciale
- Granulomatous rosacea
- Inflamed epidermal cyst
- Insect-bite reactions
- Lepromatous leprosy
- Lymphadenoma
- Lymphocytic infiltrate of Jessner
- Lymphoma cutis
- Merkel cell carcinoma
- Sarcoidosis

- Squamous cell carcinoma
- Tumid lupus erythematosus

Associations

- Acupuncture
- <u>Arthropod bite</u>
- Borreliosis
- Contact dermatitis
- Gold jewelry
- Idiopathic
- Medications
- Scabies
- Tattoo
- Trauma
- Vaccinations
- Zoster

Associated Medications

B Cell

- Amitriptyline
- Fluoxetine

T Cell

- ACE Inhibitors
- Allopurinol
- Anticonvulsants
- Antipsychotics
- Beta-blockers
- Calcium channel blockers
- Cyclosporine
- Diuretics

- Dapsone
- NSAIDs
- Phenobarbital
- Sulfa Drugs

Evaluation

- Immunophenotyping
- T or B cell gene rearrangement

Treatment Options

- Removal of underlying cause
- Intralesional corticosteroids
- Radiation
- Surgical excision

Further reading:
- Bergman R (2010) Pseudolymphoma and cutaneous lymphoma: facts and controversies. Clin Dermatol 28(5):568–574

Lymphoma, Primary Cutaneous CD30+ Anaplastic Large Cell

Uncommon type of T cell lymphoma that affects adults and is characterized by a solitary firm and violaceous tumor with or without ulceration that can occur anywhere and is associated with a good prognosis

Differential Diagnosis

- Basal cell carcinoma
- Granuloma faciale
- Granulocytic sarcoma
- Hodgkin's disease

- Jessner's benign lymphocytic infiltrate
- Leukemia cutis
- Lymphomatoid papulosis
- Keratoacanthomas
- Melanoma
- Merkel cell carcinoma
- Metastatic disease
- Orf
- Squamous cell carcinoma

Treatment Options

- Radiation therapy
- Surgical excision
- Methotrexate
- Chemotherapy

Further reading:

- Kempf W (2006) CD30+ lymphoproliferative disorders: histopathology, differential diagnosis, new variants, and simulators. J Cutan Pathol 33(Suppl 1):58–70

Lymphoma, Primary Cutaneous B Cell

Type of B cell lymphoma arising in the skin that is characterized by solitary or multiple red to plum-colored papules, nodules, or plaques most commonly on the trunk or head and neck and that carries a relatively good prognosis, except for the diffuse type which occurs on the leg

Subtypes/Variants

- Intravascular large B cell lymphoma
- Lymphomatoid granulomatosis
- Posttransplant lymphoproliferative disorder
- Primary cutaneous follicle center-cell lymphoma

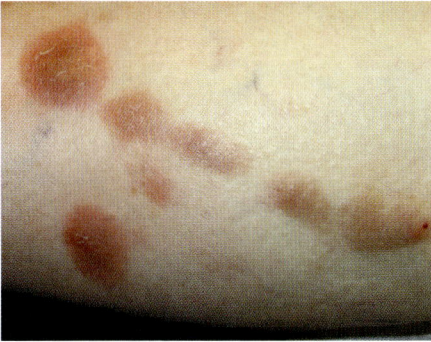

Fig. 6.68 Diffuse large B cell lymphoma, leg type

- Primary cutaneous immunocytoma/marginal zone lymphoma
- Primary cutaneous large B cell lymphoma of the leg (Fig. 6.68)
- Primary cutaneous plasmacytoma

Differential Diagnosis

- Acute myelogenous leukemia
- Amelanotic melanoma
- Basal cell carcinoma
- Chronic lymphocytic leukemia/lymphoma
- Cutaneous lymphoid hyperplasia
- Granulocytic sarcoma
- Lymphocytic infiltration of Jessner
- Merkel cell carcinoma
- Metastatic disease
- Secondary cutaneous lymphoma

Evaluation

- Calcium level
- Chest radiograph
- Complete blood count with smear
- CT scan of chest, abdomen, and pelvis

- Immunoglobulin gene rearrangement
- Immunophenotyping
- Lactate dehydrogenase level
- Lymph node exam and biopsy
- Serum/urinary protein electrophoresis
- Serum chemistry

Treatment Options

- <u>Radiation</u>
- Surgical excision
- Doxycycline
- Intralesional corticosteroids
- <u>Rituximab</u>
- Chemotherapy

Further reading:

- Bogle MA, Riddle CC, Triana EM, Jones D, Duvic M (2005) Primary cutaneous B-cell lymphoma. J Am Acad Dermatol 53(3):479–484

Lymphoma, Cutaneous T Cell

Type of T cell lymphoma arising in the skin that has several different subtypes and numerous different morphologies, some of which are indolent with a good prognosis, while others are more rapidly progressive and carry a poor prognosis

Subtypes/Variants

- Cutaneous T cell lymphoma, large cell, and CD30 negative
- Cutaneous T cell lymphoma, large cell, and CD30 positive
- Cutaneous T cell lymphoma, pleomorphic, and small/medium cell
- Granulomatous slack skin
- Lymphomatoid papulosis

- Mycosis fungoides and variants
- Pagetoid reticulosis
- Sézary's syndrome
- Subcutaneous panniculitis-like T cell lymphoma

Differential Diagnosis

- See individual subtypes.

TMN Classification

- T_1: Limited patch/plaque (involving <10% of total skin surface)
- T_2: Generalized patch/plaque (involving =10% of total skin surface)
- T_3: Tumor(s)
- T_4: Erythroderma
- N_0: No enlarged lymph nodes
- N_1: Enlarged lymph nodes, histologically uninvolved
- N_2: No enlarged lymph nodes, histologically involved
- N_3: Enlarged lymph nodes, histologically involved
- M_0: No visceral involvement
- M_1: Visceral involvement
- B_0: No circulating atypical (Sézary) cells (or <5% of lymphocytes)
- B_1: Circulating atypical (Sézary) cells (=5 of lymphocytes)

Staging

- IA: $T_1 N_0 M_0$
- IB: $T_2 N_0 M_0$
- IIA: $T_{1-2} N_1 M_0$
- IIB: $T_3 N_{0-1} M_0$
- III: $T_4 N_{0-1} M_0$
- IVA: $T_{1-4} N_{2-3} M_0$
- IVB: $T_{1-4} N_{0-3} M_1$

Evaluation

- Calcium level
- Chest radiography
- Complete blood count
- HTLV-1 serologic test
- Immunophenotyping
- Lactate dehydrogenase level
- Liver function test
- Lymph node exam and biopsy
- PET scan
- Renal function test
- Sézary cell preparation
- T cell gene rearrangement

Treatment Options

- <u>Topical corticosteroids</u>
- <u>UVB phototherapy</u>
- Topical nitrogen mustard
- <u>Total skin electron beam therapy</u>
- Methotrexate
- Interferon alpha-2a
- Topical bexarotene
- <u>Oral bexarotene</u>
- Denileukin diftitox
- Alemtuzumab
- Vorinostat
- Romidepsin
- Chemotherapy

Further reading:

- Kinney MC, Jones D (2007) Cutaneous T-cell and NK-cell lymphomas: the WHO–EORTC classification and the increasing recognition of specialized tumor types. Am J Clin Pathol 127(5):670–686

- Olsen E, Vonderheid E, Pimpinelli N et al (2007) Revisions to the staging and classification of mycosis fungoides and Sezary syndrome: a proposal of the International Society for Cutaneous Lymphomas (ISCL) and the cutaneous Lymphoma task force of the European organization of Research and Treatment of cancer (EORTC). Blood 110(6):1713–1722

Lymphoma, Intravascular (Angiotropic)
B Cell Lymphoma (Malignant Angioendotheliomatosis)

Type of B cell lymphoma affecting older patients that arises within blood vessels and is characterized by a variable clinical presentation, including vascular papules and nodules and livedo-like lesions, along with CNS disturbance due to presumed neoplastic cell-mediated infarctions, giving rise to stroke symptoms and seizures, and a poor prognosis

Differential Diagnosis

- Acroangiodermatitis
- Angiosarcoma
- Antiphospholipid antibody syndrome
- Bacillary angiomatosis
- Cryoglobulinemia
- Erythema nodosum
- Kaposi's sarcoma
- Lymphomatoid granulomatosis
- Malignant atrophic papulosis
- Panniculitis
- Perniosis (chilblains)
- Thrombophlebitis
- Phlebitis
- Reactive angioendotheliomatosis
- Sarcoidosis
- Sneddon syndrome
- Squamous cell carcinoma
- Tufted angioma
- Vasculitis

Treatment Options

- Chemotherapy
- <u>Rituximab</u>

Further reading:
- Ferreri AJ, Campo E, Seymour JF et al (2004) Intravascular lymphoma: clinical presentation, natural history, management and prognostic factors in a series of 38 cases, with special emphasis on the "cutaneous variant". Br J Haematol 127(2):173–183

Lymphoma, Natural Killer Cell (CD56+ Lymphoma)

Type of T cell lymphoma with variable clinical presentation that is associated with EBV infection; is characterized by an angiocentric, ulcerative tumor, or tumors arising most commonly in the nasal passages or on the extremities; or may resemble hydroa vacciniforme when it occurs in children

Differential Diagnosis

- Cutaneous lymphoid hyperplasia
- <u>Hydroa vacciniforme</u>
- Leishmaniasis
- Leprosy
- Lymphomatoid granulomatosis
- Nasopharyngeal carcinoma
- Paracoccidioidomycosis
- Sarcoidosis
- Subcutaneous panniculitis-like T cell lymphoma
- Syphilis
- <u>Wegener's granulomatosis</u>

Evaluation/Treatment Options

- <u>Chemotherapy</u>
- Radiation

Further reading:
- Kinney MC, Jones D (2007) Cutaneous T-cell and NK-cell lymphomas: the WHO–EORTC classification and the increasing recognition of specialized tumor types. Am J Clin Pathol 127(5):670–686

Lymphoma, Subcutaneous Panniculitis-Like T Cell Lymphoma

Type of T cell lymphoma that arises in the subcutaneous layer, resembles panniculitis clinically, and is characterized by erythematous subcutaneous nodules, constitutional symptoms, and a rapidly progressive hemophagocytic syndrome

Differential Diagnosis

- Angiocentric NK/T cell lymphoma
- Cellulitis
- Dermatomyositis panniculitis
- Erythema nodosum
- Lipodermatosclerosis
- Lupus panniculitis
- Pyoderma gangrenosum
- Scleroderma panniculitis
- Venous insufficiency ulcer

Further reading:
- Weenig RH, Ng CS, Perniciaro C (2001) Subcutaneous panniculitis-like T-cell lymphoma: an elusive case presenting as lipomembranous panniculitis and a review of 72 cases in the literature. Am J Dermatopathol 23(3):206–215

Lymphomatoid Granulomatosis

Poorly understood idiopathic lymphoma-like systemic disease with vasculitis-like features that is associated with EBV infection, affects older patients, and is characterized by pulmonary and CNS infiltration, constitutional symptoms, and erythematous papules or nodules that occasionally resemble erythema nodosum

Differential Diagnosis

- Angiocentric (NK type) lymphoma
- Churg–Strauss syndrome
- Erythema nodosum
- Hodgkin's disease
- Intravascular lymphoma
- Malignant atrophic papulosis
- Mycosis fungoides
- Sarcoidosis
- Tuberculosis
- Wegener's granulomatosis

Evaluation

- Complete blood count
- Chest radiograph
- CT/MRI scan of the brain
- Complement levels
- Renal function test
- Liver function test

Further reading:
- Muller FM, Lewis-Jones S, Morley S et al (2007) Lymphomatoid granulomatosis complicating other haematological malignancies. Br J Dermatol 157(2):426–429

Lymphomatoid Papulosis (Macaulay's Disease)

Type of CD30+ lymphoproliferative disease that predominantly affects middle-aged adults, is characterized by crops of erythematous papules with overlying pustules or vesicles which eventually necrose and heal to a small circular scar, and that has the potential to progress to CTCL or Hodgkin's disease in a small percentage of patients

Differential Diagnosis

- Aggressive epidermotropic CD8+ lymphoma
- <u>Anaplastic CD30 + large cell lymphoma</u>
- Angiocentric lymphoma
- <u>Arthropod bites</u>
- Cutaneous B cell lymphoma
- Drug eruption
- Folliculitis
- Hodgkin's disease
- Hydroa vacciniforme
- Langerhans cell histiocytosis
- Leukemia cutis
- Malignant atrophic papulosis
- Miliaria
- Papular urticaria
- <u>Pityriasis lichenoides et varioliformis acuta</u>
- Cutaneous lymphoid hyperplasia
- Scabies
- Varicella

Associations

- Anaplastic large cell lymphoma
- <u>Hodgkin's disease</u>
- <u>Mycosis fungoides</u>
- Thyroid disease

Evaluation

- Lymph node exam and biopsy
- Complete blood count
- T cell gene rearrangement

Treatment Options

- Observation
- <u>Tetracycline antibiotics</u>
- Topical corticosteroids
- Topical nitrogen mustard
- Narrowband UVB
- <u>Methotrexate</u>
- Oral bexarotene
- Radiation

Further reading:

- El Shabrawi-Caelen L, Kerl H, Cerroni L (2004) Lymphomatoid papulosis: reappraisal of clinicopathologic presentation and classification into subtypes A, B, and C. Arch Dermatol 140(4):441–447

Maffucci Syndrome

Sporadic syndrome of unknown cause characterized by venous malformations on the distal extremities and other parts of the body and enchondromas on the digits and long bones that have a potential to degenerate into chondrosarcoma

Differential Diagnosis

- Blue rubber bleb nevus syndrome
- Bockenheimer syndrome
- Gorham syndrome
- Kaposi's sarcoma
- Klippel–Trenaunay syndrome
- <u>Ollier syndrome</u>
- Proteus syndrome

Further reading:

- Shepherd V, Godbolt A, Casey T (2005) Maffucci's syndrome with extensive gastrointestinal involvement. Australas J Dermatol 46(1):33–37

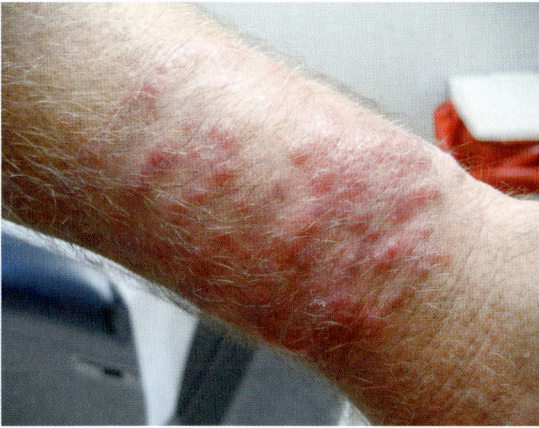

Fig. 6.69 Majocchi granuloma

Majocchi Granuloma

Refers to a deep dermatophyte folliculitis predominantly caused by *Trichophyton rubrum* that is characterized by an erythematous plaque studded with follicular papulopustules most commonly on the face or extremities (Fig. 6.69)

Differential Diagnosis

- Acne keloidalis
- Acquired perforating dermatosis
- Bacterial folliculitis
- Blastomycosis-like pyoderma
- Botryomycosis
- Coccidioidomycosis
- Cutaneous lymphoid hyperplasia
- Ecthyma
- Eosinophilic folliculitis
- Follicular mucinosis
- Herpes simplex virus infection
- Kaposi's sarcoma

- Kerion
- Lichen simplex chronicus
- Lupus erythematosus
- Pseudofolliculitis barbae
- <u>Psoriasis</u>
- Rosacea
- Scabies

Treatment Options

- <u>Terbinafine</u>
- Itraconazole
- Fluconazole
- Griseofulvin

Further reading:
- Brod C, Benedix F, Rocken M et al (2007) Trichophytic Majocchi granuloma mimicking Kaposi sarcoma. J Dtsch Dermatol Ges 5(7):591–593

Malakoplakia

Chronic inflammatory dermatosis affecting immunocompromised patients that is caused by inadequate phagolysomal activity in the immune response to bacteria (especially *E. coli*) and is characterized by an ulcerated plaque with or without draining sinus tracts in the genital, perineal, or anal areas

Differential Diagnosis

- Actinomycosis
- Botryomycosis
- <u>Furunculosis</u>
- Granular cell tumor
- Granuloma inguinale

- <u>Hidradenitis suppurativa</u>
- Langerhans cell histiocytosis
- Lymphogranuloma venereum
- Lymphoma
- Mycetoma
- Sarcoidosis
- <u>Squamous cell carcinoma</u>
- Tuberculosis

Associations

- Diabetes
- <u>Immunosuppression</u>
- Internal malignancy
- Leukemia
- Lymphoma
- Rheumatoid arthritis
- Systemic lupus erythematosus
- Transplantation

Evaluation

- Bacterial, mycobacterial, and fungal cultures of draining material

Further reading:
- Savant SR, Amladi ST, Kangle SD et al (2007) Cutaneous malakoplakia in an HIV-positive patient. Int J STD AIDS 18(6):435–436

Malignant Atrophic Papulosis (Degos Disease)

Vascular disorder of unknown cause that is associated with cutaneous infarcts with or without visceral infarcts (especially GI and CNS) and is characterized by erythematous papules on the trunk and extremities that heal to a porcelain white scar with peripheral erythema and telangiectasia

Differential Diagnosis

- Angiocentric lymphoma
- Cryoglobulinemia
- Embolic phenomenon
- Idiopathic guttate hypomelanosis
- Lichen planus, atrophic
- Lichen sclerosus et atrophicus
- <u>Livedoid vasculopathy</u>
- Lymphomatoid granulomatosis
- <u>Lymphomatoid papulosis</u>
- Polyarteritis nodosa
- Sneddon syndrome
- Thromboangiitis obliterans

Associations

- Antiphospholipid antibody syndrome
- Crohn's disease
- Dermatomyositis
- Familial
- Lupus erythematosus
- Rheumatoid arthritis
- Systemic sclerosis

Evaluation

- Anticardiolipin antibody
- Antinuclear antibodies
- Antithrombin-III level
- Beta-2 glycoprotein 1
- Chest radiograph
- Complete blood count
- Factor V Leiden mutation
- Lupus anticoagulant

- MRI scan of the brain
- Protein-C and protein-S levels
- Rheumatoid factor
- Stool for occult blood
- Upper and lower endoscopy

Treatment Options

- <u>Aspirin</u>
- <u>Dipyridamole</u>
- Heparin
- Warfarin
- Cyclosporine
- Azathioprine
- Cyclophosphamide

Further reading:

- Scheinfeld N (2007) Malignant atrophic papulosis. Clin Exp Dermatol 32(5):483–487

Malignant Fibrous Histiocytoma

Type of malignant soft tissue sarcoma that presents in older adults and is characterized as a deep mass arising from the fascia of the lower extremity, especially the thigh and buttocks, but rarely arising as a primary dermal or subcutaneous tumor

Differential Diagnosis

- <u>Atypical fibroxanthoma</u>
- Clear cell sarcoma
- <u>Dermatofibrosarcoma protuberans</u>
- Desmoid tumor
- Epithelioid sarcoma
- Leiomyosarcoma

- <u>Liposarcoma</u>
- Melanoma
- Morphea profunda

Further reading:
- Blatiere V, De Boever CM, Jacot W et al (2007) Cutaneous malignant fibrous histiocytoma in an HIV-positive patient. J Eur Acad Dermatol Venereol 21(1):106–107

Marfan Syndrome

Inherited disorder of connective tissue (AD) that is caused by mutation of the fibrillin-1 gene and is characterized by tall stature, arachnodactyly, aortic aneurysm, mitral valve prolapse, ectopia lentis, spontaneous pneumothorax, and elastosis perforans serpiginosa

Differential Diagnosis

- <u>Congenital contractural arachnodactyly</u>
- Ehlers–Danlos syndrome
- Fragile X syndrome
- Haim–Munk syndrome
- <u>Homocystinuria</u>
- Klinefelter's syndrome
- Multiple endocrine neoplasia, type IIb

Evaluation

- Echocardiography
- Aortography
- Chest radiography
- Ophthalmologic exam

Further reading:
- Judge DP, Dietz HC (2005) Marfan's syndrome. Lancet 366(9501):1965–1976

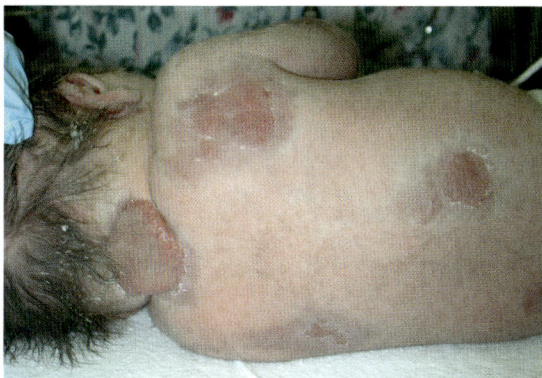

Fig 6.70 Diffuse cutaneous mastocytosis (Courtesy of A. Mistretta)

Mastocytosis

Refers to several different presentations of cutaneous and/or systemic mast cell proliferation that is most commonly characterized in children by numerous oval, erythematous to brown macules and papules on the trunk and extremities (urticaria pigmentosa) that wheal upon stroking (Darier's sign) and in adults by diffuse telangiectasias on the trunk (telangiectasia macularis eruptiva perstans) or, less commonly, by bullous lesions, diffuse cutaneous induration, erythroderma, or mast cell tumors (mastocytoma)

Subtypes/Variants

- Diffuse cutaneous mastocytosis (Fig. 6.70)
- Mast cell leukemia
- Mast cell sarcoma
- Solitary mastocytoma
- Systemic mastocytosis (indolent and aggressive types)
- Telangiectasia macularis eruptive perstans (Fig. 6.71)
- Urticaria pigmentosa

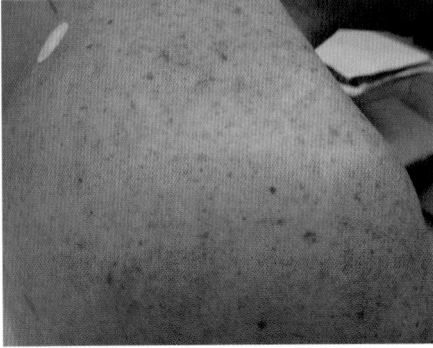

Fig. 6.71 Telangiectasia macularis eruptiva perstans

Differential Diagnosis (Urticaria Pigmentosa)

- Amyloidosis
- Arthropod bites
- Becker's nevus
- Berloque dermatitis
- Bullous pemphigoid
- Burns
- Café-au-lait macules
- Child abuse
- Congenital nevus
- Dermatographism
- Erythroderma
- Fixed drug eruption
- Generalized eruptive histiocytosis
- Granuloma annulare
- Impetigo
- Jessner's lymphocytic infiltrate
- Juvenile xanthogranuloma
- Langerhans cell histiocytosis
- Leiomyoma
- Lentigo
- Lichen planus

- Lymphoma
- Nevi
- Cutaneous lymphoid hyperplasia
- Scabies
- Secondary syphilis
- <u>Smooth muscle hamartoma</u>
- Spitz nevi
- <u>Urticaria</u>

Evaluation

- 24-h urine histamine
- Bone marrow biopsy
- Bone scan or skeletal survey
- Complete blood count
- GI tract biopsy
- Lymph node exam
- Serum tryptase level
- Urinary PGD2 level

Treatment Options

- <u>Antihistamines</u>
- Cromolyn sodium
- Topical corticosteroids
- Leukotriene inhibitors
- Cyclosporine
- Nifedipine
- Interferon alpha
- Imatinib

Further reading:
- Hannaford R, Rogers M (2001) Presentation of cutaneous mastocytosis in 173 children. Australas J Dermatol 42(1):15–21

McCune–Albright Syndrome

Sporadic syndrome that results from an activating mutation in the GNAS gene which encodes the hormone-regulating Gs alpha subunit and that is characterized by large café-au-lait macules with a "Coast of Maine" border, precocious puberty, and polyostotic fibrous dysplasia – a bony abnormality that leads to lytic lesions and subsequent fractures

Differential Diagnosis

- Ataxia–telangiectasia
- Bloom syndrome
- Congenital adrenal hyperplasia
- Fanconi anemia
- Jaffe–Campanacci syndrome
- HPA axis tumor
- Neurofibromatosis 1
- Russell–Silver syndrome
- Tuberous sclerosus

Further reading:
- Volkl TM, Dorr HG (2006) McCune–Albright syndrome: clinical picture and natural history in children and adolescents. J Pediatr Endocrinol Metab 19(Suppl 2):551–559

Measles (Rubeola)

Uncommon childhood disease of 5–7 days duration caused by a paramyxovirus and characterized by an enanthem (Koplik's spots) and later a morbilliform exanthem that starts on the forehead and neck and later generalizes in a caudal direction

Differential Diagnosis

- Enterovirus infection
- Epstein–Barr virus

- Gianotti–Crosti syndrome
- Kawasaki disease
- <u>Morbilliform drug eruption</u>
- Primary HIV infection
- <u>Rubella</u>
- Syphilis
- Toxoplasmosis
- Urticaria
- Vasculitis

Further reading:
- Carneiro SC, Cestari T, Allen SH et al (2007) Viral exanthems in the tropics. Clin Dermatol 25(2):212–220

Medallion-Like Dermal Dendrocyte Hamartoma

Hamartoma of dermal dendrocytes that is present at birth, is characterized by a circumscribed, brown plaque with a wrinkled, translucent surface, and visible vessels, and is typically located on the neck or chest (Fig. 6.72)

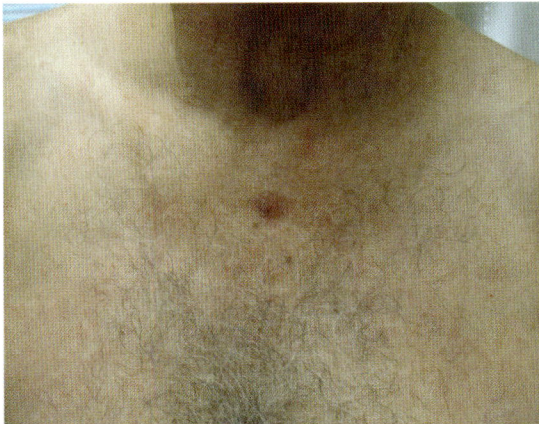

Fig. 6.72 Medallion-like dermal dendrocyte hamartoma

Differential Diagnosis

- Anetoderma
- <u>Aplasia cutis</u>
- Atrophic dermatofibroma
- Atrophic dermatofibrosarcoma protuberans
- Atrophoderma of Pasini–Pierini
- Lichen sclerosus et atrophicus
- Neurothekeoma
- <u>Scar</u>
- Smooth muscle hamartoma

Further reading:
- Rodriguez-Jurado R, Palacios C, Duran-Mckinster C et al (2004) Medallion-like dermal dendrocyte hamartoma: a new clinically and histopathologically distinct lesion. J Am Acad Dermatol 51(3):359–363

Median Nail Dystrophy (of Heller)

Type of nail dystrophy caused by trauma or various tumors around the nail matrix that is characterized by longitudinal splitting of the nail plate with a "fir tree" appearance

Differential Diagnosis

- Digital mucous cyst
- <u>Habit tic deformity</u>
- Lichen striatus
- Nail–patella syndrome
- Pterygium
- Raynaud disease
- Trachyonychia
- Trauma

Associations

- Exostosis
- Isotretinoin
- Lichen planus
- Melanoma
- Mucous cyst
- Onychomatricoma
- Onychomycosis
- Psoriasis
- Squamous cell carcinoma
- Trauma
- Wart

Further reading:
- Sweeney SA, Cohen PR, Schulze KE et al (2005) Familial median canaliform nail dystrophy. Cutis 75(3):161–165

Median Raphe Cyst

Type of columnar cyst that occurs along the midline between the anus and the urethra and is characterized by a small dermal cyst most commonly located on the glans penis near the urethral meatus

Differential Diagnosis

- Apocrine cystadenoma
- Dermoid cyst
- Epidermal inclusion cyst
- Glomus tumor
- Hidradenoma papilliferum
- Metastatic lesion
- Pilonidal cyst
- Steatocystoma
- Urethral diverticulum

Further reading:
- Park CO, Chun EY, Lee JH (2006) Median raphe cyst on the scrotum and perineum. J Am Acad Dermatol 55(5 Suppl):S114–S115

Median Rhomboid Glossitis (Brocq–Pautrier Syndrome)

Peculiar manifestation of oral candidiasis that is characterized by a rhomboid-shaped, smooth erythematous plaque on the dorsal midline tongue anterior to the circumvallate papillae and with or without erythema on the opposing aspect of the palate

Differential Diagnosis

- <u>Fixed drug eruption</u>
- <u>Geographic tongue</u>
- Granular cell tumor
- Histoplasmosis
- Lingual thyroid
- Squamous cell carcinoma
- Tertiary syphilis
- Tuberculosis

Further reading:
- Terai H, Shimahara M (2007) Partial atrophic tongue other than median rhomboid glossitis. Clin Exp Dermatol 32(4):381–384

Mediterranean Spotted Fever (Boutonneuse Fever, Tick Typhus)

Tick-borne rickettsial disease caused by *Rickettsia conorii*; transmitted by the dog tick, *Rhipicephalus sanguineus*; and characterized by "tache noir" at the site of the bite, fever, headache, and an erythematous, papular skin eruption predominantly on the lower extremities

Differential Diagnosis

- Anthrax
- Dengue fever
- Ehrlichiosis
- Infectious mononucleosis
- Kawasaki disease
- Leptospirosis
- <u>Leukocytoclastic vasculitis</u>
- Lyme disease
- Malaria
- Meningococcemia
- Relapsing fever
- <u>Rocky Mountain spotted fever</u>
- Roseola
- Rubella
- Rubeola
- Scarlet fever
- Toxic shock syndrome
- Tularemia
- Typhoid fever
- Viral exanthem

Further reading:
- Mert A, Ozaras R, Tabak F et al (2006) Mediterranean spotted fever: a review of fifteen cases. J Dermatol 33(2):103–107

Mees Lines

Type of true leukonychia with a variety of causes that is characterized by parallel white, transverse bands that grow outward with the nail plate

Differential Diagnosis

- Beau's lines
- Leukonychia
- <u>Muehrcke's lines</u>
- Onycholysis
- Onychomycosis
- Psoriasis

Associations

- <u>Arsenic ingestion</u>
- Breast cancer
- Chemotherapy
- Carbon monoxide poisoning
- Heart failure
- Hodgkin's disease
- Lead poisoning
- Leprosy
- Malaria
- Parasitic infection
- Pneumonia
- Psoriasis
- Sickle cell
- Systemic lupus erythematosus
- Transplant rejection

Further reading:
- Uede K, Furukawa F (2003) Skin manifestations in acute arsenic poisoning from the Wakayama curry-poisoning incident. Br J Dermatol 149(4):757–762

Melanoacanthoma

Refers to a benign lesion containing an increased number of both kerati-nocytes and melanocytes that presents as either a variant of seborrheic keratosis in older men (cutaneous melanoacanthoma) or a reactive lesion on the buccal mucosa of predominantly young women of African descent (oral melanoacanthoma)

Differential Diagnosis

- Actinic keratosis
- Amalgam tattoo
- Lentigo
- Melanocytic nevus
- <u>Melanoma</u>
- Mucosal melanosis
- Pigmented basal cell carcinoma
- <u>Seborrheic keratosis</u>
- Wart

Further reading:
- Fornatora ML, Reich RF, Haber S et al (2003) Oral melanoacanthoma: a report of 10 cases, review of the literature, and immunohistochemical analysis for HMB-45 reactivity. Am J Dermatopathol 25(1):12–15

Melanoma, Malignant

Malignant proliferation of melanocytes with a strong tendency for metastasis that is characterized by an irregularly hyperpigmented (less commonly, amelanotic) asymmetric papule, nodule, or plaque with or without ulceration that can occur anywhere

Subtypes/Variants

- Acral lentiginous (Fig. 6.73)
- Amelanotic (Fig. 6.74)
- Animal
- Balloon cell
- Clear cell sarcoma
- Desmoplastic (spindled, neurotropic)

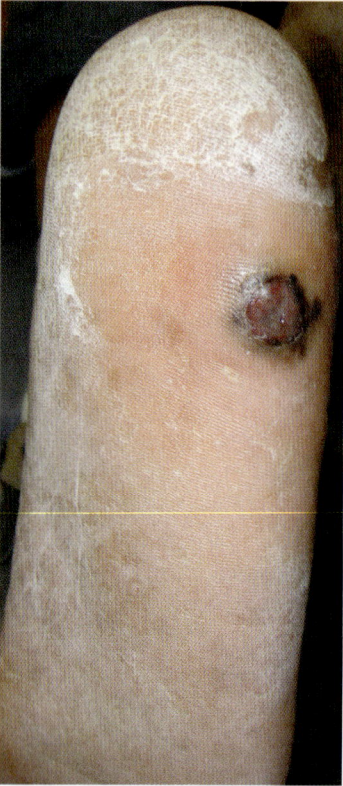

Fig. 6.73 Acral melanoma

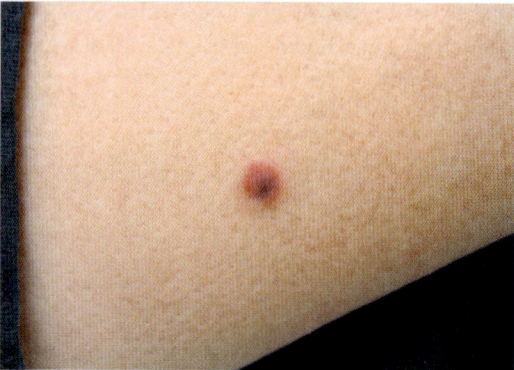

Fig. 6.74 Amelanotic melanoma

- Lentigo maligna
- Malignant blue nevus
- Mucosal
- Nevoid
- Nodular
- Ocular
- Polypoid
- Small cell
- Spitzoid
- Superficial spreading
- Verrucous

Differential Diagnosis

All Types

- Angiokeratoma
- <u>Benign melanocytic nevus</u>
- Black heel
- Blue nevus (especially cellular type)
- Bowen's disease
- Combined nevus
- <u>Congenital nevus</u>
- Cutaneous lymphoid hyperplasia
- Deep penetrating nevus
- Dermatofibroma
- <u>Dysplastic nevus</u>
- Exogenous ochronosis
- Extramammary Paget's disease
- Halo nevus
- Ink-spot lentigo
- Kaposi's sarcoma
- Lentigo simplex
- Longitudinal melanonychia
- Lymphoma

- Malignant schwannoma
- Merkel cell tumor
- Metastasis
- Oral mucosal melanosis
- Paget's disease
- Pigmented actinic keratosis
- <u>Pigmented basal cell carcinoma</u>
- Pigmented spindle cell nevus
- <u>Pyogenic granuloma</u>
- Recurrent nevus
- Seborrheic keratosis
- Spitz nevus
- Subungual hematoma
- Thrombosed or traumatized hemangioma
- Traumatic tattoo
- Tinea nigra
- Venous lake

Acral Lentiginous

- <u>Acral nevus</u>
- Chronic paronychia
- Kaposi's sarcoma
- Lentigo
- Melanonychia striata
- Poroma
- Pyogenic granuloma
- Subungual hematoma
- <u>Talon noir</u>
- <u>Tinea nigra</u>
- Traumatic tattoo
- Verruca plantaris

Amelanotic

- Actinic keratosis
- Adnexal neoplasm

- Basal cell carcinoma
- Bowen's disease
- Cutaneous lymphoid hyperplasia
- Dermatofibroma
- Keratoacanthoma
- Lymphoma cutis
- Merkel cell carcinoma
- Metastatic lesion
- Metastatic melanoma
- Poroma
- <u>Pyogenic granuloma</u>
- <u>Spitz nevus</u>
- Squamous cell carcinoma
- Verruca vulgaris

Desmoplastic

- Atypical fibroxanthoma
- <u>Basal cell carcinoma</u>
- Dermatofibroma
- Dermatofibrosarcoma protuberans
- Desmoplastic Spitz nevus
- Keloid
- Malignant schwannoma
- Neurofibroma
- Neurotized nevus
- Spindle cell squamous cell carcinoma

Oral

- Amalgam tattoo
- Blue nevus
- Drug-induced pigmentation
- Fixed drug eruption
- Foreign body granuloma
- Kaposi's sarcoma
- Laugier–Hunziker syndrome

- Melanoacanthoma
- <u>Oral melanocytic nevus</u>
- <u>Oral melanotic macule</u>
- Peutz–Jeghers syndrome
- Pyogenic granuloma
- Racial pigmentation
- Squamous cell carcinoma
- Venous lake

Associations

- Diffuse hyperpigmentation
- Melanuria
- Vitiligo-like depigmentation
- Erysipelas melanomatosum

TNM Classification

- T1: =1.0 mm (A: without ulceration and mitosis <1/mm^2; B: with ulceration and mitosis =1/mm^2)
- T2: 1.01–2.0 mm (A: without ulceration; B: with ulceration)
- T3: 2.01–4.0 mm (A: without ulceration; B: with ulceration)
- T4: >4.0 mm (A: without ulceration; B: with ulceration)
- N1: one node (A: micrometastasis; B: macrometastasis)
- N2: two to three nodes (A: micrometastasis; B: macrometastasis; C: in-transit met(s)/satellite(s) without metastatic node(s))
- N3: four or more metastatic nodes or matted nodes or in-transit met(s)/satellite(s) with metastatic node(s)
- M1a: distant skin, subcutaneous, or nodal mets, normal lactate dehydrogenase level
- M1b: lung metastases, normal lactate dehydrogenase level
- M1c: all other visceral metastases with normal lactate dehydrogenase level or any distant metastasis with elevated lactate dehydrogenase level

Staging

- Stage 0: melanoma in situ
- Stage IA: T1A
- Stage IB: T1B or T2A
- Stage IIA: T2B or T3A
- Stage IIB: T3B or T4A
- Stage IIC: T4B
- Stage IIIA: T(1–4)A/N(1–2)A
- Stage IIIB: T(1–4)B/N(1–2)A or T(1–4)A/N(1–2)(B–C)
- Stage IIIC: T(1–4)B/N(1–2)B or N3
- Stage IV: M1

Treatment Options

- <u>Wide local excision with or without sentinel node biopsy</u>
- Elective lymphadenectomy
- Therapeutic lymphadenectomy
- Interferon-alpha 2b
- Isolated limb perfusion
- Dacarbazine
- Ipilimumab
- Vemurafenib

Further reading:

- Balch CM, Gershenwald JE, Soong SJ, Thompson JF (2011) Update on the melanoma staging system: the importance of sentinel node staging and primary tumor mitotic rate. J Surg Oncol 104(4):379–385
- Beyeler M, Dummer R (2005) Cutaneous melanoma: uncommon presentations. Clin Dermatol 23(6):587–592
- Grant-Kels JM, Bason ET, Grin CM (1999) The misdiagnosis of malignant melanoma. J Am Acad Dermatol 40(4):539–548

Melasma (Chloasma)

Pigmentary disorder induced by sun exposure that predominantly affects women, may arise during pregnancy, and is characterized by tan-brown macular hyperpigmentation on the central face or around the mandible

Differential Diagnosis

- Acquired bilateral nevus of Ota-like macules
- Argyria
- Addison's disease
- Atopic dermatitis
- Berloque dermatitis
- Chronic actinic dermatitis
- Chrysiasis
- Contact dermatitis
- Cutaneous lupus erythematosus
- Drug-induced hyperpigmentation
- Erythema dyschromicum perstans
- Erythromelanosis follicularis faciei et colli
- Exogenous ochronosis
- Facial erythema ab igne
- Lentigo
- Lichen planus, actinic type
- Mastocytosis
- Minocycline pigmentation
- Photosensitive drug reaction
- Polymorphous light eruption
- Poikiloderma of Civatte
- Postinflammatory hyperpigmentation
- Riehl's melanosis

Associations

- Anticonvulsants
- <u>Oral contraception</u>
- Phototoxic drugs
- <u>Pregnancy</u>
- Retinoids, systemic
- Sun exposure

Treatment Options

- <u>Sunscreen</u>
- <u>Hydroquinone</u>
- <u>Tretinoin</u>
- Adapalene
- Azelaic
- Kojic acid
- <u>Topical corticosteroids</u>
- Glycolic acid
- Laser treatments

Further reading:
- Rigopoulos D, Gregoriou S et al (2007) Hyperpigmentation and melasma. J Cosmet Dermatol 6(3):195–202

Melkersson–Rosenthal Syndrome

Rare syndrome arising in childhood or adolescence that is characterized by facial nerve palsy, granulomatous infiltration of the face, especially the upper lip, and scrotal tongue

Differential Diagnosis

- Angioedema
- Bell's palsy
- Crohn's disease
- Intralymphatic histiocytosis
- Leprosy
- Sarcoidosis
- Solid facial edema

Treatment Options

- Intralesional corticosteroids
- Methotrexate
- Dapsone
- Systemic corticosteroids
- Infliximab
- Clofazimine
- Metronidazole
- Tetracycline antibiotics
- Azathioprine

Further reading:
- Zeng W, Geng S, Niu X, Yuan J (2010) Complete Melkersson-Rosenthal syndrome with multiple cranial nerve palsies. Clin Exp Dermatol 35(3):272–274

Meningocele, Rudimentary
(Heterotopic Meningeal Tissue, Primary Cutaneous Meningioma)

Developmental anomaly containing heterotopic meningeal tissue (but no brain tissue) that usually, but not always, has intact bone underneath, is most commonly diagnosed in the first year of life, and is characterized as a small, firm subcutaneous nodule with or without a hair collar sign which occurs most commonly on the scalp, but also on the spine or the forehead

Differential Diagnosis

- Adnexal tumors
- <u>Aplasia cutis congenita</u>
- <u>Dermoid cysts</u>
- <u>Encephalocele</u>
- Fibroma
- Hemangioma
- Melanocytic nevi
- Metastatic neuroblastoma
- Metastatic tumors
- Neurofibroma
- Nevus sebaceus
- Pigmented neuroectodermal tumor of infancy
- Pilar cyst
- Primary primitive neuroectodermal tumor
- Sinus pericranii

Evaluation

- CT/MRI scan of skull

Further reading:
- El Shabrawi-Caelen L, White WL, Soyer HP et al (2001) Rudimentary meningocele: remnant of a neural tube defect? Arch Dermatol 137(1):45–50

Meningococcemia

Blood-borne infection with *Neisseria meningitidis* that typically affects children and adolescents and is associated with meningitis, disseminated intravascular coagulation, purpura fulminans, and a high mortality (in the acute form), or with hemorrhagic lesions on the extremities and arthritis and fever (in the chronic form)

Differential Diagnosis

Acute

- <u>Bacteremia/sepsis due to a variety of bacteria</u>
- Dengue fever
- Disseminated intravascular coagulation to other causes
- Endocarditis
- Enteroviral infections
- Henoch–Schonlein purpura
- Lupus erythematosus
- Leptospirosis
- Polyarteritis nodosa
- Rocky Mountain spotted fever
- Toxic shock syndrome
- *Vibrio vulnificus* infection

Chronic

- Erythema multiforme
- Gonococcemia
- Henoch–Schonlein purpura
- Purpura
- Rat-bite fever
- Rheumatic fever
- Rickettsial infection
- <u>Subacute bacterial endocarditis</u>
- Sweet's syndrome
- <u>Vasculitis</u>
- Typhus

Associations

- Complement deficiency

Evaluation

- Blood and cerebrospinal fluid Gram stain and culture

Further reading:
- Ploysangam T, Sheth AP (1996) Chronic meningococcemia in childhood: case report and review of the literature. Pediatr Dermatol 13(6):483–487

Menkes Kinky-Hair Syndrome

Genetic disorder (XLR) of copper metabolism that is caused by a defect in the ATP7A gene, which encodes an intestinal copper transporter, and leads to low serum copper, pili torti, diffuse hypopigmentation, seizures and mental retardation, wormian bones, and death in early childhood

Differential Diagnosis

- Arginosuccinic aciduria
- Bazex syndrome
- Bjornstad syndrome
- Child abuse
- Conradi–Hunerman syndrome
- Crandall's syndrome
- Ectodermal dysplasias
- Monilethrix
- Netherton syndrome
- Phenylketonuria
- Trichothiodystrophy

Further reading:
- Gerard-Blanluet M, Birk-Moller L, Caubel I et al (2004) Early development of occipital horns in a classical Menkes patient. Am J Med Genet A 130(2):211–213

Merkel Cell Carcinoma (Primary Cutaneous Neuroendocrine Carcinoma, Trabecular Carcinoma)

Primary cutaneous malignancy of uncertain derivation that may be associated with polyoma virus infection and that has a strong tendency for metastasis and local recurrence, affects the elderly, and is characterized

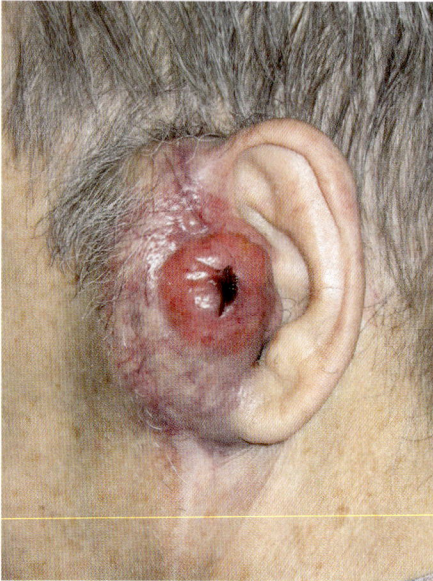

Fig. 6.75 Merkel cell carcinoma
(Courtesy of A. Record)

by a solitary erythematous or violaceous nodule on the head and neck
(Fig. 6.75)

Differential Diagnosis

- Abscess
- Angiosarcoma
- Atypical fibroxanthoma
- Basal cell carcinoma
- Cutaneous lymphoid hyperplasia
- Cutaneous metastasis
- Dermatofibroma
- Eccrine carcinoma
- Ewing's sarcoma
- Hemangioma

- Kaposi's sarcoma
- <u>Lymphoma</u>
- Malignant melanoma (especially small cell type)
- Metastatic neuroblastoma
- <u>Metastatic neuroendocrine carcinoma (small cell)</u>
- <u>Squamous cell carcinoma</u>

Diagnostic Criteria

- A – Asymptomatic
- E – Enlarging rapidly
- I – Immune suppression
- O – Older than 50
- U – UV-exposed fair skin

Associations

- Breast cancer
- Cushing's syndrome
- HIV infection
- Lambert–Eaton syndrome
- Organ transplantation
- Ovarian cancer

Treatment Options

- <u>Wide local excision</u>
- Radiation

Further reading:

- Heath M, Jaimes N, Lemos B, Mostaghimi A, Wang LC, Peñas PF, Nghiem P (2008) Clinical characteristics of Merkel cell carcinoma at diagnosis in 195 patients: the AEIOU features. J Am Acad Dermatol 58(3):375–381

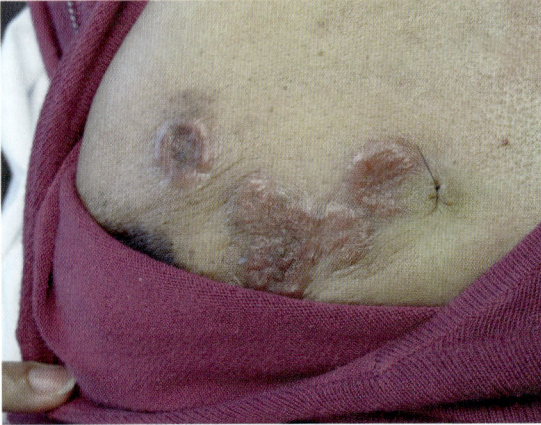

Fig. 6.76 Metastatic breast cancer

Metastasis, Cutaneous

Cutaneous manifestation of internal malignancy that is caused by distant spread of malignant cells to the skin through blood or lymphatic vessels or by direct extension from an underlying focus and that is characterized by solitary or multiple, firm, erythematous nodules with or without ulceration that are located anywhere on the skin surface

Subtypes/Variants

- Alopecia neoplastica
- Carcinoma en cuirasse
- Carcinoma erysipelatoides (inflammatory metastasis)
- Carcinoma telangiectaticum
- Incisional
- Nodular (Fig. 6.76)
- Sister Mary Joseph's nodule
- Zosteriform (Fig. 6.77)

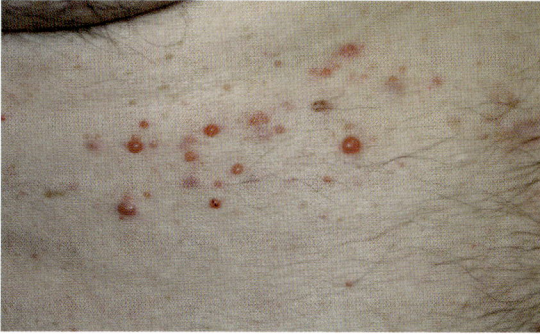

Fig. 6.77 Zosteriform melanoma metastases

Differential Diagnosis

- Aggressive digital papillary adenocarcinoma
- Alopecia areata
- Amelanotic melanoma
- Angiosarcoma
- Atypical fibroxanthoma
- Basal cell carcinoma
- Blueberry muffin baby
- Blue nevus
- Cellulitis
- Chancre
- Condyloma acuminatum
- Cutaneous lymphoid hyperplasia
- Cylindroma
- Dermatofibroma
- Endometriosis
- Epidermoid cyst
- Erysipelas
- Extramammary Paget's disease

- Furunculosis
- Granular cell tumor
- Hemangioma
- Hidradenitis suppurativa
- Kaposi's sarcoma
- Keratoacanthoma
- Kerion
- Lipoma
- Lymphedema
- Lymphangioma circumscriptum
- Merkel cell carcinoma
- Morphea/scleroderma
- Mucinous carcinoma
- Omphalomesenteric duct remnant
- Panniculitis
- Pilar cyst
- Primary cutaneous lymphoma
- Pyogenic granuloma
- Scar
- Squamous cell carcinoma
- Vasculitis
- Zoster

Evaluation

- Breast/mammography
- Chest radiography
- CT scan of chest, abdomen, and pelvis
- Stool for occult blood/colonoscopy
- Total body skin exam (for melanoma)

Further reading:
- Sariya D, Ruth K, Adams–McDonnell R et al (2007) Clinicopathologic correlation of cutaneous metastases: experience from a cancer center. Arch Dermatol 143(5):613–620

Microcystic Adnexal Carcinoma (Sclerosing Sweat Duct Carcinoma)

Uncommon malignant neoplasm of possible eccrine derivation that most commonly affects middle-aged patients; is characterized by a slow-growing, typically asymptomatic yellow-red papule, nodule, or plaque on the head and neck, especially around the nasolabial folds; and that has a high risk of local recurrence but not metastasis

Differential Diagnosis

- Adenosquamous carcinoma
- Chalazion
- Desmoplastic squamous cell carcinoma
- Desmoplastic trichoepithelioma
- Metastatic disease
- Morpheaform basal cell carcinoma
- Sebaceous carcinoma
- Seborrheic dermatitis
- Syringoma
- Trichoadenoma

Further reading:
- Snow S, Madjar DD, Hardy S et al (2001) Microcystic adnexal carcinoma: report of 13 cases and review of the literature. Dermatol Surg 27(4):401–408

Microscopic Polyangiitis

Systemic vasculitis syndrome associated with p-ANCA antibodies that is characterized by glomerulonephritis, pulmonary hemorrhage, neuropathy, inflammatory purpura, livedo reticularis, and ulcers

Differential Diagnosis

- Churg–Strauss syndrome
- Goodpasture syndrome

- Henoch–Schonlein purpura
- <u>Polyarteritis nodosa</u>
- Wegener's granulomatosis

Evaluation

- Antineutrophilic cytoplasmic antibodies
- Chest radiography
- Complete blood count
- Neurologic examination
- Renal biopsy
- Renal function test
- Sedimentation rate
- Serum chemistry
- Urinalysis

Further reading:
- Kawakami T, Soma Y, Saito C et al (2006) Cutaneous manifestations in patients with microscopic polyangiitis: two case reports and a minireview. Acta Derm Venereol 86(2):144–147

Mid-dermal Elastolysis

Acquired disorder that predominantly affects women, is caused by loss of elastic tissue in the middle dermis possibly related to ultraviolet-light exposure or tobacco smoking, and is characterized by finely wrinkled patches on the neck, trunk, and arms

Differential Diagnosis

- <u>Anetoderma</u>
- Cutis laxa
- Perifollicular elastolysis (acne scars)

- Pseudoxanthoma elasticum
- PXE-like papillary dermal elastolysis
- Solar elastosis
- <u>Striae distensae</u>

Further reading:
- Patroi I, Annessi G, Girolomoni G (2003) Mid-dermal elastolysis: a clinical, histologic, and immunohistochemical study of 11 patients. J Am Acad Dermatol 48(6):846–851

Milia

Solitary, multiple (eruptive), or clustered (milia en plaque) tiny keratinous cysts that spontaneously develop on the head and neck or in areas previously affected by blistering

Differential Diagnosis

Milia

- Acne
- Follicular mucinosis
- <u>Molluscum contagiosum</u>
- <u>Sebaceous hyperplasia</u>
- Syringoma
- Trichodiscoma
- Trichoepithelioma
- Xanthoma
- Verruca plana

Milia en Plaque

- <u>Favre–Racouchot disease</u>
- Follicular mucinosis
- Nevus comedonicus

Associations

Milia

- 5FU
- Acne
- Allergic contact dermatitis
- Basal cell carcinoma
- Bazex–Dupre–Christol syndrome
- Bullous lichen planus
- Burn
- Dermabrasion
- Epidermolysis bullosa
- Follicular mucinosis
- Gorlin's syndrome
- Leishmaniasis
- Lichen sclerosus
- Marie Unna hypotrichosis
- Naegeli–Franceshetti–Jadassohn
- Oral–facial–digital syndrome, type I
- Porphyria cutanea tarda
- Rombo syndrome
- Scar
- Topical steroids
- Zoster

Milia en Plaque

- Discoid lupus erythematosus
- Pseudoxanthoma elasticum

Further reading:
- Dogra S, Kanwar AJ (2005) Milia en plaque. J Eur Acad Dermatol Venereol 19(2):263–264

Miliaria

Dermatosis related to eccrine sweat duct obstruction at various levels that is triggered by environmental or endogenous conditions that promote sweating and that is characterized by papules, papulovesicles, pustules, or fine vesicles with a predilection for the face, trunk, and intertriginous areas

Subtypes/Variants

- Miliaria crystallina
- Miliaria profunda
- Miliaria pustulosa
- Miliaria rubra (prickly heat)

Differential Diagnosis

- Amyloidosis
- Candidiasis
- Cholinergic urticaria
- Contact dermatitis
- Drug eruption
- Erythema toxicum neonatorum
- Folliculitis
- Insect bites
- Milia
- Neonatal herpes simplex virus infection
- Papular mucinosis
- Papular sarcoidosis
- Scabies
- Syphilis
- Varicella
- Viral exanthem

Associations

- Granulosis rubra nasi
- Isotretinoin
- Pseudohypoaldosteronism

Treatment Options

- Cooling measures
- Topical corticosteroids
- Antistaphylococcal antibiotics

Further reading:
- Akcakus M, Koklu E, Poyrazoglu H et al (2006) Newborn with pseudohypoaldosteronism and miliaria rubra. Int J Dermatol 45(12):1432–1434

Mixed Connective Tissue Disease (Sharp's Syndrome)

Type of connective tissue that combines features of systemic lupus erythematosus, dermatomyositis, and systemic sclerosus, is associated with anti-U1RNP antibodies in all cases, and is characterized most commonly by Raynaud's phenomenon, digital swelling, arthritis, and myositis

Differential Diagnosis

- Dermatomyositis
- CREST syndrome
- Rheumatoid arthritis
- Systemic lupus erythematosus
- Systemic sclerosis

Evaluation

- Antinuclear antibodies
- Barium swallow

- Cardiac troponins
- Chest radiograph
- Complete blood count
- Creatine kinase and aldolase levels
- Echocardiography
- Electrocardiogram
- Pulmonary function test
- Renal function test
- Rheumatoid factor
- Urinalysis

Further reading:

- Venables PJ (2006) Mixed connective tissue disease. Lupus 15(3):132–137

Molluscum Contagiosum (Bateman's Disease)

Common viral cutaneous infection caused by the molluscum pox virus that predominantly affects children (or adults as a sexually transmitted disease) and is characterized by discrete, shiny, flesh-colored, umbilicated papules on the trunk, face, or genital area

Differential Diagnosis

- Acantholytic acanthoma
- Basal cell carcinoma
- Benign cephalic histiocytosis
- Child abuse
- Condylomata acuminata
- Cryptococcosis
- Dermatofibroma
- Elastosis perforans serpiginosa
- Fibrous papule
- Generalized eruptive histiocytosis
- Granuloma annulare

- <u>Histoplasmosis</u>
- Intradermal nevus
- Juvenile xanthogranuloma
- Lepromatous leprosy
- Lichen nitidus
- Lichen planus
- Lymphangioma circumscriptum
- Melanocytic nevi
- <u>Milia</u>
- Neurilemmomas
- Nodular basal cell carcinoma
- <u>Papular eczema</u>
- Penicilliosis
- Pneumocystosis
- Pyoderma
- Pyogenic granuloma
- Reactive perforating collagenosis
- Sebaceous hyperplasia
- Spitz nevus
- <u>Subepidermal calcified nodule</u>
- Syringoma
- Trichoepithelioma
- <u>Verruca</u>
- Xanthoma

Associations

- <u>Atopic dermatitis</u>
- HIV infection
- Immunosuppression

Treatment Options

- Observation
- <u>Cryotherapy</u>

- Curettage
- <u>Cantharidin</u>
- Podophyllin
- Salicylic acid
- Potassium hydroxide
- Imiquimod
- Electrodessication
- Tretinoin
- Tazarotene
- Cimetidine
- Griseofulvin

Further reading:
- Rogers NE (2006) The many faces of molluscum contagiosum: the fool factor. Skinmed 5(6):267–268

Mondor's Disease

Type of superficial thrombophlebitis associated with various triggers that affects the upper chest or breast of women and is characterized by a firm, tender, erythematous cord

Differential Diagnosis

- Breast abscess
- Breast cancer metastasis
- Cutaneous larva migrans
- <u>Early zoster</u>
- <u>Erysipelas/cellulitis</u>
- Interstitial granulomatous dermatitis with arthritis

Associations

- Antiphospholipid antibodies
- <u>Breast cancer</u>

- Filariasis
- Intravenous drug use
- Mastitis
- Oral contraception
- Pendulous breasts
- Pregnancy
- Protein-C deficiency
- Rheumatoid arthritis
- Surgical procedure
- Trauma

Further reading:

- Dirschka T, Winter K, Bierhoff E (2003) Mondor's disease: a rare cause of anterior chest pain. J Am Acad Dermatol 49(5):905–906

Mongolian Spots

Type of dermal melanocytosis that results from failure of migrating melanoblasts to reach the epidermis and is characterized by blue to black macular pigmentation typically localized to the lower back and buttocks which usually fades during the first few years of life

Differential Diagnosis

- Argyria
- Blue nevus
- <u>Child abuse</u>
- Contusion
- Deep hemangioma
- Dermal melanocyte hamartoma
- Drug-induced pigmentation
- Fixed drug eruption
- Nevus of Ito
- Nevus of Ota

- Ochronosis
- Port-wine stain

Associations

- Hurler and Hunter syndromes
- Phakomatosis pigmentovascularis, types II and IV

Further reading:
- Ochiai T, Suzuki Y, Kato T et al (2007) Natural history of extensive Mongolian spots in mucopolysaccharidosis type II (Hunter syndrome): a survey among 52 Japanese patients. J Eur Acad Dermatol Venereol 21(8):1082–1085

Monilethrix (Beaded Hair)

Inherited (AD or AR) hair-shaft disorder caused by defects in the genes encoding either hair keratins 1 and 6 (AD) or desmoglein 4 (AR) that is characterized by fragile periodic constrictions alternating with elliptical nodes that give the hair shaft a beaded appearance and cause variable alopecia most noticeable on the occipital scalp

Differential Diagnosis

- Pili torti
- Trichorrhexis invaginata
- Trichorrhexis nodosa

Associations

- Keratosis pilaris
- Koilonychia

Further reading:
- Schweizer J (2006) More than one gene involved in monilethrix: intracellular but also extracellular players. J Invest Dermatol 126(6):1216–1219

Monkey Pox

Self-limited, zoonotic disease predominantly found in Africa that is caused by the double-stranded DNA monkeypox virus; is acquired by contact with rodents and monkeys; is characterized by fever, headache, and a generalized vesiculopustular eruption with lesions in variable stages of evolution; and is different from smallpox in that it is milder and associated with lymphadenopathy

Differential Diagnosis

- Acute generalized exanthematous pustulosis
- Eczema herpeticum
- Pustular psoriasis
- Rickettsialpox
- Smallpox
- Tularemia
- <u>Varicella</u>

Further reading:
- Sale TA, Melski JW, Stratman EJ (2006) Monkey Pox: an epidemiologic and clinical comparison of African and US disease. J Am Acad Dermatol 55(3):478–481

Morphea

Localized form of scleroderma that is characterized by oval, linear, or guttate plaques of sclerosis which are localized to the trunk or face or in a more generalized distribution

Subtypes/Variants

- Atrophic (atrophoderma of Pasini and Pierini)
- Bullous
- Deep (morphea profunda)
- Generalized

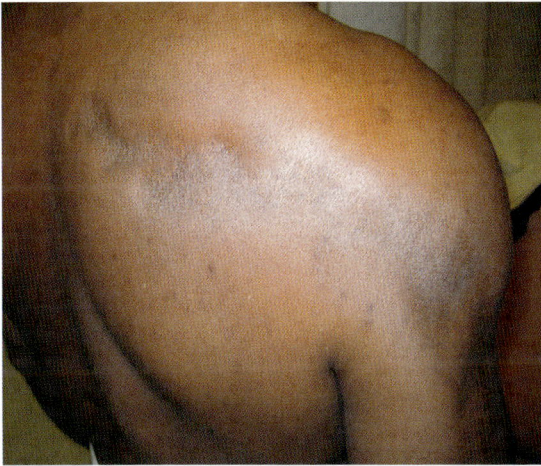

Fig. 6.78 Linear morphea

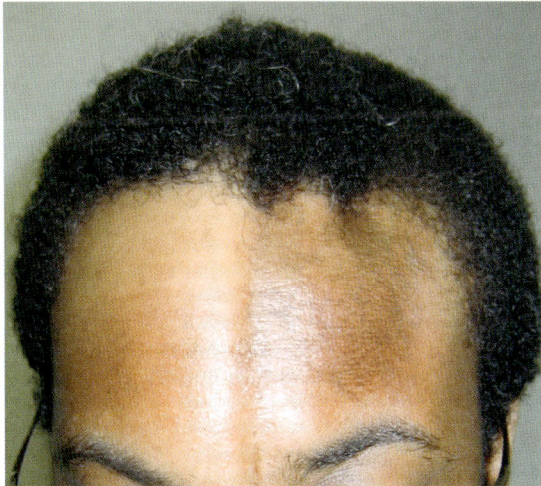

Fig. 6.79 En coup de sabre

- Guttate
- Linear (including en coup de sabre; Figs. 6.78 and 6.79)
- Nodular/keloidal
- Pansclerotic morphea of childhood
- Parry–Romberg syndrome
- Plaque (Fig. 6.80)

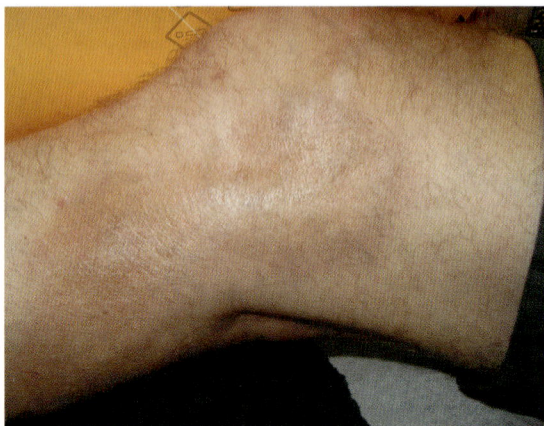

Fig. 6.80 Plaque type morphea

Differential Diagnosis

- Annular lichenoid dermatitis of youth
- Bleomycin therapy
- Carcinoma en cuirasse
- Dermatofibrosarcoma protuberans
- Dupuytren's contracture
- Eosinophilic fasciitis
- Erythema migrans (early)
- Fixed drug eruption (early)
- Graft-vs-host disease
- Granuloma annulare (patch type)
- Keloids
- Lichen sclerosus et atrophicus
- Linear atrophoderma of Moulin
- Lipodermatosclerosis
- Lupus profundus
- Paraffin or silicone injection
- Polyvinyl chloride exposure
- Porphyria cutanea tarda
- Progeria

- Radiation fibrosis
- Scleredema
- Scleromyxedema
- Silicosis
- Systemic sclerosis
- Toxic oil syndrome
- Vitamin B12 injection
- Vitamin K injection
- Waxy skin and stiff joints

Associations

- Lichen sclerosus et atrophicus
- Primary biliary cirrhosis

Evaluation

- Antinuclear antibodies (including anti-ssDNA, anti-superoxide dismutase)
- Complete blood count
- CT/MRI scan of the brain (especially Parry–Romberg syndrome)
- Lyme disease ELISA and Western blot
- Radiography of bones in the affected area (melorheostosis)
- Rheumatoid factor

Treatment Options

- <u>Topical corticosteroids</u>
- Intralesional corticosteroids
- <u>Topical vitamin D analogues</u>
- Topical tacrolimus
- <u>UVA1 phototherapy</u>
- Methotrexate
- Systemic corticosteroids
- Cyclosporine

Further reading:
- Laxer RM, Zulian F (2006) Localized scleroderma. Curr Opin Rheumatol 18(6):606–613

Mucinosis, Acral Persistent Papular

Uncommon type of mucinosis that predominantly affects women and is characterized by flesh-colored to ivory-colored papules on the dorsal hands or extensor forearms

Differential Diagnosis

- Colloid milium
- Cutaneous focal mucinosis
- Cutaneous myxoma
- Digital mucous cyst
- Erythropoietic protoporphyria
- Granuloma annulare
- Lupus erythematosus
- Molluscum contagiosum
- Reticular erythematous mucinosis
- Urticarial follicular mucinosis

Diagnostic Criteria

- 2–5 mm, few to multiple, ivory- to flesh-colored papules
- Focal, well-circumscribed mucin
- Exclusively located on back of hands, wrists, occasionally
- Distal aspect of forearms
- Persist without spontaneous resolution, may increase in number
- Predominately female patients
- No systemic disease overlap
- No associated gammopathy

Evaluation

- Antinuclear antibodies
- HIV test
- Serum/urinary protein electrophoresis

Further reading:
- Rongioletti F, Rebora A, Crovato F (1986) Acral persistent papular mucinosis: a new entity? Arch Dermatol 122:1237–1239

Mucinosis, Follicular (Alopecia Mucinosa, Pinkus Disease)

Refers to both an idiopathic, usually benign dermatosis affecting children or a potentially lymphoma-related dermatosis in older adults that is caused by deposition of hyaluronic acid in the hair follicles and is characterized by erythematous, edematous plaques with follicular accentuation on the scalp (giving rise to alopecia), face, and neck

Subtypes/Variants

- Lymphoma-related follicular mucinosis
- Benign idiopathic
- Urticarial-like follicular mucinosis

Differential Diagnosis

- Alopecia areata
- Alopecia neoplastica
- Androgenetic alopecia
- Eosinophilic folliculitis
- Granuloma faciale
- Keratosis pilaris
- Lichen planopilaris
- Lichen spinulosus

- Milia
- Pityriasis rubra pilaris, circumscribed type
- Sarcoidosis
- Telogen effluvium

Associations

- <u>Cutaneous T cell lymphoma</u>
- Eosinophilic folliculitis
- Hodgkin's disease
- Lupus erythematosus
- Pityrosporum folliculitis

Evaluation

- Complete blood count
- CT scan of chest, abdomen, and pelvis (if overt lymphoma is suspected)
- Lymph node exam
- T cell gene rearrangement and immunophenotyping

Treatment Options

- <u>Topical corticosteroids</u>
- <u>Intralesional corticosteroids</u>
- Hydroxychloroquine
- Isotretinoin
- Systemic corticosteroids
- Phototherapy
- Dapsone
- Minocycline
- Indomethacin
- Total skin electron beam therapy

Further reading:

- Cerroni L, Fink-Puches R, Back B, Kerl H (2002) Follicular mucinosis: a critical reappraisal of clinicopathologic features and association with mycosis fungoides and Sezary syndrome. Arch Dermatol 138(2):182–189

Mucinous Eccrine Carcinoma

Type of eccrine carcinoma that most commonly arises in the periorbital area of older adults and is characterized by an erythematous painless nodule with a tendency to be locally aggressive

Differential Diagnosis

- Angioma
- Basal cell carcinoma
- Chalazion
- Epidermal inclusion cyst
- Kaposi's sarcoma
- Lipoma
- Melanoma
- Metastatic adenocarcinoma (especially mucinous)
- Microcystic adnexal carcinoma
- Myxoma
- Pilomatrixoma
- Sebaceous carcinoma
- Squamous cell carcinoma

Evaluation

- Appropriate cancer screening (rule out metastatic visceral mucinous adenocarcinoma)

Further reading:

• Qureshi HS, Salama ME, Chitale D et al (2004) Primary cutaneous mucinous carcinoma: presence of myoepithelial cells as a clue to the cutaneous origin. Am J Dermatopathol 26(5):353–358

Mucocele

Cyst-like lesion on the oral mucosa that results from injury to or occlusion of the minor salivary ducts and is characterized by a solitary translucent vesicle most commonly located on the lower lip

Differential Diagnosis

- Abscess
- Adenocarcinoma of the salivary glands
- Aphthous ulcer
- Bullous lichen planus
- Cicatricial pemphigoid
- Fibroepithelial polyp
- Gingival cysts
- Hemangioma
- Irritation fibroma
- Lipoma
- Lymphangioma
- Oral lymphoepithelial cyst
- Pyogenic granuloma
- Salivary gland neoplasm
- Squamous papilloma
- Venous lake

Further reading:

• Baurmash H (2002) The etiology of superficial oral mucoceles. J Oral Maxillofac Surg 60(2):237–238

Mucosal Neuroma Syndrome
(Multiple Endocrine Neoplasia, Type IIb)

Autosomal-dominant disorder caused by a defect in the RET proto-onco-gene that is characterized by numerous small neuromas of the lips, tongue, and oral mucosa; medullary thyroid cancer; pheochromocytomas; and marfanoid body habitus

Differential Diagnosis

- Cowden disease
- Fibroma
- Gardner syndrome
- Granular cell tumor
- Marfan syndrome
- Neurofibromatosis
- Squamous cell carcinoma
- Tuberous sclerosis

Evaluation

- Calcitonin level
- CT/MRI scan of abdomen
- Thyroid function test
- Thyroid ultrasound
- Urine catecholamines

Further reading:
- Baykal C, Buyukbabani N, Boztepe H et al (2007) Multiple cutaneous neuromas and macular amyloidosis associated with medullary thyroid carcinoma. J Am Acad Dermatol 56(2 Suppl):S33–S37

Muehrcke's Lines

Type of apparent leukonychia that is caused by hypoalbuminemia-related edema of the nail bed and is characterized by two transverse and parallel white bands that fade upon pressure on the nail plate

Differential Diagnosis

- Beau's lines
- Half-and-half nails
- <u>Mees lines</u>
- Onycholysis
- Onychomycosis
- Terry's nails

Associations

- Liver disease
- Malnutrition
- Nephrotic syndrome

Evaluation

- 24-h urine protein
- Albumin level
- Liver function test
- Renal function test
- Urinalysis

Further reading:

- Alam M, Scher RK, Bickers DR (2001) Muehrcke's lines in a heart transplant recipient. J Am Acad Dermatol 44(2):316–317

Muir–Torre Syndrome

Inherited disorder (AD) that is caused by a defect in the MSH2 or MLH1 mismatch repair genes and is characterized by sebaceous adenomas, sebaceous carcinoma, keratoacanthomas, and tendency to develop visceral malignancies (most commonly colon cancer)

Differential Diagnosis

- Bannayan–Riley–Ruvulcaba syndrome
- Cowden disease
- Gardner syndrome
- Hereditary nonpolyposis colorectal cancer
- Multiple keratoacanthomas of Ferguson–Smith
- Multiple trichoepitheliomas
- Nevoid basal cell carcinoma syndrome
- Sebaceous hyperplasia
- Tuberous sclerosis

Evaluation

- Complete blood count
- Other appropriate cancer screening
- Stool for occult blood/colonoscopy

Further reading:
- Navi D, Wadhera A, Fung MA et al (2006) Muir–Torre syndrome. Dermatol Online J 12(5):4

Multicentric Reticulohistiocytosis

Idiopathic disorder of histiocytic proliferation that is characterized by red-brown papules and nodules on the face and dorsal hands and phalanges (especially on the proximal and lateral nail folds), along with

potentially mutilating polyarthritis, and in a minority of patients, internal
malignancy

Differential Diagnosis

- Cutaneous Rosai–Dorfman disease
- Dermatofibromas
- <u>Dermatomyositis</u>
- Erythema elevatum diutinum
- Farber's lipogranulomatosis
- <u>Fibroblastic rheumatism</u>
- Generalized eruptive histiocytosis
- Gouty tophi
- Granuloma annulare
- Jessner's lymphocytic infiltrate
- Juvenile xanthogranuloma
- Langerhans cell histiocytosis
- Leprosy
- Lipoid proteinosis
- Lupus miliaris disseminata faciei
- Lymphocytoma
- <u>Osteoarthritis</u>
- Progressive nodular histiocytosis
- Psoriatic arthritis
- <u>Rheumatoid arthritis</u>
- Sarcoidosis
- Xanthomas

Associations

- Hypercholesterolemia
- Hypothyroidism
- <u>Internal malignancy</u>
- Sjögren's syndrome

Evaluation

- Antinuclear antibodies
- Appropriate cancer screening
- Complete blood count
- Lipid panel
- Radiographs of the affected joints
- Rheumatoid factor
- Sedimentation rate
- Serum protein electrophoresis
- Thyroid function test

Treatment Options

- NSAIDs
- Systemic corticosteroids
- Methotrexate
- Cyclophosphamide
- TNF inhibitors
- Antimalarials

Further reading:
- Tajirian AL, Malik MK, Robinson-Bostom L et al (2006) Multicentric reticulohistiocytosis. Clin Dermatol 24(6):486–492

Multinucleate Cell Angiohistiocytoma

Uncommon, benign, reactive lesion that is characterized by multiple reddish-brown papules on the lower legs or dorsal hands of middle-aged to elderly women

Differential Diagnosis

- Acroangiodermatitis of Mali
- Angiofibroma

- Arthropod-bite reaction
- Cutaneous lymphoid hyperplasia
- <u>Dermatofibroma</u>
- Granuloma annulare
- Lichen planus
- Kaposi's sarcoma
- <u>Reactive angioendotheliomatosis</u>

Further reading:
- Perez LP, Zulaica A, Rodriguez L et al (2006) Multinucleate cell angiohistiocytoma. Report of five cases. J Cutan Pathol 33(5):349–352

Mycetoma

Chronic infection most commonly located on the distal lower extremity that is usually induced by traumatic implantation of a filamentous bacteria (actinomycetoma, most commonly *Nocardia braziliensis*) or fungus (eumycetoma, most commonly *Pseudallescheria boydii*) and is characterized by tumefaction, draining sinuses, and the diagnostic finding of grains (granular collections of the organism)

Differential Diagnosis

- <u>Actinomycetoma</u>
- Atypical mycobacterial infection
- Blastomycosis
- Botryomycosis
- <u>Chromoblastomycosis</u>
- Chronic bacterial osteomyelitis
- Coccidioidomycosis
- Elephantiasis
- <u>Factitial disease</u>
- Hidradenitis suppurativa
- Kaposi's sarcoma

- Leishmaniasis
- Leprosy
- Squamous cell carcinoma
- Sporotrichosis
- Syphilis
- Tuberculosis
- Yaws

Evaluation

- Bacterial and fungal cultures of grains and exudate
- Potassium hydroxide examination and Gram stain of grains

Further reading:

- Welsh O, Vera-Cabrera L, Salinas-Carmona MC (2007) Mycetoma. Clin Dermatol 25(2):195–202

Mycobacterium fortuitum/Mycobacterium chelonei Infection

Infection with rapidly growing mycobacteria that is capable of causing disease in immunocompetent patients and is characterized by tender, subcutaneous abscesses and cellulitis typically on the lower extremity, usually after a procedure such as injection, pedicure, implantation of a prosthetic device, or liposuction

Differential Diagnosis

- Bacterial cellulitis
- Factitial disease
- Furunculosis
- Glanders
- Mycetoma
- Nocardiosis
- Osteomyelitis

- Sporotrichosis
- Tuberculosis

Evaluation

- Bacterial, mycobacterial, and fungal cultures

Further reading:
- Uslan DZ, Kowalski TJ, Wengenack NL et al (2006) Skin and soft tissue infections due to rapidly growing mycobacteria: comparison of clinical features, treatment, and susceptibility. Arch Dermatol 142(10):1287–1292

Mycobacterium marinum **Infection**

Cutaneous infection with *Mycobacterium marinum* that is most often acquired via contact with fish tanks or swimming pools and is characterized by a slowly evolving, violaceous hyperkeratotic plaque on the hands or feet (Fig. 6.81)

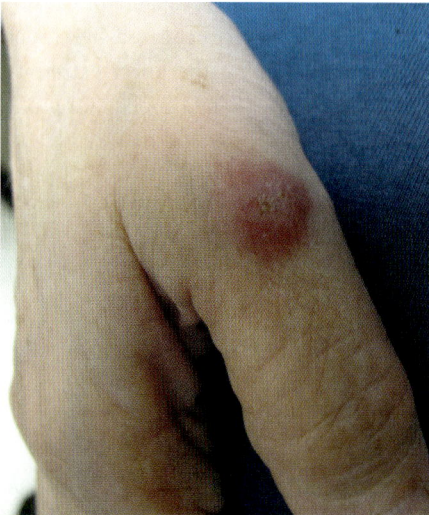

Fig. 6.81 *Mycobacterium marinum* infection

Differential Diagnosis

- Anthrax
- Bacterial pyoderma
- Botryomycosis
- Coccidioidomycosis
- Erysipeloid
- <u>Foreign body granuloma</u>
- Granuloma annulare
- Herpetic whitlow
- Leishmaniasis
- Milker's nodule
- Nocardiosis
- Orf
- Protothecosis
- Squamous cell carcinoma
- <u>Sporotrichosis</u>
- <u>Tuberculosis verrucosa cutis</u>
- Tularemia

Evaluation

- Mycobacterial culture at 30°C
- Radiograph/MRI of the affected area

Treatment Options

- <u>Minocycline</u>
- Ciprofloxacin
- Sulfomethoxazole–trimethoprim
- Rifampin
- Ethambutol

Further reading:
- Johnson RP, Xia Y, Cho S et al (2007) *Mycobacterium marinum* infection: a case report and review of the literature. Cutis 79(1):33–36

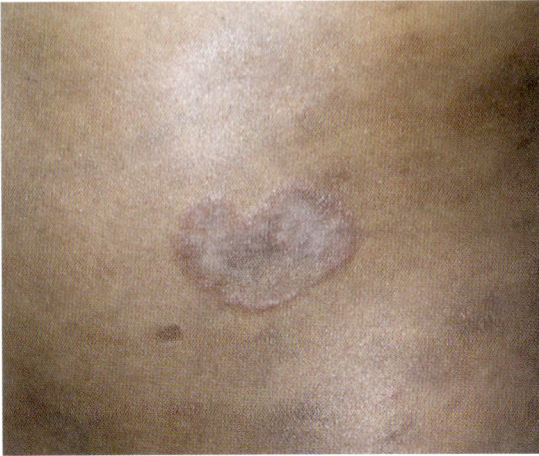

Fig. 6.82 Mycosis fungoides (Courtesy of A. Record)

Mycosis Fungoides

Type of cutaneous T cell lymphoma that predominantly affects older men; is characterized by chronic, pruritic, erythematous, scaly patches and plaques, often on the covered areas of the body such as the trunk and buttocks; and that has the potential to evolve into a tumoral or erythrodermic stage (Fig. 6.82)

Variants

- Adnexotropic
- Alopecia mucinosa
- Erythrodermic
- Follicular
- Granulomatous
- Granulomatous slack skin
- Hypopigmented
- Ichthyosiform
- Invisible

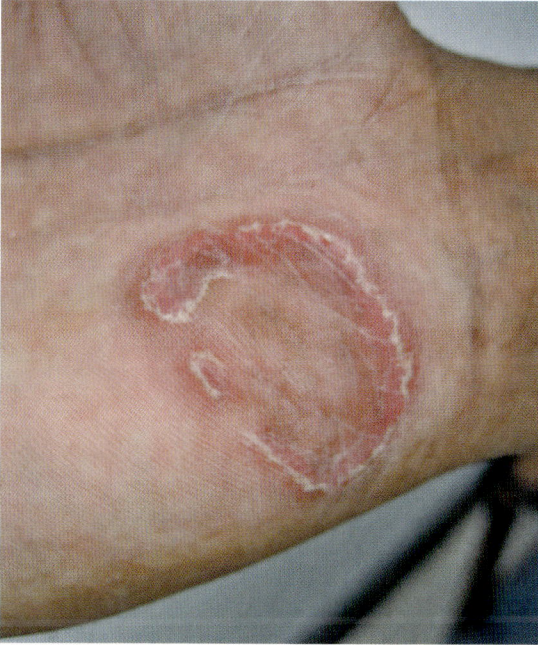

Fig. 6.83 Palmo-
plantar mycosis
fungoides

- Mucosal
- Palmoplantar (Fig. 6.83)
- Patch
- Pigmented-purpura-like
- Plaque
- Poikilodermatous
- Pustular
- Solitary
- Syringotropic
- Tumoral
- Vegetating/papillomatous
- Verrucous/hyperkeratotic
- Vesiculobullous

Differential Diagnosis

Mycosis Fungoides

- <u>Atopic dermatitis</u>
- Drug reaction
- Erythroderma
- Granuloma annulare
- Granulomatous slack skin
- Idiopathic follicular mucinosis
- <u>Large plaque parapsoriasis</u>
- Lichen planus
- Lichen sclerosus et atrophicus
- Lichenoid drug eruption
- Lupus erythematosus
- Lymphomatoid contact dermatitis
- <u>Lymphomatoid drug reaction</u>
- Lymphomatoid papulosis
- Necrobiosis lipoidica
- <u>Nummular eczema</u>
- Progressive macular hypomelanosis
- <u>Pseudomycosis fungoides</u>
- Psoriasis
- Radiodermatitis
- Reticular erythematous mucinosis
- Sarcoidosis
- Seborrheic dermatitis
- Secondary syphilis
- Small plaque parapsoriasis
- Tinea corporis
- Vitiligo

Poikiloderma Atrophicans Vasculare

- Acrodermatitis chronicum atrophicans
- Dermatoheliosis
- <u>Dermatomyositis</u>

- Erythema ab igne
- Lichen sclerosus et atrophicus
- Lupus erythematosus
- Mycosis fungoides
- Poikiloderma-like amyloidosis
- Radiation dermatitis
- Topical steroid overuse

Diagnostic Criteria (Early Mycosis Fungoides)

- Clinical
  - Persistent and/or progressive patches/thin plaques
  - Non-sun-exposed location
  - Size/shape variation
  - Poikiloderma
- Histopathologic
  - Superficial lymphoid infiltrate
  - Epidermotropism without spongiosis
  - Lymphoid atypia
- Clonal TCR gene rearrangement
- Immunopathologic
  - <50% CD2+, CD3+, and/or CD5+ T cells
  - <10% CD7+ T cells
  - Epidermal/dermal discordance of CD2, CD3, CD5, or CD7

Evaluation

- See "Lymphoma, Cutaneous T Cell"

Treatment Options

- Topical corticosteroids
- UVB phototherapy
- Topical nitrogen mustard

- <u>Total skin electron beam therapy</u>
- Methotrexate
- Interferon alpha-2a
- Topical bexarotene
- <u>Oral bexarotene</u>
- Denileukin diftitox
- Alemtuzumab
- Vorinostat
- Romidepsin
- Chemotherapy

Further reading:

- Pimpinelli N et al (2005) International Society for Cutaneous Lymphoma. Defining early mycosis fungoides. J Am Acad Dermatol 53(6):1053–1063
- Kazakov DV, Burg G, Kempf W (2004) Clinicopathological spectrum of mycosis fungoides. J Eur Acad Dermatol Venereol 18(4):397–415

Myiasis, Furuncular

Cutaneous infestation most commonly caused by larva of the botfly *Dermatobia hominis* or the tumbu fly *Cordylobia anthropophaga* that is characterized by a solitary, pruritic, furuncular nodule with serosanguineous drainage that does not respond to conventional therapy

Differential Diagnosis

- <u>Abscess</u>
- Anthrax
- Cellulitis
- Cysticercosis
- <u>Exaggerated arthropod reaction</u>
- Foreign body granuloma
- Furunculosis
- Leishmaniasis

- Lymphadenopathy
- Kerion
- Mycobacterial infection
- Nocardiosis
- Onchocerciasis
- <u>Ruptured epidermoid cyst</u>
- Tungiasis

Treatment Options

- <u>Surgical excision</u>
- Suffocation
- Ivermectin

Further reading:
- Cestari TF, Pessato S, Ramos-e-Silva M (2007) Tungiasis and myiasis. Clin Dermatol 25(2):158–164

Myxedema, Generalized

Systemic mucinosis associated with profound hypothyroidism that is characterized by xerotic, yellowish, edematous skin with periorbital infiltration, madarosis, and brittle hair

Differential Diagnosis

- <u>Anasarca</u>
- Angioedema
- Carotenoderma
- Cutaneous focal mucinosis
- Cutaneous lupus mucinosis
- Primary systemic amyloidosis
- Scleredema
- Scleromyxedema

Evaluation

- Thyroid function tests
- Serum/urinary protein electrophoresis

Further reading:
- Jackson EM, English JC III (2002) Diffuse cutaneous mucinoses. Dermatol Clin 20(3):493–501

Myxoma, Cutaneous (Superficial Angiomyxoma)

Uncommon, cutaneous stromal tumor that is either solitary or multiple (when a part of the Carney complex) and is characterized by a soft, flesh-colored cutaneous nodule on trunk, leg, or head and neck

Differential Diagnosis

- Amelanotic melanoma
- Focal cutaneous mucinosis
- Myxoid dermatofibroma
- Myxoid liposarcoma
- Myxoid malignant fibrous histiocytoma
- Neurofibroma
- Neurothekeoma
- Nodular fasciitis
- Schwannoma

Evaluation

- Echocardiography (atrial myxoma)

Further reading:
- Choi HJ, Kim YJ, Yim JH et al (2007) Unusual presentation of solitary cutaneous myxoma. J Eur Acad Dermatol Venereol 21(3):403–404

Naegeli–Franceschetti–Jadassohn Syndrome

Rare inherited (AD) ectodermal dysplasia of unknown genetic cause that is characterized by anhidrosis, absent dermatoglyphics, reticulated hyperpigmentation on the neck and trunk, palmoplantar keratoderma, and normal life expectancy, health, and intelligence

Differential Diagnosis

- Anhidrotic ectodermal dysplasia
- Confluent and reticulated papillomatosis
- Dermatopathia pigmentosa reticularis
- Dowling–Degos disease
- Dyschromatosis universalis hereditaria
- Dyskeratosis congenita
- Incontinentia pigmenti
- Macular amyloidosis
- Weary–Kindler syndrome
- Reticulate acropigmentation of Kitamura

Further reading:
- Lugassy J, Itin P, Ishida-Yamamoto A et al (2006) Naegeli–Franceschetti–Jadassohn syndrome and dermatopathia pigmentosa reticularis: two allelic ectodermal dysplasias caused by dominant mutations in KRT14. Am J Hum Genet 79(4):724–730

Nail–Patella Syndrome (Fong Syndrome)

Inherited syndrome (AD) caused by a defect in the LMX1B gene that is characterized by hypoplastic patella, nail dystrophy with triangular lunula, posterior iliac horns, pigmentation of the margin of the pupils (Lester iris), and glomerulonephropathy

Differential Diagnosis

- Coffin–Siris syndrome
- Ectodermal dysplasias
- Pachyonychia congenita
- Psoriasis

Evaluation

- Renal function test
- Radiography of the pelvis and knees
- Ophthalmologic examination
- Urinalysis

Further reading:
- Schulz-Butulis BA, Welch MD, Norton SA (2003) Nail–patella syndrome. J Am Acad Dermatol 49(6):1086–1087

Nasal Glioma (Heterotopic Brain Tissue)

Developmental anomaly that presents at birth or in early childhood, contains heterotopic CNS tissue which has lost its connection with the subarachnoid space, and is characterized by a intranasal or extranasal, noncompressible, nontransilluminating mass on the midline face near the nasal root

Differential Diagnosis

- Arteriovenous malformation
- Dermoid cyst
- Encephalocele
- Hemangioma
- Juvenile xanthogranuloma
- Nasal polyp
- Rhabdomyoma
- Venous malformation

Evaluation

- CT/MRI scan of cranium

Further reading:

- Dasgupta NR, Bentz ML (2003) Nasal gliomas: identification and differentiation from hemangiomas. J Craniofac Surg 14(5):736–738

Necrobiosis Lipoidica (Urbach–Oppenheimer Disease)

Idiopathic dermatosis that is possibly vasculopathic in etiology and is characterized by yellow, firm atrophic plaques with telangiectasias and occasional ulceration that are most commonly located on the anterior lower extremities (Fig. 6.84)

Differential Diagnosis

- Actinic granuloma
- <u>Annular elastolytic giant cell granuloma</u>
- <u>Diabetic dermopathy</u>
- Epithelioid sarcoma
- Erythema induratum
- Erythema nodosum
- Factitial disease
- <u>Granuloma annulare</u>
- Granulomatous infections
- Granulomatous mycosis fungoides
- Lichen sclerosus
- Lymphomatoid granulomatosis
- Immunodeficiency-related noninfectious granuloma
- <u>Morphea</u>
- Necrobiotic xanthogranuloma
- Palisaded neutrophilic and granulomatous dermatitis
- Plane xanthoma
- Rheumatoid neutrophilic dermatitis

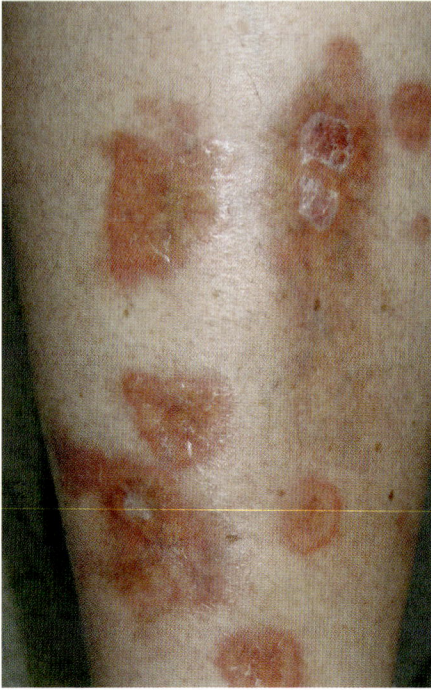

Fig. 6.84 Necrobiosis lipoidica

- Sarcoidosis
- Sclerosing lipogranuloma
- Stasis dermatitis

Associations

- <u>Diabetes mellitus</u>
- Granuloma annulare

Evaluation

- Fasting blood glucose

Treatment Options

- Topical corticosteroids
- <u>Intralesional corticosteroids</u>
- Systemic corticosteroids
- Aspirin
- Dipyridamole
- <u>Pentoxifylline</u>
- Nicotinamide
- Tretinoin
- Cyclosporine
- Heparin
- Hydroxychloroquine
- Mycophenolate mofetil
- Infliximab

Further reading:

- Wee SA, Possick P (2004) Necrobiosis lipoidica. Dermatol Online J 10(3):18

Necrobiotic Xanthogranuloma

Chronic, progressive dermatologic manifestation of monoclonal gammopathy (IgG kappa) with unknown pathogenesis that predominantly affects older adults and is characterized by bilateral, symmetric, indurated, yellow-brown, telangiectatic, occasionally ulcerated plaques on the periorbital area, and less commonly, the trunk and extremities

Differential Diagnosis

- <u>Annular elastolytic giant cell granuloma</u>
- Atypical fibroxanthoma
- Granuloma annulare
- <u>Juvenile xanthogranuloma</u>
- Multicentric reticulohistiocytosis
- <u>Necrobiosis lipoidica</u>

- Normolipemic plane xanthoma
- Sarcoidosis
- Squamous cell carcinoma
- Xanthelasma
- Xanthoma disseminatum

Evaluation

- Complement levels
- Complete blood count
- Ophthalmologic examination
- Sedimentation rate
- Serum/urinary protein electrophoresis

Treatment Options

- Systemic corticosteroids
- Intralesional corticosteroids
- Chlorambucil
- Melphalan
- Intravenous immunoglobulin
- Hydroxychloroquine
- Plasmapheresis

Further reading:
- Flann S, Wain EM, Halpern S, Andrews V et al (2006) Necrobiotic xanthogranuloma with paraproteinaemia. Clin Exp Dermatol 31(2):248–251

Necrolytic Acral Erythema

Cutaneous manifestation of hepatitis C infection that is characterized by burning or pruritic erythematous, hyperkeratotic plaques on the dorsal aspects of the feet and toes, and less commonly, the hands, with sparing of the palms and soles

Differential Diagnosis

- Acrokeratosis paraneoplastica
- <u>Allergic contact dermatitis (especially shoes)</u>
- Lichen planus
- Necrolytic migratory erythema
- <u>Psoriasis</u>
- <u>Zinc deficiency</u>

Evaluation

- CT scan of abdomen
- Liver function test
- Serum glucagon level
- Serum zinc level
- Viral hepatitis panel

Treatment Options

- Zinc supplementation
- <u>Treatment of hepatitis C</u>

Further reading:

- Abdallah M et al (2005) Necrolytic acral erythema: a cutaneous sign of hepatitis C virus infection. J Am Acad Dermatol 53:247–251

Necrolytic Migratory Erythema

Eruption associated with glucagonoma syndrome that is possibly caused by acquired amino acid deficiency and is characterized by recurrent annular, scaly, vesicular, eroded plaques most commonly located in the periorificial, intertriginous, and acral areas

Differential Diagnosis

- Candidiasis
- Darier disease
- Hailey–Hailey disease
- Kwashiorkor
- Necrolytic acral erythema
- Pemphigus
- Pellagra
- Psoriasis
- <u>Seborrheic dermatitis</u>
- Subcorneal pustular dermatosis
- <u>Zinc deficiency</u>

Associations

- Celiac disease
- Cirrhosis
- Crohn's disease
- Chronic pancreatitis
- Cystic fibrosis
- <u>Glucagon-secreting bronchial carcinoma</u>
- <u>Glucagon-secreting tumor of the pancreas</u>
- Multiple endocrine neoplasia
- Ulcerative colitis

Evaluation

- Complete blood count
- CT scan of abdomen
- Fasting plasma glucagon
- Fasting plasma glucose
- Sedimentation rate
- Serum zinc level

Treatment Options

- <u>Treat underlying cause</u>
- Octreotide
- Supplementation of amino acids, essential fatty acids, and zinc

Further reading:
- Remes-Troche JM, Garcia-de-Acevedo B, Zuniga-Varga J et al (2004) Necrolytic migratory erythema: a cutaneous clue to glucagonoma syndrome. J Eur Acad Dermatol Venereol 18(5):591–595

Necrotizing Fasciitis

Life- or limb-threatening toxin-mediated deep soft tissue bacterial infection that spreads along fascial planes and is characterized by pain out of proportion to the physical exam, rapidly advancing violaceous erythema with bullae formation, occasional crepitus, and severe sepsis or septic shock

Differential Diagnosis

- Calciphylaxis
- <u>Cellulitis</u>
- Compartment syndrome
- Disseminated intravascular coagulation
- Hematoma
- Factitial disease
- Insect-bite reaction
- Ischemic necrosis
- Polyarteritis nodosa
- Postsurgical amebiasis
- Pressure ulcer
- <u>Pyoderma gangrenosum</u>
- Pyomyositis
- <u>Spider bite</u>

- Sweet's syndrome
- Warfarin skin necrosis

Evaluation

- Bacterial culture of affected tissue
- Complete blood count
- CT/MRI scan of affected area
- Renal function
- Serum chemistry
- Surgical consultation

Treatment Options

- <u>Incision, drainage, debridement, and irrigation</u>
- Systemic antibiotics
- Amputation

Further reading:
- Kihiczak GG, Schwartz RA, Kapila R (2006) Necrotizing fasciitis: a deadly infection. J Eur Acad Dermatol Venereol 20(4):365–369

Nephrogenic Fibrosing Dermopathy (Nephrogenic Systemic Fibrosis)

Sclerotic dermatosis that most commonly affects patients on hemodialysis for chronic renal failure, may be triggered by accumulation of gadolinium in affected tissues, and is characterized by diffuse cutaneous induration involving the extremities and trunk but sparing the face

Differential Diagnosis

- Amyloidosis (especially beta-2 microglobulin type)
- <u>Anasarca</u>

- Eosinophilia–myalgia syndrome
- <u>Eosinophilic fasciitis</u>
- Calciphylaxis
- Capillary leak syndrome
- Chronic graft-vs-host disease
- Cellulitis
- Diabetic stiff skin
- Generalized myxedema
- Lipodermatosclerosis
- Morphea
- Pretibial myxedema
- Porphyria cutanea tarda
- Scleredema adultorum
- <u>Scleroderma</u>
- Scleromyxedema
- Toxic oil syndrome

Associations

- Antiphospholipid antibody
- <u>Gadolinium-based MRI scans</u>
- <u>Hemodialysis</u>
- Renal failure
- Renal transplantation

Evaluation

- Anticardiolipin antibodies
- Beta-2 glycoprotein-1 antibodies
- Lupus anticoagulant test
- Renal function
- Serum/urinary protein electrophoresis

Treatment Options

- Extracorporeal photopheresis
- UVA1 phototherapy
- Photodynamic therapy
- Plasmapheresis

Further reading:
- Chen AY, Zirwas MJ, Heffernan MP (2010) Nephrogenic systemic fibrosis: a review. J Drugs Dermatol 9(7):829–834

Netherton Syndrome

Inherited syndrome (AR) associated with mutation of the SPINK5 gene encoding the epidermal protein LEKTI that is characterized by neonatal erythroderma, the pathognomonic skin eruption known as ichthyosis linearis circumflexa (which is identified by its double-edged scale), sparse hair due to trichorrhexis invaginata, and atopic dermatitis

Differential Diagnosis

- Acrodermatitis enteropathica
- Atopic dermatitis
- Chronic mucocutaneous candidiasis
- Congenital ichthyosiform erythroderma
- Ectodermal dysplasias
- Erythrodermic psoriasis
- Erythrokeratodermia variabilis
- Hyper-IgE syndrome
- Lamellar ichthyosis
- Omenn syndrome
- Peeling skin syndrome
- Seborrheic dermatitis
- Wiskott–Aldrich syndrome

Further reading:
• Sun JD, Linden KG (2006) Netherton syndrome: a case report and review of the
  literature. Int J Dermatol 45(6):693–697

Neurilemmoma (Schwannoma)

Benign tumor of Schwann cell derivation that can be solitary or multiple
(in the setting of neurofibromatosis) and is characterized by an insidious,
occasionally painful subcutaneous nodule most commonly localized on
the head and neck or extremities

Differential Diagnosis

- Adnexal tumors
- Angiolipoma
- Dermatofibroma
- Dermoid
- Epidermoid cyst
- Ganglion cyst
- Leiomyoma
- Lipoma
- Melanocytic nevus
- Myoblastoma
- Neurofibroma
- Neuroma
- Pilar cyst
- Spiradenoma

Associations

- Carney complex (psammomatous type)
- Neurofibromatosis I
- Neurofibromatosis II
- Schwannomatosis

Further reading:
- Moon SE, Cho YJ, Kwon OS (2005) Subungual schwannoma: a rare location. Dermatol Surg 31(5):592–594

Neuroblastoma, Metastatic

Childhood neuroectodermal tumor that causes increased levels of serum and urinary catecholamines, has a propensity for metastasis to the skin, and is characterized by multiple blue dermal nodules giving the child a "blueberry muffin" appearance

Differential Diagnosis

- Adnexal tumors
- Angiolipomas
- Blueberry muffin baby
- Leukemia cutis
- Lymphoma
- Cutaneous metastasis (especially small cell)
- Mastocytoma
- Melanoma
- Merkel cell carcinoma
- Rhabdomyosarcoma

Evaluation

- Abdominal ultrasound/CT scan
- MIBG scan (metaiodobenzylguanidine)
- Skeletal surgery
- Urinary catecholamines

Further reading:
- Holland KE, Galbraith SS, Drolet BA (2005) Neonatal violaceous skin lesions: expanding the differential of the "blueberry muffin baby". Adv Dermatol 21:153–192

Neurofibroma

Benign neural tumor containing a mixture of peripheral nerve components that is characterized by a soft, button-holing, flesh-colored dermal
or subcutaneous nodule or a larger, pendulous mass that feels like a "bag
of worms" upon palpation (plexiform type), with the latter type being
congenital, pathognomonic for neurofibromatosis, and potentially degenerative into a malignant peripheral nerve sheath tumor

Differential Diagnosis

Dermal/Subcutaneous
- Dermal nevus
- Dermatofibroma
- Fibroepithelial polyp
- Leiomyoma
- Neuroma
- Neurothekeoma
- Neurotized nevus
- Nevus lipomatosus superficialis
- Schwannoma
- Skin tag
- Soft fibroma
- Trichodiscoma

Plexiform
- Deep hemangioma
- Dermatofibrosarcoma protuberans
- Neurofibrosarcoma
- Plexiform fibrohistiocytic tumor of infancy
- Plexiform schwannoma
- Rhabdomyosarcoma

Further reading:

- Barbarot S, Nicol C, Volteau C et al (2007) Cutaneous lesions in neurofibromatosis 1: confused terminology. Br J Dermatol 157(1):183–184

Neurofibromatosis

Autosomal-dominant disorder caused by a defect in the tumor suppressor gene, neurofibromin, that is characterized by café-au-lait macules, Lisch nodules, axillary freckling, optic gliomas, and cutaneous neurofibromas, along with a variety of other tumors and internal organ disease

Subtypes/Variants

- Type I: von Recklinghausen disease (Fig. 6.85)
- Type II: acoustic schwannoma

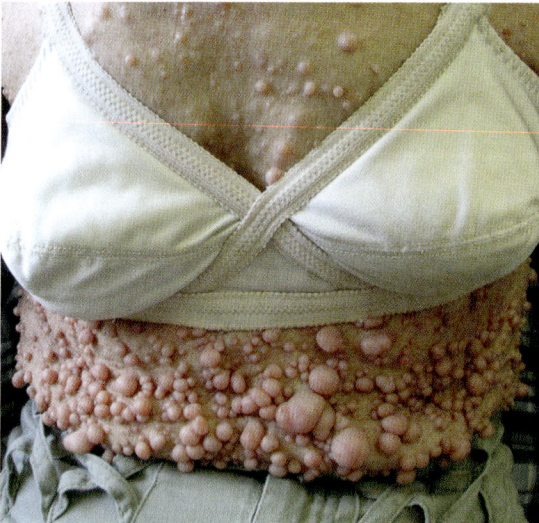

Fig. 6.85 Neurofibromatosis (Courtesy of A. Record)

- Type III: mixed
- Type IV: variant
- Type V: segmental café-au-lait macules, neurofibromas, or both
- Type VI: café-au-lait macules only
- Type VII: late onset
- Type NOS: not otherwise specified

Differential Diagnosis

- Carney's syndrome
- Cowden disease
- Cylindromatosis
- Jaffe–Campanacci syndrome
- Legius syndrome
- McCune–Albright syndrome
- Multiple endocrine neoplasia, types I and IIB
- Noonan syndrome
- Proteus syndrome
- Russell–Silver syndrome
- Tuberous sclerosis
- Watson syndrome

Diagnostic Criteria (2/7)

- Six or more café-au-lait macules over 5 mm (prepubertal) or over 15 mm (postpubertal)
- Two or more neurofibromas or one plexiform neurofibroma
- Axillary or inguinal freckling
- Optic glioma
- Two or more Lisch nodules
- Sphenoid wing dysplasia or thinning of long bone cortex (pseudoarthrosis)
- First-degree relative with NF1

Evaluation

- 24-h urine catecholamines
- Audiography
- Blood pressure
- Complete blood count
- CT/MRI scan of cranium
- Electroencephalogram
- Intelligence testing
- Psychological evaluation
- Skeletal survey
- Slit-lamp examination

Further reading:

- Mulvihill JJ, Parry DM, Sherman JL et al (1990) Neurofibromatosis 1 (Recklinghausen disease) and neurofibromatosis 2 (bilateral acoustic neurofibromatosis). An update. Ann Intern Med 113(1):39–52

Neuroma, Palisaded Encapsulated

Benign neural tumor that is characterized by a flesh-colored dome-shaped papule most commonly located on the face, especially around the nose

Differential Diagnosis

- Angiofibroma
- Basal cell carcinoma
- Fibrous papule
- Intradermal nevus
- Leiomyoma
- Myxoma
- Neurilemmoma
- Neurofibroma
- Neurothekeoma

- Traumatic neuroma
- Trichodiscoma
- Trichoepithelioma
- Tricholemmoma

Further reading:
- Golod O, Soriano T, Craft N (2005) Palisaded encapsulated neuroma: a classic presentation of a commonly misdiagnosed neural tumor. J Drugs Dermatol 4(1):92–94

Neuroma, Traumatic

Benign proliferation of nerves that arises in areas of trauma, prior surgery, or amputation (of an supernumerary digit) and is characterized by a flesh-colored painful papule on the hands or feet

Differential Diagnosis

- <u>Acquired digital fibrokeratoma</u>
- Dermatofibroma
- Foreign body granuloma
- Hypertrophic scar
- Leiomyoma
- <u>Supernumerary digit</u>
- Wart

Further reading:
- Cesinaro AM, Sighinolfi P, Monari P et al (2006) Penile condylomata? Traumatic neuromas! J Am Acad Dermatol 54(2 Suppl):S54–S55

Neurothekeoma (Nerve Sheath Myxoma)

Benign tumor of the nerve sheath that is characterized by an asymptomatic or painful, flesh-colored dermal nodule on the head and neck, trunk, or extremities and that often arises in young females

Differential Diagnosis

- <u>Clear cell sarcoma (especially cellular type)</u>
- Dermatofibroma
- Foreign body granuloma
- Hemangioma
- Keloid
- Leiomyoma
- Melanocytic nevi
- Melanoma
- <u>Myxoid neurofibroma</u>
- <u>Myxoma</u>
- Neural nevus
- Neurofibroma
- Schwannoma

Further reading:

- Fetsch JF, Laskin WB, Hallman JR et al (2007) Neurothekeoma: an analysis of 178 tumors with detailed immunohistochemical data and long-term patient follow-up information. Am J Surg Pathol 31(7):1103–1114

Neutral Lipid Storage Disease (Chanarin–Dorfman Syndrome)

Inherited (AR) disorder that is caused by a defect in the CGI-58 lipid metabolism gene and is characterized by ichthyosis, cataracts, sensorineural deafness, myopathy, lipid deposition in the liver leading to cirrhosis, and lipid vacuoles in leukocytes (Jordan's anomaly)

Differential Diagnosis

- Chondrodysplasia punctata
- Congenital ichthyosiform erythroderma
- Erythrokeratodermia variabilis
- KID syndrome
- <u>Refsum disease</u>

- Sjögren–Larsson syndrome
- X-linked ichthyosis

Further reading:
- Pujol RM, Gilaberte M, Toll A et al (2005) Erythrokeratoderma variabilis-like ichthyosis in Chanarin–Dorfman syndrome. Br J Dermatol 153(4):838–841

Neutrophilic Eccrine Hidradenitis

Neutrophilic dermatosis that is most often diagnosed in the setting of chemotherapy for leukemia (especially AML) or bacterial infection (*Serratia*, *Enterobacter*, *Nocardia*) and is characterized by self-limited, occasionally tender erythematous papules and plaques affecting the trunk or extremities

Differential Diagnosis

- Atypical pyoderma gangrenosum
- Cellulitis
- Cutaneous small vessel vasculitis
- Eccrine syringosquamous metaplasia
- Epidermal growth factor receptor inhibitor acneiform rash
- Erythema elevatum diutinum
- Erythema multiforme
- Erythema nodosum
- Folliculitis
- Graft-vs-host disease
- Idiopathic palmoplantar hidradenitis
- Leukemia cutis
- Miliaria
- Septic emboli
- Sweet's syndrome
- Urticaria
- Urticarial vasculitis

Associated Medications

- Bleomycin
- Chlorambucil
- Cisplatin
- Cyclophosphamide
- Cytarabine
- Doxorubicin
- Vincristine
- Topotecan
- 5-FU

Treatment Options

- Observation and reassurance
- NSAIDs
- Topical corticosteroids
- Systemic corticosteroids

Further reading:

- Oono T, Matsuura H, Morizane S et al (2006) A case of infectious eccrine hidradenitis. J Dermatol 33(2):142–145

Nevoid Basal Cell Carcinoma Syndrome (Gorlin's Syndrome)

Inherited syndrome (AD) that is caused by mutation of the PTCH gene and is characterized by basal cell carcinoma in childhood, palmar pits, jaw cysts, a variety of bony abnormalities, and a tendency to develop medulloblastoma

Differential Diagnosis

- Bazex–Dupre–Christol syndrome
- Basaloid follicular hamartoma
- Basal cell carcinoma with myotonic dystrophy

- <u>Multiple hereditary infundibulocystic basal cell carcinomas</u>
- Rasmussen syndrome
- Rombo syndrome
- Xeroderma pigmentosum

Diagnostic Criteria (Two Major or One Minor+Two Minor)

- Major
  - More than two BCC or one at age less than 20 years
  - Odontogenic keratocysts of jaw
  - Three or more palmar and/or plantar pits
  - Bilamellar calcification of falx
  - Fused, bifid, or splayed ribs
  - First-degree relative with Gorlin's syndrome
  - PTC gene mutation in normal tissue
- Minor
  - Macrocephaly
  - Cleft lip/palate, frontal bossing, coarse face, and hypertelorism
  - Pectus deformity or syndactyly
  - Bridging of sella turcica, rib abnormalities, vertebral anomalies, and flame-shaped lucencies of hands/feet
  - Ovarian fibroma
  - Medulloblastoma

Evaluation

- CT/MRI scan of the brain
- Panoramic radiograph of the teeth
- Pelvic ultrasound
- Radiograph of the ribs and spine

Treatment Options

- <u>Surgical excision</u>
- Mohs micrographic surgery

- <u>Electrodessication and curettage</u>
- Imiquimod
- 5FU
- Photodynamic therapy
- <u>Acitretin</u>
- CO_2 laser

Further reading:
- Pastorino L, Cusano R, Baldo C et al (2005) Nevoid basal cell carcinoma syndrome in infants: improving diagnosis. Child Care Health Dev 31(3):351–354

Nevoid Hypertrichosis

Congenital anomaly characterized by increased growth of terminal hairs in an abnormal area

Subtypes/Variants

- Anterior cervical hypertrichosis
- Auricular hypertrichosis
- Glabellar hypertrichosis
- Hairy polythelia
- Hypertrichosis cubiti

Differential Diagnosis

- Becker's nevus
- Cornelia de Lange syndrome
- <u>Hair follicle nevus (congenital vellus hamartoma)</u>
- Hypertrichosis lanuginosa

Further reading:
- Lopez-Barrantes O, Torrelo A, Mediero IG et al (2002) Nevoid hypertrichosis and hypomelanosis. Eur J Dermatol 12(6):583–585

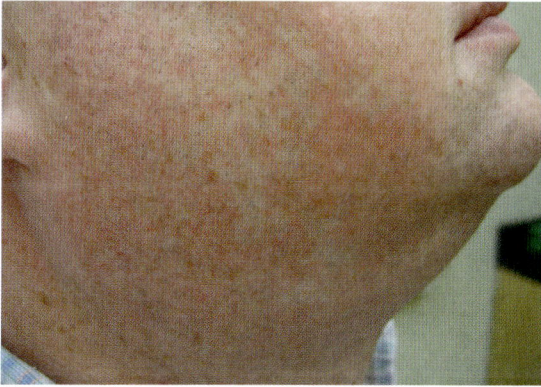

Fig. 6.86 Nevus anemicus

Nevus Anemicus (Vorner Nevus)

Congenital vascular anomaly caused by hypersensitivity to catecholamines that is characterized by localized persistently blanched macules and patches that are most commonly localized to the upper trunk (Fig. 6.86)

Differential Diagnosis

- Bier spots
- Early infantile hemangioma
- Hypomelanosis of Ito
- Leprosy
- Nevus depigmentosus
- Postinflammatory hypopigmentation
- Segmental vitiligo
- Tinea versicolor
- Tuberous sclerosis
- Vitiligo

Associations

- Lymphedema
- Neurofibromatosis

- Nevus spilus
- Phakomatosis pigmentovascularis
- Port-wine stains

Further reading:

- Sarifakioglu E, Erdal E (2006) Multiple anaemic macules of the arms: a variant of Bier's spots or naevus anemicus? J Eur Acad Dermatol Venereol 20(7):892–893

Nevus, Atypical Melanocytic (Dysplastic Nevus, Clark Nevus)

Melanocytic neoplasm with atypical clinical or histologic features that has a tendency to be familial and to be a risk factor for melanoma and is characterized by asymmetry, border irregularity, variability in color, and larger size compared with benign melanocytic nevi

Differential Diagnosis

- Basal cell carcinoma
- Irritated melanocytic nevus
- Lichenoid keratosis
- Malignant melanoma
- Myerson's nevus
- Nevus spilus
- Pigmented actinic keratoses
- Pigmented Bowen's disease
- Pigmented seborrheic keratoses
- Pigmented spindle cell nevus
- Small congenital nevi
- Solar lentigines

Further reading:

- Wick MR, Patterson JW (2005) Cutaneous melanocytic lesions: selected problem areas. Am J Clin Pathol 124(Suppl):S52–S83

Nevus, Benign Melanocytic

Very common benign neoplasm of nevus cells (melanocytes that lack dendrites and form nests) that evolve over the course of a person's life from a flat hyperpigmented macule (junctional nevus) to a dome-shaped, hyperpigmented papule (compound nevus) to a dome-shaped flesh-colored papule (intradermal nevus)

Subtypes

- Acral
- Angiomatous
- Balloon cell
- Clonal
- Cockarde
- Combined
- Compound
- Halo
- Intradermal
- Junctional
- Meyerson's nevus
- Neurotized
- Recurrent
- Verrucous

Differential Diagnosis

- Adnexal neoplasm
- Atypical nevus
- Basal cell carcinoma
- Blue nevus
- Dermatofibromas
- Fibroepithelial polyps

- Lentigo
- <u>Melanoma</u>
- Neurofibromas
- Neurothekeoma
- Seborrheic keratosis
- Traumatic tattoo

Associations (Multiple Eruptive)

- Bullous diseases
- Immunosuppression
- Sunburn

Further reading:
- Strungs I (2004) Common and uncommon variants of melanocytic naevi. Pathology 36(5):396–403

Nevus Comedonicus

Type of epidermal nevus that is characterized by localized group of open and closed comedones that are distributed linearly, segmentally, or along Blaschko's lines and most commonly located on the head and neck, trunk, or upper extremities

Differential Diagnosis

- Acne vulgaris
- Chloracne
- Favre–Racouchot syndrome
- Keratosis pilaris
- Lichen striatus
- Linear Darier's disease
- <u>Milia en plaque</u>

- Nevus lipomatosus superficialis
- <u>Porokeratotic eccrine ostial and dermal duct nevus</u>

Associations

- Cataracts
- Seizures
- Skeletal abnormalities

Further reading:

- Guldbakke KK, Khachemoune A, Deng A et al (2007) Naevus comedonicus: a spectrum of body involvement. Clin Exp Dermatol 32(5):488–492

Nevus, Congenital Melanocytic

Melanocytic nevus that is present at birth and characterized as a small (<1.5 cm), medium (>1.5 to <20 cm), or large (>20 cm) hyperpigmented papillomatous plaque occurring anywhere on the body

Differential Diagnosis

- <u>Atypical nevus</u>
- Becker's nevus
- Café-au-lait macule
- Epidermal nevus
- Large seborrheic keratosis
- <u>Melanoma</u>
- <u>Nevus sebaceus</u>
- Nevus spilus
- Neurofibromatosis
- Paget's disease
- Pigmented squamous cell carcinoma

Associations

- Melanoma
- Neurocutaneous melanosis

Further reading:

- Tannous ZS, Mihm MC Jr, Sober AJ et al (2005) Congenital melanocytic nevi: clinical and histopathologic features, risk of melanoma, and clinical management. J Am Acad Dermatol 52(2):197–203

Nevus Depigmentosus

Nevoid type of hypomelanosis with onset at birth or in the first few years of life that is characterized by a circumscribed patch of hypopigmentation in a segmental or isolated distribution, is most commonly located on the trunk, and persists for life

Differential Diagnosis

- Hypomelanosis of Ito
- Leprosy
- Nevus anemicus
- Phylloid hypomelanosis
- Postinflammatory hypopigmentation
- Segmental vitiligo
- Tinea versicolor
- Tuberous sclerosis
- Vitiligo

Diagnostic Criteria

- Leukoderma present at birth or onset early in life
- No alteration in distribution of leukoderma throughout life
- No alteration in texture, or change of sensation, in the affected area
- No hyperpigmented border around the achromic area

Further reading:

- Coupe RL (1976) Unilateral systematized achromic nevus. Dermatologica 134:19–35
- Kim SK, Kang HY, Lee ES, Kim YC (2006) Clinical and histopathologic characteristics of Nevus depigmentosus. J Am Acad Dermatol 55(3):423–428

Nevus Flammeus/Nevus Simplex (Capillary Malformation, Port-Wine Stain)

Congenital capillary malformation with variable presentation and several associated diseases that is characterized by a fading pink-to-red (nevus simplex) or a persistent red-to-purple patch (nevus flammeus) most commonly located on the occiput (stork bite), glabella (salmon patch), or unilateral face (port-wine stain), with the lateral initially smooth but becoming more pebbly or verrucous over the course of the patient's life

Differential Diagnosis (Nevus Flammeus)

- Child abuse
- Early infantile hemangioma
- Forceps injury
- Insect-bite reaction
- Telangiectatic hemangioma
- Unilateral nevoid telangiectasia

Associations

- Bannayan–Riley–Ruvulcaba syndrome
- Beckwith–Wiedemann syndrome
- Coats disease
- Cobb syndrome
- Glaucoma
- Klippel–Trenaunay syndrome
- Nevus anemicus
- Parkes Weber syndrome

- Phakomatosis pigmentovascularis
- Roberts syndrome
- Rubinstein–Taybi syndrome
- Sturge–Weber syndrome
- TAR syndrome
- von Hippel–Lindau syndrome
- Wyburn–Mason syndrome

Treatment Options

- Pulsed dye laser

Further reading:

- Garzon MC, Huang JT, Enjolras O et al (2007) Vascular malformations: part I. J Am Acad Dermatol 56(3):353–370

Nevus Lipomatosus Superficialis (Of Hoffman and Zurhelle)

Fat hamartoma that arises within the first two decades of life and is characterized by one or more soft, wrinkled, pedunculated, fleshy papules most commonly located on the buttock, hip, or thigh

Differential Diagnosis

- Agminated neurofibromas
- Angiolipoma
- Connective tissue nevus
- Cylindroma
- Epidermal nevus
- Fibroepithelial polyp
- Focal dermal hypoplasia (Goltz's syndrome)
- Melanocytic nevus
- Nevus sebaceus
- Trichoepithelioma

Associations

- Michelin tire baby appearance

Further reading:
- Lane JE, Clark E, Marzec T (2003) Nevus lipomatosus cutaneous superficialis. Pediatr Dermatol 20(4):313–314

Nevus of Ota/Nevus of Ito

Type of dermal melanocytosis that is caused by failure of melanoblasts to migrate to the epidermis and is characterized by blue-, gray-, or black-pigmented macules and patches affecting the zygomatic area of the face and sclera (Ota) or shoulder area (Ito)

Differential Diagnosis

- Acquired nevus of Ota-like macules (Sun's nevus (unilateral) or Hori's nevus (bilateral))
- Alkaptonuria
- Argyria
- Blue nevus
- Café-au-lait macule
- Congenital melanocytic nevus
- Contusion
- Drug-induced pigmentation
- Exogenous ochronosis
- Facial acanthosis nigricans
- Fixed drug eruption
- Lentigo maligna
- Melanoma
- Melasma
- Mongolian spot
- Nevus spilus

- Photosensitive drug eruption
- Riehl's melanosis

Associations

- <u>Glaucoma</u>
- Melanoma
- Neurofibromatosis
- Nevus flammeus
- Phacomatosis pigmentovascularis

Treatment Options

- Q-switched lasers (Ruby, Nd:YAG, Alexandrite)

Further reading:
- Lee CS, Lim HW (2003) Cutaneous diseases in Asians. Dermatol Clin 21(4):669–677

Nevus Sebaceus (of Jadassohn)

Type of epidermal nevus that has the potential to sprout several different adnexal neoplasms (most commonly syringocystadenoma papilliferum) later in life and is characterized by a solitary yellow, tan, or brown linear hairless plaque most commonly on the scalp or forehead (Fig. 6.87)

Differential Diagnosis

- <u>Aplasia cutis congenita</u>
- <u>Congenital melanocytic nevus</u>
- <u>Congenital triangular alopecia</u>
- Linear verrucous epidermal nevus
- Juvenile xanthogranuloma
- Mastocytoma
- Seborrheic keratosis

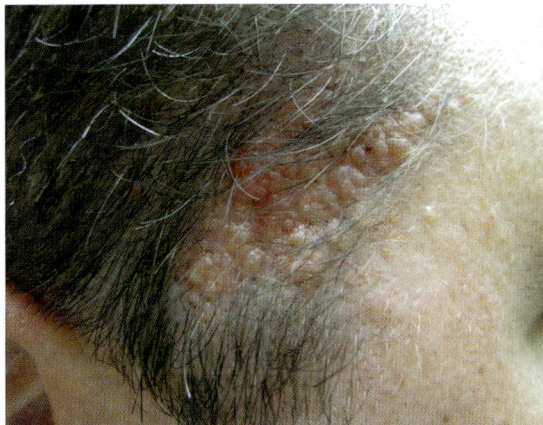

Fig. 6.87 Nevus sebaceus

Associations (Tumors Arising Within)

- Basal cell carcinoma
- Chondroid syringoma
- Hidradenoma
- Sebaceous epithelioma
- Squamous cell carcinoma
- Syringocystadenoma papilliferum
- Syringoma
- Trichilemmoma
- Trichoblastoma

Associations

- Epidermal nevus syndrome
- Nevus spilus
- Phacomatosis pigmentokeratotica

Treatment Options

- Observation
- Surgical excision

- Electrodessication and curettage
- CO_2 laser
- Photodynamic therapy

Further reading:

- Davison SP, Khachemoune A, Yu D et al (2005) Nevus sebaceus of Jadassohn revisited with reconstruction options. Int J Dermatol 44(2):145–150

Nevus Spilus (Speckled Lentiginous Nevus)

Melanocytic hamartoma of uncertain cause that is characterized by a large patch of light hyperpigmentation interspersed with more darkly pigmented macules

Differential Diagnosis

- <u>Agminated junctional melanocytic nevi</u>
- Agminated Spitz nevi
- Becker's nevus
- Café-au-lait macule
- Congenital nevus
- Linear and whorled nevoid hypermelanosis
- Nevus of Ito
- <u>Partial unilateral/segmental lentiginosis</u>

Associations

- Epidermal nevi
- FACES syndrome
- Melanoma
- Nevus sebaceus
- Phakomatosis pigmentovascularis, types III or IV

Further reading:

- Happle R (2007) Nevus spilus maculosus vs partial unilateral lentiginosis. J Eur Acad Dermatol Venereol 21(5):713

Nocardiosis

Bacterial infection with the ubiquitous and partially acid-fast *Nocardia* that has a variable presentation, including disseminated disease from an initial pulmonary focus (in immunocompromised patients, *N. asteroides*), primary cutaneous infection with sporotrichoid spread of infection (in immunocompetent patients, *N. braziliensis*), and mycetoma

Differential Diagnosis

- Acanthamebiasis
- Actinomycosis
- Atypical mycobacterium infection
- Blastomycosis
- Coccidioidomycosis
- Eumycetoma
- Glanders
- Histoplasmosis
- Leishmaniasis
- Sporotrichosis
- Tularemia
- Tuberculosis

Evaluation

- Bacterial, mycobacterial, and fungal cultures
- Chest radiography
- Complete blood count
- Gram stain of exudate

Further reading:

• Inamadar AC, Palit A (2003) Primary cutaneous nocardiosis: a case study and review. Indian J Dermatol Venereol Leprol 69(6):386–391

Nodular Fasciitis

Benign, pseudosarcomatous condition that is associated with trauma, affects predominantly young adults, and is characterized by a firm, subcutaneous nodule predominantly located on the upper extremity, or around the cranium in young children (cranial fasciitis) (Fig. 6.88)

Differential Diagnosis

- Dermatofibrosarcoma protuberans
- Desmoid tumor
- Enchondroma
- Epidermal inclusion cyst
- Epithelioid sarcoma
- Fibrosarcoma
- Leiomyoma

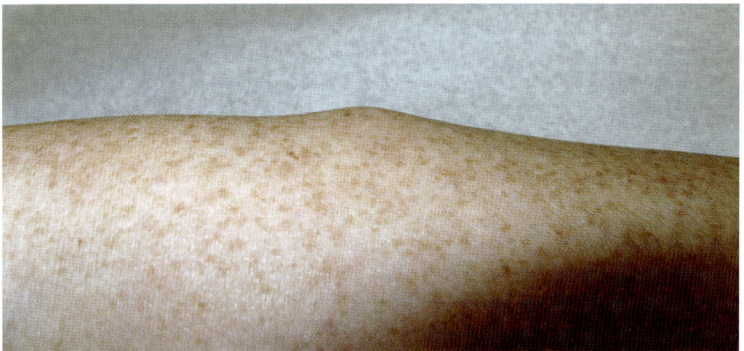

Fig. 6.88 Nodular fasciitis

- Leiomyosarcoma
- Lipoma
- Malignant fibrous histiocytoma
- Myxoma
- Neurilemmoma
- Neurothekeoma

Further reading:
- Nishi SP, Brey NV, Sanchez RL (2006) Dermal nodular fasciitis: three case reports of the head and neck and literature review. J Cutan Pathol 33(5):378–382

Nodular Vasculitis (Erythema Induratum of Whitfield)

Idiopathic type of panniculitis with predilection for young females that is characterized by erythematous tender nodules that occasionally ulcerate, drain, and scar and that are most commonly located on the posterior aspect of the lower extremity

Differential Diagnosis

- Antitrypsin deficiency panniculitis
- Chilblains
- Erythema nodosum leprosum
- Erythema nodosum
- Factitial panniculitis
- Infectious panniculitis
- Lupus panniculitis
- Pancreatic panniculitis
- Perniosis
- Polyarteritis nodosa
- Subcutaneous lymphoma
- Subcutaneous sarcoidosis
- Thrombophlebitis

Evaluation

- Bacterial, mycobacterial, and fungal cultures of blood and lesional tissue
- Chest radiograph
- Complete blood count
- PCR of lesional skin
- Sedimentation rate
- Tuberculin skin test

Treatment Options

- <u>Antituberculosis therapy</u>
- <u>Potassium iodide</u>
- Dapsone
- Colchicine
- Hydroxychloroquine
- Mycophenolate mofetil
- Systemic corticosteroids
- NSAIDs

Further reading:
- Requena L, Sanchez Yus E (2001) Panniculitis. Part II. Mostly lobular panniculitis. J Am Acad Dermatol 45(3):325–361

Noonan Syndrome

Autosomal-dominant or sporadic syndrome that resembles Turner syndrome but can affect males, is caused by a defect in the PTPN11 gene, and is characterized by many features, including keratosis pilaris atrophicans faciei, short stature, cryptorchidism, pulmonic stenosis, cubitis valgus, and lymphedema

Differential Diagnosis

- Cardiofaciocutaneous syndrome
- Costello syndrome
- Fetal alcohol syndrome
- Legius syndrome
- LEOPARD syndrome
- Neurofibromatosis
- Turner syndrome
- Watson syndrome

Evaluation

- Echocardiography

Further reading:
- Fox LP, Geyer AS, Anyane-Yeboa K et al (2005) Cutis verticis gyrata in a patient with Noonan syndrome. Pediatr Dermatol 22(2):142–146

Notalgia Paresthetica

Neurocutaneous disorder that may be caused by nerve root irritation of thoracic nerves and is characterized by the sensation of burning pain or itch on one side of the back, inferior to the scapula, with or without hyperpigmentation in the affected area and possible associated macular amyloidosis

Differential Diagnosis

- Atopic dermatitis
- Contact dermatitis
- Elastofibroma dorsi
- Fixed drug eruption
- Intercostal neuralgia

- Leprosy
- Lichen amyloidosis
- Lichen simplex chronicus
- Macular amyloidosis
- Postherpetic neuralgia
- Thoracic outlet syndrome
- Tinea incognito
- Xerosis
- Zoster

Treatment Options

- Lidocaine patches
- Capsaicin cream
- Doxepin cream
- Pramoxine cream
- Gabapentin
- Amitriptyline
- Topiramate
- Carbamazepine
- Physical therapy
- Transcutaneous electric nerve stimulation
- Spinal surgery

Further reading:
- Savk O, Savk E (2005) Investigation of spinal pathology in notalgia paresthetica. J Am Acad Dermatol 52(6):1085–1087

Nummular Eczema

Idiopathic type of eczema that predominantly affects adults and is characterized by coin-shaped, pruritic eczematous plaques with a predilection for the dorsal extremities, shoulders, breasts, and buttocks

Differential Diagnosis

- Asteatotic eczema
- Atopic dermatitis
- <u>Autosensitization dermatitis</u>
- Bowen's disease
- <u>Contact dermatitis</u>
- Dermatitis herpetiformis
- Lichen simplex chronicus
- Mycosis fungoides
- <u>Nummular-eczema-like drug eruption</u>
- Parapsoriasis
- Pityriasis rosea
- <u>Psoriasis</u>
- Scabies
- Tinea corporis

Treatment Options

- Emollients
- <u>Topical corticosteroids</u>
- <u>Systemic antibiotics</u>
- <u>Systemic corticosteroids</u>
- Cyclosporine
- Tar
- Tacrolimus ointment
- Narrowband UVB phototherapy
- Methotrexate

Further reading:

- Krupa Shankar DS, Shrestha S (2005) Relevance of patch testing in patients with nummular dermatitis. Indian J Dermatol Venereol Leprol 71(6):406–408

Ochronosis, Exogenous

Localized pigmentary disturbance caused by application of various chemicals, such as hydroquinone, with subsequent inhibition of homogentisic acid oxidase that is characterized by blue-black patches on the exposed area, most commonly the face

Differential Diagnosis

- Acanthosis nigricans
- Alkaptonuria
- Argyria
- Drug-induced hyperpigmentation
- Fixed drug eruption
- Melasma
- Nevus of Ota
- Photosensitive drug reaction
- Pigmented contact dermatitis
- Postinflammatory hyperpigmentation
- Riehl's melanosis
- Sarcoidosis

Further reading:
- Huerta Brogeras M, Sanchez-Viera M (2006) Exogenous ochronosis. J Drugs Dermatol 5(1):80–81

Oculocutaneous Albinism

Refers to several different pigmentary disorders (oculocutaneous albinism, types I–IV) that are characterized by failure to produce or distribute melanin in the skin and eyes and are characterized by variable pigmentary dilution of the skin, hair, and eyes, increased sensitivity to ultraviolet radiation with skin cancers early in life, visual defects, and numerous other defects

Differential Diagnosis

- <u>Chediak–Higashi syndrome</u>
- <u>Griscelli syndrome</u>
- <u>Hermansky–Pudlak syndrome</u>
- Homocystinuria
- Menkes syndrome
- Phenylketonuria
- Tietze syndrome

Associations

- Angelman syndrome
- Prader–Willi syndrome

Further reading:
- Okulicz JF, Shah RS, Schwartz RA, Janniger CK (2003) Oculocutaneous albinism. J Eur Acad Dermatol Venereol 17(3):251–256

Olmsted Syndrome

Keratinization disorder with uncertain inheritance pattern and cause that is characterized by a severe, mutilating, and painful type of palmoplantar keratoderma with pseudoainhum, nail dystrophy, and periorificial hyperkeratotic plaques

Differential Diagnosis

- Acrodermatitis enteropathica
- Chronic mucocutaneous candidiasis
- Giant verruca
- <u>Keratitis–ichthyosis–deafness syndrome</u>
- <u>Mal de Meleda</u>
- Pachyonychia congenita

- Psoriasis
- Verrucous carcinoma
- <u>Vohwinkel syndrome</u>

Further reading:
- Mevorah B, Goldberg I, Sprecher E et al (2005) Olmsted syndrome: mutilating palmoplantar keratoderma with periorificial keratotic plaques. J Am Acad Dermatol 53(5 Suppl 1):S266–S272

Onchocerciasis (Robles Disease)

Tropical infestation that is caused by the microfilarial form of *Onchocerca volvulus*, is transmitted by the *Simulium* blackfly, and is characterized by cutaneous nodules, lichenification (sowda), atrophy (lizard skin), ichthyosis, a papular eruption, lymphedema, pruritus, and hypopigmentation (leopard skin)

Differential Diagnosis

- Acquired ichthyosis
- Allergic contact dermatitis
- <u>Atopic dermatitis</u>
- Chemical leukoderma
- <u>Chronic eczema</u>
- Dermatophytosis
- Insect bites
- Leprosy
- Leukoderma of scleroderma
- Lichen planus
- Lichen sclerosus et atrophicus
- <u>Loaiasis</u>
- Pityriasis lichenoides
- Postinflammatory hypopigmentation
- Scabies

- <u>Syphilitic leukoderma</u>
- Vitiligo

Further reading:
- Udall DN (2007) Recent updates on onchocerciasis: diagnosis and treatment. Clin Infect Dis 44(1):53–60

Onychomatricoma

Benign filiform tumor of the nail matrix that causes thickening of the nail plate, longitudinal ridging, transverse overcurvature, splinter hemorrhages, yellow discoloration, and longitudinal cavities within the nail plate

Differential Diagnosis

- Acral fibrokeratoma
- Bowen's disease
- Onychomycosis
- Osteochondroma
- Porocarcinoma
- <u>Squamous cell carcinoma</u>
- <u>Subungual exostosis</u>
- Subungual keratoacanthoma
- <u>Wart</u>

Further reading:
- Piraccini BM, Antonucci A, Rech G et al (2007) Onychomatricoma: first description in a child. Pediatr Dermatol 24(1):46–48

Oral Florid Papillomatosis (Ackerman Tumor)

Type of verrucous carcinoma that affects the oral cavity of older patients, is caused most commonly by HPV types VI and XI, and is characterized by a white verrucous plaque on the buccal mucosa or gums

Differential Diagnosis

- Darier's disease
- Granular cell tumor
- Fibromas
- Focal epithelial hyperplasia (Heck's disease)
- Leukoplakia
- Lymphangioma
- Malignant acanthosis nigricans
- Proliferative verrucous leukoplakia
- Squamous cell carcinoma
- White sponge nevus

Further reading:
- Wenzel K, Saka B, Zimmermann R et al (2003) Malignant conversion of florid oral and labial papillomatosis during topical immunotherapy with imiquimod. Med Microbiol Immunol 192(3):161–164

Orf (Ecthyma Contagiosum)/Milker's Nodule

Two zoonotic viral infections with similar clinical features that are caused by parapoxviruses, occur after contact with a sheep's or goat's mouth (orf), or a cow's udder (milker's nodule), and are characterized by a evolving, solitary hemorrhagic and purulent nodule on the digits or hands

Differential Diagnosis

- Anthrax
- Cowpox
- Erysipeloid
- Herpetic whitlow
- Keratoacanthoma
- Leishmaniasis
- Milker's nodule

- Molluscum contagiosum
- Mycobacterial infection
- Nocardiosis
- <u>Pyoderma gangrenosum</u>
- Pyogenic granuloma
- Squamous cell carcinoma
- Sporotrichosis
- Sweet's syndrome
- Syphilitic chancre, extragenital
- Tuberculosis
- Tularemia
- *Vibrio vulnificus* infection

Stages

- I: Maculopapular
- II: Targetoid
- III: Acute
- IV: Regenerative
- V: Papillomatous
- VI: Regressive

Associations

- Erythema multiforme
- Erythema nodosum

Treatment Options

- <u>Observation and wound care</u>
- Surgical excision
- Cryotherapy
- Cidofovir

Further reading:
- Ballanger F, Barbarot S, Mollat C et al (2006) Two giant orf lesions in a heart/lung transplant patient. Eur J Dermatol 16(3):284–286

Osteoma Cutis

Deposition of bone within the skin that can occur as a primary or secondary process and is characterized by a hard nodule or plaque anywhere on the body

Differential Diagnosis

- Calcinosis cutis
- Cartilaginous tumors
- Foreign body reaction
- Gouty tophus
- Metastatic lesion
- Pilomatricoma
- Rheumatoid nodule

Associations

- Acne (miliary osteomas)
- Albright's hereditary osteodystrophy
- Fibrodysplasia ossificans progressiva
- Plate-like osteoma cutis
- Progressive osseous heteroplasia

Further reading:
- Thielen AM, Stucki L, Braun RP et al (2006) Multiple cutaneous osteomas of the face associated with chronic inflammatory acne. J Eur Acad Dermatol Venereol 20(3):321–326

Oxalosis, Cutaneous

Cutaneous manifestation of primary hyperoxaluria that is characterized by Raynaud's phenomenon, acral necrosis and gangrene, livedo reticularis, and erythematous subcutaneous nodules in a patient with a history of recurrent kidney stones

Differential Diagnosis

- <u>Antiphospholipid antibody syndrome</u>
- Calciphylaxis
- <u>Cholesterol emboli syndrome</u>
- <u>Cryoglobulinemia</u>
- Disseminated intravascular coagulation
- Warfarin necrosis
- Scleroderma

Associations (Secondary Oxalosis)

- Crohn's disease
- Ethylene glycol poisoning
- Excessive ascorbic acid
- Glycerol infusion
- Hemodialysis
- Methoxyflurane anesthesia
- Pyridoxine deficiency

Evaluation

- 24-h urine studies for oxalate
- Renal function

Further reading:

- Blackmon JA, Jeffy BG, Malone JC, Knable AL Jr (2011) Oxalosis involving the skin: case report and literature review. Arch Dermatol 147(11):1302–1305

Pachydermodactyly

Rare, benign, idiopathic digital fibromatosis arising predominantly in younger males that is characterized by symmetric swelling of soft tissue on the lateral aspects of the second through fifth proximal interphalangeal joints

Differential Diagnosis

- Gout
- Juvenile fibromatosis
- Juvenile rheumatoid arthritis
- Knuckle pads
- Pachydermoperiostosis
- Rheumatoid arthritis
- Sarcoidosis
- Xanthomas

Further reading:

- Sandobal C, Kuznietz A, Varizat A, Roverano S, Paira S (2007) Pachydermodactyly: four additional cases. Clin Rheumatol 26(6):962–964

Pachydermoperiostosis (Primary Hypertrophic Osteoarthropathy, Touraine–Solente–Golé Syndrome)

Inherited disorder (AD) of unknown cause that is characterized by cutis verticis gyrata and thickening of the skin (pachyderma), clubbing and periosteal swelling, hyperhidrosis, and acromegalic features

Differential Diagnosis

- <u>Acromegaly</u>
- Clubbing
- <u>Pachydermodactyly</u>
- Psoriatic arthritis
- Scleromyxedema
- Secondary hypertrophic osteoarthropathy
- Thyroid acropachy

Associations

- Crohn's disease
- Myelofibrosis
- Protein-losing enteropathy

Further reading:
- Seyhan T, Ozerdem OR, Aliagaoglu C (2005) Severe complete pachydermoperiostosis (Touraine–Solente–Gole syndrome). Dermatol Surg 31(11 Pt 1):1465–1467

Pachyonychia Congenita

Inherited disorder (AD) that is caused by gene defects in keratin 6a and keratin 16 (type I, Jadassohn–Lewandowski type) and keratin 6b and keratin 17 (type II, Jackson–Lawler) and that is characterized by markedly thickened nails with subungual hyperkeratosis, palmoplantar keratoderma, follicular keratotic papules on the face and extensors, oral leukokeratosis, and steatocystoma multiplex (type II)

Differential Diagnosis

- Chronic mucocutaneous candidiasis
- Dyskeratosis congenita

- <u>Hidrotic ectodermal dysplasia</u>
- Lichen planus
- Onychomycosis
- <u>Palmoplantar keratodermas, hereditary</u>
- Psoriasis
- Weber–Cockayne syndrome
- White sponge nevus

Further reading:
- Leachman SA, Kaspar RL, Fleckman P et al (2005) Clinical and pathological features of pachyonychia congenita. J Investig Dermatol Symp Proc 10(1):3–17

Paget's Disease of Breast

Cutaneous eruption overlying an intraductal breast carcinoma that is possibly caused by metastasis of malignant cells through the lactiferous or lymphatic ducts to the epidermis and is characterized by a unilateral, recalcitrant, scaly, and eczematous eruption on the nipple and areola

Differential Diagnosis

- Allergic contact dermatitis
- Atopic dermatitis
- <u>Bowen's disease</u>
- <u>Clear cell papulosis</u>
- <u>Erosive adenomatosis</u>
- Fixed drug eruption
- Irritant dermatitis
- Melanoma
- Mycosis fungoides
- Nipple adenoma
- <u>Nipple eczema</u>
- Parapsoriasis
- Psoriasis

- Seborrheic dermatitis
- Tinea mammae

Treatment Options

- <u>Surgical excision</u>
- Radiation
- Chemotherapy

Further reading:

- Kanitakis J (2007) Mammary and extramammary Paget's disease. J Eur Acad Dermatol Venereol 21(5):581–590

Pagetoid Reticulosis (Woringer–Kolopp Disease)

Uncommon localized lymphoproliferative disorder with uncertain relationship to mycosis fungoides (unlike classic mycosis fungoides, infiltrates can be predominantly CD8+ and the disease more often arises in younger patients) that is characterized by a solitary, indolent, hyperkeratotic, erythematous plaque on the extremities, especially the palms or soles, or less commonly, multiple disseminated lesions (Ketron–Goodman variant)

Differential Diagnosis

- <u>CD8± epidermotropic cutaneous T cell lymphoma</u>
- Cutaneous lymphoid hyperplasia
- Erythema annulare centrifugum
- Hand eczemas
- Lichen planus
- Lichen simplex chronicus
- Lymphomatoid papulosis, type B
- <u>Mycosis fungoides palmaris et plantaris</u>
- <u>Psoriasis</u>
- Stasis dermatitis

- Tinea corporis
- Unilesional mycosis fungoides

Treatment Options

- Topical corticosteroids
- Topical nitrogen mustard
- Phototherapy
- Surgical excision
- Radiation

Further reading:
- Steffen C (2005) Ketron-Goodman disease, Woringer-Kolopp disease, and pagetoid reticulosis. Am J Dermatopathol 27(1):68–85

Palisaded Neutrophilic and Granulomatous Dermatosis (Rheumatoid Papules)

Poorly defined, probably vasculitic dermatosis that is associated with autoimmunity, may be related to interstitial granulomatous dermatitis, and is characterized by symmetric, umbilicated, or eroded papules, nodules, and plaques predominantly on the extensor surface of the extremities (Fig. 6.89)

Differential Diagnosis

- Churg–Strauss syndrome
- Granuloma annulare
- Granulomatous drug reaction
- Interstitial granulomatous dermatitis with arthritis
- Methotrexate-induced papular eruption
- Necrobiosis lipoidica
- Perforating disorder
- Rheumatic fever nodule

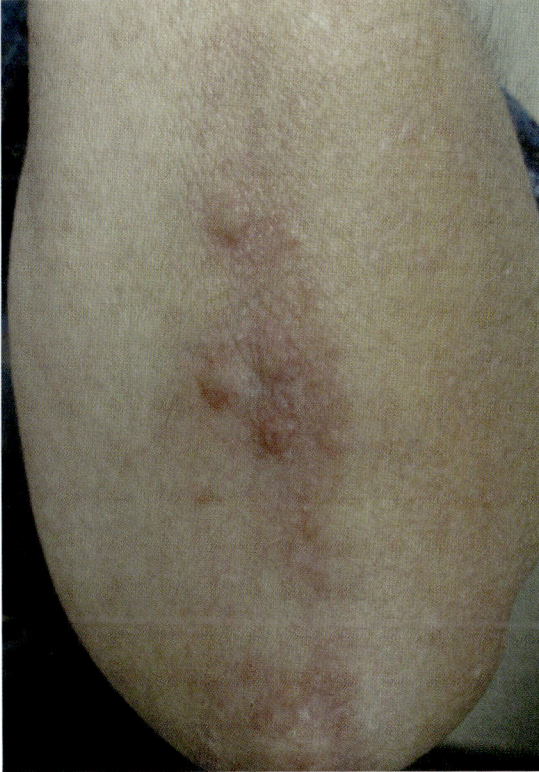

Fig. 6.89 Palisaded neutrophilic and granulomatous dermatitis

- <u>Rheumatoid neutrophilic dermatosis</u>
- Rheumatoid nodules
- Wegener's granulomatosis
- Vasculitis

Associations

- HUS/TTP
- Inflammatory bowel disease
- Myelodysplastic syndrome

- Raynaud's disease
- <u>Rheumatoid arthritis</u>
- Sulfa drugs
- Systemic lupus erythematosus
- Thyroiditis
- Vasculitis syndromes

Treatment Options

- Topical corticosteroids
- Intralesional corticosteroids
- <u>Systemic corticosteroids</u>
- <u>Hydroxychloroquine</u>
- <u>Methotrexate</u>
- Dapsone
- Colchicine
- Cyclosporine
- Infliximab

Further reading:

- Sayah A, English JC (2005) Rheumatoid arthritis: a review of the cutaneous manifestations. J Am Acad Dermatol 53(2):191–209

Palmoplantar Pustulosis

Chronic dermatosis of the palms and soles that predominantly affects smokers and is characterized by erythematous plaques with dry, keratotic pustules in various stages of evolution

Differential Diagnosis

- Acrodermatitis continua of Hallopeau
- <u>Allergic contact dermatitis</u>
- <u>Dyshidrotic eczema</u>
- Keratoderma blennorrhagicum

- Mycosis fungoides palmaris et plantaris
- Orf/milker's nodules
- Secondary syphilis
- Tinea manuum/pedis

Associations

- Psoriasis
- SAPHO syndrome
- Smoking
- Thyroiditis

Treatment Options

- Topical corticosteroids
- Tetracycline antibiotics
- Acitretin
- Methotrexate
- Cyclosporine
- Sulfasalazine
- Colchicine
- TNF inhibitors
- Ustekinumab

Further reading:
- Yamamoto T, Yokozeki H, Tsuboi R (2007) Koebner's phenomenon associated with palmoplantar pustulosis. J Eur Acad Dermatol Venereol 21(7):990–992

Pancreatic Panniculitis

Type of panniculitis associated with both pancreatitis and pancreatic cancer that is caused by lipase-induced liquefactive necrosis of the subcutaneous layer and is characterized by tender, erythematous nodules on the lower extremity that occasionally break down and discharge an oily exudate

Differential Diagnosis

- <u>Antitrypsin deficiency panniculitis</u>
- <u>Erythema induratum</u>
- <u>Erythema nodosum</u>
- Factitial panniculitis
- <u>Infectious panniculitis</u>
- Lipodermatosclerosis
- Lupus panniculitis
- Mucormycosis
- Mycetoma
- Subcutaneous lymphoma
- Traumatic panniculitis

Evaluation

- Abdominal CT scan
- Amylase level
- Calcium level
- Chest radiograph
- Complete blood count
- Joint-fluid examination
- Lipase level
- Liver function test
- Renal function test

Treatment Options

- Treat the underlying cause

Further reading:
- Requena L, Sanchez Yus E (2001) Panniculitis. Part II. Mostly lobular panniculitis. J Am Acad Dermatol 45(3):325–361

Panniculitis, Poststeroid

Uncommon type of panniculitis that predominantly affects children shortly after rapid withdrawal of systemic glucocorticosteroids and is characterized by indurated erythematous subcutaneous nodules on the adipose-rich areas of the body, especially the cheeks

Differential Diagnosis

- Atopic dermatitis
- Cellulitis/erysipelas
- Cold panniculitis
- Erythema infectiosum
- Erythema nodosum
- Lupus erythematosus
- Periapical dental abscess
- Sclerema neonatorum
- Subcutaneous fat necrosis of the newborn

Further reading:
- Requena L, Sanchez Yus E (2001) Panniculitis. Part II. Mostly lobular panniculitis. J Am Acad Dermatol 45(3):325–361

Papular and Purpuric Gloves and Stockings Syndrome

Cutaneous manifestation of viral infection, especially parvovirus infection, that typically affects young, healthy adults and is characterized by a sharply marginated eruption of edema, erythematous papules, and petechiae on the hands and feet

Differential Diagnosis

- Contact dermatitis
- Erythema multiforme

- Erythromelalgia
- Gianotti–Crosti syndrome
- Kawasaki disease
- <u>Hand–foot–mouth syndrome</u>
- Lichen planus
- Psoriasis
- Rocky Mountain spotted fever

Treatment Options

- Observation and reassurance

Further reading:
- Carlesimo M, Palese E, Mari E et al (2006) Gloves and socks syndrome caused by parvovirus B19 infection. Dermatol Online J 12(6):19

Papular Elastorrhexis

Uncommon, idiopathic disorder of elastic tissue that is characterized by the development in adolescence of multiple, white, firm, nonfollicular papules on the trunk and extremities (a variant of papular elastorrhexis that is localized to the trunk is called nevus anelasticus)

Differential Diagnosis

- Anetoderma
- Collagenomas
- Idiopathic guttate hypomelanosis
- Middermal elastolysis
- <u>Papular acne scars (perifollicular elastolysis)</u>

Further reading:
- Choi Y, Jin SY, Lee JH et al (2011) Papular elastorrhexis: a case and differential diagnosis. Ann Dermatol 23 Suppl 1:S53–S56

Papular Urticaria

Pruritic hypersensitivity reaction to arthropod bites that predominantly affects atopic children and is characterized by erythematous, excoriated, and impetiginized papules and nodules that are most commonly located on the lower extremity

Differential Diagnosis

- Atopic dermatitis
- Autosensitization dermatitis
- Dermatitis herpetiformis
- Drug eruption
- Furunculosis
- Gianotti–Crosti syndrome
- Grover's disease
- Id reaction
- Impetigo
- Lymphomatoid papulosis
- Mastocytosis
- Pityriasis lichenoides et varioliformis acuta
- Prurigo nodularis
- Pruritic papular eruption of HIV
- Scabies
- Urticaria
- Varicella

Treatment Options

- Topical corticosteroids
- Tacrolimus ointment
- Antihistamines
- Menthol, camphor, and pramoxine lotions
- Insect repellants

Further reading:

- Stibich AS, Schwartz RA (2001) Papular urticaria. Cutis 68(2):89–91

Papuloerythroderma of Ofuji

Rare disease affecting older men, especially those of Asian descent, that is possibly a precursor to cutaneous T cell lymphoma and that is characterized by widespread pruritic, erythematous papules and plaques with sparing the folds of the trunk (deck-chair sign)

Differential Diagnosis

- Atopic dermatitis
- Bullous pemphigoid
- Contact dermatitis
- Cutaneous lymphoid hyperplasia
- Cutaneous T cell lymphoma
- Dermatitis herpetiformis
- Drug eruption
- Grover's disease
- Hypereosinophilic syndrome
- Idiopathic erythroderma
- Pityriasis rubra pilaris
- Prurigo
- Psoriasis
- Scabies
- Urticarial dermatitis

Treatment Options

- Topical corticosteroids
- Systemic corticosteroids
- Acitretin

- Phototherapy
- Cyclosporine

Further reading:
- Martinez-Barranca ML, Munoz-Perez MA, Garcia-Morales I et al (2005) Ofuji papuloerythroderma evolving to cutaneous T-cell lymphoma. J Eur Acad Dermatol Venereol 19(1):104–106

Papulonecrotic Tuberculid

Type of tuberculid affecting patients with active tuberculosis that is characterized by recurrent crops of asymptomatic, erythematous, necrotic papules affecting the extensor extremities and resolving to varioliform scars

Differential Diagnosis

- Churg–Strauss granuloma
- Drug reaction
- Endocarditis
- Erythema multiforme
- Leukocytoclastic vasculitis
- Lymphomatoid papulosis
- Miliary tuberculosis
- Papular eczema
- Papular urticaria
- Perforating granuloma annulare
- Pityriasis lichenoides et varioliformis acuta
- Prurigo nodularis
- Reactive perforating collagenosis
- Secondary syphilis

Further reading:
- Akhras V, McCarthy G (2007) Papulonecrotic tuberculid in an HIV-positive patient. Int J STD AIDS 18(9):643–644

Paracoccidioidomycosis
(South American Blastomycosis, Lutz Disease)

Respiratory mycosis with secondary dissemination to the skin that predominantly affects men, is caused by *Paracoccidioides brasiliensis*, and is characterized by lymphadenopathy and erythematous ulcerated papules and nodules on mucocutaneous surfaces, especially on the gingiva, tongue, lips, and nose

Differential Diagnosis

- Actinomycosis
- Blastomycosis
- Coccidioidomycosis
- Histoplasmosis
- Hodgkin's disease
- Mucocutaneous leishmaniasis
- NK cell lymphoma
- Oral squamous cell carcinoma
- Rhinoscleroma
- Rhinosporidiosis
- Sporotrichosis
- Syphilis
- Tuberculosis
- Wegener's granulomatosis

Evaluation

- Chest radiograph
- Fungal culture
- Potassium hydroxide examination of lesional tissue
- Serologic immunodiffusion assay for antibodies

Further reading:
- Lupi O, Tyring SK, McGinnis MR (2005) Tropical dermatology: fungal tropical diseases. J Am Acad Dermatol 53(6):931–951

Parakeratosis Pustulosa

Nail disorder with uncertain association to psoriasis, eczema, and other inflammatory skin diseases that predominantly affects one or multiple digits of the hands and feet of young children and is characterized by nontender, erythematous, periungual changes with fine scale, onycholysis, and onychorrhexis

Differential Diagnosis

- <u>Acrodermatitis continua</u>
- Acrodermatitis enteropathica
- Atopic dermatitis
- Blistering distal dactylitis
- Chronic mucocutaneous candidiasis
- Dermatophytosis
- Ectodermal dysplasia
- Epidermolysis bullosa
- Herpetic whitlow
- Kawasaki disease
- Langerhans cell histiocytosis
- Lichen nitidus
- Lichen planus
- Lichen striatus
- Onychophagia
- Paronychia
- <u>Psoriasis</u>

Treatment Options

- <u>Topical corticosteroids</u>
- Topical retinoids
- Topical vitamin D analogues
- Tacrolimus ointment

Further reading:

- Pandhi D, Chowdhry S, Grover C et al (2003) Parakeratosis pustulosa: a distinct but less familiar disease. Indian J Dermatol Venereol Leprol 69(1):48–50

Paraneoplastic Pemphigus (Paraneoplastic Autoimmune Multiorgan Syndrome)

Paraneoplastic autoimmune blistering disease that is caused by autoantibodies directed against several different epidermal and basement membrane zone antigens and is characterized by intractable stomatitis and a polymorphous lichenoid, bullous, or erythrodermatous eruption

Differential Diagnosis

- Bullous pemphigoid
- Candidiasis
- Chemotherapy-related stomatitis
- Cicatricial pemphigoid
- Epidermolysis bullosa acquisita
- Erythema multiforme
- Graft-vs-host disease
- Lichen planus
- Lichenoid drug eruption
- Pemphigus vulgaris
- Persistent herpes simplex virus infection
- Stevens–Johnson syndrome

Diagnostic Criteria

- Painful progressive stomatitis with preferential tongue involvement
- Histologic features of acantholysis, lichenoid, or interface dermatitis

- Demonstration of antiplakin antibodies
- Demonstration of underlying lymphoproliferative disorder

Associations

- Bronchogenic squamous cell carcinoma
- Castleman's disease
- <u>Chronic lymphocytic leukemia</u>
- Liposarcoma
- <u>Non-Hodgkin's lymphoma</u>
- Sarcoma
- Thymoma
- Waldenstrom's macroglobulinemia

Evaluation

- Appropriate cancer screening
- Chemistry panel
- Complete blood count
- CT scan of chest, abdomen, and pelvis
- Direct immunofluorescence
- Indirect immunofluorescence on monkey esophagus and rat bladder
- Lymph node exam
- Serum protein electrophoresis

Treatment Options

- Treat the underlying cause

Further reading:

- Park GT, Lee JH, Yun SJ et al (2007) Paraneoplastic pemphigus without an underlying neoplasm. Br J Dermatol 156(3):563–566

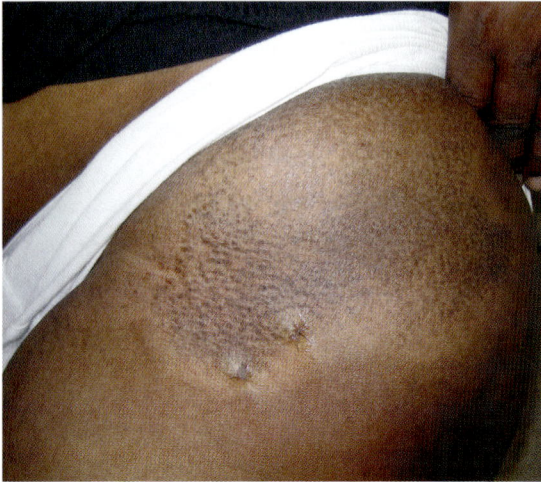

Fig. 6.90 Large plaque parapsoriasis

Parapsoriasis, Large Plaque

Chronic inflammatory skin disease affecting older adults that may represent a precursor to cutaneous T cell lymphoma and is characterized by large scaly, atrophic, or poikilodermatous plaques on the lower trunk, buttocks, and proximal lower extremities (Fig. 6.90)

Differential Diagnosis

- Chronic radiation dermatitis
- Contact dermatitis
- Dermatomyositis
- Dermatophytosis
- Lupus erythematosus
- Lichen planus
- <u>Mycosis fungoides</u>
- <u>Nummular eczema</u>
- Poikilodermatous genodermatoses
- Pityriasis rosea

- Psoriasis
- Seborrheic dermatitis
- Small plaque parapsoriasis
- Syphilis
- <u>Topical steroid atrophy</u>

Treatment Options

- Topical corticosteroids
- <u>Narrowband UVB</u>
- Topical nitrogen mustard

Further reading:

- Vakeva L, Sarna S, Vaalasti A et al (2005) A retrospective study of the probability of the evolution of parapsoriasis en plaques into mycosis fungoides. Acta Derm Venereol 85(4):318–323

Parapsoriasis, Small Plaque

Idiopathic, benign inflammatory skin disease with no potential to progress to cutaneous T cell lymphoma that is characterized by pink, often digitate, finely scaly plaques on the trunk (especially the flanks) and extremities

Differential Diagnosis

- Contact dermatitis
- Leprosy
- Lichen planus
- Lupus erythematosus
- Mycosis fungoides
- <u>Nummular eczema</u>
- Pityriasis alba
- <u>Pityriasis rosea</u>

- Pityriasis-rosea-like drug eruption
- Psoriasis
- Secondary syphilis
- Tinea versicolor
- Xerosis

Treatment Options

- Topical corticosteroids
- <u>Narrowband UVB</u>

Further reading:
- Aydogan K, Karadogan SK, Tunali S et al (2006) Narrowband UVB phototherapy for small plaque parapsoriasis. J Eur Acad Dermatol Venereol 20(5):573–577

Paronychia

Acute or chronic inflammatory process affecting the proximal and/or lateral nail folds that is most often caused by an acute staphylococcal infection or a chronic *Candida* superinfection (after cuticular separation from the nail plate) and is characterized by pain, swelling, purulent material, and thickening of the nail fold

Differential Diagnosis

- <u>Acrodermatitis continua</u>
- Acrodermatitis enteropathica
- Acrokeratosis paraneoplastica
- Aggressive digital papillary adenocarcinoma
- Bowen's disease
- Herpetic whitlow
- Hypoparathyroidism
- Indinavir therapy
- <u>Irritant contact dermatitis</u>

- Keratoacanthoma
- Leukemia cutis
- Onychomycosis
- Parakeratosis pustulosa
- Pemphigus vulgaris
- Periungual melanoma
- Periungual metastasis
- Psoriatic nail disease
- Reiter syndrome
- Retinoid therapy
- Squamous cell carcinoma
- Syphilitic chancre
- Tuberculosis
- Verrucous carcinoma

Treatment Options

- Incision and drainage (acute)
- Topical antibiotics
- Systemic antibiotics
- Topical corticosteroids (chronic)
- Nystatin
- Fluconazole (chronic)
- Thymol in chloroform

Further reading:
- Luther J, Glesby MJ (2007) Dermatologic adverse effects of antiretroviral therapy: recognition and management. Am J Clin Dermatol 8(4):221–233

Paroxysmal Nocturnal Hemoglobinuria

Rare stem-cell disorder associated with hemolytic anemia, hypercoagulability, and bone marrow failure that has uncommon cutaneous manifestations, including pyoderma-gangrenosum-like lesions and hemorrhagic bullae

Differential Diagnosis

- Cryoglobulinemia
- Felty syndrome
- Leukemia cutis
- Lymphoma
- Polyarteritis nodosa
- Purpura fulminans
- <u>Pyoderma gangrenosum</u>
- Septic vasculitis
- Sweet's syndrome
- Wegener's granulomatosis

Further reading:
- White JM, Watson K, Arya R et al (2003) Haemorrhagic bullae in a case of paroxysmal nocturnal haemoglobinuria. Clin Exp Dermatol 28(5):504–505

Pearly Penile Papules

Benign penile angiofibromas that are characterized by a row of pearly, smooth dome-shaped papules on the coronal sulcus of the penis

Differential Diagnosis

- <u>Condyloma acuminata</u>
- Lichen nitidus
- Lichen planus
- Molluscum contagiosum
- Papular mucinosis
- Scabies

Further reading:
- Agrawal SK, Bhattacharya SN, Singh N (2004) Pearly penile papules: a review. Int J Dermatol 43(3):199–201

Pediculosis Capitis

Infestation of scalp hair that predominantly affects children, is caused by *Pediculus humanus* var. *capitis,* and is characterized by nits attached to the hair follicles, scalp pruritus, and, occasionally, an associated id reaction

Differential Diagnosis

- Acne keloidalis
- Delusions of parasitosis
- Folliculitis decalvans
- Hair casts
- Impetigo
- Piedra
- Pityriasis amiantacea
- Plica polonica
- Psoriasis
- Scalp dysesthesia
- Seborrheic dermatitis
- Tinea capitis

Treatment Options

- Topical permethrin 1% and 5%
- Malathion lotion
- Lindane shampoo
- Ivermectin
- Sulfamethoxazole–trimethoprim
- Benzyl alcohol 5% lotion
- Carbaryl shampoo
- Spinosad

Further reading:
- Ko CJ, Elston DM (2004) Pediculosis. J Am Acad Dermatol 50(1):1–12

Pediculosis Corporis/Pubis

Infestation of the body or pubic area caused by *Pediculus humanus var corporis* or the sexually transmitted *Phthirus pubis,* respectively, that is characterized by macula cerulea, excoriations, nits on the pubic hair, eyelashes, clothing, and bedding

Differential Diagnosis

- <u>Delusions of parasitosis</u>
- Drug reaction
- Ephelid
- <u>Formication</u>
- Hair casts
- Irritant dermatitis
- Neurodermatitis
- Pigmented purpuric dermatosis
- <u>Scabies</u>
- Trichomycosis axillaris

Associations

- Epidemic typhus
- Id reaction
- Relapsing fever
- Trench fever

Treatment Options

- <u>Laundering of all clothing and bedsheets (body lice)</u>
- <u>Topical permethrin 1% and 5%</u>
- <u>Malathion lotion</u>
- Lindane shampoo

- Ivermectin
- Sulfamethoxazole–trimethoprim
- <u>Benzyl alcohol 5% lotion</u>
- Carbaryl shampoo
- Spinosad

Further reading:
- Ko CJ, Elston DM (2004) Pediculosis. J Am Acad Dermatol 50(1):1–12

Peeling Skin Syndrome

Rare, life-long keratinization disorder (probably AR) with onset at birth or early childhood that is characterized by asymptomatic, spontaneous intracorneal or subcorneal, nonvesicular peeling without inflammation (type A) or with inflammation (type B) in a generalized distribution or, less commonly, in an acral or facial distribution

Differential Diagnosis

- Bullous mastocytosis
- Collodion baby
- <u>Nonbulloua congenital ichthyosiform erythroderma</u>
- <u>Epidermolysis bullosa simplex (especially superficialis type)</u>
- Kawasaki disease
- <u>Ichthyosis bullosa of Siemens</u>
- Viral infections
- Netherton syndrome
- Scarlet fever
- Staphylococcal scalded-skin syndrome
- Sunburn

Further reading:
- Janjua SA, Hussain I, Khachemoune A (2007) Facial peeling skin syndrome: a case report and a brief review. Int J Dermatol 46(3):287–289

Pellagra

Potentially fatal disorder associated with a variety of causes of niacin deficiency that is characterized by a photodistributed, hyperpigmented, scaly eruption around the neck (Casal's necklace), face, and arms along with dementia and diarrhea

Differential Diagnosis

- Chronic actinic dermatitis
- Contact dermatitis
- Erythropoietic protoporphyria
- Hartnup syndrome
- Kwashiorkor
- Lupus erythematosus
- Pemphigus erythematosus
- Porphyria cutanea tarda
- Photosensitive drug reaction
- Polymorphous light eruption
- Seborrheic dermatitis
- Variegate porphyria

Associations

- 6MP/Azathioprine
- Alcoholism
- Anorexia nervosa
- Carcinoid syndrome
- Corn-rich diet
- Niacin deficiency
- Gastrointestinal diseases
- Hartnup disease
- Isoniazid

- Pyridoxine deficiency
- Total parenteral nutrition

Evaluation

- Complete blood count
- Liver function test
- Serum niacin and tryptophan levels
- Urinary 5-HIAA

Further reading:

- Hegyi J, Schwartz RA, Hegyi V (2004) Pellagra: dermatitis, dementia, and diarrhea. Int J Dermatol 43(1):1–5

Pemphigoid, Bullous

Subepidermal autoimmune blistering disorder caused by the production of antibodies against BPAgs1 and 2 that affects the elderly most commonly and is characterized by pruritic urticarial skin lesions and tense inflammatory bullae located on the lower trunk, flexures, and proximal extremities

Subtypes/Variants

- Childhood
- Cicatricial
- Dyshidrosiform
- Erythrodermic
- Gestational
- Nonbullous
- Pemphigoid nodularis
- Pemphigoid vegetans
- Polymorphic
- Pretibial
- Seborrheic
- Vulvar

Differential Diagnosis

- Arthropod-bite reaction
- <u>Bullous drug reaction</u>
- Bullous impetigo
- Bullous mastocytosis
- <u>Cicatricial pemphigoid</u>
- <u>Contact dermatitis</u>
- <u>Drug reaction</u>
- Epidermolysis bullosa acquisita
- Erythema multiforme
- <u>Linear IgA bullous dermatosis</u>
- Pemphigoid gestationis
- Porphyria cutanea tarda
- Pompholyx
- Prurigo simplex
- Pseudoporphyria
- <u>Scabies</u>
- <u>Urticaria</u>
- Urticarial vasculitis
- Vasculitis

Associated Medications

- ACE inhibitors
- Amiodarone
- Benzodiazepines
- Furosemide
- Influenza vaccine
- Nalidixic Acid
- NSAIDs
- Penicillin
- Penicillamine
- Sulfasalazine

Evaluation

- Direct immunofluorescence

Treatment Options

- Topical corticosteroids
- Systemic corticosteroids
- Tetracycline
- Nicotinamide
- Dapsone
- Azathioprine
- Mycophenolate mofetil
- Methotrexate
- Cyclophosphamide
- Cyclosporine
- Plasmapheresis
- Intravenous immunoglobulin

Further reading:
- Lamb PM, Abell E, Tharp M et al (2006) Prodromal bullous pemphigoid. Int J Dermatol 45(3):209–214

Pemphigoid, Cicatricial (Mucosal Pemphigoid, Lortat–Jacob Disease)

Scarring type of autoimmune blistering disease affecting predominantly the elderly that is caused by the production of autoantibodies against one of several basement membrane proteins and that is characterized by subepidermal blister formation involving mostly mucosal surfaces, which leads to oral or genital erosions, desquamative gingivitis, synechiae, and symblepharon

Subtypes/Variants

- Ocular type
- Localized (Brunsting–Perry) type
- Antiepiligrin (antilaminin 5, malignancy-associated) type

Differential Diagnosis

- Angina bullosa hemorrhagica
- Bullous pemphigoid
- Infectious conjunctivitis
- Epidermolysis bullosa acquisita
- Erosive lichen planus
- Erythema multiforme
- Linear IgA bullous dermatosis
- Ocular pseudopemphigoid (drug-induced)
- Ophthalmic zoster
- Paraneoplastic pemphigus
- Pemphigus vulgaris
- Stevens–Johnson syndrome

Associated Medications

- Timolol

Evaluation

- Direct immunofluorescence
- Indirect immunofluorescence (with salt split skin)
- Appropriate cancer screening (especially if antiepilegrin)

Treatment Options

- Systemic corticosteroids
- Dapsone

- Azathioprine
- Mycophenolate mofetil
- <u>Cyclophosphamide</u>
- Rituximab
- Plasmapheresis
- Intravenous immunoglobulin

Further reading:

- Chan LS, Ahmed AR, Anhalt GJ (2002) The first international consensus on mucous membrane pemphigoid: definition, diagnostic criteria, pathogenic factors, medical treatment, and prognostic indicators. Arch Dermatol 138(3):370–379

Pemphigoid Gestationis

Subepidermal autoimmune blistering disease associated with pregnancy that is caused by autoantibodies directed against BPAg2 and is characterized by pruritic urticarial plaques and tense bullae most commonly located on the abdomen (including the umbilicus)

Differential Diagnosis

- Allergic contact dermatitis
- Autoimmune progesterone dermatitis
- Bullous scabies
- <u>Cholestasis of pregnancy</u>
- Dermatitis herpetiformis
- Drug eruption
- <u>Erythema multiforme</u>
- Herpes simplex virus infection
- Impetigo herpetiformis
- Linear IgA bullous dermatosis
- Prurigo of pregnancy
- <u>Pruritic urticarial papules and plaques of pregnancy</u>
- <u>Urticaria</u>

Associations

- Graves' disease

Evaluation

- Complete blood count
- Direct immunofluorescence
- Indirect immunofluorescence
- Thyroid function tests

Treatment Options

- Topical corticosteroids
- <u>Systemic corticosteroids</u>
- Antihistamines
- Dapsone
- Cyclophosphamide
- Cyclosporine
- Plasmapheresis
- Intravenous immunoglobulin

Further reading:
- Al-Fouzan AW, Galadari I, Oumeish I et al (2006) Herpes gestationis (pemphigoid gestationis). Clin Dermatol 24(2):109–112

Pemphigus

Family of intraepidermal autoimmune blistering diseases of which there are several different types with variable clinical features depending on the epidermal antigen targeted

Subtypes/Variants

- Drug-induced pemphigus
- IgA pemphigus

- Paraneoplastic pemphigus
- Pemphigus erythematosus
- Pemphigus foliaceus
- Pemphigus herpetiformis
- Pemphigus vegetans
- Pemphigus vulgaris

Associations

- Foods
- Hormones
- Infectious agents
- Malignancy
- Medications
- Pesticides
- Stress
- Thymoma
- Ultraviolet light

Associated Medications

- ACE inhibitors (especially captopril)
- Beta-blockers
- Heroin
- IL-2
- Penicillamine
- Penicillin
- Progesterone
- Rifampin
- Sulfa drugs

Evaluation

- Direct immunofluorescence
- Indirect immunofluorescence

- Antidesmoglein antibody titers
- Chest radiograph

Treatment Options

- Topical corticosteroids
- Systemic corticosteroids
- Azathioprine
- Mycophenolate mofetil
- Methotrexate
- Cyclophosphamide
- Rituximab
- Plasmapheresis
- Intravenous immunoglobulin

Further reading:

- Brenner S, Mashiah J, Tamir E et al (2003) PEMPHIGUS: an acronym for a disease with multiple etiologies. Skinmed 2(3):163–167
- Grando SA (2006) Pemphigus in the XXI century: new life to an old story. Autoimmunity 39(7):521–530

Pemphigus Erythematosus (Senear–Usher Syndrome)

Type of sunlight-associated pemphigus that is caused by IgG autoantibodies directed against desmoglein 1 and is characterized by flaccid vesiculobullous lesions and crusts on the malar portion of the face, the chest, and the back (Fig. 6.91)

Differential Diagnosis

- Acute lupus erythematosus
- Chronic actinic dermatitis
- Pellagra
- Pemphigus foliaceus

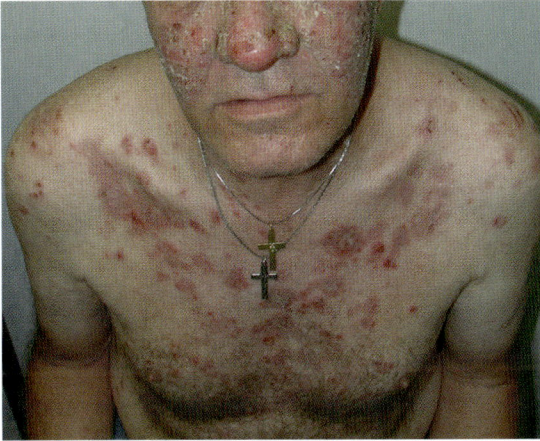

Fig. 6.91 Pemphigus erythematosus (Courtesy of K. Guidry)

- Photocontact dermatitis
- Photosensitive drug reaction
- Rosacea
- Subacute lupus erythematosus
- Seborrheic dermatitis

Evaluation/Treatment Options

- See "Pemphigus"

Further reading:

- Scheinfeld NS, Howe KL, di Costanzo DP et al (2003) Pemphigus erythematosus associated with anti-DNA antibodies and multiple anti-ENA antibodies: a case report. Cutis 71(4):303–306

Pemphigus Foliaceus (Cazenave's Disease)

Type of pemphigus that is caused by IgG autoantibodies against desmoglein 1 and is characterized by flaccid vesiculobullous lesions and crusts primarily on the scalp, face, upper chest, and upper back

Differential Diagnosis

- Bullous impetigo
- Contact dermatitis
- Darier's disease
- Dermatitis herpetiformis
- Dermatophytosis
- Erythema multiforme
- Exfoliative erythroderma
- Friction blister
- Fogo selvagem
- Grover's disease
- Hailey–Hailey disease
- IgA pemphigus
- Impetiginized dermatitis
- Lupus erythematosus
- Linear IgA dermatosis
- Necrolytic migratory erythema
- Nummular eczema
- Pemphigus erythematosus
- Pemphigus vulgaris
- Seborrheic dermatitis
- Subcorneal pustular dermatosis
- Staphylococcal scalded-skin syndrome

Evaluation/Treatment Options

- See "Pemphigus"

Further reading:
- Zaraa I, Mokni M, Hsairi M et al (2007) Pemphigus vulgaris and pemphigus foliaceus: similar prognosis? Int J Dermatol 46(9):923–926

Pemphigus, IgA

Type of pemphigus that is caused by IgA autoantibodies directed against desmocollin 1 (SPD type) or desmoglein 1 or 3 (IEN type) and is characterized by flaccid vesiculopustules [occasionally in a sunflower configuration (IEN type)] on the scalp, trunk, and extremities

Subtypes/Variants

- Intraepidermal neutrophilic (IEN) type
- Subcorneal pustular dermatosis (SPD) type

Differential Diagnosis

- Acute generalized exanthematous pustulosis
- Bullous impetigo
- Paraneoplastic pemphigus
- Pemphigus foliaceus
- Pemphigus herpetiformis
- Pemphigus vulgaris
- Pustular psoriasis
- Subcorneal pustular dermatosis

Associations

- IgA monoclonal gammopathy
- Pyoderma gangrenosum

Evaluation/Treatment Options

- See "Pemphigus"
- Serum protein electrophoresis
- Immunoglobulin levels

Further reading:

- Aste N, Fumo G, Pinna AL et al (2003) IgA pemphigus of the subcorneal pustular dermatosis type associated with monoclonal iga gammopathy. J Eur Acad Dermatol Venereol 17(6):725–727

Pemphigus Vegetans

Type of pemphigus caused by IgG autoantibodies directed against desmoglein 3 that is characterized by moist, vegetating, eroded plaques most commonly in the flexural areas

Differential Diagnosis

- Acute generalized exanthematous pustulosis
- Axillary granular parakeratosis
- Blastomycosis
- Botryomycosis
- Chromoblastomycosis
- Condyloma lata
- Darier's disease
- Granuloma inguinale
- Hailey–Hailey disease
- Halogenoderma
- Subcorneal pustular dermatosis

Evaluation/Treatment Options

- See "Pemphigus"

Further reading:

- Markopoulos AK, Antoniades DZ, Zaraboukas T (2006) Pemphigus vegetans of the oral cavity. Int J Dermatol 45(4):425–428

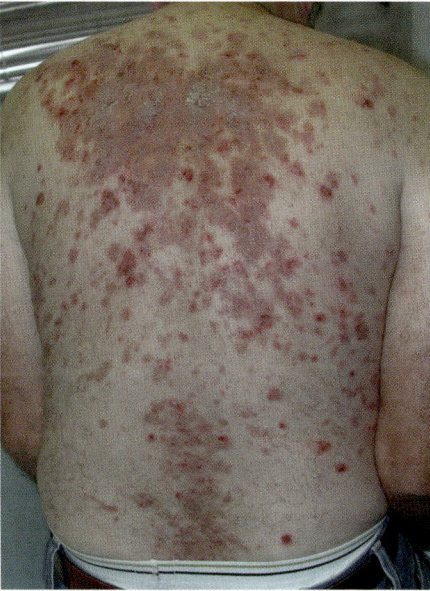

Fig. 6.92 Pemphigus vulgaris
(Courtesy of K. Guidry)

Pemphigus Vulgaris

Type of pemphigus caused by IgG autoantibodies directed against desmogleins 1 and 3 that is characterized by erosions arising in the mucosal areas with or without skin involvement; when the skin is involved, flaccid vesiculobullous lesions occur on the scalp, trunk, and intertriginous areas (Fig. 6.92)

Differential Diagnosis

- Acute herpetic stomatitis
- Aphthous stomatitis
- Bullous pemphigoid
- Cicatricial pemphigoid
- Drug-induced pemphigus

- Erythema multiforme
- Grover's disease
- <u>Hailey–Hailey disease</u>
- Linear IgA dermatosis
- <u>Oral erosive lichen planus</u>
- Paraneoplastic pemphigus
- <u>Pemphigus foliaceus</u>
- Stevens–Johnson syndrome

Associations

- Myasthenia gravis
- Thymoma

Evaluation/Treatment Options

- See "Pemphigus"

Further reading:
- Espana A, Fernandez S, del Olmo J et al (2007) Ear, nose and throat manifestations in pemphigus vulgaris. Br J Dermatol 156(4):733–737

Perforating Calcific Elastosis (Periumbilical Pseudoxanthoma Elasticum)

Acquired elastic tissue disorder affecting primarily obese, multiparous women that is characterized by periumbilical, yellow, reticulated, keratotic papules that can be confluent in cobblestone-like plaques

Differential Diagnosis

- Acquired perforating dermatosis
- <u>Calcinosis cutis</u>
- Elastosis perforans serpiginosa

- <u>Eruptive xanthomas</u>
- Nodular scabies
- Perforating granuloma annulare
- <u>Prurigo nodularis</u>
- Pseudoxanthoma elasticum
- Reactive perforating collagenosis

Further reading:
- Lopes LC, Lobo L, Bajanca R (2003) Perforating calcific elastosis. J Eur Acad Dermatol Venereol 17(2):206–207

Perforating Dermatosis, Acquired

Collective term that refers to a group of perforating disorders that are characterized by folliculocentric, hyperkeratotic papules or nodules with a predilection for extensor surfaces that are possibly self-induced in the setting of pruritus of chronic renal failure

Differential Diagnosis

- Acne
- Elastosis perforans serpiginosa
- Familial dyskeratotic comedones
- <u>Folliculitis</u>
- Insect-bite reaction
- Perforating granuloma annulare
- Perforating pseudoxanthoma elasticum
- Pseudofolliculitis barbae
- <u>Prurigo nodularis</u>
- Reactive perforating collagenosis

Associations

- Herpes zoster healed areas
- HIV infection

- Hyperparathyroidism
- Hypothyroidism
- Liver disease
- Laser hair removal
- <u>Renal failure</u>
- Sclerosing cholangitis
- Xerosis

Evaluation

- Calcium and phosphorus level
- Fasting blood glucose
- Liver function test
- Parathyroid hormone level
- Renal function test
- Thyroid function test

Treatment Options

- <u>Antihistamines and itch control</u>
- <u>Narrowband UVB</u>
- Topical retinoids
- Systemic retinoids
- Cryosurgery
- Tetracycline antibiotics

Further reading:
- Saray Y, Seckin D, Bilezikci B (2006) Acquired perforating dermatosis: clinicopathological features in twenty-two cases. J Eur Acad Dermatol Venereol 20(6):679–688

Perioral Dermatitis

Idiopathic eruption and possible variant of rosacea that affects the face of women and occasionally children, may arise after application of topical steroids to the affected area, and is characterized by erythematous papules and pustules in a perioral (with an area of sparing around the lips) and/or periocular distribution and characteristic involvement of the nasolabial fold

Differential Diagnosis

- <u>Acne vulgaris</u>
- Allergic dermatitis
- Atopic dermatitis
- Contact dermatitis
- Demodicosis
- Haber syndrome
- Histoplasmosis
- Lupus erythematosus
- Lip-licker dermatitis
- Lupus miliaris disseminata faciei
- Lymphocytoma cutis
- Molluscum
- <u>Granulomatous periorificial dermatitis</u>
- <u>Rosacea</u>
- Sarcoidosis
- <u>Seborrheic dermatitis</u>
- Tinea faciei
- Verruca plana

Treatment Options

- Emollients
- Topical metronidazole
- Topical calcineurin inhibitors
- Topical clindamycin
- Topical erythromycin
- <u>Oral tetracycline antibiotics</u>
- Azithromycin

Further reading:
- Hafeez ZH (2003) Perioral dermatitis: an update. Int J Dermatol 42(7):514–517

Perniosis (Chilblains)

Vascular disorder affecting acral areas of the body that is triggered by cold exposure and characterized by tender or pruritic, erythematous papules and nodules most commonly on the fingers and toes

Differential Diagnosis

- Achenbach syndrome
- Acrocyanosis
- Acrokeratosis paraneoplastica
- Chilblains lupus erythematous
- Cold urticaria
- Contact urticaria
- Coumadin blue-toe syndrome
- Crack-cocaine abuse
- Cryofibrinogenemia
- Cryoglobulinemia
- Endocarditis
- Erythema multiforme
- Erythema nodosum
- Erythromelalgia
- Granuloma annulare
- Hemolytic anemia
- Leukemia cutis
- Lupus pernio
- Monoclonal gammopathy
- Nodular vasculitis
- Paronychia
- Polycythemia vera
- Raynaud's phenomenon

- Sarcoidosis
- Septic emboli
- <u>Vasculitis</u>

Associations

- Anorexia nervosa
- Antiphospholipid antibody syndrome
- Crack-cocaine abuse
- Leukemia
- Lupus erythematosus
- Oral contraceptive pills
- Paraproteinemia

Evaluation

- Antinuclear antibodies
- Anticardiolipin antibody test
- Lupus anticoagulant antibody
- Complete blood count
- Serum protein electrophoresis

Treatment Options

- Warming measures, such as gloves
- <u>Nifedipine</u>
- Topical corticosteroids
- Systemic corticosteroids
- Aspirin
- Pentoxifylline

Further reading:
- McCleskey PE, Winter KJ, Devillez RL (2006) Tender papules on the hands. Idiopathic chilblains (perniosis). Arch Dermatol 142(11):1501–1506

- Payne-James JJ, Munro MH, Rowland Payne CM (2007) Pseudosclerodermatous triad of perniosis, pulp atrophy and "parrot-beaked" clawing of the nails: a newly recognized syndrome of chronic crack cocaine use. J Forensic Leg Med 14(2):65–71

Peutz–Jeghers Syndrome

Inherited syndrome (AD) that is caused by mutation of the STK11 tumor suppressor gene and is characterized by perioral and intraoral hyperpigmented macules, hamartomatous polyps of the small intestine with intussusception and gastrointestinal bleeding, and an increased risk of colon cancer, pancreatic cancer, breast cancer, and several other visceral cancers

Differential Diagnosis

- Addison's disease
- Bannayan–Riley–Ruvulcaba syndrome
- Cowden syndrome
- Cronkhite–Canada syndrome
- Inherited patterned lentiginosis
- Juvenile polyposis syndrome
- Laugier–Hunziker syndrome
- Smoker's melanosis
- Turcot syndrome

Evaluation

- Breast exam/mammography
- Colonoscopy
- Complete blood count
- Contrast endoscopy with small bowel follow-through
- CT scan of abdomen and pelvis
- Iron studies

Further reading:
- Heymann WR (2007) Peutz–Jeghers syndrome. J Am Acad Dermatol 57(3):513–514

Peyronie's Disease

Fibrosing disorder of the penile shaft that affects middle-aged men, is possibly traumatic in etiology, and is characterized by erection-related pain, curvature of the penis, and a midline firm, fibrous plaque

Differential Diagnosis

- Balanitis xerotica obliterans
- Congenital penile curvature
- Dorsal vein thrombosis
- Leukemia cutis
- Lymphogranuloma venereum
- Penile fracture
- Scleroderma/morphea
- Sclerosing lymphangiitis
- Syphilis

Associations

- Diabetes mellitus
- Dupuytren's contracture
- Erectile dysfunction
- Knuckle pads
- Plantar fibromatosis
- Scleroderma

Treatment Options

- Surgery
- Colchicine
- Pentoxifylline
- NSAIDs
- Vitamin E

- Potaba
- L-carnitine
- Intralesional verapamil
- Intralesional interferon
- Tamoxifen

Further reading:
- Briganti A, Salonia A, Deho F et al (2003) Peyronie's disease: a review. Curr Opin Urol 13(5):417–422

Phaeohyphomycosis

Term for mycotic infection caused by one of several dematiaceous fungi (including *Exophiala jeanselmei*, *Alternaria*, *Bipolaris*, and *Curvularia*) that is most commonly characterized by a cyst-like trauma-related subcutaneous abscess in immunocompetent patients and CNS or disseminated disease in immunocompromised patients

Differential Diagnosis

- <u>Atypical mycobacterial infection</u>
- Chromoblastomycosis
- Cutaneous leishmaniasis
- <u>Epidermal cyst</u>
- Foreign body granuloma
- Invasive aspergillosis
- Lipoma
- Mycetoma
- Nodular fasciitis

Treatment Options

- Surgical excision

Further reading:

• Revankar SG (2006) Phaeohyphomycosis. Infect Dis Clin North Am 20(3):609–620

Phakomatosis Pigmentovascularis

Group of hamartomatous disorders associated with twin spotting that are characterized by the combination of a vascular lesion (either a port-wine stain (flammea), rose-colored vascular stain (rosea), or cutis marmorata telangiectatica congenita (marmorata)) and a pigmented lesion either mongolian spots (cesio = blue spot) or nevus spilus (spilo) and several other less consistent features

Differential Diagnosis

- Adams–Oliver syndrome
- Bannayan–Riley–Ruvulcaba syndrome
- Klippel–Trenaunay syndrome
- Phakomatosis pigmentokeratotica
- Proteus syndrome
- Sturge–Weber syndrome

Subtypes

New Classification
- Phakomatosis cesioflammea
- Phacomatosis spilorosa
- Phacomatosis cesiomarmorata

Old Classification
- Type I: nevus flammeus+epidermal nevus
- Type II: nevus flammeus+mongolian spots
- Type III: nevus flammeus+nevus spilus
- Type IV: nevus flammeus+nevus spilus+mongolian spots
- Type V: nevus flammeus+mongolian spots+cutis marmorata telangiectatica congenita

Associations

- Granular cell tumors (spilorosa)
- Klippel–Trenaunay syndrome
- Ocular anomalies
- Renal anomalies
- Scoliosis
- Seizures
- Sturge–Weber syndrome

Further reading:
- Happle R (2005) Phacomatosis pigmentovascularis revisited and reclassified. Arch Dermatol 141(3):385–388

Photosensitive Drug Reaction

Type of drug reaction induced by ultraviolet light that is caused by either phototoxicity (the drug or a metabolite is directly toxic after photoactivation) or photoallergy (type IV hypersensitivity reaction to a photoactivated hapten) that is characterized by a severe sunburn-like reaction (phototoxicity) or eczematous plaques on the sun-exposed areas (photoallergy)

Differential Diagnosis

- <u>Airborne contact dermatitis</u>
- Chronic actinic dermatitis
- Lichenoid drug eruption
- <u>Lupus erythematosus</u>
- Pellagra
- <u>Photoallergic contact dermatitis</u>
- Polymorphous light eruption
- Porphyria

Associated Medications

Photoallergy

- Antimalarials
- <u>Chlorpromazine</u>
- Enoxacin
- Gold
- Griseofulvin
- Ketoprofen
- NSAIDs
- Phenothiazines
- Promethazine
- Pyridoxine
- Quinidine
- <u>Sulfonamides</u>
- Tricyclic antidepressants

Phototoxicity

- Amiodarone
- Fluoroquinolones
- Furocoumarins
- Furosemide
- NSAIDS
- Phenothiazines
- Psoralens
- <u>Tetracyclines</u>

Further reading:
- Stein KR, Scheinfeld NS (2007) Drug-induced photoallergic and phototoxic reactions. Expert Opin Drug Saf 6(4):431–443

Phrynoderma

Cutaneous eruption that is now considered a nonspecific eruption of a variety of malnutrition-related deficiencies and is characterized by widespread xerosis along with numerous papules containing central keratin-filled plugs on the extensor aspects of the extremities, shoulders, and buttocks

Differential Diagnosis

- Acquired perforating dermatosis
- Darier's disease
- Familial dyskeratotic comedones
- Keratosis pilaris
- Lichen nitidus
- Lichen spinulosus
- Pityriasis rubra pilaris
- Scurvy

Associations

- Alcoholism
- Cholestasis
- Crohn's disease
- Cystic fibrosis
- Fat malabsorption
- Liver disease
- Measles
- Nutritional deficiency

Further reading:
- Heath ML, Sidbury R (2006) Cutaneous manifestations of nutritional deficiency. Curr Opin Pediatr 18(4):417–422

Piebaldism

Inherited pigmentary disorder (AD) that is caused by absence of melanocytes due to mutation of the c-kit proto-oncogene and is characterized by
a white forelock, depigmentation on the central chest and the middle portion of the arms and legs, with sparing of the back, and hyperpigmented
macules within the areas of depigmentation

Differential Diagnosis

- Albinism
- Chemical leukoderma
- Hypomelanosis of Ito
- Leprosy
- Nevus depigmentosus
- Onchocerciasis
- Pinta
- Pityriasis alba
- Tinea versicolor
- Vitiligo
- Vogt–Koyanagi–Harada syndrome
- Waardenburg syndrome
- Ziprkowski–Margolis syndrome

Evaluation

- Hearing test
- Ophthalmologic examination

Further reading:
- Hazan C (2005) Piebaldism. Dermatol Online J 11(4):18

Piedra (Beigel's Disease)

Fungal infection of the external portion of hair shaft that is caused by *Piedra hortae* (black piedra) or *Trichosporon asahii* (white piedra) that is characterized by black, hard, fixed nodules on the hair shafts of the scalp (black) or soft, white, less adherent nodules on the hair shafts of the axillary or pubic areas (white)

Differential Diagnosis

- Hair casts
- Monilethrix
- Pediculosis
- Psoriasis
- Seborrheic dermatitis
- Tinea capitis/corporis
- Trichomycosis axillaris
- Trichorrhexis nodosa

Treatment Options

- Removal of hair
- Terbinafine
- Selenium sulfide
- Itraconazole
- Ciclopirox

Further reading:
- Kiken DA, Sekaran A, Antaya RJ et al (2006) White piedra in children. J Am Acad Dermatol 55(6):956–961

Piezogenic Pedal Papules

Term for pressure-related fat herniations on the lateral aspects of the feet that are only noticeable while standing and characterized by occasionally tender, fleshy protuberant papules

Differential Diagnosis

- Cerebriform plantar collagenoma
- Fascial herniation
- Infantile pedal papules
- Nevus lipomatosus superficialis
- Plantar lipomas

Associations

- Ehlers–Danlos syndrome
- Obesity
- Pseudoxanthoma elasticum

Further reading:

- Redbord KP, Adams BB (2006) Piezogenic pedal papules in a marathon runner. Clin J Sport Med 16(1):81–83

Pigmented Purpuric Dermatosis (Benign Pigmented Purpura)

Group of purpuric disorders that are associated with capillaritis and that are characterized by purpuric lesions on the lower extremities with variable features, including occasional pruritus, eczematous changes, or cayenne pepper-like petechiae

Subtypes/Variants

- Eczematid-like purpura of Doucas and Kapetanakis (itchy purpura, disseminated pruriginous angiodermatitis)
- Granulomatous pigmented purpura
- Lichen aureus (Fig. 6.93)
- Pigmented purpuric lichenoid dermatosis of Gougerot and Blum
- Progressive pigmentary dermatosis (Schamberg's disease)
- Purpura annularis telangiectodes (Majocchi's disease)
- Unilateral linear capillaritis

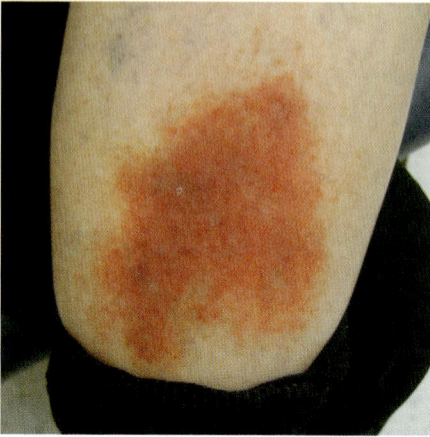

Fig. 6.93 Lichen aureus

Differential Diagnosis

- Acroangiodermatitis of Mali
- Angioma serpiginosum
- Benign hypergammaglobulinemic purpura of Waldenstrom
- Clotting disorders
- Cryoglobulinemia
- Exercise-related purpura
- Henoch–Schonlein purpura
- Kaposi's sarcoma
- Leukocytoclastic vasculitis
- Pigmented-purpuric-dermatosis-like mycosis fungoides
- Scurvy
- Stasis pigmentation
- Thrombocytopenia
- Purpuric contact dermatitis

Associations

- Drugs
- Exercise
- Venous stasis

Associated Medications

- Acetaminophen
- Captopril
- Carbamazepine
- Carbromal
- Carbutamide
- Chlordiazepoxide
- Furosemide
- Glipizide
- Medroxyprogesterone
- Nitroglycerin
- Thiamine

Treatment Options

- Rest
- <u>Vitamin C</u>
- Rutoside
- <u>Topical corticosteroids</u>
- Antihistamines
- Griseofulvin
- Narrowband UVB

Further reading:
- Magro CM, Schaefer JT, Crowson AN et al (2007) Pigmented purpuric dermatosis: classification by phenotypic and molecular profiles. Am J Clin Pathol 128(2):218–229

Pilar Cyst (Trichilemmal Cyst)

Common benign cyst that is derived from the outer root sheath and is characterized by an asymptomatic, firm subcutaneous nodule predominantly on the scalp

Differential Diagnosis

- Adnexal neoplasm
- Arteriovenous malformation
- Dermoid cyst
- Epidermal inclusion cyst
- Hematoma
- Lipoma
- Lymphadenopathy
- Metastatic lesion
- Osteoma
- Pilomatrixoma
- Subcutaneous neurofibroma
- Subcutaneous schwannoma

Further reading:

- Golden BA, Zide MF (2005) Cutaneous cysts of the head and neck. J Oral Maxillofac Surg 63(11):1613–1619

Pilar Tumor, Proliferating

Rare neoplasm derived from the outer root sheath that arises in a pilar cyst, is controversial with regard to its malignant potential, and is characterized by a rapidly growing, ulcerated nodule on the scalp

Differential Diagnosis

- Adnexal neoplasm
- Angiosarcoma
- Basal cell carcinoma
- Cylindroma
- Dermatofibrosarcoma protuberans
- Epidermoid cyst
- Lipoma
- Merkel cell carcinoma
- Metastasis
- Pilar cyst
- Squamous cell carcinoma

Further reading:
- Satyaprakash AK, Sheehan DJ, Sangueza OP (2007) Proliferating trichilemmal tumors: a review of the literature. Dermatol Surg 33(9):1102–1108

Pili Bifurcati

Hair-shaft abnormality characterized by the bifurcation of the hair shaft into two parts, each with its own cuticle, which rejoin into one shaft distally

Differential Diagnosis

- Pili multigemini
- Trichoptilosis

Further reading:
- Camacho FM, Happle R, Tosti A et al (2000) The different faces of pili bifurcati. A review. Eur J Dermatol 10(5):337–340

Pili Multigemini

Hair-shaft abnormality predominantly identified on the beard in men or on the scalp in children that is characterized by a matrix which is divided and gives rise to multiple hair shafts within a single follicle

Differential Diagnosis

- Ingrown hair
- Pili bifurcati
- Pseudofolliculitis barbae
- Trichofolliculoma
- Trichoptilosis
- Trichostasis spinulosa
- Tufted folliculitis

Further reading:
- Lester L, Venditti C (2007) The prevalence of pili multigemini. Br J Dermatol 156(6):1362–1363

Pili Torti

Hair-shaft abnormality associated with a variety of syndromes that is caused by twisting of the hair shaft on its own axis and is characterized by sparse, fragile hair and alopecia

Differential Diagnosis

- Menke's kinky-hair syndrome
- Monilethrix
- Uncombable hair syndrome
- Woolly hair

Associations

- Anorexia
- Bazex–Dupre–Christol syndrome
- Bjornstad's syndrome
- Citrullinemia
- Crandall's syndrome
- EEC syndrome
- Menkes syndrome
- Netherton's syndrome
- Pachyonychia congenita, type II
- Rapp–Hodgkin syndrome
- Retinoid therapy
- Trichothiodystrophy

Further reading:

- Richards KA, Mancini AJ (2002) Three members of a family with pili torti and sensorineural hearing loss: the Bjornstad syndrome. J Am Acad Dermatol 46(2):301–303

Pilomatricoma (Calcifying Epithelioma of Malherbe)

Benign neoplasm that predominantly affects children, is derived from the matrix of the hair follicle, and is characterized by a hard, calcified subcutaneous nodule most commonly on the face that reveals "tenting" upon stretching of the overlying skin

Differential Diagnosis

- Basal cell carcinoma
- Branchial cleft cyst
- Calcinosis cutis
- Cutaneous tuberculosis

- Dermatofibroma
- Dermatofibrosarcoma protuberans
- Epidermal inclusion cyst
- Foreign body granuloma
- Granuloma annulare
- Idiopathic facial aseptic granuloma
- Keratoacanthoma
- Merkel cell carcinoma
- Metastasis
- Osteoma cutis
- Sarcoidosis
- Schwannoma
- Subepidermal calcified nodule
- Trichilemmoma
- Trichoepithelioma

Associations

- Gardner syndrome
- Myotonic dystrophy
- Rubinstein–Taybi syndrome
- Turner syndrome

Further reading:

- Kumaran N, Azmy A, Carachi R et al (2006) Pilomatrixoma: accuracy of clinical diagnosis. J Pediatr Surg 41(10):1755–1758

Pilonidal Sinus/Cyst

Acquired cyst or sinus that is associated with the follicular occlusion triad, most commonly arises in the sacrococcygeal area, and is possibly caused by entry of hair shafts into the skin with subsequent foreign body reaction, deep abscess formation, and chronic sinus tract

Differential Diagnosis

- <u>Bacterial abscess</u>
- Crohn's disease
- Decubitus ulcer
- Dermoid cyst
- <u>Epidermal inclusion cyst</u>
- Fissure
- Hidradenitis suppurativa
- Pyogenic granuloma

Further reading:
- Hull TL, Wu J (2002) Pilonidal disease. Surg Clin North Am 82(6):1169–1185

Pinta

Treponemal infection caused by *Treponema pallidum carateum* in which there is a primary stage characterized by a solitary scaly plaque on the lower extremity that slowly expands and does not ulcerate, a secondary stage with an eruption of highly infectious, scaly psoriasiform papules called pintids, and a tertiary stage characterized by vitiligo-like hypopigmentation on the extremities

Differential Diagnosis

- Atrophic lichen planus
- Eczema
- <u>Endemic syphilis</u>
- Leprosy
- Lupus erythematosus
- Onchocerciasis
- Pityriasis alba
- Psoriasis
- Sclerodermal dyschromia

- Tinea corporis
- Tinea versicolor
- <u>Syphilis</u>
- <u>Vitiligo</u>
- Yaws

Further reading:
- Farnsworth N, Rosen T (2006) Endemic treponematosis: review and update. Clin Dermatol 24(3):181–190

Pitted Keratolysis

Superficial bacterial infection of the soles of the feet caused by *Kytococcus sedentarius* and characterized by shallow discrete and coalescent pits, hyperhidrosis, and malodor (Fig. 6.94)

Differential Diagnosis

- Arsenical keratoses
- Basal cell nevus syndrome
- Dyshidrotic eczema
- Essential hyperhidrosis
- Focal acral hypokeratosis
- Juvenile plantar dermatosis
- <u>Keratolysis exfoliativa</u>

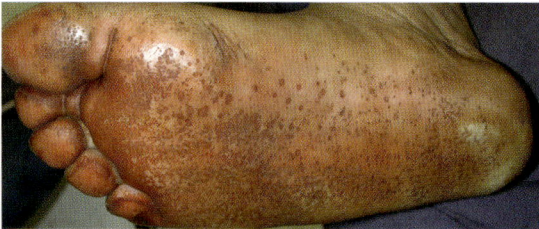

Fig. 6.94 Pitted keratolysis (Courtesy of K. Guidry)

- <u>Punctate palmoplantar keratoderma</u>
- Tinea pedis

Treatment Options

- <u>Topical clindamycin</u>
- Topical gentamycin
- Aluminum chloride
- Mupirocin cream
- Benzoyl peroxide
- Oral erythromycin

Further reading:

- Lee PL, Lemos B, O'Brien SH et al (2007) Cutaneous diphtheroid infection and review of other cutaneous Gram-positive *Bacillus* infections. Cutis 79(5):371–377

Pityriasis Alba

Dermatosis affecting children, especially atopics, that is likely a low-grade form of eczema and manifests as patchy hypopigmentation with or without fine scale on the cheeks, trunk, or upper arms

Differential Diagnosis

- Chemical leukoderma
- <u>Hypopigmented mycosis fungoides</u>
- Leprosy
- Nummular eczema
- Pityriasis lichenoides chronica
- Progressive macular hypomelanosis
- Psoriasis
- Seborrheic dermatitis
- Tinea corporis

- <u>Tinea versicolor</u>
- Vitiligo

Treatment Options

- <u>Emollients</u>
- Topical corticosteroids
- <u>Tacrolimus ointment</u>
- Narrowband UVB phototherapy
- Sun exposure

Further reading:
- Lin RL, Janniger CK (2005) Pityriasis alba. Cutis 76(1):21–24

Pityriasis Amiantacea (Tinea Amiantacea)

Scalp finding that occasionally accompanies psoriasis, seborrheic dermatitis, or tinea capitis, is caused by secondary infection, and is characterized by yellow-white crusts and scales that have matted and encased hairs

Differential Diagnosis

- Erosive pustular dermatosis
- Hair casts
- Favus
- Folliculitis decalvans
- <u>Impetigo</u>
- Pediculosis capitis
- Plica polonica/plica neuropathica

Evaluation

- Fungal culture
- Bacterial culture

Treatment Options

- Salicylic acid
- Urea
- Topical corticosteroids
- Topical antibiotics
- Systemic antibiotics
- Ketoconazole shampoo
- Terbinafine
- Ciclopirox

Further reading:

- Abdel-Hamid IA, Agha SA, Moustafa YM et al (2003) Pityriasis amiantacea: a clinical and etiopathologic study of 85 patients. Int J Dermatol 42(4):260–264

Pityriasis Lichenoides et Varioliformis Acuta (Mucha–Haberman Disease)

Acute form of pityriasis lichenoides that predominantly affects children and young adults; is characterized by crops of asymptomatic erythematous papules which evolve over a period of days to weeks to vesicular and hemorrhagic, crusted, scarring papules; and most commonly involves the trunk and extremities (Fig. 6.95)

Differential Diagnosis

- Arthropod-bite reactions
- Cutaneous small vessel vasculitis
- Dermatitis herpetiformis
- Drug eruption
- Erythema multiforme
- Folliculitis
- Gianotti–Crosti syndrome
- Hydroa vacciniforme

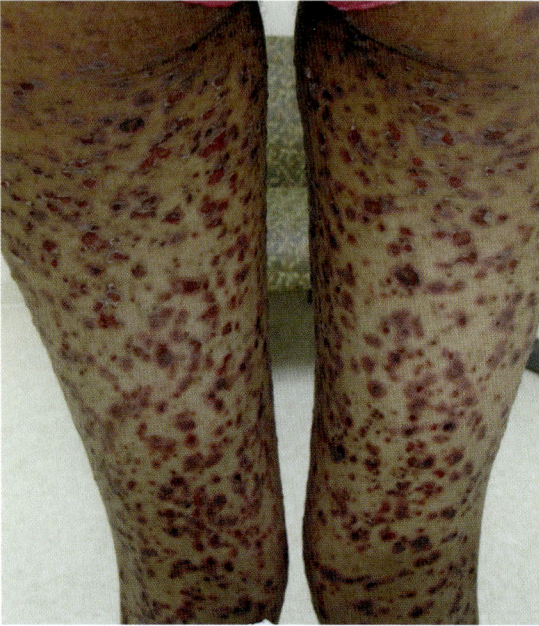

Fig. 6.95 Pityriasis lichenoides et varioliformis acuta

- Lupus erythematosus
- Lymphomatoid papulosis
- Papulonecrotic tuberculid
- Pityriasis rosea
- Scabies
- Secondary syphilis
- Varicella
- Viral exanthem

Associations

- EBV infection
- HIV infection
- Toxoplasmosis

Treatment Options

- <u>Oral tetracycline antibiotics</u>
- Oral erythromycin
- UVB phototherapy
- Systemic corticosteroids
- <u>Methotrexate</u>
- Acitretin
- Pentoxifylline
- Dapsone
- Cyclosporine

Further reading:

- Khachemoune A, Blyumin ML (2007) Pityriasis lichenoides: pathophysiology, classification, and treatment. Am J Clin Dermatol 8(1):29–36

Pityriasis Lichenoides Chronica

Persistent, chronic form of pityriasis lichenoides that predominantly affects adults; is characterized by superficial, pink-brown or hypopigmented, mildly pruritic, scaly papules and small plaques; and predominantly involves the trunk and proximal extremities

Differential Diagnosis

- Arthropod bites
- Drug eruption
- <u>Guttate psoriasis</u>
- Lupus erythematosus
- Lichen planus
- Lymphomatoid papulosis
- <u>Papular eczema</u>
- <u>Pityriasis rosea</u>
- Secondary syphilis

- Small plaque parapsoriasis
- Tinea corporis
- Viral exanthem

Treatment Options

- <u>UVB phototherapy</u>
- Tetracycline antibiotics
- Methotrexate
- Acitretin
- Cyclosporine

Further reading:
- Khachemoune A, Blyumin ML (2007) Pityriasis lichenoides: pathophysiology, classification, and treatment. Am J Clin Dermatol 8(1):29–36

Pityriasis Rosea (Gibert Disease)

Self-limited papulosquamous eruption that is probably viral in origin, predominantly affects adolescents and young adults, and is characterized first by a large oval erythematous macule with a peripheral collarette of scale (herald patch) and then a generalized eruption of erythematous scaly papules and plaques on the trunk (following skin lines in a Christmas-tree-like distribution) and extremities but rarely the face

Subtypes/Variants

- Cervicocephalic
- Circinate and confluent
- Classic
- Gigantea
- Herald patch absent
- Herald patch only
- Inverse

- Oral
- Papular
- Persistent (HIV-related)
- Purpuric
- Pustular
- Unilateral
- Urticarial
- Vesicular

Differential Diagnosis

- Disseminated contact dermatitis
- Drug eruption
- Erythema annulare centrifugum
- Erythema dyschromicum perstans
- Erythema multiforme
- Exfoliative dermatitis
- Gianotti–Crosti syndrome
- Guttate psoriasis
- Henoch–Schonlein purpura
- HIV exanthem
- Id reaction
- Leukemia (especially purpuric type)
- Lichen planus
- Lupus erythematosus
- Mycosis fungoides
- Nummular eczema
- Pityriasis lichenoides chronica
- Pityriasis-rosea-like drug eruption
- Purpura
- Scabies
- Seborrheic dermatitis
- Secondary syphilis
- Small plaque parapsoriasis

- <u>Tinea corporis</u>
- Tinea versicolor
- Viral exanthem

Associated Medications (PR-Like Drug Reaction)

- ACE inhibitors
- Barbiturates
- Beta-blockers
- Clonidine
- D-penicillamine
- Gold
- Griseofulvin
- Imatinib mesylate
- Isotretinoin
- Metronidazole
- Omeprazole

Treatment Options

- <u>Observation and reassurance</u>
- Topical corticosteroids
- Oral antihistamines
- UVB phototherapy
- Acyclovir
- Systemic corticosteroids

Further reading:

- Atzori L, Pinna AL, Ferreli C et al (2006) Pityriasis rosea-like adverse reaction: review of the literature and experience of an Italian drug-surveillance center. Dermatol Online J 12(1):1
- Bernardin RM, Ritter SE, Murchland MR (2002) Papular pityriasis rosea. Cutis 70(1):51–55
- Chuh A, Zawar V, Lee A (2005) Atypical presentations of pityriasis rosea: case presentations. J Eur Acad Dermatol Venereol 19(1):120–126

Pityriasis Rotunda (Toyama Syndrome)

Uncommon, idiopathic papulosquamous eruption that is occasionally familial or associated with systemic illness and is characterized by multiple, circular hyperpigmented or hypopigmented plaques with fine scale on the trunk or extremities

Differential Diagnosis

- Erythrasma
- Fixed drug eruption
- Ichthyosis vulgaris
- Large plaque parapsoriasis
- Leprosy
- Mycosis fungoides
- Pityriasis alba
- Porokeratosis of Mibelli
- Progressive macular hypomelanosis
- Tinea corporis
- Tinea versicolor

Associations

- Cirrhosis
- Hepatoma and other cancers
- Favism
- Leukemia
- Malnutrition
- Tuberculosis

Further reading:
- Hasson I, Shah P (2003) Pityriasis rotunda. Indian J Dermatol Venereol Leprol 69(1):50–51

Pityriasis Rubra Pilaris (Devergie's Disease)

Chronic papulosquamous disorder of unknown cause that affects children and adults and is characterized first by scaly plaques on the scalp and neck followed by generalized "nutmeg-grater-like" keratotic papules that become confluent in large orange-red scaly plaques with islands of sparing and a waxy yellow-orange palmoplantar keratoderma

Subtypes/Variants

- Type I: classic adult
- Type II: atypical adult
- Type III: classic juvenile
- Type IV: circumscribed juvenile
- Type V: atypical juvenile
- Type VI: HIV associated

Differential Diagnosis

Adult
- Contact dermatitis
- Crusted scabies
- Cutaneous T cell lymphoma
- Darier's disease
- Dengue fever eruption
- Dermatomyositis (Wong-type PRP)
- Eczema
- Erythrokeratoderma variabilis
- Erythroderma
- Lichen spinulosus
- Peeling skin syndrome
- Phrynoderma
- Psoriasiform drug eruption
- Psoriasis

- Seborrheic dermatitis
- Subacute lupus erythematosus
- Tinea versicolor

Child

- Eczema
- Erythroderma variabilis
- Kawasaki disease
- Lichen spinulosus
- Nummular eczema
- Peeling skin syndrome
- Phrynoderma
- Pityriasis lichenoides chronica
- Pityriasis rosea
- Pityriasis-rosea-like drug eruption
- Progressive symmetric erythrokeratodermia
- Psoriasis
- Seborrheic dermatitis
- Secondary syphilis

Evaluation

- Complete blood count
- Serum electrolyte studies
- Thyroid function test

Treatment Options

- Acitretin
- Isotretinoin
- Methotrexate
- Azathioprine
- Cyclosporine
- Infliximab

- Adalimumab
- Etanercept

Further reading:
- Sehgal VN, Srivastava G (2006) (Juvenile) Pityriasis rubra pilaris. Int J Dermatol 45(4):438–446

Pityrosporum Folliculitis

Type of folliculitis that is characterized by pruritic follicular-based papules and pustules on the trunk and proximal upper extremities with absence of comedones and absence of response to acne treatments

Differential Diagnosis

- Acne mechanica
- Acne vulgaris
- Candidiasis
- Drug-induced acne
- Eosinophilic folliculitis
- Steroid acne
- Gram-negative folliculitis
- *Pseudomonas* folliculitis

Associations

- Antibiotics
- Cushing's syndrome
- Diabetes mellitus
- Down syndrome
- HIV infection
- Immunosuppression
- Seborrheic dermatitis
- Tinea versicolor

Treatment Options

- Ketoconazole cream
- <u>Oral ketoconazole</u>
- Fluconazole

Further reading:
- Gupta AK, Batra R, Bluhm R et al (2004) Skin diseases associated with *Malassezia* species. J Am Acad Dermatol 51(5):785–798

Plague, Bubonic

Zoonotic bacterial infection caused by *Yersinia pestis* that is transmitted by the rat flea, *Xenopsylla cheopis*, and is characterized by fever, shock, purpuric lesions, and painful lymphadenopathy (buboes) most commonly in the inguinal area

Differential Diagnosis

- Atypical mycobacterial infection
- Cat-scratch disease
- Filariasis
- Lymphogranuloma venereum
- Primary inoculation tuberculosis
- Sporotrichosis
- Streptococcal cellulitis
- Suppurative lymphadenitis
- Syphilis
- <u>Tularemia</u>
- Typhus, Endemic

Evaluation

- Chest radiography
- Complete blood count
- Direct fluorescent antibody for *Y. pestis*

- Gram stain and culture of blood, bubo aspirate, and cerebrospinal fluid
- Liver function test

Further reading:
- Prentice MB, Rahalison L (2007) Plague. Lancet 369(9568):1196–1207

Plantar Fibromatosis (Ledderhose Disease)

Idiopathic fibromatosis that affects the plantar surface of the foot of men and is characterized by bilateral firm subcutaneous nodules on the medial aspect of the sole of the foot

Differential Diagnosis

- Calcinosis cutis
- Cerebriform plantar collagenoma
- Desmoid tumor
- Dermatofibrosarcoma protuberans
- Gout
- Granuloma annulare
- Hypertrophic scar
- Keloid
- Melanoma
- Neurofibroma
- Neuroma, traumatic
- Osteoma
- Plantar fasciitis
- Plantar lipoma/fibrolipoma
- Sarcoma

Associations

- Dupuytren's contracture
- Knuckle pads
- Peyronie's disease

Further reading:

- Graells Estrada J, Garcia Fernandez D, Badia Torroella F et al (2003) Familial plantar fibromatosis. Clin Exp Dermatol 28(6):669–670

Plasma Cell Balanitis (Zoon Balanitis, Balanitis Circumscripta Plasmacellularis)

Uncommon benign, inflammatory dermatosis affecting uncircumcised, older men that is characterized by a solitary, circumscribed, brightly erythematous, occasionally erosive plaque on the prepuce and glans penis

Differential Diagnosis

- <u>Candida balanitis</u>
- Erosive lichen planus
- <u>Erythroplasia of Queyrat</u>
- Extramammary Paget's disease
- <u>Fixed drug eruption</u>
- Herpes simplex virus
- Lupus erythematosus
- Mucosal pemphigoid
- Plasmacytoma
- Primary syphilis
- Pseudoepitheliomatous keratotic and micaceous balanitis
- Psoriasis
- Squamous cell carcinoma

Treatment Options

- <u>Tacrolimus ointment</u>
- Topical corticosteroids
- Imiquimod cream

Further reading:

- Weyers W, Ende Y, Schalla W, Diaz-Cascajo C (2002) Balanitis of Zoon: a clinicopathologic study of 45 cases. Am J Dermatopathol 24(6):459–467

Pneumocystis, Cutaneous

Rare manifestation of disseminated pulmonary *Pneumocystis jiroveci* infection that affects the profoundly immunocompromised patient and is characterized by erythematous to blue papules and nodules with or without ulceration that are mostly commonly located around the external auditory canal

Differential Diagnosis

- Acanthamebiasis
- Angiolymphoid hyperplasia with eosinophilia
- *Aspergillus* otomycosis
- Disseminated opportunistic fungal infection
- Kaposi sarcoma
- Mucormycosis
- Otitis externa (including malignant)
- Ramsay Hunt syndrome

Further reading:
- Bundow DL, Aboulafia DM (1997) Skin involvement with pneumocystis despite dapsone prophylaxis: a rare cause of skin nodules in a patient with AIDS. Am J Med Sci 313(3):182–186

Poikiloderma of Civatte

Acquired changes in the skin of fair-skinned individuals that are caused by chronic sun exposure and characterized by reticular erythematous to brown patches with atrophy and telangiectasia on the central chest, sides of neck, and face with sparing of the anterior neck just inferior to the chin

Differential Diagnosis

- Berloque dermatitis
- Bloom syndrome

- Cutaneous T cell lymphoma
- Dermatomyositis (shawl sign)
- Erythromelanosis follicularis faciei et colli
- Large plaque parapsoriasis
- Lupus erythematosus
- Melasma
- Poikiloderma atrophicans vasculare
- Riehl's melanosis
- Rothmund–Thomson syndrome

Treatment Options

- Topical retinoids
- Hydroquinone cream
- Pulsed dye laser
- Intense pulsed light

Further reading:

- Katoulis AC, Stavrianeas NG, Georgala S et al (2005) Poikiloderma of Civatte: a clinical and epidemiological study. J Eur Acad Dermatol Venereol 19(4):444–448

Poison Ivy Dermatitis (Rhus Dermatitis)

Common type of allergic contact dermatitis that is caused by various species of the *Toxicodendron* family of urushiol-containing plants and is characterized by intensely pruritic, streaky, linear, vesicular plaques on the exposed areas

Differential Diagnosis

- Allergic contact dermatitis (other types)
- Bullous pemphigoid
- Burn
- Dermatitis herpetiformis
- Phytophotodermatitis

- Scabies
- Zoster

Treatment Options

- Topical corticosteroids
- Systemic corticosteroids

Further reading:
- Mcgovern TW, Lawarre SR, Brunette C (2000) Is it, or isn't it? Poison ivy look-a-likes. Am J Contact Dermat 11(2):104–110

Polyarteritis Nodosa, Cutaneous

Variant of polyarteritis nodosa (Kussmaul–Maier syndrome) that lacks systemic features of vasculitis and is characterized by erythematous subcutaneous nodules and ulcers with surrounding livedo reticularis and a predilection for the lower extremities

Differential Diagnosis

- Cryoglobulinemia
- Erythema nodosum
- Henoch–Schonlein purpura
- Infectious endocarditis
- Livedoid vasculopathy
- Lupus erythematosus
- Malignancy
- Microscopic polyangiitis
- Nodular vasculitis
- Panniculitis
- Rheumatoid vasculitis
- Sjögren's syndrome
- Subcutaneous T cell lymphoma

Associations

- Crohn's disease
- Hepatitis B infection
- Hepatitis C infection
- Lupus erythematosus
- Relapsing polychondritis
- Streptococcal infections
- Takayasu arteritis
- Tuberculosis

Evaluation

- Anticardiolipin antibodies
- Antineutrophilic cytoplasmic antibodies
- Chest radiograph
- Complement levels
- Lupus anticoagulant
- Neurologic examination
- Renal function test
- Stool for occult blood
- Urinalysis
- Viral hepatitis panel

Treatment Options

- <u>Systemic corticosteroids</u>
- Methotrexate
- Azathioprine
- Mycophenolate mofetil
- Intravenous immunoglobulin
- Pentoxifylline
- Infliximab
- <u>Cyclophosphamide</u>

Further reading:

- Diaz-Perez JL, De Lagran ZM, Luis Diaz-Ramon J et al (2007) Cutaneous polyarteritis nodosa. Semin Cutan Med Surg 26(2):77–86

Polymorphous Light Eruption

Idiopathic photosensitivity disorder that predominantly affects young to middle-aged women and is characterized by a polymorphous eruption comprised of edematous erythematous papules, papulovesicles, and plaques on the sun-exposed portions of the face, chest, and arms

Subtypes

- Eczematous
- Erythematous
- Papular
- Papulovesicular
- Plaque-like

Differential Diagnosis

- Actinic lichen nitidus
- Actinic prurigo
- Airborne contact dermatitis
- Atopic dermatitis, photoexacerbated
- Chronic actinic dermatitis
- Erythema multiforme
- Erythropoietic protoporphyria
- Hydroa vacciniforme
- Jessner's lymphocytic infiltrate
- Lupus erythematosus
- Miliaria
- Photoallergic contact dermatitis

- <u>Photosensitive drug eruption</u>
- Psoriasis
- Rosacea
- Seborrheic dermatitis
- Solar urticaria

Associations

- Lupus erythematosus
- Positive ANA

Evaluation

- Antinuclear antibodies (including SS-A and SS-B)
- Phototesting

Treatment Options

- <u>Sun avoidance measures</u>
- <u>Narrowband UVB phototherapy</u>
- Topical corticosteroids
- <u>Systemic corticosteroids</u>
- Tacrolimus ointment
- <u>Hydroxychloroquine</u>
- Nicotinamide
- Azathioprine
- Cyclosporine
- Mycophenolate mofetil

Further reading:

- Naleway AL, Greenlee RT, Melski JW (2006) Characteristics of diagnosed polymorphous light eruption. Photodermatol Photoimmunol Photomed 22(4):205–207

Porocarcinoma, Eccrine

Malignant eccrine neoplasm that arises in the elderly and is characterized by a red, blue, or black ulcerated, vegetating nodule predominantly on the lower extremities but rarely on the palms and soles

Differential Diagnosis

- Basal cell carcinoma
- Bowen's disease
- Melanoma, amelanotic
- Leiomyosarcoma
- Merkel cell carcinoma
- <u>Pyogenic granuloma</u>
- Seborrheic keratosis
- <u>Squamous cell carcinoma</u>
- Verrucous carcinoma
- Verruca vulgaris

Further reading:
- de Giorgi V, Sestini S, Massi D et al (2007) Eccrine porocarcinoma: a rare but sometimes fatal malignant neoplasm. Dermatol Surg 33(3):374–377

Porokeratosis

Autosomal-dominant or sporadic disorder of keratinization affecting children and adults that is caused by an abnormal clone of keratinocytes which form a column of parakeratosis (cornoid lamella) and is characterized by discrete, circular, or linear atrophic plaques with a keratotic ridge

Subtypes/Variants

- Porokeratosis of Mibelli
- Linear porokeratosis

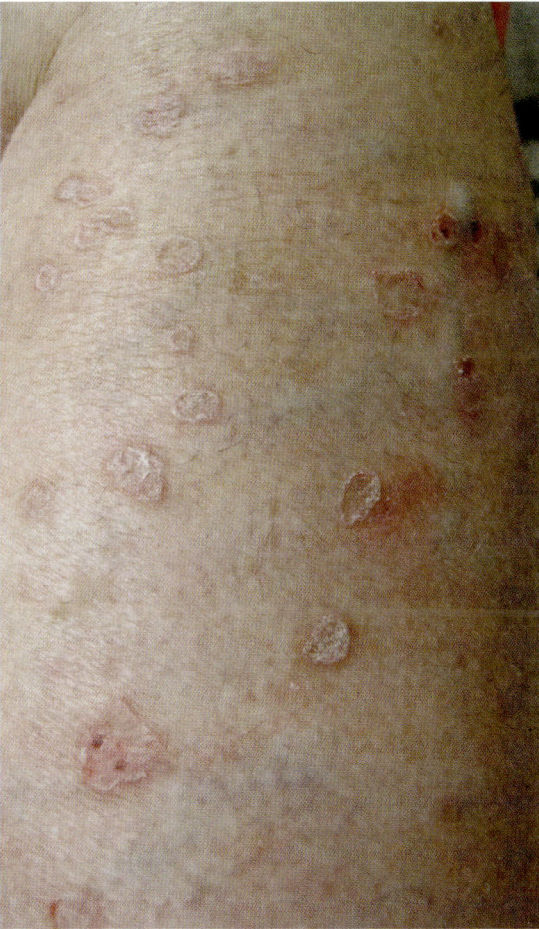

Fig. 6.96 Disseminated superficial porokeratosis

- Disseminated superficial porokeratosis (Fig. 6.96)
- Disseminated superficial actinic porokeratosis
- Porokeratosis palmaris et plantaris et disseminata (Fig. 6.97)
- Porokeratosis ptychotropica (flexural)
- Punctate porokeratosis

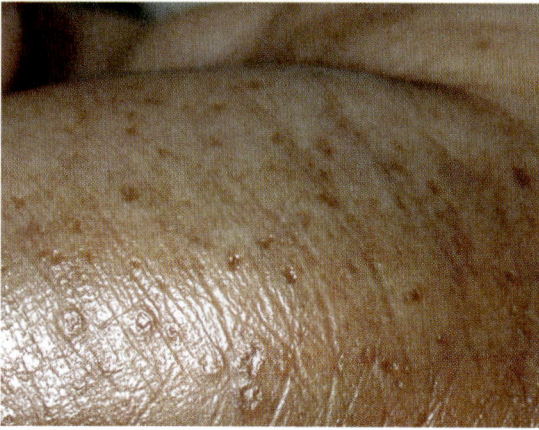

Fig. 6.97 Porokeratosis punctata palmaris et plantaris (Courtesy of K. Guidry)

Differential Diagnosis

Disseminated Superficial

- Acrokeratosis verruciformis of Hopf
- Actinic keratoses
- Cutaneous T cell lymphoma
- Epidermodysplasia verruciformis
- Hyperkeratosis lenticularis perstans (Flegel's disease)
- Lichen sclerosus et atrophicus
- Stucco keratoses
- Verruca plana

Linear

- Incontinentia pigmenti (stage II)
- Inflammatory linear verrucous epidermal nevus
- Lichen striatus
- Linear Darier's disease
- Linear lichen planus
- Linear psoriasis

- <u>Linear verruca</u>
- <u>Porokeratotic eccrine ostial and dermal duct nevus</u>

Mibelli

- Actinic keratosis
- <u>Annular atrophic lichen planus</u>
- Elastosis perforans serpiginosa
- Granuloma annulare
- Pityriasis rotunda
- Psoriasis
- Squamous cell carcinoma
- Superficial basal cell carcinoma

Porokeratosis Punctata

- Arsenical keratoses
- Corns
- Palmar pits
- Pitted keratolysis
- <u>Punctate keratoderma</u>
- Spiny keratoderma
- Verruca

Treatment Options

- <u>Observation</u>
- <u>Cryotherapy</u>
- <u>5FU cream</u>
- Acitretin
- Imiquimod
- Vitamin D analogues
- Tazarotene

Further reading:

- Kim C (2005) Linear porokeratosis. Dermatol Online J 11(4):22

Porokeratotic Eccrine Ostial and Dermal Duct Nevus

Eccrine type of epidermal nevus that is present at birth or arises in early childhood and is characterized by multiple comedo-like keratotic papules in a linear pattern on the flexural aspects of one hand or foot

Differential Diagnosis

- Eccrine syringofibroadenoma
- Ichthyosis hystrix
- Inflammatory linear verrucous epidermal nevus
- Lichen planus
- Lichen striatus
- Linear Darier's disease
- Linear epidermal nevus
- Linear porokeratosis
- Music-box spiny keratoderma
- Nevus comedonicus
- Punctate keratoderma

Further reading:
- Cambiaghi S, Gianotti R, Caputo R (2007) Widespread porokeratotic eccrine ostial and dermal duct nevus along Blaschko lines. Pediatr Dermatol 24(2):162–167

Poroma

Benign neoplasm of eccrine or apocrine derivation that is characterized by a slow-growing, flesh-colored nodule that occasionally has a verrucous or ulcerated surface and is most commonly located on the palms or soles (Fig. 6.98)

Differential Diagnosis

- Acrospiroma
- Callus

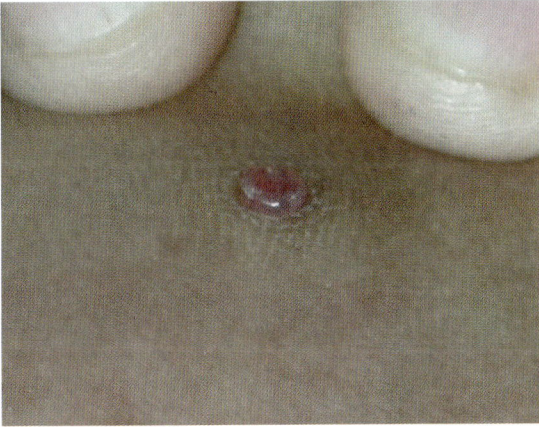

Fig. 6.98 Poroma
(Courtesy of
K. Guidry)

- Eccrine syringofibroadenoma
- Foreign body reaction
- Hidradenoma
- Hidroacanthoma simplex
- Melanoma
- Porocarcinoma
- Pyogenic granuloma
- Squamous cell carcinoma
- Trichilemmoma
- Verruca

Associations

- Hidrotic ectodermal dysplasia (multiple)

Further reading:

- Altamura D, Piccolo D, Lozzi GP, Peris K (2005) Eccrine poroma in an unusual site: a clinical and dermoscopic simulator of amelanotic melanoma. J Am Acad Dermatol 53(3):539–541

Porphyria

Group of metabolic disorders that are caused by variety of inherited or acquired enzyme defects in the heme biosynthesis pathway and that are characterized by the accumulation of phototoxic or neurotoxic porphyrins, the building blocks of heme

Subtypes (with Skin Findings)

- Congenital erythropoietic porphyria
- Erythropoietic protoporphyria
- Hepatoerythropoietic porphyria
- Hereditary coproporphyria
- Porphyria cutanea tarda
- Variegate porphyria

Differential Diagnosis

- See "Erythropoietic Protoporphyria"
- See "Porphyria Cutanea Tarda"
- See "Porphyria, Congenital Erythropoietic"

Evaluation

- Urine, stool, erythrocyte, and plasma porphyrins
- Liver function test
- Ophthalmologic exam
- Renal function test

Further reading:
- Norman RA (2005) Past and future: porphyria and porphyrins. Skinmed 4(5):287–292

Porphyria, Congenital Erythropoietic (Gunther's Disease)

Type of porphyria (AR) that is caused by deficiency of the enzyme, uroporphyrinogen III synthase, and is characterized by photosensitivity, vesiculobullous lesions in the sun-exposed areas, scarring, hypertrichosis, erythrodontia, pink urine, scleral and corneal disease, and hemolytic anemia

Differential Diagnosis

- Bloom syndrome
- Erythropoietic protoporphyria
- Hepatoerythropoietic porphyria
- Porphyria cutanea tarda
- Polymorphous light eruption
- Variegate porphyria
- Xeroderma pigmentosum

Further reading:
- Bari AU (2007) Congenital erythropoietic porphyria in three siblings. Indian J Dermatol Venereol Leprol 73(5):340–342

Porphyria Cutanea Tarda

Familial or acquired (more common) type of porphyria caused by decreased activity of hepatic uroporphyrinogen decarboxylase that is characterized by skin fragility, bullae on the dorsal hands and face, facial hypertrichosis, photodistributed hyperpigmentation, and in chronic, untreated cases, scleroderma-like skin changes (Fig. 6.99)

Differential Diagnosis

- Bullous amyloidosis
- Bullous diabeticorum

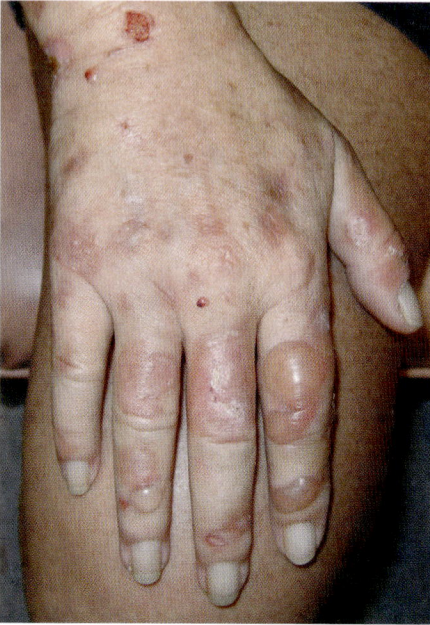

Fig. 6.99 Porphyria cutanea tarda

- Bullous lupus erythematosus
- Bullous pemphigoid
- Congenital erythropoietic porphyria
- Epidermolysis bullosa acquisita
- Hepatoerythropoietic porphyria
- Hydroa vacciniforme
- Melasma
- Photoallergic contact dermatitis
- Photoallergic drug eruption
- Phototoxic drug eruption
- Polymorphous light eruption
- Pseudoporphyria
- Variegate porphyria

Associations

- Alcoholism
- Chloracne
- CREST syndrome
- Cytomegalovirus
- Diabetes mellitus
- Dialysis
- Hematologic malignancy
- <u>Hemochromatosis</u>
- Hepatitis B
- <u>Hepatitis C</u>
- Hepatocellular carcinoma
- HIV infection
- Lupus erythematosus
- Myelofibrosis
- Renal failure
- Thalassemia
- Wilson's disease

Exacerbating Medications

- Alcohol
- Barbiturates
- Chlorinated hydrocarbons
- Estrogens
- Griseofulvin
- Iron
- Nalidixic Acid
- NSAIDs
- Phenytoin
- Pravastatin
- Rifampin
- Sulfa Drugs

- Tamoxifen
- Tetracyclines
- Vitamin B12

Evaluation

- 24-h urine porphyrins
- Complete blood count
- Fasting blood glucose
- HFE gene mutation analysis
- HIV test
- Iron studies
- Liver biopsy
- Liver function test
- Viral hepatitis panel

Treatment Options

- <u>Phlebotomy</u>
- Treat underlying cause
- Hydroxychloroquine
- Cimetidine

Further reading:

- Sams H, Kiripolsky MG, Bhat L et al (2004) Porphyria cutanea tarda, hepatitis C, alcoholism, and hemochromatosis: a case report and review of the literature. Cutis 73(3):188–190

Postinflammatory Hyperpigmentation

Hyperpigmentation associated with a preceding inflammatory dermatosis that is caused by either increased melanin transfer to keratinocytes or melanin dropping into the dermis and is characterized by brown-to-black pigmented macules coalescent into patches that coincide with areas affected by the dermatosis

Differential Diagnosis

- Acanthosis nigricans
- Addison's disease
- Amyloidosis
- Black dermographism
- Bleomycin flagellate pigmentation
- <u>Drug-induced hyperpigmentation</u>
- <u>Erythema dyschromicum perstans</u>
- Lupus erythematosus
- <u>Lichen planus pigmentosus</u>
- Melasma
- Mushroom dermatitis
- Nevoid hypermelanosis
- <u>Tinea versicolor</u>
- Traumatic tattoo

Associations

- Acne vulgaris
- Atopic dermatitis
- Atrophoderma of Pasini and Perini
- Discoid lupus erythematosus
- Erythema dyschromicum perstans
- Erythroderma
- Fixed drug eruption
- Idiopathic eruptive macular pigmentation
- Impetigo
- Insect bites
- Interface dermatoses
- <u>Lichen planus</u>
- Lichen simplex chronicus
- Lichenoid drug eruption
- Morbilliform drug eruption
- Morphea

- Pityriasis rosea
- Psoriasis
- Transient neonatal pustular melanosis

Treatment Options

- Observation and reassurance

Further reading:
- Ruiz-Maldonado R, Orozco-Covarrubias ML (1997) Postinflammatory hypopigmentation and hyperpigmentation. Semin Cutan Med Surg 16(1):36–43

Postinflammatory Hypopigmentation

Hypopigmentation that results from either inflammatory disruption of melanin production or destruction of melanocytes and is characterized by hypopigmentation and, less commonly, depigmentation, in the area affected by the dermatosis, often an eczematous process

Differential Diagnosis

- Atopic dermatitis
- Bier spots
- Chemical leukoderma
- Lichen sclerosus
- Lichen striatus
- Lupus erythematosus
- Mycosis fungoides
- Pityriasis alba
- Pityriasis lichenoides chronica
- Progressive macular hypomelanosis
- Psoriasis
- Sarcoidosis

- Seborrheic dermatitis
- Steroid-induced hypopigmentation
- Vitiligo

Associations

- Atopic dermatitis
- Blistering dermatoses
- Eczema
- Leprosy (especially tuberculoid)
- Pityriasis lichenoides
- Psoriasis
- Sarcoidosis
- Syphilis
- Tinea versicolor

Treatment Options

- Observation and reassurance
- Address the underlying cause
- Narrowband UVB therapy

Further reading:
- Vachiramon V, Thadanipon K (2011) Postinflammatory hypopigmentation. Clin Exp Dermatol 36(7):708–714

Preauricular Pit (Preauricular Sinus)

Developmental anomaly caused by incomplete fusion of the hillocks derived from the first and second branchial arches that is characterized by a small depression anterior to the superior insertion of the helix

Differential Diagnosis

- Basal cell carcinoma
- Branchial cleft cyst
- Dermoid sinus
- <u>Dilated pore</u>
- <u>Epidermal inclusion cyst</u>
- Parotid tumor

Associations

- Branchio-otic syndrome
- Branchio-oto-renal syndrome
- Hemifacial microsomia syndrome
- Goldenhar's syndrome
- Renal dysplasia
- Treacher Collins–Franceschetti syndrome

Evaluation

- Hearing test
- Renal ultrasound

Further reading:
- Huang XY, Tay GS, Wansaicheong GK, Low WK (2007) Preauricular sinus: clinical course and associations. Arch Otolaryngol Head Neck Surg 133(1):65–68

Pretibial Myxedema

Idiopathic mucinosis affecting patients with thyroid disease (especially after definitive treatment for Graves' disease) that is caused by deposition of hyaluronic acid in the dermis and characterized by indurated, nonpitting plaques or nodules on the bilateral anterior lower extremities, or rarely, on the upper extremities (Fig. 6.100)

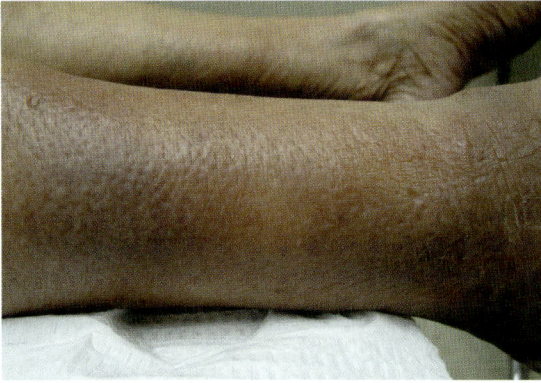

Fig. 6.100 Pretibial myxedema

Differential Diagnosis

- Acral ichthyosiform mucinosis
- B cell lymphoma of the leg
- Dermatomyositis
- Elephantiasis verrucosa
- Erythema nodosum
- Hypertrophic lichen planus
- Lichen amyloidosis
- Lichen myxedematosus
- Lichen simplex chronicus
- Lipodermatosclerosis
- Lymphedema
- Nephrogenic fibrosing dermopathy
- Scleromyxedema
- Venous stasis changes

Evaluation

- Antithyroid antibodies
- Thyroid function test

- Thyroid-stimulating antibodies
- Thyroid ultrasound

Treatment Options

- Topical corticosteroids
- Intralesional corticosteroids
- Pentoxifylline
- Systemic corticosteroids

Further reading:
- Jabbour SA (2003) Cutaneous manifestations of endocrine disorders: a guide for dermatologists. Am J Clin Dermatol 4(5):315–331

Progeria (Hutchinson–Gilford Progeria)

Rare premature aging syndrome (AD) that is caused by mutation of the lamin A gene and is characterized by death in the first two decades of life due to coronary atherosclerosis, dwarfism, paucity of subcutaneous fat, markedly enlarged head with characteristic facies, atrophic skin with prominent subcutaneous veins, and sclerodermatous changes on the extremities

Differential Diagnosis

- Acrogeria (Gottron syndrome)
- Ataxia–telangiectasia
- Berardinelli–Seip syndrome
- Cockayne syndrome
- Donahue syndrome
- Hallermann–Streiff syndrome
- Kindler syndrome
- Metageria
- Rothmund–Thomson syndrome

- Seckel syndrome
- Systemic sclerosis
- Werner syndrome

Further reading:

- Mazereeuw–Hautier J, Wilson LC, Mohammed S et al (2007) Hutchinson–Gilford progeria syndrome: clinical findings in three patients carrying the G608G mutation in LMNA and review of the literature. Br J Dermatol 156(6):1308–1314

Progesterone Dermatitis, Autoimmune

Rare cutaneous eruption with variable age of onset that is caused by an allergic reaction to endogenous progesterone and is characterized by a polymorphous recurrent eruption of erythema-multiforme-like plaques, urticaria-like plaques, or vesiculobullous lesions predominantly on the trunk

Differential Diagnosis

- Atopic dermatitis
- Bullous pemphigoid
- Contact dermatitis
- Erythema annulare centrifugum
- Erythema multiforme
- Dermatitis herpetiformis
- Dyshidrotic eczema
- Pemphigoid gestationis
- Pruritic urticarial papules and plaques of pregnancy
- Urticaria
- Urticarial dermatitis

Evaluation

- Progesterone intradermal skin test

Treatment Options

- Topical corticosteroids
- <u>Antihistamines</u>
- <u>Systemic corticosteroids</u>
- Danazol
- Stanozolol
- <u>Tamoxifen</u>

Further reading:
- Rasi A, Khatami A (2004) Autoimmune progesterone dermatitis. Int J Dermatol 43(8):588–590

Progressive Macular Hypomelanosis

Acquired dermatosis predominantly affecting young females of African descent or from tropical areas that is possibly caused by *Propionibacterium acnes* and is characterized by nummular, ill-defined nonscaly, asymptomatic hypopigmented macules and patches predominantly on the trunk, without preceding inflammation

Differential Diagnosis

- Hypopigmented mycosis fungoides
- Pityriasis alba
- Pityriasis lichenoides chronica
- Postinflammatory hypopigmentation
- <u>Tinea versicolor</u>
- Tuberculoid leprosy

Treatment Options

- Topical clindamycin
- <u>Benzoyl peroxide wash</u>

- Tetracycline antibiotics
- Narrowband UVB phototherapy

Further reading:
- Relyveld GN, Menke HE, Westerhof W (2007) Progressive macular hypomelanosis: an overview. Am J Clin Dermatol 8(1):13–19

Proliferative Verrucous Leukoplakia

Distinct type of aggressive leukoplakia that arises in elderly patients that has a high recurrence rate after adequate therapy and a high incidence of evolving to squamous cell carcinoma and that is characterized by multifocal, white, verrucous plaques on any surface of the oral mucosa, but most commonly the buccal mucosa or tongue

Differential Diagnosis

- Candidiasis
- Cheek-bite keratosis
- Focal epithelial hyperplasia
- Leukoedema
- Lichen planus
- Oral leukoplakia
- Smoker's palate
- Squamous cell carcinoma
- Verrucous carcinoma
- White sponge nevus

Further reading:
- Cabay RJ, Morton TH Jr, Epstein JB (2007) Proliferative verrucous leukoplakia and its progression to oral carcinoma: a review of the literature. J Oral Pathol Med 36(5):255–261

Proteus Syndrome

Idiopathic sporadic syndrome with protean features that presents at birth or in the first year of life and is characterized by epidermal nevi, capillary malformations, lymphangiomas, plantar cerebriform collagenomas, lipomas, hemihypertrophy, and a variety of other cutaneous, ocular, skeletal, and CNS defects

Differential Diagnosis

- <u>Bannayan–Riley–Ruvulcaba syndrome</u>
- <u>Encephalocraniocutaneous lipomatosis</u>
- Epidermal nevus syndrome
- Klippel–Trenaunay syndrome
- Maffucci syndrome
- Neurofibromatosis

Diagnostic Criteria

- Mandatory general criteria
  - Mosaic distribution of lesions
  - Progressive course
  - Sporadic occurrence
- Specific criteria (A, or two from group B, or three from group C)
  - Group A
    - Connective tissue nevus
  - Group B
    - Epidermal nevus
    - Disproportionate overgrowth of limbs, skull, external auditory meatus, vertebra, or viscera (spleen and/or thymus)
    - Bilateral ovarian cystadenomas or parotid monomorphic adenoma before the end of the second decade

— Group C
  — Lipoma or regional absence of fat
  — Capillary, venous, and/or lymphatic malformation
  — Dolichocephaly, long face, minor downslanting of palpebral fissures, and/or minor ptosis, low nasal bridge, wide or anteverted nares, and open mouth at rest

Further reading:

- Biesecker LG, Happle R, Mulliken JB et al (1999) Proteus syndrome: diagnostic criteria, differential diagnosis, and patient evaluation. Am J Med Genet 84(5):389–395
- Nguyen D, Turner JT, Olsen C et al (2004) Cutaneous manifestations of proteus syndrome: correlations with general clinical severity. Arch Dermatol 140(8):947–953

Protothecosis

Trauma-related cutaneous infection caused by the algae, *Prototheca wickerhamii*, that is characterized by olecranon bursitis or a chronic verrucous nodule or plaque on the extremities

Differential Diagnosis

- Anthrax
- Blastomycosis-like pyoderma
- Deep fungal infection
- *Mycobacterium marinum* infection
- Nocardiosis
- Olecranon bursitis
- Orf
- Pyoderma
- Pyoderma gangrenosum
- Sporotrichosis

Further reading:

- Lass-Florl C, Mayr A (2007) Human protothecosis. Clin Microbiol Rev 20(2):230–242

Prurigo Nodularis

Chronic neurodermatitis associated with pruritus with or without an underlying cause that leads to repeated rubbing, picking, and scratching of the itchy areas and is characterized by solitary or multiple hyperpigmented scaly nodules with overlying excoriation that are most commonly located on the extensor aspects of the extremities

Differential Diagnosis

- Actinic keratosis
- Arthropod bites
- Cutaneous metastasis
- Cutaneous T cell lymphoma
- Disseminated superficial porokeratosis
- Halogenoderma
- Hypertrophic lichen planus
- Lichen simplex chronicus
- Lymphomatoid papulosis
- Molluscum contagiosum
- Multiple dermatofibromas
- Multiple granular cell tumors
- Multiple keratoacanthomas
- Nodular amyloidosis
- Nodular scabies
- Pemphigoid nodularis
- Perforating diseases
- Pruriginous epidermolysis bullosa
- Sarcoidosis
- Trichotillomania
- Xanthoma

Evaluation

- Complete blood count
- HIV test

- Liver function test
- Renal function test
- Serum chemistry, including calcium level
- Thyroid function

Treatment Options

- Topical corticosteroids
- Antihistamines
- Intralesional corticosteroids
- Cryotherapy
- Gabapentin
- UVB phototherapy
- Cyclosporine
- Thalidomide

Further reading:

- Lee MR, Shumack S (2005) Prurigo nodularis: a review. Australas J Dermatol 46(4):211–218

Prurigo Pigmentosa

Idiopathic pruritic disorder most commonly described in young Japanese women that is characterized by a recurrent eruption of erythematous macules, papules, and papulovesicles that are symmetrically located on the upper back, chest, and sacral area and that heal to leave behind a reticulate pattern of hyperpigmentation

Differential Diagnosis

- Confluent and reticulated papillomatosis
- Contact dermatitis
- Dermatitis herpetiformis
- Excoriations
- Lupus erythematosus

- Macular amyloidosis
- Neurodermatitis
- Pityriasis lichenoides
- <u>Subacute prurigo</u>
- Terra firma–forme dermatosis
- Urticarial dermatitis

Treatment Options

- <u>Minocycline</u>
- Dapsone

Further reading:
- Asgari M, Daneshpazhooh M, Chams Davatchi C et al (2006) Prurigo pigmentosa: an underdiagnosed disease in patients of Iranian descent? J Am Acad Dermatol 55(1):131–136

Prurigo Simplex (Subacute Prurigo, Papular Dermatitis, and Itchy Red Bump Disease)

Idiopathic chronic pruritic disorder that affects middle-aged to elderly individuals and that is characterized by erythematous dome-shaped papules with a central vesicle that is quickly excoriated

Differential Diagnosis

- Atopic dermatitis
- <u>Bullous pemphigoid</u>
- Contact dermatitis
- <u>Dermatitis herpetiformis</u>
- Dermatographism
- Galli–Galli disease
- Grover's disease

- Hypereosinophilic syndrome
- Id reaction
- <u>Insect-bite reactions</u>
- Linear IgA disease
- Papular urticaria
- Papuloerythroderma of Ofuji
- Pityriasis lichenoides et varioliformis acuta
- <u>Scabies</u>
- Urticaria
- Urticarial dermatitis

Treatment Options

- <u>Topical corticosteroids</u>
- <u>Systemic corticosteroids</u>
- <u>UVB phototherapy</u>
- <u>Antihistamines</u>
- Methotrexate
- Mycophenolate mofetil
- Gabapentin
- Cyclosporine
- Olanzapine

Further reading:
- Wallengren J (2004) Prurigo: diagnosis and management. Am J Clin Dermatol 5(2):85–95

Pruritic Urticarial Papules and Plaques of Pregnancy

Idiopathic, benign dermatosis of pregnancy that primarily affects primigravida patients in the third trimester and is characterized by erythematous, urticarial, papules and plaques predominantly on the abdomen, with sparing of the periumbilical area and preferential involvement of abdominal striae

Differential Diagnosis

- Allergic contact dermatitis
- Autoimmune progesterone dermatitis
- Cholestasis of pregnancy
- Drug eruptions
- Erythema multiforme
- Impetigo herpetiformis
- Insect bites
- Pemphigoid gestationis
- Scabies
- Urticaria
- Viral exanthem

Treatment Options

- Topical corticosteroids
- Systemic corticosteroids
- Antihistamines
- Induction of labor

Further reading:
- Matz H, Orion E, Wolf R (2006) Pruritic urticarial papules and plaques of pregnancy: polymorphic eruption of pregnancy (PUPPP). Clin Dermatol 24(2):105–108

Pseudoatrophoderma Colli

Uncommon dermatosis of unknown cause that is characterized by atrophic-like hyperpigmented or hypopigmented macules on the neck, shoulders, and upper trunk

Differential Diagnosis

- <u>Acanthosis nigricans</u>
- Anetoderma
- Confluent and reticulated papillomatosis
- Erythema dyschromicum perstans
- Lichen sclerosus et atrophicus
- <u>Middermal elastolysis</u>
- Poikiloderma of Civatte
- Small plaque parapsoriasis
- <u>Tinea versicolor</u>
- Vitiligo

Associations

- Acanthosis nigricans
- Confluent and reticulated papillomatosis

Further reading:
- Kauh YC, Knepp ME, Luscombe HA (1980) *Pseudoatrophoderma colli*. A familial case. Arch Dermatol 116(10):1181–1182

Pseudocyst of the Auricle

Idiopathic, possibly trauma-related, fluid-filled cyst-like dilatation between the two embryonic layers of auricular cartilage that is characterized by a unilateral, noninflammatory swelling of the ear (Fig. 6.101)

Differential Diagnosis

- Cutaneous B cell lymphoma
- Relapsing polychondritis
- <u>Traumatic auricular hematoma</u>

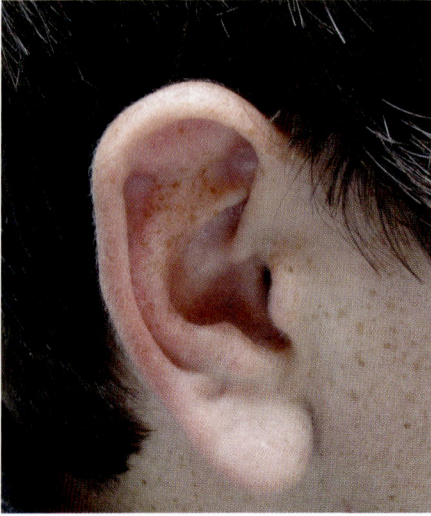

Fig. 6.101 Pseudocyst of the auricle

Further reading:

- Ng W, Kikuchi Y, Chen X, Hira K et al (2007) Pseudocysts of the auricle in a young adult with facial and ear atopic dermatitis. J Am Acad Dermatol 56(5):858–861

Psuedoepitheliomatous Keratotic and Micaceous Balanitis

Premalignant disorder that may progress to verrucous carcinoma (but not associated with human papillomavirus) that affects older men and is characterized by a psoriasiform, micaceous, or verrucous plaque on the glans penis, with fissures and ulceration

Differential Diagnosis

- Bowenoid papulosis
- Condyloma acuminatum
- Deep fungal infection
- Erythroplasia of Queyrat

- Granular cell tumor
- Lichen planus
- <u>Psoriasis</u>
- <u>Squamous cell carcinoma</u>
- Verrucous carcinoma
- Zoon balanitis

Further reading:
- Child FJ, Kim BK, Ganesan R et al (2000) Verrucous carcinoma arising in pseudoepitheliomatous keratotic and micaceous balanitis, without evidence of human papillomavirus. Br J Dermatol 143(1):183–187

Pseudofolliculitis Barbae

Inflammatory disorder of the beard follicles that predominantly affects men of African descent, is caused by a inflammatory reaction to follicle-penetrating hair shafts after a close shave, and is characterized by numerous follicular papules and pustules, with a tendency for scarring or keloid formation

Differential Diagnosis

- <u>Acne vulgaris</u>
- Herpetic sycosis
- Rosacea
- Sarcoidosis
- <u>Sycosis barbae</u>
- Tinea barbae
- Trichostasis spinulosa

Associations

- Acne keloidalis nuchae

Treatment Options

- <u>Education regarding shaving technique</u>
- Topical clindamycin
- Topical corticosteroids
- Topical retinoids
- Glycolic acid peels, lotions, or cleansers
- Tetracycline antibiotics

Further reading:
- Perry PK, Cook-Bolden FE, Rahman Z et al (2002) Defining pseudofolliculitis barbae in 2001: a review of the literature and current trends. J Am Acad Dermatol 46:S113–S119

Pseudomonas **Hot-Foot Syndrome**

Type of eccrine hidradenitis caused by *Pseudomonas aeruginosa* that is associated with community outbreaks among children exposed to high concentrations of *Pseudomonas* in swimming pools and is characterized by erythematous tender nodules on the plantar surfaces

Differential Diagnosis

- Contact urticaria
- Delayed pressure urticaria
- Erythema nodosum
- Infectious panniculitis
- Piezogenic pedal papules
- <u>Recurrent idiopathic palmoplantar hidradenitis</u>

Further reading:
- Fiorillo L, Zucker M, Sawyer D, Lin AN (2001) The pseudomonas hot-foot syndrome. N Engl J Med 345(5):335–338

Pseudoporphyria

Porphyria-cutanea-tarda-like eruption associated with medications, ultraviolet-light therapy, or hemodialysis that is probably an exaggerated phototoxic reaction and is characterized by fragile skin, scarring, and vesiculobullous lesions on the dorsal hands and forearms but without the hypertrichosis, hyperpigmentation, sclerodermatous skin changes, and elevated porphyrin levels seen in its namesake

Differential Diagnosis

- Bullous amyloidosis
- Cutaneous lupus erythematosus
- Epidermolysis bullosa acquisita
- Hydroa vacciniforme
- Pemphigus erythematosus
- Phototoxic drug reaction
- Polymorphous light eruption
- Porphyria cutanea tarda
- Toxic epidermal necrolysis

Associated Medications

- Acitretin
- Alcohol
- Amiodarone
- Barbiturates
- Cyclosporine
- Dapsone
- Dialysis
- Estrogen
- Furosemide
- Griseofulvin
- Imatinib

- Isotretinoin
- Naproxen
- NSAIDs
- Oral contraception
- Sulfonamides
- Tetracyclines
- Voriconazole

Further reading:

- Tolland JP, Mckeown PP, Corbett JR (2007) Voriconazole-induced pseudoporphyria. Photodermatol Photoimmunol Photomed 23(1):29–31

Pseudoverrucous Papules and Nodules

Uncommon manifestation of irritant contact dermatitis that occurs predominantly in the perianal area of infants and that is characterized by small erythematous, round, flat-topped papules

Differential Diagnosis

- Candidiasis
- Condyloma acuminatum
- Cutaneous Crohn's disease
- Granuloma gluteale infantum
- Jacquet's erosive diaper dermatitis
- Langerhans cell histiocytosis
- Lichen simplex chronicus

Treatment Options

- Management of incontinence
- Barrier creams
- Low potency topical corticosteroids

Further reading:

- Robson KJ, Maughan JA, Purcell SD et al (2006) Erosive papulonodular dermatosis associated with topical benzocaine: a report of two cases and evidence that granuloma gluteale, pseudoverrucous papules, and Jacquet's erosive dermatitis are a disease spectrum. J Am Acad Dermatol 55(5 Suppl):S74–S80

Pseudoxanthoma Elasticum

Autosomal-recessive disorder caused by a defect in the ABCC6 (ATP-binding cassette transporter C6) that leads to multisystem calcification and fragmentation of elastic fibers and is characterized by redundant, yellow pebbly skin folds of the flexures (plucked chicken skin), angioid streaks in the eye with possible blindness, hypertension, and gastrointestinal hemorrhage (Fig. 6.102)

Differential Diagnosis

- Actinic elastosis
- Amyloid elastosis

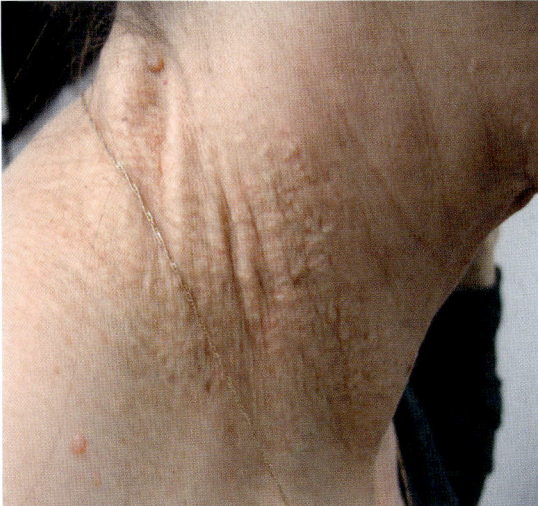

Fig. 6.102 Pseudoxanthoma elasticum

- Buschke–Ollendorf syndrome
- Calcinosis cutis
- Cutis laxa
- D-Penicillamine therapy
- Ehlers–Danlos syndrome
- Eosinophilia–myalgia syndrome
- Fibroelastolytic papulosis of the neck
- Fox–Fordyce disease
- Granulomatous slack skin
- Juxtaclavicular beaded lines
- Late-onset focal dermal elastosis
- Lupus erythematosus, chronic cutaneous
- Marfan syndrome
- Normolipemic plane xanthomas
- Papular elastorrhexis
- Perforating calcific elastosis
- Saltpeter exposure
- Scleromyxedema
- Xanthoma disseminatum

Diagnostic Criteria

- Major criteria
  - Characteristic skin involvement
  - Characteristic histologic features in lesional skin
  - Characteristic ocular disease
- Minor criteria
  - Characteristic features in nonlesional skin
  - Family history of PXE in first-degree relatives

Associations

- Elastosis perforans serpiginosa
- Hereditary spherocytosis

- Sickle cell anemia
- Thalassemia

Evaluation

- Cardiovascular evaluation
- CT/MRI of the brain
- Lipid panel
- Liver function test
- Ophthalmologic exam
- Renal function test
- Serum chemistry profile including calcium and phosphate
- Stool for occult blood
- Urinalysis

Further reading:

- Lebwohl M, Neldner K, Pope FM et al (1994) Classification of pseudoxanthoma elasticum: report of a consensus conference. J Am Acad Dermatol 30:103–107
- Ringpfeil F (2005) Selected disorders of connective tissue: pseudoxanthoma elasticum, cutis laxa, and lipoid proteinosis. Clin Dermatol 23(1):41–46

Psoriasis

Common, immune-mediated disorder of epidermal proliferation that is characterized by variably sized pink to erythematous plaques with overlying silvery scale, has pinpoint bleeding with removal of scale (Auspitz sign), displays the Koebner phenomenon, has an occasional pustular or erythrodermic presentation, and typically affects the scalp, elbows, knees, and nails, with the potential to involve widespread areas of the body

Subtypes/Variants

- Annular
- Discoid
- Erythrodermic

- Facial
- Figurate
- Follicular
- Genital
- Guttate
- Gyrate
- Inverse
- Nail
- Ostraceous
- Palmoplantar
- Plaque
- Pustular
- Rupial
- Scalp

Differential Diagnosis

Erythrodermic
- Atopic dermatitis
- Drug reaction
- Erythrodermic mycosis fungoides
- Generalized contact dermatitis
- Pityriasis rubra pilaris
- Sezary syndrome

Facial
- Acrokeratosis paraneoplastica
- Allergic contact dermatitis
- Lupus erythematosus
- Seborrheic dermatitis
- Tinea faciei

Genital
- Candidiasis
- Contact dermatitis

- Erythroplasia of Queyrat
- Extramammary Paget's disease
- Fixed drug eruption
- <u>Lichen planus</u>
- Lichen simplex chronicus
- Psuedoepitheliomatous keratotic and micaceous balanitis
- Reiter syndrome
- Seborrheic dermatitis
- Tinea cruris

Guttate

- Disseminated histoplasmosis
- <u>Eruptive lichen planus</u>
- <u>Pityriasis lichenoides chronica</u>
- <u>Pityriasis rosea</u>
- Psoriasiform drug eruption
- Scabies
- Scarlet fever
- <u>Secondary syphilis</u>
- Small plaque parapsoriasis
- Viral exanthem (especially resolving)

Inverse

- Baboon syndrome
- Candidiasis
- Contact dermatitis
- Extramammary Paget's disease
- <u>Intertrigo</u>
- Langerhans cell histiocytosis
- Lichen planus pigmentosus–inversus
- Lichen simplex chronicus
- Pemphigus foliaceus
- <u>Seborrheic dermatitis</u>
- Tinea cruris

Nail

- Acrokeratosis paraneoplastica
- Alopecia areata
- Contact dermatitis
- Idiopathic onycholysis
- Keratoderma blennorrhagicum
- Lichen planus
- <u>Onychomycosis</u>
- Parakeratosis pustulosa
- Pityriasis rubra pilaris
- Scabies
- Sezary syndrome
- Traumatic onycholysis

Plaque, Including Palmoplantar

- Bowen's disease
- Crusted scabies
- Dermatomyositis
- Discoid lupus erythematosus
- Erythema annulare centrifugum
- Erythema gyratum repens
- Lichen planus
- Lichen simplex chronicus
- Mycosis fungoides
- <u>Nummular eczema</u>
- Pemphigus foliaceus
- Pityriasis rosea
- Porokeratosis of Mibelli
- Reiter's syndrome
- Sarcoidosis
- Seborrheic dermatitis
- Small plaque parapsoriasis
- Subacute cutaneous lupus

- Tertiary syphilis
- Tinea corporis

Pustular

- <u>Acute generalized exanthematous pustulosis</u>
- Amicrobial pustulosis with autoimmunity
- Candidiasis
- Folliculitis
- <u>IgA pemphigus</u>
- Miliaria pustulosa
- Pemphigus foliaceus
- Reiter's syndrome
- <u>Subcorneal pustular dermatosis</u>

Scalp

- Atopic dermatitis
- Dermatomyositis
- Lichen simplex chronicus
- <u>Seborrheic dermatitis</u>
- Tinea capitis

Associations

- Alcohol abuse
- Arthritis (especially nail)
- <u>Coronary artery disease</u>
- Hypocalcemia (especially pustular)
- Medications
- <u>Obesity</u>
- SAPHO syndrome (especially pustular)
- Smoking
- Streptococcal infection (especially guttate)
- Stress
- Viral infection

Exacerbating Medications

- Antimalarials
- Beta-blockers
- Calcium channel blockers
- Captopril
- G-CSF
- Glyburide
- Interferons
- Lipid-lowering drugs
- Lithium
- NSAIDs
- Terbinafine

Treatment Options

- Topical corticosteroids
- Anthralin
- Tar
- Salicylic acid
- Vitamin D analogues
- Tacrolimus ointment
- UVB phototherapy
- Acitretin
- Methotrexate
- Sulfasalazine
- Etanercept
- Adalimumab
- Alefacept
- Infliximab
- Ustekinumab
- Hydroxyurea
- Cyclosporine
- Mycophenolate mofetil
- Azathioprine

Further reading:

- Griffiths CE, Barker JN (2007) Pathogenesis and clinical features of psoriasis. Lancet 370(9583):263–271

Psoriatic Arthritis

Inflammatory type of arthritis that has several different subtypes and is associated with psoriasis

Subtypes/Variants

- Arthritis mutilans
- Ankylosing-spondylitis-like
- Asymmetric oligoarthritis
- Distal interphalangeal joint only
- Rheumatoid-arthritis-like

Differential Diagnosis

- Gouty arthritis
- Juvenile rheumatoid arthritis
- Multicentric reticulohistiocytosis
- Osteoarthritis
- Reactive arthritis with urethritis and conjunctivitis
- Rheumatoid arthritis

Diagnostic Criteria

- Inflammatory articular disease (joint, spine, or entheseal) with three points from the following five categories:
  - Evidence of current psoriasis, a personal history of psoriasis, or a family history of psoriasis
  - Typical psoriatic nail dystrophy including onycholysis, pitting, and hyperkeratosis

- A negative test result for the presence of rheumatoid factor by any method except latex
- Either current dactylitis, defined as swelling of an entire digit, or a history of dactylitis
- Radiographic evidence of juxtaarticular new bone formation on plain radiographs of the hand or foot

Further reading:
- Taylor W, Gladman D, Helliwell P et al (2006) Classification criteria for psoriatic arthritis: development of new criteria from a large international study. Arthritis Rheum 54(8):2665–2673

Purpura, Actinic (Bateman's Purpura)

Purpura on the extensor surface of the forearms that affects the elderly, is caused by blood vessel fragility related to photoaging, and is characterized by large purpura and ecchymoses with or without a history of trauma to the affected area

Differential Diagnosis

- AL amyloidosis
- Anticoagulant therapy
- Coagulation disorder
- Elder abuse
- Psychogenic purpura
- Steroid-induced purpura
- Trauma
- Vitamin K deficiency

Further reading:
- Carlson JA, Chen KR (2007) Cutaneous pseudovasculitis. Am J Dermatopathol 29(1):44–55

Pyoderma Faciale (Rosacea Fulminans)

Uncommon acneiform condition of the face of young women characterized by facial erythema, papulopustules, confluent nodules, and draining
sinuses, but no comedones

Differential Diagnosis

- <u>Acne conglobata</u>
- <u>Cutaneous Rosai–Dorfman disease</u>
- Deep inflammatory tinea faciei
- Jessner's lymphocytic infiltrate
- Lupus erythematosus tumidus
- Leukemia cutis
- Lymphoma
- Pyoderma gangrenosum
- Solid facial edema
- Staphylococcal furunculosis
- <u>Sweet's syndrome</u>
- Wegener's granulomatosis

Associations

- Erythema nodosum
- Inflammatory bowel disease

Treatment Options

- <u>Systemic corticosteroids</u>
- <u>Isotretinoin</u>
- Systemic tetracyclines
- Azithromycin
- Dapsone

Further reading:

- Akhyani M, Daneshpazhooh M, Ghandi N (2007) The association of pyoderma faciale and erythema nodosum. Clin Exp Dermatol 32(3):275–277

Pyoderma Gangrenosum

Idiopathic neutrophilic dermatosis associated with internal disease that is characterized by erythematous nodules on the lower extremity or elsewhere that rapidly ulcerate and expand outward with a violaceous undermined, overhanging border and central purulent, necrotic material

Subtypes/Variants

- Bullous
- Neutrophilic dermatosis of the dorsal hands (Fig. 6.103)

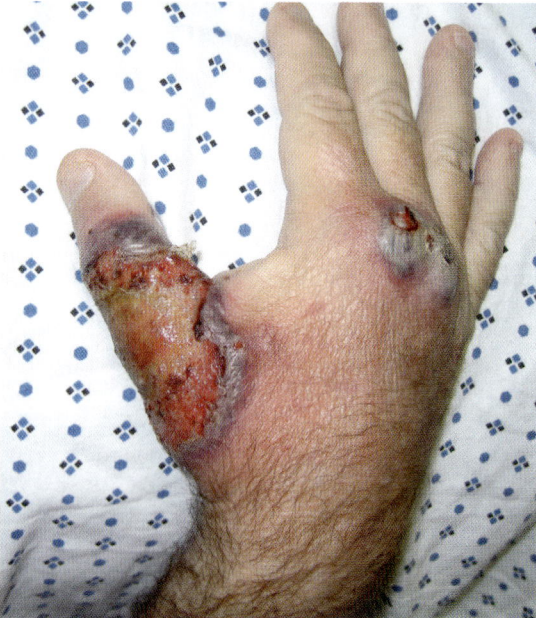

Fig. 6.103 Neutrophilic dermatosis of the dorsal hands

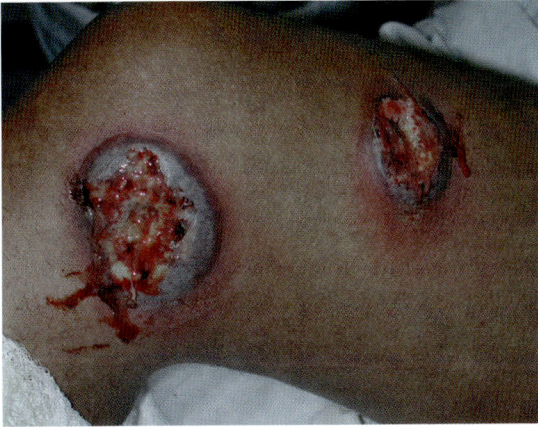

Fig. 6.104 Pyoderma gangrenosum (Courtesy of K. Guidry)

- Peristomal
- Pustular
- Ulcerative (classic; Fig. 6.104)
- Vegetative (superficial granulomatous)

Differential Diagnosis

- Amebiasis
- Anthrax
- Antiphospholipid antibody syndrome
- Arterial insufficiency ulcer
- Basal cell carcinoma
- Behçet's disease
- Bowel-associated dermatosis–arthritis syndrome
- Brown recluse spider bite
- Cellulitis
- Chancriform pyoderma
- Churg–Strauss syndrome
- Cutaneous polyarteritis nodosa
- Deep fungal infection (especially blastomycosis)
- Ecthyma

- Ecthyma gangrenosum
- <u>Factitial disease</u>
- <u>Felty syndrome</u>
- Follicular infections
- Gummatous treponemal ulcers
- Halogenoderma
- Hemoglobinopathies
- Herpes simplex virus infection
- Insect-bite reaction
- Leishmaniasis
- Lymphoma
- <u>Mycobacterial infections</u>
- Orf/milker's nodule
- Panniculitides
- Pemphigus vegetans
- Rheumatoid vasculitis
- Schistosomiasis
- Septic emboli
- Sporotrichosis
- Squamous cell carcinoma
- Streptococcal synergistic gangrene
- <u>Sweet's syndrome</u>
- Thrombosis
- Ulcerative necrobiosis lipoidica
- Venous stasis ulcer
- Wegener's granulomatosis

Associations

- Acne conglobata
- <u>Acute myelogenous leukemia</u>
- Ankylosing spondylitis
- Behçet's disease
- Chronic active hepatitis

- Connective tissue disease
- Diabetes mellitus
- Erythema elevatum diutinum
- Hairy-cell leukemia
- Hidradenitis suppurativa
- HIV infection
- Inflammatory bowel disease
- IgA gammopathy
- IgA pemphigus
- Myelofibrosis
- Myeloma
- Paroxysmal nocturnal hemoglobinuria
- Polycythemia vera
- Primary biliary cirrhosis
- Rheumatoid arthritis
- Sarcoidosis
- SAPHO syndrome
- Seronegative arthritis
- Spondylitis
- Subcorneal pustular dermatosis
- Sweet's syndrome
- Takayasu's disease
- Thyroid disease

Evaluation

- Antinuclear antibodies
- Immunoglobulin panel
- Antineutrophilic cytoplasmic antibodies
- Antiphospholipid antibodies
- Bone marrow examination
- Complete blood count with smear
- Colonoscopy with biopsy
- Chest radiography

- Liver function test
- Rheumatoid factor
- Serum/urinary protein electrophoresis
- Stool for occult blood
- Urinalysis

Treatment Options

- Topical corticosteroids
- Tacrolimus ointment
- Dapsone
- Minocycline
- Systemic corticosteroids
- Nicotine replacement
- Cyclosporine
- Azathioprine
- Mycophenolate mofetil
- Methotrexate
- Infliximab
- Sulfasalazine

Further reading:

- Ahmadi S, Powell FC (2005) Pyoderma gangrenosum: uncommon presentations. Clin Dermatol 23(6):612–620

Pyogenic Granuloma

Reactive vascular neoplasm of uncertain pathogenesis that is often associated with trauma and is characterized by a small, solitary (or multiple, eruptive) friable vascular papule or nodule that bleeds easily, is often covered with a bandage by the patient (band-aid sign), and is located on the periungual area, the digits, the palms, or any other area, including the oral cavity (Fig. 6.105)

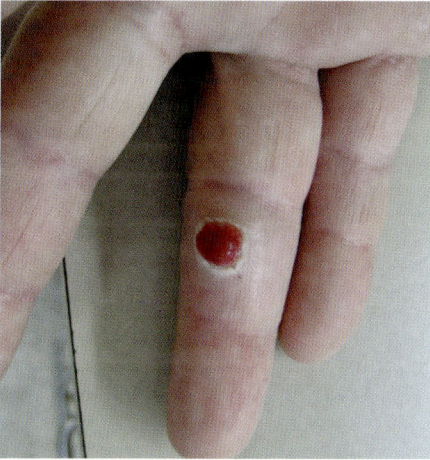

Fig. 6.105 Pyogenic granuloma

Differential Diagnosis

- Adnexal carcinoma
- Atypical fibroxanthoma
- Amelanotic melanoma
- Angioendothelioma
- Angiolymphoid hyperplasia
- Angiosarcoma
- Atypical fibroxanthoma
- Bacillary angiomatosis
- Clear cell acanthoma
- Eccrine acrospiroma
- Epithelioid fibrous histiocytoma
- Glomus tumors
- Granulation tissue
- Hemangiomas
- Irritated nevi
- Kaposi's sarcoma
- Merkel cell carcinoma

- <u>Metastatic lesion</u>
- Orf
- Poroma
- Spitz nevus
- Traumatized angioma
- Wart

Associations

- Medications
- Pregnancy (granuloma gravidarum)
- Trauma

Associated Medications

- Capecitabine
- 5FU
- EGF receptor inhibitors
- Indinavir
- Isotretinoin
- Mitoxantrone
- Oral contraceptives

Further reading:
- Scheinfeld NS (2008) Pyogenic granuloma. Skinmed 7(1):37–39

Pyostomatitis Vegetans

Idiopathic, eosinophil-rich, inflammatory disorder of the oral cavity that is predominantly associated with inflammatory bowel disease, especially ulcerative colitis, but also liver disease, and is characterized by multiple pustules on the labial and buccal mucosa, which erode to form "snail-track" ulcers and vegetating lesions, along with peripheral eosinophilia

Differential Diagnosis

- <u>Behçet's disease</u>
- Bullous drug eruption
- Bullous pemphigoid
- <u>Eosinophilic ulcer</u>
- Epidermolysis bullosa acquisita
- Erythema multiforme
- Herpes simplex virus infection
- <u>Pemphigus vegetans</u>
- Syphilis

Further reading:

- Hegarty AM, Barrett AW, Scully C (2004) Pyostomatitis vegetans. Clin Exp Dermatol 29(1):1–7

Pyridoxine Deficiency

Deficiency of vitamin B6 that is characterized by peripheral neuropathy, seizures, confusion, a seborrheic-dermatitis-like rash, a pellagra-like eruption (because of secondary niacin deficiency), glossitis, and cheilitis

Differential Diagnosis

- Acrodermatitis enteropathica
- Essential fatty acid deficiency
- B12 deficiency
- Necrolytic migratory erythema
- Pellagra
- Riboflavin deficiency
- <u>Seborrheic dermatitis</u>

Associations

- Alcoholism
- Cirrhosis
- Hydralazine
- Isoniazid
- Malnutrition
- Oral contraception
- Penicillamine
- Uremia

Further reading:

- Friedli A, Saurat JH (2004) Images in clinical medicine. Oculo-orogenital syndrome: a deficiency of vitamins B2 and B6. N Engl J Med 350(11):1130

Radiation Dermatitis

Acute or chronic cutaneous changes caused by exposure to ionizing radiation that is characterized by erythema, swelling, and blistering (acute, arises within the first month) or atrophic, scarring, hyperpigmentation, hypopigmentation, and telangiectasia (chronic, arises 6 months after radiation), with the latter having the potential to ulcerate or develop basal cell and squamous cell carcinomas, angiosarcomas, and other soft tissue sarcomas

Differential Diagnosis

- Basal cell carcinoma
- Contact dermatitis
- Decubitus ulcer
- <u>Erythema ab igne</u>
- Lichen sclerosus et atrophicus
- Metastatic disease

- <u>Morphea</u>
- Poikiloderma vasculare atrophicans
- Resolved infantile hemangioma
- Squamous cell carcinoma
- <u>Steroid atrophy</u>
- Traumatic ulceration
- Unilateral nevoid telangiectasia

Further reading:

- Franchi A, Massi D, Gallo O et al (2006) Radiation-induced cutaneous carcinoma of the head and neck: is there an early role for p53 mutations? Clin Exp Dermatol 31(6):793–798

Ranula

Large type of mucocele that is caused by mucus extravasating out of a major salivary duct into the submucosal space and characterized by a blue, translucent submucosal swelling involving the floor of the mouth or neck

Differential Diagnosis

- Abscess
- Blue rubber bleb nevus
- Dermoid cyst
- Hemangioma
- Lipoma
- <u>Lymphangioma</u>
- Plexiform neurofibroma
- Salivary gland neoplasm
- Venous malformation

Further reading:

- Chidzonga MM, Mahomva L (2007) Ranula: experience with 83 cases in Zimbabwe. J Oral Maxillofac Surg 65(1):79–82

Rat-Bite Fever (Haverhill Fever, Sodoku)

Infectious disease that is acquired by rat bite, that is caused by either
Streptobacillus moniliformis (Haverhill fever; major cause in the West) or
Spirillum minus (Sodoku, major cause in the East), and is characterized
by fever, arthralgias, and a morbilliform or petechial skin eruption
(*S. moniliformis*), or fever, no arthralgias, lymphadenopathy, and an eruption of violaceous to erythematous indurated or urticarial plaques on the
trunk (*S. minus*)

Differential Diagnosis

- Brucellosis
- Ehrlichiosis
- Epstein–Barr virus infection
- Erythema multiforme
- Gonococcemia
- Leptospirosis
- Lyme disease
- Malaria
- Meningococcemia
- Relapsing fever
- Rheumatic fever
- Rocky Mountain spotted fever
- Secondary syphilis
- Serum sickness
- Sweet's syndrome
- Syphilis
- Systemic lupus erythematosus
- Typhoid fever
- Viral exanthem

Evaluation

- Blood cultures

Further reading:

- Elliott SP (2007) Rat-bite fever and *Streptobacillus moniliformis*. Clin Microbiol Rev 20(1):13–22

Raynaud's Phenomenon/Raynaud's Disease

Multifactorial vascular disorder that can accompany a variety of connective tissue diseases (phenomenon) or occur as a solitary complaint (disease) and is characterized by recurrent, cold-induced episodes of peripheral vasoconstriction leading to pain, numbness, and color change cycling from white (pallor) to blue (cyanosis) to red (hyperemia) in one or more asymmetric digits and, if chronic, the digits suffer from complications such as tip necrosis, ulceration, and gangrene

Differential Diagnosis

- Achenbach syndrome
- Acrocyanosis
- Acrodynia
- Arteriosclerosis
- Bleomycin therapy
- Buerger's disease
- Carcinoid syndrome
- Carpal tunnel syndrome
- Chemotherapy induced
- Cholesterol emboli syndrome
- Cold agglutinin disease
- Cold injury
- Cryofibrinogenemia
- Cryoglobulinemia
- Dermatomyositis
- Erythromelalgia
- Frostbite
- Paraproteinemia
- Paroxysmal nocturnal hemoglobinuria

- Perniosis
- Pheochromocytoma
- Polycythemia vera
- Polyvinyl chloride exposure
- <u>Peripheral vascular disease</u>
- <u>Scleroderma</u>
- Systemic lupus erythematosus
- Takayasu's arteritis
- Thoracic outlet syndrome
- Vibration disease

Diagnostic Criteria (For Primary Raynaud's Disease)

- Absence of gangrene or gangrene limited to fingertips
- Bilateral extremity involvement
- Negative antinuclear antibodies
- Normal sedimentation rate
- Normal vascular exam with symmetric pulses and normal nail-fold capillary microscopy
- Symptoms for at least 2 years
- Vasospastic attacks precipitated by exposure to cold or emotional stimuli

Associations

- Arteriosclerosis
- Cryoglobulins and cryofibrinogens
- Idiopathic
- <u>Lupus erythematosus</u>
- Medications
- Nerve compression
- Nicotine
- Paraneoplastic acral vascular syndrome
- Polyarteritis nodosa

- <u>Scleroderma</u>
- Stenosis
- Thoracic outlet syndrome
- Thrombotic disorders
- Trauma
- Vasculitis
- Vibration white finger
- Vinyl chloride

Associated Medications

- Amphetamines
- Beta-blockers
- Bleomycin
- Bromocriptine
- Clonidine
- Cyclosporine
- Fluoxetine
- Interferon alpha
- Oral contraceptives
- Vinblastine

Evaluation

- Anticardiolipin antibodies
- Antinuclear antibodies
- Chest radiograph
- Complete blood count
- Cryoglobulins
- Lupus anticoagulant
- Rheumatoid factor
- Sedimentation rate
- Serum protein electrophoresis

Treatment Options

- Warming measures/gloves
- <u>Nifedipine</u>
- Diltiazem
- <u>Topical nitroglycerin</u>
- Aspirin
- Dipyridamole
- Fluoxetine
- Prostacyclin
- <u>Sildenafil</u>
- Sympathectomy

Further reading:

- Pope JE (2007) The diagnosis and treatment of Raynaud's phenomenon: a practical approach. Drugs 67(4):517–525
- Leroy EC, Medsger TA Jr (1992) Raynaud's phenomenon: a proposal for classification. Clin Exp Rheumatol 10(5):485–488

Reactive Angioendotheliomatosis

Benign reactive disorder of endothelial proliferation that is associated with several vasoocclusive triggers and is characterized by erythematous or hemorrhagic papules and nodules on the trunk or lower extremities

Differential Diagnosis

- Bacillary angiomatosis
- Diffuse dermal angiomatosis
- Dabska's tumor
- Glomeruloid hemangioma
- Kaposi's sarcoma
- <u>Intravascular large B cell lymphoma (malignant angioendotheliomatosis)</u>
- Intravascular histiocytosis

- <u>Intravascular papillary endothelial hyperplasia</u>
- Intravascular pyogenic granuloma
- Livedo reticularis
- Multinucleate cell angiohistiocytoma
- Polyarteritis nodosa
- Vasculitis, cutaneous small vessel

Associations

- Amyloidosis
- Antiphospholipid antibody syndrome
- Atherosclerosis
- Cirrhosis
- Cryoglobulinemia
- Endocarditis
- Paraproteinemia
- Rheumatoid arthritis
- Systemic infection
- Tuberculosis

Evaluation

- Anticardiolipin antibodies
- Blood cultures
- Cryoglobulins
- Echocardiography
- Liver function test
- Lupus anticoagulant
- Renal function test
- Serum protein electrophoresis
- Tuberculin skin test

Further reading:

- Kirke S, Angus B, Kesteven PJ, Calonje E, Simpson N (2007) Localized reactive angioendotheliomatosis. Clin Exp Dermatol 32(1):45–47

Reactive Arthritis with Urethritis and Conjunctivitis (Reiter Syndrome)

Idiopathic syndrome predominantly affecting HLA-B27+ young men that is most commonly associated with *Chlamydia* infections (or dysentery in young children) and is characterized by hyperkeratotic pustular skin lesions on the palms and soles (keratoderma blennorrhagicum, Vidal–Jacquet syndrome), circinate balanitis, dystrophic nails, arthritis affecting the large joints, such as knees or sacroiliac joint, and urethritis and conjunctivitis

Differential Diagnosis

- Acute generalized exanthematous pustulosis
- Ankylosing spondylitis
- Atopic dermatitis
- Behçet's disease
- Chronic mucocutaneous candidiasis
- Dermatomyositis
- Gonococcemia
- Juvenile rheumatoid arthritis
- Kawasaki disease
- Lupus erythematosus
- Lichen planus
- Lyme disease
- Mycosis fungoides
- Pityriasis rubra pilaris
- Psoriasis
- Rheumatic fever
- Scabies
- Septic arthritis
- Serum sickness
- Subcorneal pustular dermatosis
- Trench fever

Evaluation

- Antinuclear antibodies
- Blood cultures
- *Chlamydia* serologic test
- HIV test
- HLA-B27 assay
- Joint-fluid analysis
- Ophthalmologic examination
- Radiograph of affected joints
- Rheumatoid factor
- Sedimentation rate
- Stool cultures
- Urethral/cervical culture
- Urinalysis and culture

Treatment

- Treat underlying cause
- Topical corticosteroids
- Tazarotene cream
- Acitretin
- Methotrexate
- Cyclosporine
- Infliximab

Further reading:
- Schneider JM, Matthews JH, Graham BS (2003) Reiter's syndrome. Cutis 71(3):198–200

Reactive Perforating Collagenosis

Hereditary perforating disorder with onset in childhood that is characterized by trauma-induced, erythematous papules with central keratotic plugs that are most commonly located on the extensor aspect of the extremities

Differential Diagnosis

- <u>Acquired perforating dermatosis</u>
- Arthropod bites
- Dermatofibromas
- <u>Elastosis perforans serpiginosa</u>
- Erythema elevatum diutinum
- Familial dyskeratotic comedones
- Folliculitis
- Molluscum contagiosum
- Multiple keratoacanthomas
- <u>Perforating granuloma annulare</u>
- Perforating pseudoxanthoma elasticum
- Prurigo nodularis

Further reading:
- Ramesh V, Sood N, Kubba A et al (2007) Familial reactive perforating collagenosis: a clinical, histopathological study of 10 cases. J Eur Acad Dermatol Venereol 21(6):766–770

Refsum Disease

Inherited disorder (AR) caused by mutation of the phytanoyl-CoA hydroxylase gene that leads to excessive amounts of dietary plant or animal-derived phytanic acid and is characterized by ichthyosis, cerebellar ataxia, sensory and motor polyneuropathy, and retinitis pigmentosa

Differential Diagnosis

- Acute intermittent porphyria
- Guillain–Barre syndrome
- Hereditary motor neuropathies
- Ichthyosis vulgaris
- Lamellar ichthyosis
- <u>Neonatal adrenal leukodystrophy</u>

- Rhizomelic chondrodysplasia punctata
- Sjögren–Larsson syndrome
- X-linked ichthyosis
- Zellweger syndrome

Further reading:

- Horn MA, van den Brink DM, Wanders RJ et al (2007) Phenotype of adult Refsum disease due to a defect in peroxin 7. Neurology 68(9):698–700

Relapsing Fever

Epidemic louse-borne (northeast Africa) or endemic tick-borne disease (United States) that is caused by either *Borrelia recurrentis* (louse only) or several other species of *Borrelia*, including *Borrelia hermsii or Borrelia duttonii* (tick); is transmitted either by the human body louse, *Pediculus humanus*, or the soft-bodied tick, *Ornithodoros*; and is characterized by recurrent febrile episodes with headaches, myalgias, and a morbilliform or petechial skin eruption

Differential Diagnosis

- Brucellosis
- Chronic meningococcemia
- Colorado tick fever
- Dengue fever
- Juvenile rheumatoid arthritis
- Leptospirosis
- Lyme disease
- Lymphocytic choriomeningitis
- Malaria
- Rat-bite fever
- Rocky Mountain spotted fever
- Trench fever
- Yellow fever

Further reading:

* McGinley-Smith DE, Tsao SS (2003) Dermatoses from ticks. J Am Acad Dermatol 49(3):363–392

Relapsing Polychondritis

Autoimmune disease caused by autoantibodies against type II collagen that is associated with inflamed cartilage in the ears, nose, or trachea and is characterized by auricular inflammation that spares the lobule, saddle-nose deformity, and a potential for airway compromise, along with an inflammatory arthritis and vasculitis affecting the skin and internal organs

Differential Diagnosis

* Alkaptonuria
* Cellulitis
* Chondrodermatitis nodularis helicis
* Chronic external otitis
* Cogan syndrome
* Congenital syphilis
* Erysipelas
* Erythromelalgia (otomelalgia)
* Infectious perichondritis
* Jessner's lymphocytic infiltrate
* Malignant otitis externa
* NK cell lymphoma
* Polyarteritis nodosa
* Polymorphous light eruption
* Postsurgical chondritis
* Pseudocyst of the auricle
* Rheumatoid arthritis
* Sarcoidosis

- Sjögren's syndrome
- Syphilis
- Traumatic auricular calcification
- Traumatic chondritis
- Wegener's granulomatosis

Diagnostic Criteria (3/6)

- Bilateral auricular chondritis
- Nonerosive seronegative inflammatory polyarthritis
- Nasal chondritis
- Ocular inflammation
- Respiratory tract chondritis
- Audiovestibular damage

Associations

- <u>Behçet's disease (MAGIC syndrome)</u>
- Dermatomyositis
- Erythema elevatum diutinum
- Erythema nodosum
- Goserelin therapy
- Inflammatory bowel disease
- Leukocytoclastic vasculitis
- Livedo reticularis
- <u>Myelodysplastic syndrome</u>
- Polyarteritis nodosa
- Pyoderma-gangrenosum-like lesions
- Sjögren's syndrome
- Systemic vasculitis syndromes
- Sweet's syndrome
- Thyroiditis

Evaluation

- Antinuclear antibodies
- Chest CT/MRI
- Complete blood count
- Echocardiogram
- Electrocardiogram
- Ophthalmologic examination
- Pulmonary function test
- Renal function
- Rheumatoid factor
- Urinalysis

Treatment Options

- <u>Systemic corticosteroids</u>
- NSAIDs
- <u>Dapsone</u>
- Azathioprine
- Cyclosporine
- <u>Methotrexate</u>
- <u>Cyclophosphamide</u>
- Colchicine
- Minocycline
- Pentoxifylline
- Plasmapheresis
- <u>Infliximab</u>

Further reading:

- McAdam LP, O'Hanlan MA, Bluestone R, Pearson CM (1976) Relapsing polychondritis: prospective study of 23 patients and a review of the literature. Medicine (Baltimore) 55(3):193–215
- Rapini RP, Warner NB (2006) Relapsing polychondritis. Clin Dermatol 24(6):482–485

Reticular Erythematous Mucinosis

Idiopathic mucinosis that predominantly affects middle-aged women, may arise after sun exposure, and is characterized by erythematous macules or flat papules and plaques in a reticular pattern on the upper chest or upper back

Differential Diagnosis

- Alopecia mucinosa
- Dermatomyositis
- Erythema annulare centrifugum (deep type)
- Focal mucinosis
- Jessner's lymphocytic infiltrate
- Lupus erythematosus (especially tumid type)
- Mycosis fungoides
- Myxedema
- Nevus mucinosis
- Papular mucinosis
- Polymorphous light eruption
- Scleredema
- Scleromyxedema
- Seborrheic dermatitis

Associations

- Diabetes mellitus
- Graves' disease
- Hashimoto's thyroiditis
- Lupus erythematosus
- Thrombocytopenic purpura

Treatment Options

- Sunscreen
- Topical corticosteroids
- Hydroxychloroquine
- Tacrolimus ointment
- Systemic corticosteroids

Further reading:
- Adamski H, Le Gall F, Chevrant-Breton J (2004) Positive photobiological investigation in reticular erythematous mucinosis syndrome. Photodermatol Photoimmunol Photomed 20(5):235–238

Reticulate Acropigmentation of Kitamura

Inherited pigmentary disorder of unknown cause that is characterized by hyperpigmented macules on both sides of the hands and feet and pits on the volar surface

Differential Diagnosis

- Acropigmentation of Dohi (dyschromatosis symmetrica hereditaria)
- Dowling–Degos disease
- Dyschromatosis universalis hereditaria
- Solar lentigines
- Universal acquired melanosis

Further reading:
- Al Hawsawi K, Al Aboud K, Alfadley A et al (2002) Reticulate acropigmentation of Kitamura–Dowling Degos disease overlap: a case report. Int J Dermatol 41(8):518–520

Reticulohistiocytoma, Solitary (Epithelioid Histiocytoma)

Benign reactive histiocytic lesion arising in young adults, especially males, that is characterized by solitary, firm, dome-shaped, dermal nodule on any body area, but uncommonly on the face or hands, as in multicentric reticulohistiocytosis

Differential Diagnosis

- Adnexal tumor
- Atypical fibroxanthoma
- Dermatofibroma
- Epithelioid fibrous histiocytoma
- Epithelioid sarcoma
- Histiocytic sarcoma
- Infectious granulomas
- Juvenile xanthogranuloma
- Melanocytic nevus
- Rosai–Dorfman disease

Further reading:
- Miettinen M, Fetsch JF (2006) Reticulohistiocytoma (solitary epithelioid histiocytoma): a clinicopathologic and immunohistochemical study of 44 cases. Am J Surg Pathol 30(4):521–528

Rhabdomyomatous Mesenchymal Hamartoma

Congenital striated muscle hamartoma in which striated muscle is ectopically located in the deep dermis and subcutaneous layers and is characterized by a flesh-colored, often mobile, pedunculated nodule or finger-like projection on the face

Differential Diagnosis

- <u>Accessory tragus</u>
- <u>Acrochordon</u>
- Fibrous hamartoma of infancy
- Infantile myofibromatosis
- Nasal glioma
- Nevus lipomatosus superficialis
- Rhabdomyoma
- Rhabdomyosarcoma
- Smooth muscle hamartoma

Associations

- Amniotic band syndrome
- Delleman syndrome

Further reading:
- Rosenberg AS, Kirk J, Morgan MB (2002) Rhabdomyomatous mesenchymal hamartoma: an unusual dermal entity with a report of two cases and a review of the literature. J Cutan Pathol 29(4):238–243

Rhabdomyosarcoma

Malignant soft tissue neoplasm that is derived from the embryonal mesenchymal cells that give rise to striated muscle, arises in childhood, and is characterized by a subcutaneous, protruding, exophytic mass on the head and neck, often the face (or when congenital, as a blueberry muffin baby presentation)

Differential Diagnosis

- Ewing sarcoma
- Leiomyosarcoma

- Leukemia cutis
- Liposarcoma
- Lymphoma
- Malignant fibrous histiocytoma
- Neuroblastoma
- <u>Rhabdomyoma</u>
- Rhabdomyomatous mesenchymal hamartoma

Further reading:
- Brecher AR, Reyes-Mugica M, Kamino H et al (2003) Congenital primary cutaneous rhabdomyosarcoma in a neonate. Pediatr Dermatol 20(4):335–338

Rheumatoid Neutrophilic Dermatosis

Dermatosis that is associated with rheumatoid arthritis and characterized by erythematous papules, plaques, nodules, and urticarial wheals that occur over the extremities and trunk

Differential Diagnosis

- Atypical mycobacterium infection
- Behçet's disease
- Bullous lupus erythematosus
- Bowel bypass dermatosis–arthrosis syndrome
- Churg–Strauss syndrome
- Cutaneous Crohn's disease
- Dermatitis herpetiformis
- <u>Erythema elevatum diutinum</u>
- Granuloma annulare
- <u>Interstitial granulomatous dermatitis with arthritis</u>
- <u>Methotrexate-induced papular eruption</u>
- <u>Palisaded neutrophilic and granulomatous dermatitis</u>
- Pyoderma gangrenosum
- Sweet's syndrome

- Urticaria
- Vasculitis
- Wegener's granulomatosis

Treatment Options

- Treatment of rheumatoid arthritis
- Systemic corticosteroids
- Dapsone
- Methotrexate
- Infliximab

Further reading:

- Bevin AA, Steger J, Mannino S (2006) Rheumatoid neutrophilic dermatitis. Cutis 78(2):133–136

Rheumatoid Nodule

Cutaneous manifestation of rheumatoid arthritis that occurs in patients with severe disease and high rheumatoid factor levels and is characterized by subcutaneous nodules over the bony prominences and tendons, especially on the dorsal hands, around the olecranon, or over the Achilles tendon

Differential Diagnosis

- Epidermoid cyst
- Epithelioid sarcoma
- Ganglion cyst
- Gouty tophi
- Foreign body granuloma
- Necrobiosis lipoidica
- Necrobiotic xanthogranuloma
- Nodular amyloidosis
- Palisaded neutrophilic and granulomatous dermatosis

- Rheumatic fever nodule
- Sarcoidosis
- Subcutaneous granuloma annulare
- Synovial cyst
- Tumoral calcinosis
- Xanthoma (tuberous)

Further reading:
- Sayah A, English JC (2005) Rheumatoid arthritis: a review of the cutaneous manifestations. J Am Acad Dermatol 53(2):191–209

Rhinophyma (Phymatous Rosacea)

Deforming process of the nose caused by marked sebaceous overgrowth that arises predominantly in older men with or without a history of rosacea and is characterized by bulbous protrusion of the nose, with lumpy surface changes, sebaceous hyperplasia, and fibrosis

Differential Diagnosis

- Angiofibromas
- Angiosarcoma
- B cell lymphoma
- Basal cell carcinoma
- Chronic fibrosing vasculitis
- Cutaneous lymphoid hyperplasia
- Granuloma faciale
- Leishmaniasis
- Melanoma
- Metastatic disease
- Microcystic adnexal carcinoma
- Rhinoscleroma
- Sarcoidosis
- Sebaceous adenoma

Treatment Options

- Surgical excision
- Dermabrasion
- Electrosurgery
- CO_2 laser
- Isotretinoin

Further reading:
- Powell FC (2005) Clinical practice. Rosacea. N Engl J Med 352(8):793–803

Rhinoscleroma

Chronic infection of the nose and nasal passages that is caused by *Klebsiella rhinoscleromatis* and is characterized by chronic nasal inflammation with epistaxis, nasal obstruction, indurated nodules on the nasal mucosa, and eventual sclerosis and destruction of the nasal airway (Hebra nose)

Differential Diagnosis

- Actinomycosis
- Blastomycosis
- Coccidioidomycosis
- Histoplasmosis
- Keloid
- Langerhans cell histiocytosis
- Leprosy
- Lymphoma
- Mucocutaneous leishmaniasis
- Nasal tuberculosis
- Nasopalatine duct cyst
- Paracoccidioidomycosis
- Rhinoentoophthoromycosis

- <u>Rhinosporidiosis</u>
- Rosai–Dorfman disease
- <u>Sarcoidosis</u>
- Tertiary syphilis
- Verrucous carcinoma
- Wegener's granulomatosis
- Yaws

Evaluation

- Bacterial culture of affected tissue

Further reading:

- Fernandez-Vozmediano JM, Armario Hita JC et al (2004) Rhinoscleroma in three siblings. Pediatr Dermatol 21(2):134–138

Rhinosporidiosis

Chronic granulomatous infection of the nasal passages with the aquatic protistan parasite, *Rhinosporidia seeberi*, that is characterized by vascular, friable, nasal-polyp-like masses with resulting epistaxis and nasal obstruction, and accompanying polyps on the conjunctiva in some patients

Differential Diagnosis

- Foreign body
- Mucocele
- <u>Myospherulosis</u>
- <u>Nasal polyp</u>
- Paracoccidioidomycosis
- <u>Pyogenic granuloma</u>
- Metastatic disease
- <u>Rhinoscleroma</u>
- Sarcoidosis

- Squamous cell carcinoma
- Verrucous carcinoma

Evaluation

- Potassium hydroxide examination of tissue

Further reading:
- Ghorpade A (2006) Polymorphic cutaneous rhinosporidiosis. Eur J Dermatol 16(2):190–192

Riboflavin Deficiency
(Oculo-Oro-Genital Syndrome, Jacobs Syndrome)

Deficiency of vitamin B2 that is most commonly caused by malnutrition in the setting of alcoholism and is characterized by angular cheilitis, atrophic glossitis, dermatitis of the face and groin, and blepharoconjunctivitis

Differential Diagnosis

- Acrodermatitis enteropathica
- Behçet's disease
- Candidiasis
- Necrolytic migratory erythema
- Pellagra
- Pyridoxine deficiency
- Seborrheic dermatitis

Associations

- Alcoholism
- Hypothyroidism

- Low-cereal diet
- Low-vegetable diet
- Neonatal hyperbilirubinemia

Further reading:
- Friedli A, Saurat JH (2004) Images in clinical medicine. Oculo-orogenital syndrome: a deficiency of vitamins B2 and B6. N Engl J Med 350(11):1130

Rickettsialpox

Febrile illness caused by *Rickettsia akari* that is transmitted by the mite of the house mouse and characterized by an initial tache noir and later a generalized vesiculopustular exanthem

Differential Diagnosis

- Aspergillosis
- Cutaneous anthrax
- Ecthyma gangrenosum
- Enterovirus infection
- Factitial dermatitis
- Hand, foot, and mouth disease
- Monkeypox
- Pityriasis lichenoides et varioliformis acuta
- Pustular drug eruption
- Scrub typhus
- Smallpox
- Spider bite
- Trauma
- Varicella

Further reading:
- Walker DH (2007) Rickettsiae and rickettsial infections: the current state of knowledge. Clin Infect Dis 45(Suppl 1):S39–S44

Riehl's Melanosis (Pigmented Contact Dermatitis)

Acquired pigmentary disorder predominantly affecting patients of Asian descent that is caused by a low-grade allergic contact dermatitis to fragrances and other cosmetic products and that is characterized by hyperpigmentation on the face in areas that came into contact with the triggering chemical

Differential Diagnosis

- Acanthosis nigricans
- Acquired brachial cutaneous dyschromatosis
- <u>Berloque dermatitis</u>
- Drug-induced pigmentation
- Lupus erythematosus
- <u>Lichen planus pigmentosus</u>
- <u>Melasma</u>
- Nevus of Ota
- Phytophotodermatitis
- Poikiloderma of Civatte
- Polymorphous light eruption
- <u>Postinflammatory hyperpigmentation</u>
- Tar melanosis (melanodermatitis toxica)

Further reading:
- Ebihara T, Nakayama H (1997) Pigmented contact dermatitis. Clin Dermatol 15(4):593–599

Rocky Mountain Spotted Fever

Potentially fatal febrile illness caused by *Rickettsiae rickettsii*, transmitted by *Dermacentor* and *Amblyomma* ticks, and characterized by a petechial eruption that starts acrally and spreads in a centripetal pattern (sometimes with a spotless variant), fever and chills, severe headache, vasculitis, disseminated intravascular coagulation, and cardiovascular collapse

Differential Diagnosis

- Atypical measles
- Babesiosis
- <u>Bacterial sepsis</u>
- Dengue fever
- Drug reaction
- Ehrlichiosis
- <u>Encephalitis</u>
- Erythema multiforme
- Immune thrombocytopenic purpura
- Leptospirosis
- Lyme disease
- Malaria
- Measles
- <u>Meningococcemia</u>
- Mononucleosis
- Rat-bite fever
- Rubella
- Secondary syphilis
- <u>Small vessel leukocytoclastic vasculitis</u>
- Thrombotic thrombocytopenic purpura
- Toxic shock syndrome
- Toxoplasmosis
- Tularemia
- Typhoid fever
- Viral infection

Evaluation

- Cerebrospinal fluid analysis
- Complete blood count
- CT/MRI scan of brain
- Indirect immunofluorescence antibody test
- Liver function test

- Renal function test
- Serum chemistry

Further reading:

- Lacz NL, Schwartz RA, Kapila R (2006) Rocky Mountain spotted fever. J Eur Acad Dermatol Venereol 20(4):411–417

Rosacea

Chronic acneiform condition of the central face characterized by erythema, telangiectasias, papules, and pustules, but no comedones

Subtypes/Variants

- Erythematotelangiectatic
- Granulomatous
- Ocular
- Papulopustular
- Perioral dermatitis
- Phymatous
- Pyoderma faciale
- Steroid-induced

Differential Diagnosis

- Acne vulgaris
- Acute cutaneous lupus erythematosus
- Angiosarcoma
- Carcinoid syndrome
- Cutaneous sinus histiocytosis (Rosai–Dorfman disease)
- Demodicosis
- Granuloma faciale
- Granulomatous periorificial dermatitis
- Haber syndrome

- Halogenoderma
- Lupus miliaris disseminata faciei
- Lupus vulgaris
- Lymphedema
- Mastocytosis
- <u>Perioral dermatitis</u>
- Pheochromocytoma
- Photosensitive drug reaction
- Polymorphous light eruption
- Recurrent erysipelas
- <u>Sarcoidosis</u>
- <u>Seborrheic dermatitis</u>
- Syringomas
- Tinea faciei
- Trichoepitheliomas

Associations

- Alcohol
- <u>*Demodex folliculorum*</u>
- Flushing
- Heat
- *Helicobacter pylori* infection
- Migraine
- Oral contraception
- Sun exposure

Treatment Options

- Topical metronidazole
- Oral metronidazole
- <u>Azelaic acid</u>
- <u>Oral tetracyclines</u>
- Oral macrolides

- Topical clindamycin
- Benzoyl peroxide
- Sulfur/sulfacetamide
- Spironolactone
- Isotretinoin
- <u>Ivermectin</u>
- <u>Permethrin</u>
- <u>Sunscreen</u>
- Nicotinamide
- Clonidine
- Beta-blockers
- <u>Pulsed dye laser</u>
- Intense pulse light

Further reading:
- Powell FC (2005) Clinical practice. Rosacea. N Engl J Med 352(8):793–803

Rosai–Dorfman Disease (Sinus Histiocytosis with Massive Lymphadenopathy)

Non-Langerhans type of histiocytosis that is possibly viral in etiology, arises in the first or second decade of life, and is characterized by lymphadenopathy (often massive), fever, anemia, leukocytosis and, uncommonly, extranodal disease and skin lesions, which are typically red-brown or red-yellow papules and nodules on variable locations of the body. Less commonly and in older patients, Rosai–Dorfman disease can present only on the skin, where the lesions show a predilection for the face

Differential Diagnosis

- Acne conglobata
- Benign cephalic histiocytosis
- Cutaneous lymphoid hyperplasia
- Dermatofibroma

- Deep fungal infection
- EBV infection
- Generalized eruptive histiocytoma
- Granuloma annulare
- <u>Granuloma faciale</u>
- Indeterminate cell histiocytosis
- Lepromatous leprosy
- Lupus erythematosus
- Lupus miliaris disseminata faciei
- Lymphoma
- Kikuchi–Fujimoto disease
- Papular xanthomas
- Reticulohistiocytosis
- <u>Rosacea</u>
- <u>Sarcoidosis</u>
- Tuberculosis

Further reading:

- Frater JL, Maddox JS, Obadiah JM et al (2006) Cutaneous Rosai–Dorfman disease: comprehensive review of cases reported in the medical literature since 1990 and presentation of an illustrative case. J Cutan Med Surg 10(6):281–290

Roseola Infantum (Exanthem Subitum)

Common illness affecting children in the first year of life that is caused by human herpes virus 6 and characterized by a prodrome of extremely high fever (with possible febrile seizures) followed by a morbilliform eruption predominantly affecting the neck and trunk

Differential Diagnosis

- Adenovirus infection
- Dengue
- <u>Enterovirus infection</u>

- Epstein–Barr virus
- Erythema infectiosum
- Kawasaki disease
- Measles
- Medication reaction
- Meningococcemia
- Rocky Mountain spotted fever
- Rubella
- Scarlet fever

Treatment Options

- Observation and reassurance

Further reading:
- Dyer JA (2007) Childhood viral exanthems. Pediatr Ann 36(1):21–29

Rothmund–Thomson Syndrome (Poikiloderma Congenitale)

Autosomal-recessive disorder caused by a defect in the DNA repair helicase, RECQL4, that is characterized by photodistributed erythema and telangiectasia, hypoplastic radius and thumbs, short stature, cataracts, and tendency to develop osteosarcoma

Differential Diagnosis

- Acrogeria
- Bloom syndrome
- Cockayne syndrome
- Dermatomyositis
- Dyskeratosis congenita
- Erythropoietic protoporphyria
- Fanconi's anemia

- Kindler syndrome
- Lupus erythematosus
- Poikiloderma atrophicans vasculare
- <u>Progeria</u>
- <u>Weary–Kindler syndrome</u>
- Werner syndrome
- Xeroderma pigmentosum

Further reading:
- Kumar P, Sharma PK, Gautam RK et al (2007) Late-onset Rothmund–Thomson syndrome. Int J Dermatol 46(5):492–493

Rubella (German Measles)

Uncommon viral disease caused by the rubella togavirus that affects children and young adults and is characterized by a morbilliform eruption which lasts 3 days and begins on the face and neck but generalizes caudally, as well as petechiae of the soft palate (Forschheimer spots) and suboccipital and postauricular lymphadenopathy

Differential Diagnosis

- Drug eruption
- Erythema infectiosum
- Juvenile rheumatoid arthritis
- Kawasaki disease
- <u>Measles</u>
- Roseola
- Scarlet fever
- Viral exanthem

Further reading:
- Carneiro SC, Cestari T, Allen SH et al (2007) Viral exanthems in the tropics. Clin Dermatol 25(2):212–220

Sarcoidosis (Besnier–Boeck Disease)

Acquired immune-mediated disease of uncertain cause that is marked by granulomatous inflammation in the skin, lungs, and other organs; is possibly a foreign body reaction in individuals susceptible to an infectious or noninfectious exogenous antigen; and is characterized (cutaneously) by red-brown papules, nodules, and plaques on the face, especially the nose and periorbital areas, as well as the trunk and extremities

Subtypes/Variants

- Angiolupoid
- Annular
- Cicatricial alopecia (discoid-lupus-like; Fig. 6.106)
- Exfoliative/erythrodermic
- Granulomatous cheilitis
- Hypopigmented
- Ichthyosiform
- Lupus pernio
- Micropapular (lichenoid)
- Morpheaform
- Mucosal
- Nail

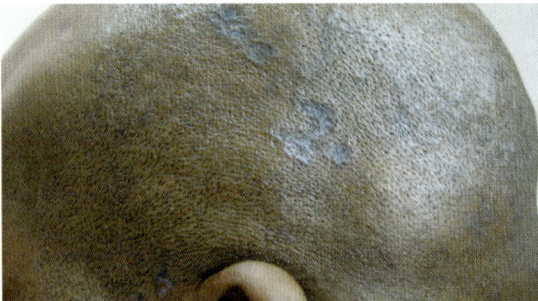

Fig. 6.106 Discoid-lupus-like sarcoidosis

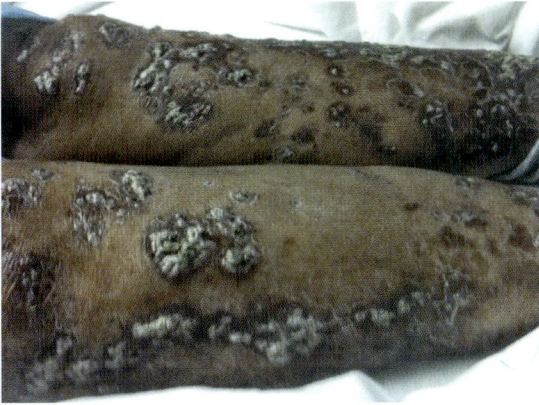

Fig. 6.107 Verrucous sarcoidosis

- Nodular
- Papular
- Perforating
- Plaque
- Psoriasiform
- Scar
- Subcutaneous (Darier–Roussy sarcoid)
- Systemic
- Tattoo
- Ulcerative
- Verrucous (Fig. 6.107)

Differential Diagnosis

Papular, Micropapular, Plaques, Verrucous Plaques, Ulcers, and Alopecia

- Acne
- Actinic granuloma
- Amyloidosis
- Angiofibromas
- Annular elastolytic giant cell granuloma

- Atypical mycobacteria
- Berylliosis
- Blau syndrome
- Cheilitis granulomatosis
- Crohn's disease, cutaneous
- Cutaneous lymphoid hyperplasia
- Cutaneous T cell lymphoma
- Epithelioid sarcoma
- Erythema multiforme
- Folliculitis
- Foreign body granuloma
- Gouty tophus
- Granuloma annulare
- Granuloma faciale
- Granulomatous mycosis fungoides
- Granulomatous periorificial dermatitis
- Granulomatous rosacea
- Granulomatous skin lesions associated with systemic lymphoma
- Histiocytoses
- Immunodeficiency-related noninfectious granuloma
- Interstitial granulomatous drug reaction
- Kaposi's sarcoma
- Leprosy
- Lichen nitidus
- Lichen planus, hypertrophic
- Lichen sclerosus
- Lichen scrofulosorum
- Lichen simplex
- Lipodermatosclerosis
- Lupus erythematosus
- Lupus miliaris disseminata faciei
- Lupus vulgaris
- Lymphocytoma cutis
- Lymphoma
- Lymphomatoid granulomatosis

- Morphea
- Multinucleate cell angiohistiocytoma
- <u>Necrobiosis lipoidica</u>
- Necrobiotic xanthogranuloma
- Pityriasis rosea
- Psoriasis
- Pyoderma gangrenosum
- Rosai–Dorfman disease
- Scabies
- Sporotrichosis
- Syphilis
- Syringomas
- Tinea corporis
- Trichoepitheliomas
- <u>Tuberculosis</u>
- Verruca plana
- Whipple's disease
- Xanthomas

Hypopigmented

- Chemical leukoderma
- Discoid lupus erythematosus
- <u>Hypopigmented mycosis fungoides</u>
- Idiopathic guttate hypomelanosis
- Leishmaniasis
- Leprosy
- Tinea versicolor
- Vitiligo
- Pinta
- <u>Postinflammatory hypopigmentation</u>
- Syphilis

Lupus Pernio

- Lupus erythematosus
- Lupus vulgaris

- <u>Rosacea</u>
- <u>Rhinophyma</u>
- Rhinoscleroma
- Tertiary syphilis
- Wegener's granulomatosis

Subcutaneous

- Epidermoid cyst
- Gouty tophi
- Interstitial granulomatous dermatitis
- Lipoma
- Lymphadenopathy
- Metastasis
- Morphea
- <u>Panniculitis</u>
- Rheumatoid nodule
- <u>Subcutaneous granuloma annulare</u>
- Subcutaneous lymphoma

Associations

- Autoimmune hemolytic anemia
- Dermatitis herpetiformis
- Exogenous ochronosis
- Heerfordt's syndrome
- Interferon-alpha therapy
- Lofgren's syndrome
- Mikulicz syndrome
- Sweet's syndrome
- Systemic sclerosis
- Tattoos
- Thyroiditis
- Vitiligo

Evaluation

- ACE level
- Calcium level
- Chest radiograph
- Complete blood count (lymphopenia)
- Cultures for bacteria, mycobacteria, and fungus
- Electrocardiography
- Hepatic function test
- Neurologic exam
- Opththalmologic exam
- Pulmonary function test
- Serum protein electrophoresis
- Tuberculin skin test (with controls)

Treatment Options

- Topical corticosteroids
- Intralesional corticosteroids
- Systemic corticosteroids
- Hydroxychloroquine
- Quinacrine
- Methotrexate
- Allopurinol
- Minocycline
- Isotretinoin
- Thalidomide
- Azathioprine
- Infliximab

Further reading:

- Tchernev G, Patterson JW, Nenoff P et al (2010) Sarcoidosis of the skin--a dermatological puzzle: important differential diagnostic aspects and guidelines for clinical and histopathological recognition. J Eur Acad Dermatol Venereol 24(2):125–137

Scabies

Superficial cutaneous infestation with the *Sarcoptes scabiei* female mite and characterized by extremely pruritic excoriated papules and vesicles, eczematous dermatitis, and burrows predominantly in the acral areas, web spaces, and groin that can become severely crusted (Norwegian type) in the immunosuppressed

Differential Diagnosis

Classic

- Atopic dermatitis
- Bedbug bites
- Bullous pemphigoid
- Cheyletiella dermatitis
- Chigger bites
- Cocaine abuse
- Contact dermatitis
- Cutaneous lymphoid hyperplasia
- Delusions of parasitosis
- Dermatitis herpetiformis
- Dyshidrotic eczema
- Eosinophilic folliculitis
- Erythroderma
- Fiberglass dermatitis
- Formication
- Gianotti–Crosti syndrome
- Grover's disease
- Harvest-mite bites
- Id reaction
- Impetigo
- Infantile acropustulosis
- Langerhans cell histiocytosis
- Lichen planus

- <u>Neurotic excoriations</u>
- <u>Papular dermatitis</u>
- Papular urticaria
- <u>Pediculosis corporis</u>
- Pityriasis lichenoides
- Pityriasis rosea
- <u>Prurigo simplex</u>
- <u>Pruritus of internal disease</u>
- Psoriasis
- Pyoderma
- Sabra dermatitis
- Seborrheic dermatitis
- Secondary syphilis
- Urticaria
- Urticaria pigmentosum
- Xerotic eczema

Norwegian Crusted Type

- Acquired ichthyosis
- Drug eruption
- Eczema
- Exfoliative dermatitis
- Langerhans cell histiocytosis
- Pityriasis rubra pilaris
- Psoriasis
- Seborrheic dermatitis

Treatment Options

- <u>Permethrin cream</u>
- Malathion lotion
- Benzyl benzoate
- Lindane
- Precipitated sulfur

- Crotamiton
- Ivermectin

Further reading:
- Hengge UR, Currie BJ, Jager G et al (2006) Scabies: a ubiquitous neglected skin disease. Lancet Infect Dis 6(12):769–779

Scarlet Fever

Toxin-mediated syndrome that is associated with infection of the oropharynx by group A beta-hemolytic *Streptococcus* and is characterized by fever, cervical lymphadenopathy, strawberry-like tongue, a diffuse sandpaper-like erythematous eruption, linear petechiae in the intertriginous folds (Pastia's lines), and eventual acral desquamation

Differential Diagnosis

- Drug eruption
- Epstein–Barr virus infection
- Erythema infectiosum
- Gianotti–Crosti syndrome
- Juvenile rheumatoid arthritis
- Kawasaki disease
- Lupus erythematosus
- Measles
- Rat-bite fever
- Rheumatic fever
- Rubella
- Secondary syphilis
- Serum-sickness-like reaction
- Staphylococcal scalded-skin syndrome (abortive form)
- Toxic shock syndrome
- Urticaria
- Viral exanthem

Treatment Options

- Antistreptococcal antibiotics

Further reading:
- Aber C, Alvarez Connelly E, Schachner LA (2007) Fever and rash in a child: when to worry? Pediatr Ann 36(1):30–38

Schnitzler Syndrome

Acquired syndrome of uncertain pathogenesis that is characterized by IgM monoclonal gammopathy, chronic urticaria, febrile episodes, arthralgias and bone pain, and lymphadenopathy

Differential Diagnosis

- Adult Still's disease
- Chronic immune urticaria
- Episodic angioedema with eosinophilia
- Familial Mediterranean fever
- Hepatitis virus infection
- Lupus erythematosus
- Muckle–Wells syndrome
- Multiple myeloma
- Serum-sickness-like drug reaction
- Urticarial vasculitis
- Waldenstrom macroglobulinemia

Evaluation

- Complete blood count
- Radiography of painful bones
- Sedimentation rate
- Serum/urinary protein electrophoresis

Further reading:

• Almerigogna F, Giudizi MG, Cappelli F et al (2002) Schnitzler's syndrome: what's new? J Eur Acad Dermatol Venereol 16(3):214–219

Scleredema

Idiopathic mucinosis affecting children or adults that is characterized by mucin deposition in the dermis that leads to poorly defined mildly erythematous indurated plaques with a "peau d'orange" appearance on the upper back or less commonly the face and extremities (Fig. 6.108)

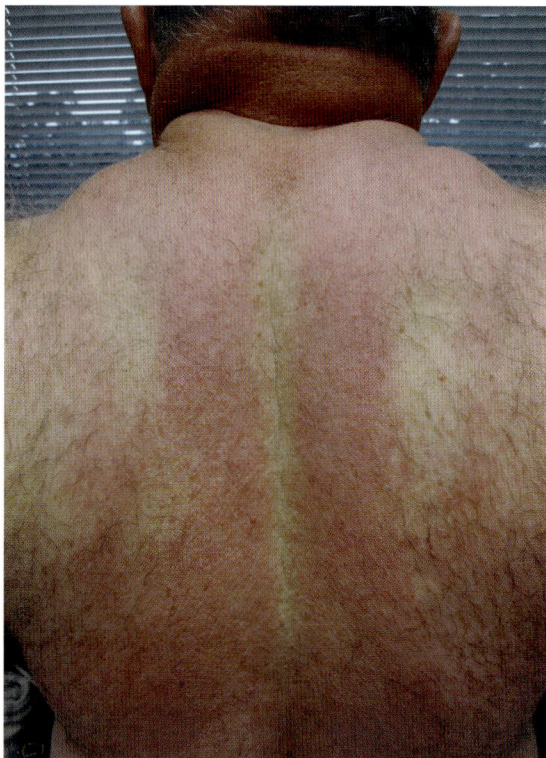

Fig. 6.108 Scleredema

Subtypes/Variants

- Type I (adultorum of Buschke): poststreptococcal
- Type II: monoclonal gammopathy associated
- Type III: (diabeticorum): diabetes associated

Differential Diagnosis

- Amyloidosis
- Cardiovascular edema
- Cellulitis
- Dermatomyositis
- Erysipelas
- Generalized myxedema
- Lymphedema
- Reticular erythematous mucinosis
- Sclerema neonatorum
- Scleromyxedema
- Systemic sclerosis
- Trichinosis

Evaluation

- Antistreptolysin O titer
- Fasting blood glucose
- Serum/urinary protein electrophoresis

Treatment Options

- Treat underlying cause
- Radiation
- Cyclosporine

Further reading:
- Beers WH, Ince A, Moore TL (2006) Scleredema adultorum of Buschke: a case report and review of the literature. Semin Arthritis Rheum 35(6):355–359

Sclerema Neonatorum (Underwood Disease)

Very rare panniculitis that affects preterm neonates because of a higher melting point of subcutaneous fat (higher saturated to unsaturated fat ratio) and is characterized by generalized induration of the skin along with flexion contractures and a high mortality

Differential Diagnosis

- Congenital lymphedema
- Poststeroid panniculitis
- Restrictive dermopathy
- Scleredema
- Scleroderma
- Subcutaneous fat necrosis of the newborn
- Turner syndrome

Associations

- Hypothermia
- Neonatal infections
- Prematurity

Treatment Options

- Supportive care
- Systemic antibiotics
- Systemic corticosteroids

Further reading:
- Battin M, Harding J, Gunn A (2002) Sclerema neonatorum following hypothermia. J Paediatr Child Health 38(5):533–534

Scleromyxedema (Arndt–Gottron Syndrome)

Diffuse sclerotic variant of lichen myxedematosus that is associated with IgG-lambda monoclonal gammopathy and that is characterized by a generalized eruption of waxy, flesh-colored papules that coalesce into indurated plaques with eventual diffuse sclerosis of the skin and, occasionally, the internal organs, especially the gastrointestinal tract

Differential Diagnosis

- Diffuse papular granuloma annulare
- Eosinophilic fasciitis
- Generalized eruptive histiocytoma
- Generalized morphea
- Lichen myxedematosus
- Lipoid proteinosis
- Micropapular sarcoidosis
- Mycosis fungoides
- Nephrogenic fibrosing dermopathy
- Scleredema
- Systemic sclerosis

Diagnostic Criteria

- Generalized papular and sclerodermoid eruption
- Microscopic triad of mucin, fibroblasts, and fibrosis
- Monoclonal gammopathy
- Absence of thyroid disease

Evaluation

- Antinuclear antibodies
- Serum protein electrophoresis
- Thyroid function tests

Treatment Options

- Topical corticosteroids
- Intralesional corticosteroids
- Acitretin
- Isotretinoin
- Melphalan
- <u>Plasmapheresis</u>
- <u>Intravenous immunoglobulin</u>
- Methotrexate
- Cyclosporine
- Radiation
- Extracorporeal photopheresis
- Thalidomide
- Cyclophosphamide
- Chlorambucil

Further reading:
- Rongioletti F, Rebora A (2001) Updated classification of papular mucinosis, lichen myxedematosus, and scleromyxedema. J Am Acad Dermatol 44(2):273–281

Sclerosis, Diffuse Systemic (Scleroderma)

Autoimmune disease that is caused by immune-mediated vascular damage and excessive production of profibrotic cytokines (TGF-B and PDGF) that leads to cutaneous and systemic fibrosis and that has the major clinical features of Raynaud phenomenon, progressive tightening and thickening of the skin (especially involving the hands, face, and upper chest and neck), salt-and-pepper-like dyschromia, pulmonary fibrosis, esophageal dysmotility, arthritis, and renal disease

Differential Diagnosis

- Amyloidosis
- Aromatic hydrocarbon exposure

- Bleomycin toxicity
- Carcinoid syndrome
- Chronic graft-vs-host disease
- Congenital erythropoietic porphyria
- <u>CREST syndrome</u>
- Diabetic cheiroarthropathy
- <u>Eosinophilia myalgia syndrome</u>
- <u>Eosinophilic fasciitis</u>
- Generalized morphea
- Hepatoerythropoietic porphyria
- Huriez syndrome
- <u>Mixed connective tissue disease</u>
- Nephrogenic fibrosing dermopathy
- Phenylketonuria
- POEMS syndrome
- Porphyria cutanea tarda
- Progeria
- Radiation exposure
- Reflex sympathetic dystrophy
- Scleredema
- <u>Scleromyxedema</u>
- Silicosis
- Toxic oil syndrome
- Trichinosis
- Tumid lupus erythematosus
- Vibration white finger
- Vinyl chloride toxicity
- Vitamin K injection
- Werner syndrome

Associations

- Primary biliary cirrhosis

Associated Medications (Scleroderma-Like Drug Reaction)

- Bleomycin
- Carbidopa
- Cocaine
- Docetaxel
- Fosinopril
- Penicillamine
- Vinyl chloride
- Taxanes

Evaluation

- Antinuclear antibodies (including anticentromere and Scl-70)
- Barium swallow
- Chest radiography
- Complete blood count
- Creatine kinase and aldolase levels
- Echocardiography
- Pulmonary function test
- Renal function test

Treatment Options

- <u>ACE inhibitor</u>
- Nifedipine
- Methotrexate
- <u>Cyclophosphamide</u>
- <u>Systemic corticosteroids</u>
- Acitretin
- UVA1 phototherapy
- Cyclosporine
- Thalidomide
- Etanercept
- Mycophenolate mofetil

Further reading:

- Mori Y, Kahari VM, Varga J (2002) Scleroderma-like cutaneous syndromes. Curr Rheumatol Rep 4(2):113–122

Scrotal Tongue (Lingua Plicata, Fissured Tongue)

Idiopathic textural change of the dorsal tongue that is associated with several diseases and characterized by furrows or grooves giving the tongue a cerebriform or rugous appearance (Fig. 6.109)

Differential Diagnosis

- <u>Amyloid infiltration</u>
- Geographic tongue
- <u>Herpetic geometric glossitis</u>
- Lymphedema
- Lymphangioma
- <u>Macroglossia</u>
- Mucosal neuroma syndrome
- Syphilitic glossitis

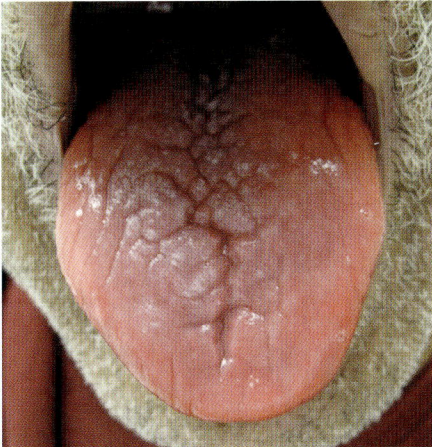

Fig. 6.109 Scrotal tongue

Associations

- Acrodermatitis continua
- Bazex–Dupre–Christol syndrome
- Cowden syndrome
- Down syndrome
- Melkersson–Rosenthal syndrome
- Pachyonychia congenita
- Pemphigus vegetans

Further reading:
- Zargari O (2006) The prevalence and significance of fissured tongue and geographical tongue in psoriatic patients. Clin Exp Dermatol 31(2):192–195

Scurvy

Disorder caused by vitamin C deficiency, which is essential for collagen synthesis, that is characterized by follicular hyperkeratosis with corkscrew hairs, perifollicular purpura, anemia, impaired wound healing, peridontal disease with bleeding gums, and intraarticular or subperiosteal hemorrhage

Differential Diagnosis

- Coagulation abnormality
- Cutaneous small vessel vasculitis
- Ehlers–Danlos syndrome
- Folliculitis
- Keratosis pilaris
- Langerhans cell histiocytosis
- Leukemia
- Phrynoderma
- Physical abuse
- Platelet abnormality
- Pigmented purpuric dermatosis
- Pityriasis rubra pilaris

Further reading:
- Heymann WR (2007) Scurvy in children. J Am Acad Dermatol 57(2):358–359

Seabather's Eruption

Acute, pruritic skin eruption that is caused by contact with the nemato-cysts of the thimble jellyfish and is characterized by erythematous mac-ules and papules in the covered areas that develop shortly after aquatic activity

Differential Diagnosis

- Autoeczematization dermatitis
- Bedbug bites
- Contact dermatitis
- Drug eruption
- Eosinophilic folliculitis
- Folliculitis
- Insect-bite reaction
- Jellyfish sting
- Papular urticaria
- Pityriasis rosea
- Psoriasis, guttate
- Scabies
- Swimmer's itch
- Urticaria
- Varicella
- Viral exanthem

Treatment Options

- Topical corticosteroids
- Systemic corticosteroids
- Antihistamines

Further reading:

• Segura-Puertas L, Ramos ME, Aramburo C et al (2001) One Linuche mystery solved: all 3 stages of the coronate scyphomedusae *Linuche unguiculata* cause seabather's eruption. J Am Acad Dermatol 44(4):624–628

Sebaceous Adenoma

Benign sebaceous neoplasm that affects older patients and is character-ized by a large yellow, occasionally polypoid, papule or nodule with cen-tral umbilication that is located on the head and neck, including the scalp

Differential Diagnosis

• Basal cell carcinoma (with sebaceous differentiation)
• Cylindroma
• Keratoacanthoma
• Molluscum contagiosum
• Nevus sebaceus
• Nodular hidradenoma (eccrine acrospiroma)
• Sebaceous carcinoma
• Sebaceous hyperplasia
• Syringocystadenoma papilliferum
• Trichoepithelioma
• Xanthelasma
• Xanthoma

Associations

• Muir–Torre syndrome

Further reading:

• Singh AD, Mudhar HS, Bhola R et al (2005) Sebaceous adenoma of the eyelid in Muir–Torre syndrome. Arch Ophthalmol 123(4):562–565

Sebaceous Carcinoma

Malignant neoplasm of sebaceous gland derivation that affects the elderly and is characterized by a slow-growing, asymptomatic nodule most commonly on the eyelid and less commonly on other areas of the head and neck or the genitalia

Differential Diagnosis

- Adnexal tumor
- Atypical fibroxanthoma
- Basal cell carcinoma (with sebaceous differentiation)
- Chalazion
- Chronic blepharitis
- Clear cell hidradenocarcinoma
- Hordeolum
- Melanoma (especially balloon cell type)
- Merkel cell carcinoma
- Metastasis
- Mucinous carcinoma
- Ocular pemphigoid
- Ocular rosacea
- Pyogenic granuloma
- Sarcoidosis
- Squamous cell carcinoma (especially clear cell type)

Associations

- Chalazion
- Muir–Torre syndrome

Further reading:

- Tan O, Ergen D, Arslan R (2006) Sebaceous carcinoma on the scalp. Dermatol Surg 32(10):1290–1293

Sebaceous Hyperplasia

Hyperplasia of the sebaceous glands that commonly affects middle-aged patients, is caused by decreased cell turnover of sebocytes, and is characterized by yellow papules on the face with central umbilication

Differential Diagnosis

- Angiofibroma
- Basal cell carcinoma
- Calcinosis cutis
- Colloid milium
- Favre–Racouchot disease
- Fibrous papule
- Granuloma annulare
- Lipoid proteinosis
- Lymphadenoma
- Milia
- Molluscum contagiosum
- Nevus
- Rhinophyma
- Sarcoidosis
- Sebaceous adenoma
- Sebaceous carcinoma
- Solar elastosis
- Squamous cell carcinoma
- Syringoma
- Trichilemmoma
- Trichodiscoma
- Trichoepithelioma
- Xanthelasma
- Xanthoma

Associations

- Anhidrotic ectodermal dysplasia
- Cyclosporine therapy

Further reading:
- Salim A, Reece SM, Smith AG et al (2006) Sebaceous hyperplasia and skin cancer in patients undergoing renal transplant. J Am Acad Dermatol 55(5):878–881

Seborrheic Dermatitis (Unna Disease)

Type of dermatitis that affects all age groups and is characterized by erythematous plaques with greasy scale, in the areas of the body with numerous sebaceous glands, including the scalp, central face, chest, and intertriginous areas

Subtypes/Variants

- Annular
- Cradle cap
- Erythrodermic
- Facial
- Hypopigmented
- Intertriginous
- Petaloid
- Pityriasiform
- Scalp
- Sebopsoriasis

Differential Diagnosis

Adult

- Actinic keratosis
- Atopic dermatitis
- <u>Candidiasis</u>
- <u>Contact dermatitis</u>
- Darier's disease
- Dermatomyositis
- <u>Erythrasma</u>
- External otitis media
- Extramammary Paget's disease
- Grover's disease
- Hailey–Hailey disease
- Infectious eczematoid dermatitis
- <u>Intertrigo</u>
- Keratosis lichenoides chronica
- Langerhans cell histiocytosis
- Lichen simplex chronicus
- Lupus erythematosus
- Malabsorption disorders
- Necrolytic migratory erythema
- Pellagra
- Pemphigus erythematosus
- <u>Pemphigus foliaceus</u>
- Pityriasis rosea
- Pityriasis lichenoides chronica
- Pityriasis rubra pilaris
- <u>Psoriasis</u>
- Pyridoxine deficiency
- Riboflavin deficiency
- <u>Rosacea</u>
- Subacute cutaneous lupus erythematosus
- Superficial basal cell carcinoma
- Syphilis

- Tinea barbae
- Tinea capitis
- Tinea faciei
- <u>Tinea versicolor</u>
- Zinc deficiency

Infantile

- Acrodermatitis enteropathica
- Atopic dermatitis
- Biotin deficiency
- <u>Candidiasis</u>
- Essential fatty acid deficiency
- Infantile psoriasis
- Infectious eczematoid dermatitis
- Infective dermatitis
- <u>Irritant-diaper dermatitis</u>
- Langerhans cell histiocytosis
- Leiner disease
- Malabsorption syndrome
- Netherton syndrome
- Omenn syndrome
- Riboflavin deficiency
- Wiskott–Aldrich syndrome

Scalp

- Atopic dermatitis
- <u>Contact dermatitis</u>
- Dermatomyositis
- Lupus erythematosus
- Lichen planus
- Pemphigus foliaceus
- Pityriasis amiantacea
- Pityriasis rubra pilaris
- <u>Psoriasis</u>

- Scalp dysesthesia
- Tinea capitis

Associations

- Acquired zinc deficiency
- Bell's palsy
- HIV infection
- Parkinson's disease
- Pityriasis amiantacea
- Stroke

Treatment Options

- Topical corticosteroids
- Topical ketoconazole
- Ciclopirox cream
- Topical calcineurin inhibitors
- Oral ketoconazole
- Benzoyl peroxide
- Zinc pyrithione
- Selenium sulfide
- Salicylic acid
- Tar

Further reading:

- Schwartz RA, Janusz CA, Janniger CK (2006) Seborrheic dermatitis: an overview. Am Fam Physician 74(1):125–130

Seborrheic Keratosis

Benign epidermal neoplasm that affects middle-aged to elderly patients and is characterized by a "stuck-on" verrucous or papillomatous, greasy hyperpigmented papule on the head and neck, trunk, or extremities

Subtypes (Histologic)

- Acanthotic
- Clonal
- Hyperkeratotic
- Irritated
- Melanoacanthoma
- Reticulated (adenoid)

Differential Diagnosis

Seborrheic Keratosis

- Acrochordon
- Acrokeratosis verruciformis of Hopf
- <u>Actinic keratosis</u>
- Arsenical keratosis
- <u>Basal cell carcinoma</u>
- Benign lichenoid keratosis
- Bowen's disease
- Bowenoid papulosis
- Condyloma acuminatum
- Confluent and reticulated papillomatosis
- Cutaneous horn
- Dermatosis papulosa nigra
- Eccrine poroma
- <u>Epidermal nevus</u>
- Epidermodysplasia verruciformis
- Granular cell tumor
- Hidroacanthoma simplex
- Inverted follicular keratosis
- Lentigo
- Malignant melanoma
- <u>Melanocytic nevus</u>
- <u>Melanoma</u>

- Nevus sebaceus
- Pemphigus erythematosus
- Pinkus tumor
- Porokeratosis
- Prurigo nodularis
- Psoriasis, guttate
- Sign of Leser–Trelat
- Solar lentigo
- <u>Squamous cell carcinoma</u>
- Stucco keratosis
- Syringocystadenoma papilliferum
- Tumor of the follicular infundibulum
- Verruca plana
- <u>Verruca vulgaris</u>
- Warty dyskeratoma

Sign of Leser–Trelat

- Acrokeratosis verruciformis of Hopf
- Chemotherapy-induced reaction in seborrheic keratoses
- Epidermodysplasia verruciformis
- Erythroderma-related eruptive seborrheic keratoses
- Florid cutaneous papillomatosis
- Verrucous mycosis fungoides
- Warts

Associations

Multiple Eruptive

- Erythroderma
- Internal malignancy
- Pregnancy

Sign of Leser–Trelat

- Acanthosis nigricans
- Hypertrichosis lanuginosa

- Internal malignancy
- Pruritus
- Weight loss

Further reading:

- Duque MI, Jordan JR, Fleischer AB Jr et al (2003) Frequency of seborrheic keratosis biopsies in the United States: a benchmark of skin lesion care quality and cost effectiveness. Dermatol Surg 29(8):796–801

Serum-Sickness-Like Drug Reaction

Type of drug reaction that resembles serum sickness but lacks any evidence of immune complex deposition and is characterized by fever, arthralgias, periarticular edema, and urticaria, angioedema, or erythema-multiforme-like skin lesions

Differential Diagnosis

- Cryoglobulinemia
- Erythema marginatum
- Erythema multiforme
- Henoch–Schonlein purpura
- Hepatitis B infection
- Sweet's syndrome
- Still's disease
- Urticaria
- Urticarial drug eruption
- Urticarial vasculitis
- Vasculitis

Associated Medications

- Beta-lactam antibiotics
- Bupropion

- Carbamazepine
- Cefaclor
- Ciprofloxacin
- Clopidogrel
- Co-trimoxazole
- Fluoxetine
- Infliximab
- Minocycline
- Phenytoin
- Rifampin

Treatment Options

- Discontinue offending medication
- Antihistamines
- Systemic corticosteroids

Further reading:
- Yerushalmi J, Zvulunov A, Halevy S (2002) Serum sickness-like reactions. Cutis 69(5):395–397

Severe Combined Immunodeficiency

Syndrome of combined T cell and B cell deficiency with variable cause and presentation that is most commonly caused by an X-linked mutation of the common gamma chain of the T cell receptor and is characterized by recurrent visceral and cutaneous infections with *Candida* and various other fungal or bacteria pathogens, a severe seborrheic-dermatitis-like eruption (Leiner's disease), failure to thrive, and early death

Subtypes/Variants

- Adenosine deaminase (ADA) deficiency
- IL-7 receptor deficiency
- JAK3 deficiency

- MHC class II deficiency
- Omenn syndrome
- Purine nucleoside phosphorylase (PNP) deficiency
- T cell receptor deficiency
- X-linked severe combined immunodeficiency
- ZAP-70 deficiency

Differential Diagnosis

- <u>Chronic mucocutaneous candidiasis</u>
- DiGeorge syndrome
- Good syndrome
- HIV infection
- Leukemia
- Nezelof syndrome
- Wiskott–Aldrich syndrome
- X-linked agammaglobulinemia

Evaluation

- Chest radiograph
- Complete blood count
- Immunoglobulin levels
- Lymphocyte flow cytometry
- *Trichophytin* or *Candida* skin testing

Further reading:
- Buckley RH (2004) The multiple causes of human SCID. J Clin Invest 114(10):1409–1411

Sezary Syndrome

Leukemic variant of cutaneous T cell lymphoma with a poor prognosis that is characterized by erythroderma, lymphadenopathy, and Sezary cells in the blood, skin, and lymph nodes, along with severe pruritus, palmoplantar keratoderma, alopecia, and nail dystrophy

Differential Diagnosis

- Atopic dermatitis
- Congenital ichthyosiform erythroderma
- <u>Drug reaction</u>
- <u>Erythrodermic mycosis fungoides</u>
- <u>Idiopathic erythroderma</u>
- Paraneoplastic erythroderma
- Pityriasis rubra pilaris
- Psoriasis

Diagnostic Criteria (One or More)

- Aberrant expression of pan T cell markers
- Absolute Sezary cell count of 1,000 cells/mm^3
- CD4/CD8 ratio of 10 or higher
- Chromosomal abnormality in T cell clone
- Increased lymphocyte counts with evidence of a T cell clone by Southern blot or PCR

Evaluation

- Bone marrow biopsy
- Chest radiograph
- Complete blood count with peripheral blood Sezary cell prep
- CT scan of chest, abdomen, and pelvis
- Lactate dehydrogenase level
- Liver function test
- Lymph node exam and biopsy
- Lymphocyte flow cytometry
- Serum chemistry

Treatment Options

- <u>Methotrexate</u>
- <u>Extracorporeal photochemotherapy</u>
- Bexarotene
- Systemic antibiotics
- Antihistamines
- Vorinostat
- Alemtuzumab
- Gemcitabine
- Single or multiagent chemotherapy

Further reading:

- Vonderheid EC, Bernengo MG, Burg G et al (2002) Update on erythrodermic cutaneous T-cell lymphoma: report of the International Society for Cutaneous Lymphomas. J Am Acad Dermatol 46(1):95–106

Sinus Pericranii

Acquired or congenital anomalous connection (possibly trauma related) between an extracranial blood-filled nodule and the intracranial dural sinuses that is characterized by a soft, compressible mass near the midline of the frontal, parietal, or occipital scalp that increases in size with increased intracranial pressure

Differential Diagnosis

- Aplasia cutis congenita
- <u>Arteriovenous fistula</u>
- Cutaneous meningioma
- Cylindroma
- Dermoid cyst

- En coupe de sabre
- Eosinophilic granuloma
- Hemangioma
- Heterotopic brain tissue
- Meningoencephalocele
- Venous malformation

Further reading:
- Sheu M, Fauteux G, Chang H et al (2002) Sinus pericranii: dermatologic considerations and literature review. J Am Acad Dermatol 46(6):934–941

Sjögren's Syndrome

Autoimmune disease of unknown cause that predominantly affects women and is characterized by dry skin, dry eyes, dry mouth, salivary gland enlargement, arthritis, an annular papulosquamous eruption, SS-A or SS-B antibodies, and other concomitant autoimmune diseases

Differential Diagnosis

- Amyloidosis
- Burning mouth syndrome
- Cheilitis granulomatosis
- Drug reaction or adverse effect
- Graft-vs-host disease
- HIV infection
- Lupus erythematosus
- Lymphoma
- Mucosal pemphigoid
- Rheumatoid arthritis
- Sarcoidosis
- Viral infection

Diagnostic Criteria (4/6)

- Salivary gland biopsy reveals aggregation of at least 50 mononuclear cells around intralobular duct
- Antibodies to SS-B and/or SS-A, positive ANA, or RF
- Daily dry eyes for more than 3 months
- Daily dry mouth for more than 3 months
- Salivary scintigraphy, parotid sialography test positive, or reduced salivary flow test
- Schirmer's test positive (<5 mm in 5 min)

Associations

- Acral ichthyosiform myxedema
- B cell lymphoma
- Benign hypergammaglobulinemic purpura of Waldenstrom
- Other autoimmune diseases
- Salivary gland enlargement
- Thyroiditis

Evaluation

- Antinuclear antibodies (including SS-A and SS-B)
- Chest radiograph
- Complete blood count
- Liver function test
- Ophthalmologic exam (Schirmer's test)
- Renal function test
- Rheumatoid factor
- Urinalysis

Further reading:
- Vitali C, Bombardieri S, Jonsson R et al (2002) Classification criteria for Sjogren's syndrome: a revised version of the European criteria proposed by the American–European Consensus Group. Ann Rheum Dis 61(6):554–558

Sjögren–Larsson Syndrome

Inherited metabolic disorder (AR) that is caused by deficiency of fatty aldehyde dehydrogenase (FALDH) and is characterized by flexure-predominant ichthyosis, photophobia, "glistening dot"-type retinitis pigmentosa, spastic diplegia, mental retardation, and seizures

Differential Diagnosis

- Ataxia–telangiectasia
- Congenital ichthyosiform erythroderma
- IFAP syndrome
- Lamellar ichthyosis
- Multiple sulfatase deficiency
- Neutral lipid storage disease
- Refsum disease
- Severe ichthyosis vulgaris
- Trichothiodystrophy
- X-linked recessive ichthyosis

Further reading:
- Alio AB, Bird LM, McClellan SD et al (2006) Sjogren–Larsson syndrome: a case report and literature review. Cutis 78(1):61–65

Smallpox (Variola)

Viral infection caused by the smallpox virus that is characterized by erythematous macules that erupt first on the face, spread to the trunk and extremities, evolve simultaneously to become monomorphic vesiculopustules with central umbilication, and eventually crust and scar

Differential Diagnosis

- Acute generalized exanthematous pustulosis
- Contact dermatitis
- Coxsackievirus infection
- Disseminated zoster
- Eczema herpeticum
- <u>Enteroviral infection</u>
- Erythema multiforme
- <u>Herpes simplex virus infection</u>
- Impetigo
- Infectious mononucleosis
- Kaposi's varicelliform eruption
- Kawasaki disease
- Leukemia
- Meningococcemia
- <u>Monkeypox</u>
- Molluscum contagiosum
- Parvovirus infection
- Rat-bite fever
- Rickettsialpox
- Rocky Mountain spotted fever
- Rubella
- Rubeola
- Scarlet fever
- Syphilis
- <u>Varicella</u>

Evaluation

- Viral culture of the oropharynx
- Electron microscopy or PCR of lesional tissue

Further reading:

- Moore ZS, Seward JF, Lane JM (2006) Smallpox. Lancet 367(9508):425–435

Smooth Muscle Hamartoma

Congenital or acquired hamartoma of smooth muscle that becomes more indurated with rubbing (pseudo-Darier's sign), is associated with Becker's nevus (acquired) or the Michelin tire baby presentation (congenital and generalized variant), and is characterized by a firm plaque with or without hyperpigmentation and hypertrichosis on the trunk, especially the lumbosacral area, or the proximal extremities

Differential Diagnosis

- Accessory nipple
- Becker's nevus
- Café-au-lait macule
- Congenital melanocytic nevus
- Connective tissue nevus
- Dermatofibrosis lenticularis disseminata
- Fibrous hamartoma of infancy
- Infantile myofibromatosis
- Leiomyoma
- Neurofibroma
- Rhabdomyoma
- Solitary mastocytoma

Further reading:
- Morales-Callaghan A, Vila JB, Cardenal EA, Bernier MA, Fraile HA, Miranda-Romero A (2005) Acquired cutaneous smooth muscle hamartoma. J Eur Acad Dermatol Venereol 19(1):142–143

Solar Elastosis

Common acquired disorder of elastic tissue that affects the elderly, is associated with chronic cumulative sun exposure, and is characterized by multiple yellow papules which coalesce into plaques on the sun-exposed areas, especially the face and neck

Subtypes/Variants

- Actinic elastotic plaque or papule (Dubreuil elastoma)
- Bullous solar elastosis
- Cutis rhomboidalis nuchae
- Favre–Racouchot syndrome
- Fibroelastolytic papulosis of the neck
- Juxtaclavicular beaded lines

Differential Diagnosis

- Basal cell carcinoma
- Carotenoderma
- Colloid milium
- Comedonal acne
- Epidermoid cysts
- Granuloma annulare
- Lupus erythematosus
- Papular mucinosis
- Polymorphous light eruption
- Pseudoxanthoma elasticum
- Sebaceous hyperplasia
- Squamous cell carcinoma

Further reading:

- Heras JA, Jimenez F, Soguero ML et al (2007) Bullous solar elastosis. Clin Exp Dermatol 32(3):272–274

Solid Facial Edema

Variant or complication of acne vulgaris that is characterized by tender, nonpitting erythematous edema of the glabella, nasal bridge, and cheeks

Differential Diagnosis

- Angioedema
- Cellulitis
- Erysipelas
- Melkersson–Rosenthal syndrome
- Rosacea fulminans
- <u>Rosacea-related lymphedema (Morbihan disease)</u>

Treatment Options

- Tetracycline antibiotics
- Isotretinoin
- Systemic corticosteroids
- Compression and massage

Further reading:

- Manolache L, Benea V, Petrescu-Seceleanu D (2009) A case of solid facial oedema successfully treated with isotretinoin. J Eur Acad Dermatol Venereol 23(8):965–966

Spider Angioma (Nevus Araneus)

Benign acquired vascular ectasia that is characterized by a blanching vascular papule with a central feeding arteriole from which numerous tiny vessels extend radially and is most commonly located on the trunk, but also the face or extremities

Differential Diagnosis

- Angioma serpiginosum
- Arteriovenous malformation

- Arthropod-bite reaction
- Cherry angioma
- Rosacea
- <u>Telangiectatic mat</u>

Associations

- Hyperestrogenemia
- Liver disease (especially alcoholic)
- Oral contraception
- Pregnancy
- Thyrotoxicosis

Further reading:
- Requena L, Sangueza OP (1997) Cutaneous vascular anomalies. Part I. Hamartomas, malformations, and dilation of preexisting vessels. J Am Acad Dermatol 37(4):523–549

Spiny Keratoderma (Music-Box Spine Dermatosis)

Uncommon subtype of focal palmoplantar keratoderma characterized by miniscule digitate hyperkeratoses of the palms and soles, with occasional association with internal malignancy

Differential Diagnosis

- Arsenical keratoses
- Darier's disease
- Filiform warts
- Hyperkeratotic spicules of myeloma
- Keratosis punctata
- Multiple minute digitate hyperkeratosis
- Porokeratosis punctata

Further reading:

- Torres G, Behshad R, Han A, Castrovinci AJ, Gilliam AC (2008) "I forgot to shave my hands": a case of spiny keratoderma. J Am Acad Dermatol 58(2):344–348

Spitz Nevus

Tumor of epithelioid and/or spindle cell melanocytes that is confused histologically with melanoma, arises in children and young adults, and is characterized by a red, orange, or brown dome-shaped papule (or, occasionally, a darkly pigmented papule, also known as a pigmented spindle cell nevus of Reed) on the face or extremities

Differential Diagnosis

- Adnexal tumors
- Arthropod-bite reaction
- Blue nevus
- Dermatofibroma
- Hemangioma
- Juvenile xanthogranuloma
- Idiopathic facial aseptic granuloma
- Keloid
- Malignant melanoma
- Mastocytoma
- Melanoacanthoma
- Melanocytic nevus
- Molluscum contagiosum
- Pigmented basal cell carcinoma
- Pyogenic granuloma
- Traumatic tattoo
- Verruca

Further reading:

- Sulit DJ, Guardiano RA, Krivda S (2007) Classic and atypical Spitz nevi: review of the literature. Cutis 79(2):141–146

Sporotrichosis (Schenck's Disease)

Chronic deep fungal infection caused by contamination of traumatized skin with the dimorphic fungus, *Sporothrix schencki,* and that is characterized most commonly by erythematous nodules and ulcers along the lines of lymphatic drainage of an extremity

Subtypes/Variants

- Disseminated
- Fixed
- Lymphocutaneous

Differential Diagnosis

- Anthrax
- Atypical mycobacterial infection
- Cat-scratch disease
- Cellulitis
- Chromoblastomycosis
- Dimorphic fungi
- Erysipeloid
- Leishmaniasis
- Mycetoma
- Nocardiosis
- Protothecosis
- Pyoderma gangrenosum
- Pyogenic lesions
- Sarcoidosis

- Syphilis
- Tuberculosis
- Tularemia

Evaluation

- Bacterial, mycobacterial, and fungal culture of affected tissue
- Chest radiograph

Treatment Options

- <u>Itraconazole</u>
- Surgical excision
- Potassium iodide

Further reading:
- Ramos-e-Silva M, Vasconcelos C, Carneiro S et al (2007) Sporotrichosis. Clin Dermatol 25(2):181–187

Squamous Cell Carcinoma

Malignant epidermal neoplasm that most commonly arises in the chronically sun-exposed areas of elderly patients and is characterized by an erythematous, indurated, hyperkeratotic papule, nodule, or plaque with central ulceration and crust

Subtypes (Histologic)

- Acantholytic
- Adenosquamous
- Angiosarcoma-like
- Basosquamous
- Clear cell
- Desmoplastic

- Keratoacanthoma
- Metaplastic carcinoma
- Spindle cell
- Verrucous

Differential Diagnosis

General

- Adnexal tumor
- <u>Atypical fibroxanthoma</u>
- <u>Actinic keratosis</u>
- <u>Basal cell carcinoma</u>
- Blastomycosis
- Bromoderma
- Eccrine poroma
- Granular cell tumor
- Halogenoderma
- Inverted follicular keratosis
- Keratoacanthoma
- Leishmaniasis
- Lymphoepithelioma-like carcinoma
- Melanoma (especially amelanotic)
- <u>Merkel cell carcinoma</u>
- <u>Metastatic squamous cell carcinoma</u>
- Paget's disease
- Porocarcinoma
- Proliferating pilar cyst
- Pseudoepitheliomatous hyperplasia
- Pyoderma gangrenosum
- Pyogenic granuloma
- Sebaceous carcinoma
- <u>Seborrheic keratosis</u>
- Syphilis
- Tuberculosis
- Trichilemmal carcinoma

- Verrucous carcinoma
- Wart
- Warty dyskeratoma

Penile
- Bowen's disease
- Buschke–Lowenstein tumor
- Chronic herpes simplex virus infection
- Condyloma acuminatum
- Genital ulcer
- Metastatic disease
- Pseudoepitheliomatous keratotic and micaceous balanitis
- Verruciform xanthoma
- Warty dyskeratoma

Periungual/Subungual
- Keratoacanthoma
- Metastatic carcinoma
- Onychomatricoma
- Porocarcinoma
- Verrucous carcinoma
- Viral warts

Associations

- Acne conglobata
- Actinic keratosis
- Arsenical keratosis
- Burn scars
- Chromomycosis
- Dental sinus
- Discoid lupus erythematosus
- Environmental carcinogen exposure
- Epidermodysplasia verruciformis

- Epidermolysis bullosa (especially dystrophic)
- Erythema ab igne
- Ferguson–Smith syndrome
- Granuloma inguinale
- Hailey–Hailey disease
- Hidradenitis suppurativa
- HPV infection
- Leprosy
- Lichen sclerosus et atrophicus
- Lupus vulgaris
- Marjolin ulcer
- Morphea
- Muir–Torre syndrome
- Necrobiosis lipoidica
- Oculocutaneous albinism
- Oral erosive lichen planus
- Osteomyelitis
- Perianal pyoderma
- Pilonidal cyst
- Porokeratosis
- Radiation dermatitis
- Scars
- Snake-bite ulcer
- Venous ulcers
- Xeroderma pigmentosum

Associations (Penile)

- Chronic irritation and inflammation
- Granuloma inguinale
- Human papilloma virus infection
- Immunosuppression
- Lack of circumcision
- Lichen sclerosus
- Poor hygiene
- Pseudoepitheliomatous keratotic and micaceous balanitis

Treatment Options

- <u>Simple surgical excision</u>
- <u>Mohs micrographic surgery</u>
- 5FU cream
- Imiquimod
- Electrodessication and curettage
- Intralesional 5FU
- Intralesional methotrexate
- Intralesional interferon
- Acitretin
- Isotretinoin
- Radiation

Further reading:

- Cassarino DS, Derienzo DP, Barr RJ (2006) Cutaneous squamous cell carcinoma: a comprehensive clinicopathologic classification. J Cutan Pathol 33(3):191–206

Staphylococcal Scalded-Skin Syndrome (Ritter's Disease)

Superficial blistering disorder of children and adults that is caused by release of epidermolytic toxin from a distal focus of infection and is characterized by tender erythema and superficial flaccid bullae most commonly noted around the mouth and intertriginous areas

Differential Diagnosis

- Bullous congenital ichthyosiform erythroderma
- Bullous impetigo
- Child abuse
- Diffuse cutaneous mastocytosis
- <u>Drug reaction</u>
- Epidermolysis bullosa
- Graft-vs-host disease

- Ichthyosis bullosa of Siemens
- <u>Kawasaki disease</u>
- Peeling skin syndrome
- Pemphigus foliaceus
- Scarlet fever
- Sunburn reaction
- Thermal burn
- <u>Toxic epidermal necrolysis</u>
- Toxic shock syndrome
- Viral exanthem

Associations

- <u>Chronic renal failure</u>
- HIV infection
- Wound infections
- Occult infections

Treatment Options

- Treat the underlying cause
- Antistaphylococcal antibiotics

Further reading:
- Stanley JR, Amagai M (2006) Pemphigus, bullous impetigo, and the staphylococcal scalded-skin syndrome. N Engl J Med 355(17):1800–1810

Stasis Dermatitis

Type of dermatitis that arises on the ankle, dorsal foot, and/or tibial area of patients with chronic venous insufficiency and is characterized by pruritic, scaly, erythematous eczematous, or lichenified plaques with surrounding lipodermatosclerosis, hemisiderosis, edema, venous varicosities, or other features of venous stasis

Differential Diagnosis

- Acroangiodermatitis of Mali
- Asteatotic eczema
- Atopic dermatitis
- Cellulitis
- Contact dermatitis
- Dermatophytosis
- Elephantiasis
- Kaposi's sarcoma
- Lichen planus
- Lipodermatosclerosis
- Livedoid vasculopathy
- Mycosis fungoides
- Necrobiosis lipoidica
- Nummular eczema
- Pigmented purpuric dermatosis
- Pretibial myxedema
- Psoriasis

Associations

- Acroangiodermatitis
- Atrophie blanche
- Lipodermatosclerosis
- Venous leg ulcers

Treatment Options

- Compression, elevation, and rest
- Topical corticosteroids
- Systemic corticosteroids
- Systemic antibiotics
- Pentoxifylline
- Diuresis

Further reading:

- Barron GS, Jacob SE, Kirsner RS (2007) Dermatologic complications of chronic venous disease: medical management and beyond. Ann Vasc Surg 21(5):652–662

Steatocystoma Multiplex

Inherited disorder (AD) associated with mutation of keratin 17 that is characterized by multiple yellow to flesh-colored superficial cutaneous cysts containing an oily fluid on the upper chest or proximal upper extremities

Differential Diagnosis

- Acne conglobata
- Acne vulgaris
- Chloracne
- Dermoid cyst
- Epidermal inclusion cysts
- Eruptive vellus hair cysts
- Gardner syndrome
- Milia
- Syringoma
- Trichilemmal cyst

Associations

- Hidradenitis suppurativa
- LEOPARD syndrome
- Natal teeth
- Pachyonychia congenita, type II
- Preauricular pits

Treatment Options

- Incision and drainage
- Surgical excision

- Tetracycline antibiotics
- Isotretinoin

Further reading:
- Chu DH (2003) Steatocystoma multiplex. Dermatol Online J 9(4):18

Stevens–Johnson Syndrome/Toxic Epidermal Necrolysis

Related life-threatening syndromes that are caused by immune-mediated epithelial apoptosis, are associated with a variety of medicinal and infectious triggers, and that clinically fall on spectrum with Stevens–Johnson syndrome having more erosions of the mucosal surfaces along with atypical target lesions affecting <10% of the body surface area while toxic epidermal necrolysis is characterized by more widespread (>30% BSA) epidermal sloughing and necrosis (Fig. 6.110)

Differential Diagnosis

Stevens–Johnson Syndrome

- Aphthous stomatitis
- Behçet's disease

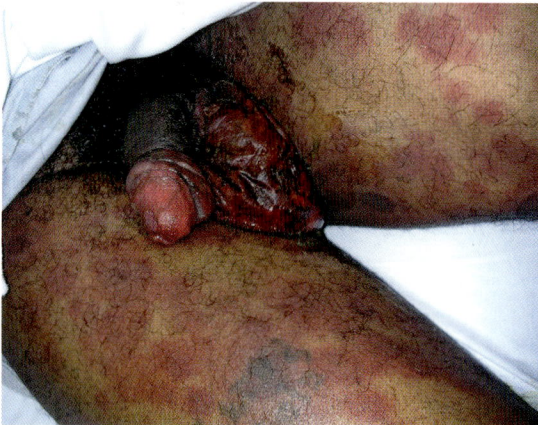

Fig. 6.110 Stevens–Johnson syndrome

- Erosive lichen planus
- Erythema multiforme
- <u>Fixed drug eruption</u>
- Henoch–Schonlein purpura
- Herpes simplex virus infection
- <u>Kawasaki disease</u>
- <u>Linear IgA bullous dermatosis</u>
- Mucosal pemphigoid
- Paraneoplastic pemphigus
- Pemphigus vulgaris
- Rowell's syndrome
- Toxic epidermal necrolysis

Toxic Epidermal Necrolysis
- Acute graft-vs-host disease
- <u>Acute generalized exanthematous pustulosis</u>
- Drug-induced pemphigoid
- Drug-induced pemphigus
- <u>Drug-induced linear IgA bullous dermatosis</u>
- Paraneoplastic pemphigus
- Pseudoporphyria
- <u>Severe presentation of acute lupus erythematosus (ASAP syndrome)</u>
- Severe phototoxicity
- <u>Staphylococcal scalded-skin syndrome</u>
- Stevens–Johnson syndrome
- Subacute cutaneous lupus erythematosus
- Thermal burns
- Widespread fixed drug eruption

Associations

- Bone marrow transplant
- HIV infection
- Medications
- *Mycoplasma* infection

Associated Medications

- Allopurinol
- Aminopenicillins
- Antiretroviral medications
- Barbiturates
- Carbamazepine
- Lamotrigine
- Phenytoin
- Piroxicam
- Sulfonamides
- Tetracycline

Staging (SCORTEN: Predicts Mortality)

- Age >40 years
- Bicarbonate <20 mmol/l
- Blood urea nitrogen >10 mmol/l
- Glucose >14 mmol/l
- HR >120
- Initial epidermal detachment of >10% BSA
- Malignancy

Evaluation

- Bacterial culture of affected tissues
- Chest radiograph
- Liver function test
- Ophthalmology consultation
- Renal function test
- Serum chemistry/glucose

Treatment Options

- <u>Supportive care</u>
- <u>Intravenous immunoglobulins</u>
- Systemic corticosteroids
- Cyclosporine

Further reading:
- Pereira FA, Mudgil AV, Rosmarin DM (2007) Toxic epidermal necrolysis. J Am Acad Dermatol 56(2):181–200

Stomatitis Nicotina

Heat-induced inflammation of the minor salivary glands of the palate that is associated with tobacco smoking and is characterized by white papules with central erythema on the hard palate

Differential Diagnosis

- <u>Aphthous stomatitis</u>
- Forschheimer spots
- Herpangina
- Orolabial herpes infection
- Thermal burn

Further reading:
- Taybos G (2003) Oral changes associated with tobacco use. Am J Med Sci 326(4):179–182

Streptococcal Perianal Disease

Superficial infection of the perianal area caused by group A beta-hemolytic streptococcus that is most commonly seen in children and is characterized by bright-red erythema surrounding the anus

Differential Diagnosis

- <u>Candidiasis</u>
- Chafing
- Child abuse
- Inflammatory bowel disease
- <u>Intertrigo (diaper dermatitis)</u>
- <u>Pinworm infection</u>
- <u>Psoriasis</u>
- Seborrheic dermatitis

Associations

- Guttate psoriasis

Treatment Options

- Antistreptococcal antibiotics

Further reading:
- Herbst R (2003) Perineal streptococcal dermatitis/disease: recognition and management. Am J Clin Dermatol 4(8):555–560

Striae Distensae

Atrophy of the dermis caused by stretching of the skin during pregnancy, weight gain, or muscle building that is characterized by linear atrophic erythematous bands on the trunk or proximal extremities

Differential Diagnosis

- <u>Anetoderma</u>
- Linear focal elastosis
- Marfan syndrome

- Middermal elastolysis
- Steroid-induced striae
- Trauma

Associations

- Corticosteroids
- Cushing's syndrome
- Obesity
- Pregnancy
- Puberty
- Weight loss

Treatment Options

- Observation
- <u>Topical tretinoin</u>
- Pulsed dye laser
- Glycolic acid
- Intense pulsed light

Further reading:
- Yosipovitch G, Devore A, Dawn A (2007) Obesity and the skin: skin physiology and skin manifestations of obesity. J Am Acad Dermatol 56(6):901–916

Stucco Keratosis

Benign hyperkeratotic papules of unknown cause that commonly affect middle-aged to elderly patients and are characterized by white, scaly, papules on the anterior lower extremities and occasionally the dorsal hands

Differential Diagnosis

- Acrokeratosis verruciformis
- Disseminated actinic porokeratosis

- Epidermodysplasia verruciformis
- Flegel's disease
- Hyperkeratotic seborrheic keratosis
- <u>Verruca plana</u>

Further reading:
- Stockfleth E, Rowert J, Arndt R et al (2000) Detection of human papillomavirus and response to topical 5% imiquimod in a case of stucco keratosis. Br J Dermatol 143(4):846–850

Subcorneal Pustular Dermatosis (Sneddon–Wilkinson Disease)

Idiopathic pustular psoriasis-like eruption affecting middle-aged to elderly patients that is characterized by superficial flaccid pustules, often in annular or serpiginous patterns that are located predominantly in the flexures

Differential Diagnosis

- <u>Acute generalized exanthematous pustulosis</u>
- Amicrobial pustulosis with autoimmunity
- Bullous impetigo
- Candidiasis
- Dermatophytosis
- Dermatitis herpetiformis
- Eosinophilic pustular folliculitis
- Folliculitis
- Hailey–Hailey disease
- <u>IgA pemphigus, subcorneal pustular dermatosis type</u>
- Necrolytic migratory erythema
- Pemphigus foliaceus
- Pemphigus vulgaris
- <u>Pustular psoriasis</u>
- Tinea corporis

Associations

- Crohn's disease
- Hyperthyroidism
- IgA paraproteinemia
- Morphea
- Multiple sclerosis
- Pyoderma gangrenosum
- Rheumatoid arthritis
- SAPHO syndrome
- Systemic lupus erythematosus

Evaluation

- Complete blood count
- Direct immunofluorescence
- Gram stain and potassium hydroxide examination of pustule
- Serum/urinary protein electrophoresis

Treatment Options

- Dapsone
- Systemic corticosteroids
- Acitretin
- Tetracycline
- Narrowband UVB
- Infliximab

Further reading:
- Iobst W, Ingraham K (2005) Sneddon–Wilkinson disease in a patient with rheumatoid arthritis. Arthritis Rheum 52(12):3771

Subcutaneous Fat Necrosis of the Newborn

Uncommon panniculitis affecting term newborns that is possibly caused by an increased ratio of saturated to unsaturated subcutaneous fat and is characterized by hypercalcemia along with erythematous, edematous plaques predominantly located on the cheeks, buttocks, and thighs

Differential Diagnosis

- Cellulitis
- Erythema nodosum
- Farber's lipogranulomatosis
- Hemangioma
- Neurofibromatosis
- Poststeroid panniculitis
- Sarcoma
- Sclerema neonatorum

Associations

- Complicated delivery
- Hypothermia
- Meconium aspiration

Treatment Options

- Supportive care
- Management of hypercalcemia

Further reading:
- Mahe E, Girszyn N, Hadj-Rabia S et al (2007) Subcutaneous fat necrosis of the newborn: a systematic evaluation of risk factors, clinical manifestations, complications and outcome of 16 children. Br J Dermatol 156(4):709–715

Subepidermal Calcified Nodule

Type of idiopathic calcinosis cutis that arises in childhood and is characterized by a solitary, hard, yellow-white or erythematous, protuberant dermal nodule on the head and neck, especially the face or ear

Differential Diagnosis

- Chondroid syringoma
- Cutaneous horn
- Dermatofibroma
- Epidermal inclusion cyst
- Milia-like calcinosis cutis
- Molluscum contagiosum
- Pilomatricoma
- Verruca vulgaris

Further reading:
- Juzych LA, Nordby CA (2001) Subepidermal calcified nodule. Pediatr Dermatol 18(3):238–240

Submucous Fibrosis of Oral Cavity

Fibrosing disorder of the oral cavity that is associated with various irritating substances and is characterized first by a progressive thickening of the palate and tonsillar pillars with later involvement of the entire oral cavity, which can eventually become ulcerated or associated with trismus, or develop squamous cell carcinoma

Differential Diagnosis

- Amyloidosis
- Gingival fibromatosis
- Leukoplakia

- Lichen planus
- Lipoid proteinosis
- Mucosal pemphigoid
- Oral fibroma
- Salivary gland neoplasm
- Scleroderma
- Squamous cell carcinoma

Associations

- Betel nuts (areca nuts)
- Chili peppers
- Iron deficiency
- Malnutrition
- Vitamin deficiency

Further reading:
- Hazarey VK, Erlewad DM, Mundhe KA et al (2007) Oral submucous fibrosis: study of 1000 cases from central India. J Oral Pathol Med 36(1):12–17

Subungual Exostosis

Uncommon, solitary, cartilaginous tumor that is likely caused by trauma, arises most commonly on the great toe in the first two decades of life, and is characterized by a hard, painful, raised subungual nodule with or without overlying nail dystrophy and surrounding callus formation

Differential Diagnosis

- Enchondroma
- Glomus tumor
- Koenen tumor
- Melanoma
- Metastatic lesion

- <u>Osteochondroma</u>
- Pterygium inversus unguis
- <u>Squamous cell carcinoma of nail bed</u>
- Subungual wart
- Traumatic nail dystrophy

Further reading:
- Guarneri C, Guarneri F, Risitano G et al (2005) Solitary asymptomatic nodule of the great toe. Int J Dermatol 44(3):245–247
- Suga H, Mukouda M (2005) Subungual exostosis: a review of 16 cases focusing on postoperative deformity of the nail. Ann Plast Surg 55(3):272–275

Supernumerary Digit (Rudimentary Polydactyly)

Developmental anomaly caused by erroneous duplication of digital soft tissue or intrauterine amputation of a superfluous digit that is characterized by a solitary or bilateral flesh-colored pedunculated nodule most commonly located on the ulnar aspect of the fifth digit

Differential Diagnosis

- <u>Acquired digital fibrokeratoma</u>
- Epidermal inclusion cyst
- Fibroma
- Neurofibroma
- Pyogenic granuloma
- <u>Traumatic neuroma</u>
- Wart

Associations

- Basal cell nevus syndrome
- Bardet–Biedl syndrome
- Down syndrome

- EEC syndrome
- Ellis–van Creveld syndrome
- Oral–facial–digital syndrome
- Rubinstein–Taybi syndrome
- VATER association

Further reading:
- Leber GE, Gosain AK (2003) Surgical excision of pedunculated supernumerary digits prevents traumatic amputation neuromas. Pediatr Dermatol 20(2):108–112

Supernumerary Nipple

Developmental anomaly characterized by the development of an additional nipple or areola with or without underlying mammary tissue along the mammary (milk) line, the line of ectodermal differentiation along which the breasts develop that runs from the axilla to the groin

Differential Diagnosis

- Acrochordon
- Café-au-lait macule
- Congenital melanocytic nevus
- Dermatofibroma
- Lipoma
- Lymphangioma
- Neurofibroma
- Nevus
- Scar
- Wart

Associations

- Ectodermal dysplasias
- Fanconi anemia

- Ipsilateral Becker's nevi
- Urinary tract malformations
- Simpson–Golabi–Behmel syndrome
- Trichoodontoonychial dysplasia
- Turner syndrome

Further reading:
- Brown J, Schwartz RA (2004) Supernumerary nipples and renal malformations: a family study. J Cutan Med Surg 8(3):170–172

Sweet's Syndrome (Acute Febrile Neutrophilic Dermatosis)

Idiopathic reactive inflammatory syndrome associated with several triggers that is characterized by fever, leukocytosis, and neutrophil-rich, erythematous, edematous plaques with central pustules (and, occasionally, vesiculation) on the face and extremities (Fig. 6.111)

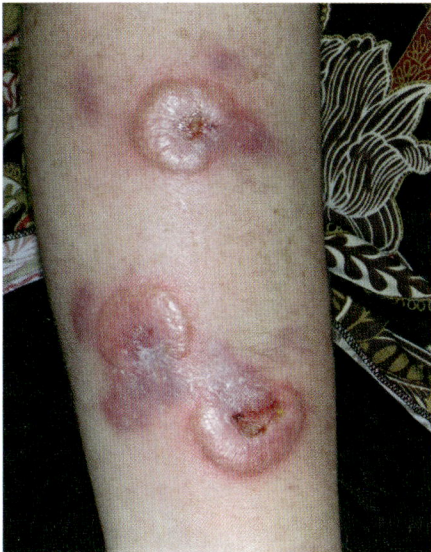

Fig. 6.111 Sweet's syndrome (Courtesy of A. Record)

Differential Diagnosis

- Acne fulminans
- Acral erythema
- Acute hemorrhagic edema of infancy
- Behçet's disease
- Bowel-associated dermatosis–arthritis syndrome
- <u>Cellulitis</u>
- Chloroma
- Cutaneous small vessel vasculitis
- Deep fungal infection
- Eccerine syringosquamous metaplasia
- Erythema elevatum diutinum
- Erythema multiforme
- Erythema nodosum
- Familial Mediterranean fever
- Fixed drug eruption, neutrophilic type
- Granuloma annulare
- Granuloma faciale
- Halogenoderma
- Hyper-IgD syndrome
- Lupus erythematosus
- Leishmaniasis
- <u>Leukemia cutis</u>
- Lymphoma cutis
- Metastatic disease
- Mycobacterial infection (including leprosy)
- <u>Neutrophilic dermatosis of the dorsal hands</u>
- Neutrophilic eccrine hidradenitis
- Panniculitis
- Pyoderma
- <u>Pyoderma gangrenosum (especially bullous type)</u>
- <u>Rheumatoid neutrophilic dermatosis</u>
- Rosacea fulminans

- Sarcoidosis
- Septic vasculitis
- Syphilis
- TNF-receptor-associated periodic fever syndrome
- Urticarial vasculitis

Diagnostic Criteria (Two Major and Two Minor)

- Major criteria
  - Abrupt onset of typical cutaneous lesions
  - Histopathology consistent with Sweet's syndrome
- Minor criteria
  - Preceded by one of the associated infections or vaccinations, or accompanied by one of the associated malignancies, inflammatory disorders, or pregnancy
  - Presence of fever and constitutional signs and symptoms
  - Leukocytosis
  - Excellent response to systemic corticosteroids

Associations

- Behçet's disease
- Hematologic malignancy
- Hepatitis B infection
- Inflammatory bowel disease
- Medications
- Polycythemia
- Pregnancy
- Rheumatoid arthritis
- Sarcoidosis
- Sjögren's syndrome
- Solid tumors
- Streptococcal upper respiratory illness

- Thyroid disease
- Tuberculosis
- Vaccination (influenza)
- Yersiniosis

Associated Medications

- All-trans retinoic acid
- Carbamazepine
- Celecoxib
- Clozapine
- Diazepam
- G-CSF
- Furosemide
- Hydralazine
- Isotretinoin
- Minocycline
- Nitrofurantoin
- Oral contraception
- Sulfamethoxazole–trimethoprim

Evaluation

- Antinuclear antibodies
- Antistreptolysin O titers
- Appropriate cancer screening
- Bacterial, mycobacterial, and fungal cultures
- Complete blood count
- Liver function test
- Pregnancy test
- Rheumatoid factor
- Sedimentation rate
- Thyroid function test
- Urinalysis

Treatment Options

- <u>Systemic corticosteroids</u>
- <u>Dapsone</u>
- <u>Colchicine</u>
- Potassium iodide
- Tetracycline
- Metronidazole
- Cyclosporine
- Clofazimine
- Cyclophosphamide

Further reading:

- Neoh CY, Tan AW, Ng SK (2007) Sweet's syndrome: a spectrum of unusual clinical presentations and associations. Br J Dermatol 156(3):480–485

Swimmer's Itch

Acute pruritic eruption that is caused by aquatic contact with cercarial forms of avian schistosomes and is characterized by pruritic erythematous papules on the uncovered areas of the body

Differential Diagnosis

- Allergic contact dermatitis
- Aquagenic urticaria
- Cholinergic urticaria
- Cold urticaria
- Creeping eruption
- Dermatographism
- Harvest-mite infestation
- Marine plant allergy
- <u>Insect bites</u>
- Scabies

- <u>Seabather's eruption</u>
- Urticaria

Treatment Options

- Observation and reassurance
- <u>Antihistamines</u>
- Topical corticosteroids
- Systemic corticosteroids

Further reading:
- Folster-Holst R, Disko R, Rowert J et al (2001) Cercarial dermatitis contracted via contact with an aquarium: case report and review. Br J Dermatol 145(4):638–640

Syphilis, Acquired

Sexually transmitted multistage infection that is caused by *Treponema pallidum* and is characterized by a painless, firm, well-defined genital ulcer (primary), a papulosquamous eruption involving the face, trunk, and extremities, including the palms and soles (secondary), and gummatous lesions along with cerebral and cardiovascular effects (tertiary)

Subtypes/Variants

- Annular
- Condyloma lata
- Corymbose
- Corona veneris
- Lues maligna
- Lues maligna (Fig. 6.112)
- Moth-eaten alopecia
- Mucous patches
- Rupial (Fig. 6.113)
- Split papules

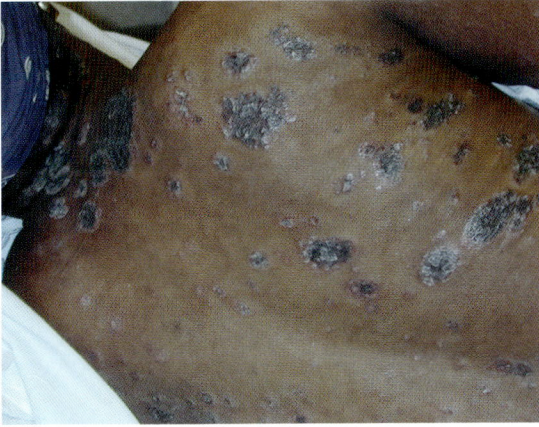

Fig. 6.112 Lues maligna (Courtesy of A. Record)

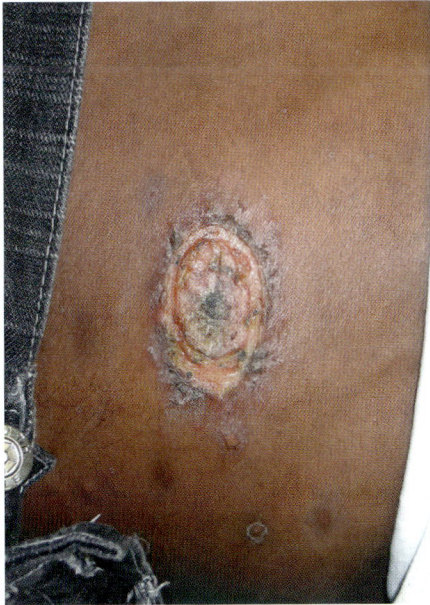

Fig. 6.113 Rupial syphilis

Differential Diagnosis

Primary

- Aphthous stomatitis
- Behçet's disease
- Chancroid
- Fixed drug eruption
- Genital herpes
- Genital trauma
- Granuloma inguinale
- Lymphogranuloma venereum
- Lymphoma
- Squamous cell carcinoma
- Trauma

Secondary

- Alopecia areata
- Bowenoid papulosis
- Chronic aphthous ulcers
- Condyloma acumination
- Cutaneous plasmacytosis
- Drug eruption
- Erythema multiforme
- Eruptive syringomas
- Folliculitis
- Granuloma annulare
- Guttate psoriasis
- Hand–foot–mouth disease
- Herpangina
- Lupus erythematosus
- Lichen planus, eruptive
- Nummular eczema
- Perleche
- Pityriasis lichenoides chronica
- Pityriasis rosea

- Pityriasis rubra pilaris
- Primary HIV infection
- Scabies
- Squamous cell carcinoma
- <u>Viral exanthem</u>
- Warts

Tertiary

- <u>Deep fungal infection</u>
- Leishmaniasis
- Leprosy
- Lupus erythematosus
- Lupus vulgaris
- Mycosis fungoides
- Sarcoidosis
- Venous ulcer

Treatment Options

- <u>Penicillin</u>
- Azithromycin
- Doxycycline
- Ceftriaxone

Further reading:
- Lautenschlager S (2006) Cutaneous manifestations of syphilis: recognition and management. Am J Clin Dermatol 7(5):291–304

Syphilis, Congenital

Intrauterine infection of the fetus with *Treponema pallidum* that gives rise to numerous birth and developmental defects, including rhagades (parrot lines), snuffles (rhinitis), mucous patches, bullous lesions, hepatospleno-megaly, lymphadenopathy, saddle-nose deformity, Hutchinson's triad

(VIII cranial nerve deafness, keratitis, peg-shaped teeth), mulberry molars, pseudoparalysis, and frontal bossing

Differential Diagnosis

- Congenital CMV
- Congenital rubella
- Ectodermal dysplasia
- Hurler syndrome
- Neonatal herpes simplex virus infection
- Neonatal lupus
- Neonatal pemphigus
- Staphylococcal scalded-skin syndrome
- Toxoplasmosis

Treatment Options

- Penicillin

Further reading:
- Lugo A, Sanchez S, Sanchez JL (2006) Congenital syphilis. Pediatr Dermatol 23(2):121–123

Syringocystadenoma Papilliferum (of Werther)

Benign neoplasm of apocrine derivation (a type of apocrine adenoma) that most often arises in a nevus sebaceus (and less commonly on normal skin) and is characterized by a cluster of erythematous papules that are occasionally oozing, crusted, or verrucous

Differential Diagnosis

- Apocrine adenoma
- Basal cell carcinoma

- Eccrine acrospiroma
- Metastatic adenocarcinoma
- <u>Pyogenic granuloma</u>
- Trichadenoma
- Trichoblastoma
- Trichilemmoma
- Warty dyskeratoma
- Verruca

Further reading:

- Laxmisha C, Thappa DM, Mishra MM et al (2007) Linear syringocystadenoma papilliferum of the scalp. J Eur Acad Dermatol Venereol 21(2):275–276

Syringofibroadenoma of Mascaro, Eccrine (Acrosyringeal Nevus of Weedon and Lewis)

Benign tumor of acrosyringeal derivation that is characterized by a flesh-colored or erythematous, hyperkeratotic, occasionally linear, nodule or plaque most commonly on the distal extremities, including the palms and soles

Differential Diagnosis

- Clear cell acanthoma
- Fibroepithelioma of Pinkus
- Hidroacanthoma simplex
- Irritated seborrheic keratosis
- Palmoplantar keratoderma
- Porocarcinoma
- <u>Porokeratotic eccrine ostial dermal duct nevus</u>
- Poroma
- Spiradenoma
- Tumor of the follicular infundibulum
- <u>Verruca</u>

- Verrucous carcinoma
- Verrucous xanthoma

Associations

- Bullous pemphigoid
- Burns
- Chronic ulcer
- Ectodermal dysplasias
- Epidermolysis bullosa
- Erosive lichen planus
- Schopf–Schulz–Passarge syndrome (multiple)
- Squamous cell carcinoma
- Venous stasis

Further reading:
- Kawaguchi M, Takeda H, Mitsuhashi Y et al (2003) Eccrine syringofibroadenoma with diffuse plantar hyperkeratosis. Br J Dermatol 149(4):885–886

Syringoma

Benign neoplasm of eccrine ductal derivation that is characterized by multiple, small, flesh-colored, slightly translucent papules on the face, especially the lower eyelid and infraorbital cheek, or elsewhere in an eruptive fashion, on the neck, chest, arms, or periumbilical area

Differential Diagnosis

Facial
- Basal cell carcinoma
- Eruptive vellus hair cysts
- Granulomatous rosacea

- Lupus miliaris disseminata faciei
- Microcystic adnexal carcinoma
- Milium
- Molluscum contagiosum
- Periocular dermatitis
- Sarcoidosis
- Secondary syphilis
- Steatocystoma multiplex
- Trichodiscoma
- Trichoepithelioma
- <u>Verruca plana</u>
- Xanthelasma

Eruptive

- Acne vulgaris
- Eruptive xanthomas
- Lichen nitidus
- <u>Lichen planus</u>
- Papular pityriasis rosea
- Papular sarcoidosis
- <u>Verruca plana</u>

Associations

- Brooke–Spiegler syndrome
- Carbamazepine
- <u>Diabetes (clear cell type)</u>
- <u>Down syndrome</u>
- Nicolau–Balus syndrome

Further reading:
- Teixeira M, Ferreira M, Machado S et al (2005) Eruptive syringomas. Dermatol Online J 11(3):34

Tache Noir

Refers to the "black spot" or eschar that results from a tick bite and is associated with several rickettsial diseases, especially scrub typhus, rickettsialpox, and Mediterranean fever

Differential Diagnosis

- Anthrax
- Arthropod-bite reaction
- Aspergillosis
- Brown recluse spider bite
- Cigarette burn
- <u>Ecthyma</u>
- Ecthyma gangrenosum
- Fusariosis
- Pyoderma gangrenosum
- Squamous cell carcinoma
- Tularemia

Further reading:
- Kim DM, Won KJ, Park CY et al (2007) Distribution of eschars on the body of scrub typhus patients: a prospective study. Am J Trop Med Hyg 76(5):806–809

Takayasu's Arteritis (Pulseless Disease)

Large vessel type of vasculitis that predominantly occurs in Asia and is characterized by aortitis leading to absent pulses and impaired circulation, generalized pyoderma-gangrenosum-like skin lesions, erythema nodosum, and other features

Differential Diagnosis

- Atherosclerosis
- Behçet's disease

- Buerger's disease
- Coarctation of the aorta
- Cogan's syndrome
- Hodgkin's disease
- <u>Pyoderma gangrenosum</u>
- Sarcoidosis
- Syphilitic aortitis
- Temporal arteritis
- Viral myocarditis

Diagnostic Criteria (ACR; 3/6)

- Age <40 years at onset
- Arteriogram abnormal
- BP >10 mmHg difference between two arms
- Bruits
- Decreased brachial artery pulses
- Limb claudication

Evaluation

- Antinuclear antibodies
- Chest radiograph
- Complete blood count
- Echocardiography
- Liver function tests
- MR angiography/MRI of chest
- Renal function tests
- Rheumatoid factor level
- Sedimentation rate
- Urinalysis

Further reading:

- Fiorentino DF (2003) Cutaneous vasculitis. J Am Acad Dermatol 48(3):311–340

Talon Noir (Black Heel)

Dark discoloration of the heel or palm that is caused by shearing forces on the skin (often sports-related) which lead to hemorrhage into the epidermis and is characterized by an asymptomatic black macule

Differential Diagnosis

- Achenbach syndrome
- Fixed drug eruption
- Foreign body
- Lentigo
- Melanoma
- Nevus
- Wart
- Tinea nigra
- Traumatic tattoo

Further reading:
- Mailler-Savage EA, Adams BB (2006) Skin manifestations of running. J Am Acad Dermatol 55(2):290–301

Targetoid Hemosiderotic Hemangioma (Hobnail Hemangioma)

Benign vascular neoplasm that is often induced by trauma; is characterized by a nodule or plaque with a violaceous center and a brown, erythematous, or hemorrhagic periphery (giving it a targetoid appearance); and is typically located on the trunk or extremities of a young to middle-aged adult (Fig. 6.114)

Differential Diagnosis

- Angiokeratoma
- Angiosarcoma

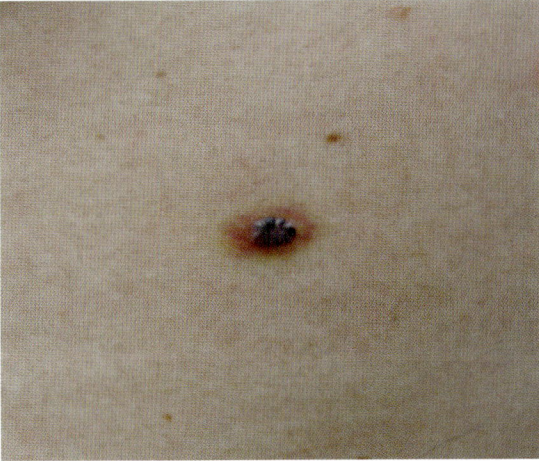

Fig. 6.114 Targetoid hemosiderotic hemangioma

- Benign hemangioma
- Benign lymphangiomatosis
- Cutaneous endometriosis
- Dabska's tumor
- Dermatofibroma
- Erythema multiforme
- Granuloma annulare
- Kaposi's sarcoma
- Melanoma
- Nevus
- Retiform hemangiomaendothelioma
- Spider angioma
- <u>Traumatized cherry angioma</u>
- Traumatized lymphangiectasis
- Venous lake

Further reading:

- Morales-Callaghan AM, Martinez-Garcia G, Aragoneses-Fraile H et al (2007) Targetoid hemosiderotic hemangioma: clinical and dermoscopical findings. J Eur Acad Dermatol Venereol 21(2):267–269

Telangiectasia, Generalized Essential

Idiopathic, acquired disorder with onset in adult life that predominantly affects women and is characterized by persistent telangiectasias that initially erupt on the lower extremities and then spread to encompass the upper extremities and trunk

Differential Diagnosis

- Angiokeratoma corporis diffusum
- Carcinoma telangiectaticum
- CREST syndrome
- Drug-induced telangiectasia
- Hereditary benign telangiectasia
- Hereditary hemorrhagic telangiectasia
- Spider angiomas (especially in liver disease)
- Telangiectasia macularis eruptive perstans
- Universal angiomatosis

Further reading:
- Blume JE (2005) Generalized essential telangiectasia: a case report and review of the literature. Cutis 75(4):223–224

Telangiectasia, Hereditary Hemorrhagic (Osler–Weber–Rendu Disease)

Inherited vascular disorder (AD) caused by defects in the endoglin or activin-like kinase genes that is characterized by epistaxis, telangiectasias of the skin and oral mucosa, pulmonary arteriovenous malformations, and gastrointestinal bleeding

Differential Diagnosis

- Angiokeratoma corporis diffusum
- Ataxia–telangiectasia
- Carcinoma telangiectaticum
- Coats disease
- Cockayne syndrome
- <u>CREST syndrome</u>
- Dermatomyositis
- Generalized essential telangiectasia
- Hereditary benign telangiectasia
- Rosacea
- Rothmund–Thomson syndrome
- Scleroderma
- Telangiectasia macularis eruptive perstans
- Universal angiomatosis

Diagnostic Criteria (3/4)

- Epistaxis: spontaneous and recurrent
- Telangiectasias: multiple at characteristic sites
- Visceral lesions: gastrointestinal telangiectasia, pulmonary, hepatic, cerebral, or spinal AVM
- Family history: one affected first-degree relative

Evaluation

- Chest radiography
- Complete blood count
- Iron studies
- Prothrombin time and partial thromboplastin time
- Stool for occult blood
- Upper and lower endoscopy

Further reading:

- Garzon MC, Huang JT, Enjolras O, Frieden IJ (2007) Vascular malformations. Part II: associated syndromes. J Am Acad Dermatol 56(4):541–564

Telangiectasia Macularis Eruptiva Perstans

Rare subtype of cutaneous mastocytosis that affects adults and is characterized by numerous mildly pruritic, reddish-brown, blanchable macules with telangiectasias that are Darier's sign negative and predominantly located on the trunk (Fig. 6.71)

Differential Diagnosis

- Angioma serpiginosum
- Carcinoid syndrome
- Carcinoma telangiectaticum
- Corticosteroids
- CREST syndrome
- Dermatomyositis
- Drug-induced telangiectasia
- Generalized essential telangiectasia
- Hereditary benign telangiectasia
- Liver disease
- Lupus erythematosus
- Mycosis fungoides
- Osler–Weber–Rendu disease
- Radiodermatitis
- Spider angiomas
- Unilateral nevoid telangiectasia

Evaluation

- Complete blood count
- Serum tryptase level

Treatment Options

- Observation and reassurance
- Antihistamines
- Pulsed dye laser

Further reading:
- Nguyen NQ (2004) Telangiectasia macularis eruptiva perstans. Dermatol Online J 10(3):1

Telangiectasia, Unilateral Nevoid

Congenital or acquired vascular nevus that is characterized by a linear, segmental distribution of telangiectasias involving a dermatome, most commonly on the neck, upper chest, or shoulder

Differential Diagnosis

- Angioma serpiginosum
- Carcinoma telangiectaticum
- Erythema ab igne
- Generalized essential telangiectasia
- Poikiloderma atrophicans vasculare
- Port-wine stain
- Radiation-induced telangiectasias
- Steroid-induced telangiectasias

Further reading:
- Sharma VK, Khandpur S (2006) Unilateral nevoid telangiectasia: response to pulsed dye laser. Int J Dermatol 45(8):960–964

Telogen Effluvium

Type of alopecia that is often associated with a stressful event which triggers a large number of hairs to enter telogen simultaneously and is characterized by the acute onset (or less commonly, a more chronic process) of diffuse, nonscarring, noninflammatory alopecia

Differential Diagnosis

- <u>Alopecia areata, diffuse pattern</u>
- Anagen effluvium
- <u>Androgenetic alopecia</u>
- Androgen-induced alopecia
- Loose anagen hair
- Lupus hair
- Syphilitic alopecia
- Thyrotoxicosis
- Tinea capitis
- Trichorrhexis nodosa
- Trichotillomania

Associations

- Allergic contact dermatitis
- Anticoagulants
- Antithyroid antibodies
- <u>Extreme dieting</u>
- Flare of systemic lupus erythematosus
- <u>High fever</u>
- Hyperthyroidism
- <u>Hypothyroidism</u>
- <u>Medications</u>
- Newborn
- <u>Postpartum period</u>
- <u>Postoperative period</u>
- <u>Profound blood loss</u>
- <u>Rapid weight loss</u>
- Retinoids
- Seborrheic dermatitis
- Severe chronic illness
- <u>Severe infection</u>
- Severe prolonged stress
- Trichodynia

Associated Medications

- ACE inhibitors
- Albendazole
- <u>Anticoagulants</u>
- Antimitotic agents
- <u>Beta-blockers</u>
- Bromocriptine
- Carbamazepine
- Danazol
- Heparin
- Interferon alpha
- Lipid-lowering drugs
- Lithium
- Nicotinic acid
- Nitrofurantoin
- <u>Oral contraception</u>
- Retinoids
- Valproate

Treatment Options

- <u>Observation and reassurance</u>
- Minoxidil

Further reading:
- Harrison S, Sinclair R (2002) Telogen effluvium. Clin Exp Dermatol 27(5):389–395

Temporal Arteritis (Giant Cell Arteritis)

Large vessel vasculitis syndrome of unknown cause that affects the elderly and is characterized by jaw claudication, headaches or scalp tenderness, visual disturbance, polymyalgia rheumatica, and rarely, ulceration of the scalp

Differential Diagnosis

- Amyloidosis
- Behçet's disease
- Cogan's syndrome
- Headache (other causes)
- Idiopathic facial pain syndrome
- Lupus erythematosus
- Polyarteritis nodosa
- Rheumatoid arthritis
- Sarcoidosis
- Takayasu's arteritis
- <u>Trigeminal neuralgia</u>
- Wegener's granulomatosis

Diagnostic Criteria (3/5)

- Abnormal temporal artery on clinical examination (tenderness to palpation or decreased pulsation)
- Age >50 years at onset
- Elevated erythrocyte sedimentation rate
- New type of headache
- Temporal artery biopsy showing vasculitis

Evaluation

- Complete blood count
- CT scan/angiography of affected vessels
- Ophthalmologic examination
- Renal function test
- Sedimentation rate
- Temporal artery biopsy

Further reading:

- Fiorentino DF (2003) Cutaneous vasculitis. J Am Acad Dermatol 48(3):311–340

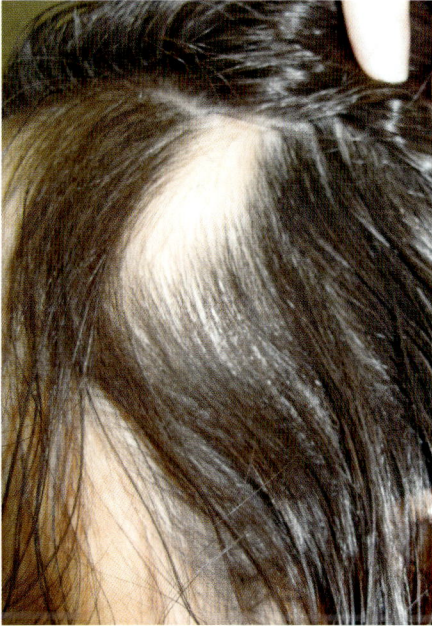

Fig. 6.115 Triangular temporal alopecia

Temporal Triangular Alopecia (Brauer Nevus)

Idiopathic, usually acquired, localized type of alopecia that develops in early childhood and is characterized by a triangular, nonscarring patch of alopecia on the frontotemporal portion of the scalp (Fig. 6.115)

Differential Diagnosis

- Alopecia areata
- Aplasia cutis congenita
- Nevus sebaceus
- Tinea capitis
- Traction alopecia
- Trichotillomania

Associations

- Epilepsy
- Mental retardation
- Phakomatosis pigmentovascularis

Further reading:
- Elmer KB, George RM (2002) Congenital triangular alopecia: a case report and review. Cutis 69(4):255–256

Terra Firma–Forme Dermatosis

Cutaneous discoloration of uncertain cause that is characterized by dirty-brown macular hyperpigmentation that cannot be removed with routine cleaning but can be removed with isopropyl alcohol

Differential Diagnosis

- <u>Acanthosis nigricans</u>
- Atopic dermatitis
- Confluent and reticulated papillomatosis
- <u>Dermatosis neglecta</u>
- Postinflammatory hyperpigmentation
- Prurigo pigmentosa
- X-linked ichthyosis

Further reading:
- Browning J, Rosen T (2005) Terra firma–forme dermatosis revisited. Dermatol Online J 11(2):15

Thromboangiitis Obliterans (Buerger's Disease)

Idiopathic vascular disorder that is associated with smoking, occurs predominantly in young to middle-aged adult men, and is characterized by digital pain, ischemic necrosis, and gangrene of the hands and feet

Differential Diagnosis

- Achenbach syndrome
- <u>Antiphospholipid antibody syndrome</u>
- Arteriosclerosis obliterans
- Cannabis arteritis
- Cocaine abuse
- CREST syndrome
- <u>Cryoglobulinemia</u>
- Neuropathic ulcers
- Peripheral artery disease
- Raynaud's disease
- Reflex sympathetic dystrophy
- Scleroderma
- <u>Systemic vasculitis syndromes</u>
- Takayasu's arteritis

Diagnostic Criteria

- Age younger than 45 years
- Current (or recent) history of tobacco use
- Presence of distal extremity ischemia documented by noninvasive vascular testing such as ultrasound
- Exclusion of autoimmune diseases, hypercoagulable states, and diabetes mellitus by laboratory tests
- Exclusion of a proximal source of emboli by echocardiography and arteriography
- Consistent arteriographic findings in the clinically involved and noninvolved limbs

Evaluation

- Anticardiolipin antibodies
- Antinuclear antibodies (including Scl-70 antibodies)

- Arteriography
- Complete blood count
- Echocardiography
- Lupus anticoagulant
- Rheumatoid factor
- Sedimentation rate

Treatment Options

- <u>Cessation of tobacco use</u>
- Iloprost
- Pain control
- Antibiotics
- Amputation

Further reading:
- Olin JW, Shih A (2006) Thromboangiitis obliterans (Buerger's disease). Curr Opin Rheumatol 18(1):18–24

Thrombophlebitis, Superficial

Inflammation of the superficial veins that is caused by various hypercoagulable disorders, infection, or trauma and is characterized by a tender linear erythematous subcutaneous cord

Differential Diagnosis

- Bacterial infection
- Behçet's disease
- Candidiasis
- <u>Cellulitis</u>
- Cutaneous larva migrans
- <u>Deep venous thrombosis</u>
- Erythema induratum
- Erythema nodosum

- Factitial
- Hypercoagulable
- Internal malignancy
- Interstitial granulomatous dermatitis (rope sign)
- Lupus panniculitis
- Lymphangiitis
- Mondor's disease
- Oral contraception
- Pancreatic panniculitis
- Polyarteritis nodosa
- Pregnancy
- Secondary syphilis

Associations

- Buerger's disease
- Hormonal therapy
- Hypercoagulable state
- Internal malignancy
- Pregnancy
- Prolonged immobilization
- Sickle cell disease
- Surgery
- Trauma

Further reading:
- Luis Rodriguez-Peralto J, Carrillo R, Rosales B et al (2007) Superficial thrombophlebitis. Semin Cutan Med Surg 26(2):71–76

Thyroglossal Duct Cyst

Developmental anomaly that is caused by failure of the thyroglossal duct to involute and is characterized by a recurrently inflamed subcutaneous mass in the anterior midline neck located between the thyroid gland and the posterior tongue

Differential Diagnosis

- Branchial cleft cyst
- Bronchogenic cyst
- Congenital midline cervical cleft
- Dermoid cyst
- Epidermal inclusion cyst
- Infantile hemangioma
- Lipoma
- Thyroid cancer
- Venous malformation

Further reading:
- Acierno SP, Waldhausen JH (2007) Congenital cervical cysts, sinuses and fistulae. Otolaryngol Clin North Am 40(1):161–176, vii–viii

Tinea Barbae

Dermatophyte infection of the beard area that can be superficial and noninflammatory or deeper and inflammatory (kerion type) and is characterized by scaly, annular plaques with pustules and broken-off hairs (superficial; most commonly caused by *T. rubrum* or *T. violaceum*) or a deep inflammatory nodule or plaque with pustules and sinus tracts (deep; most commonly by *T. mentagrophytes* or *T. verrucosum*)

Differential Diagnosis

- Acne vulgaris
- Actinomycosis
- Bacterial folliculitis
- Blastomycosis
- Blastomycosis-like pyoderma
- *Candida* folliculitis
- Dental sinus
- Halogenoderma

- <u>Herpetic sycosis</u>
- Impetigo
- Lupus vulgaris
- Perioral dermatitis
- <u>Pseudofolliculitis barbae</u>
- Pyoderma faciale
- Ruptured epidermal inclusion cyst
- Seborrheic dermatitis
- Sweet's syndrome
- <u>Sycosis barbae</u>
- Syphilis

Treatment Options

- <u>Terbinafine</u>
- Griseofulvin
- Itraconazole

Further reading:

- Maeda M, Nakashima T, Satho M et al (2002) Tinea barbae due to *Trichophyton verrucosum*. Eur J Dermatol 12(3):272–274

Tinea Capitis

Dermatophyte infection of the scalp caused most commonly by *Trichophyton tonsurans* that predominantly affects African–American children and is characterized by gray patches of hair loss, stubs of broken hairs (black-dot pattern), pustules, fine seborrheic scale, kerion formation (inflammatory, boggy nodule caused by hypersensitivity to dermatophyte), and accompanying regional lymphadenopathy (Fig. 6.116)

Subtypes/Variants

- Black dot
- Favus

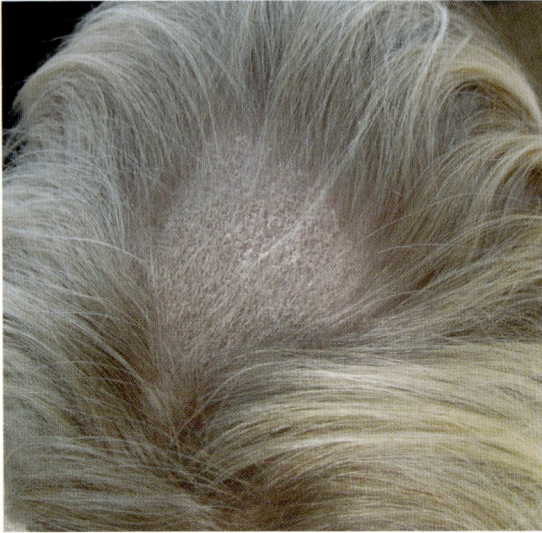

Fig. 6.116 Tinea capitis

- Gray patch
- Kerion
- Seborrheic-dermatitis-like

Differential Diagnosis

Classic

- <u>Alopecia areata</u>
- Bacterial pyoderma
- Demodicosis
- Dermatomyositis
- Folliculitis
- Folliculitis decalvans
- Impetigo
- Lichen simplex
- Lupus erythematosus
- Pediculosis

- Pemphigus foliaceus
- Pityriasis amiantacea
- Psoriasis
- Seborrheic dermatitis
- Secondary syphilis
- Traction alopecia
- Triangular temporal alopecia
- Trichotillomania

Kerion

- Bacterial pyoderma/furuncle
- Botryomycosis
- Dissecting cellulitis
- Folliculitis decalvans
- Inflammed cyst
- Metastatic lesion
- Myiasis

Treatment Options

- Terbinafine
- Griseofulvin
- Itraconazole

Further reading:
- Seebacher C, Abeck D, Brasch J et al (2007) Tinea capitis: ringworm of the scalp. Mycoses 50(3):218–226

Tinea Corporis

Dermatophyte infection of the trunk and extremities that is most commonly caused by *Trichophyton rubrum* and is characterized by pruritic, erythematous, annular scaly plaques (Fig. 6.117)

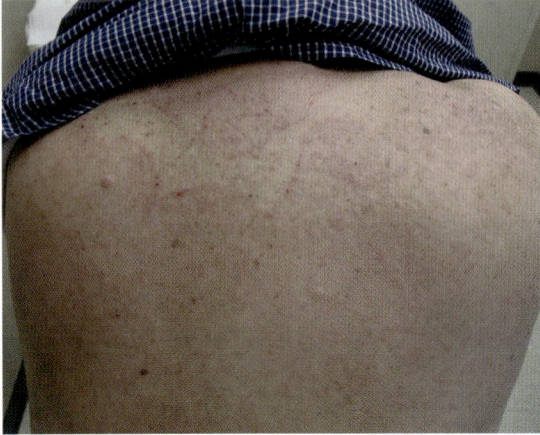

Fig. 6.117 Tinea corporis

Subtypes/Variants

- Tinea corporis, classic
- Tinea gladiatorum
- Tinea imbricata
- Tinea profunda (Majocchi's granuloma)

Differential Diagnosis

- Candidiasis
- Contact dermatitis
- Cutaneous T cell lymphoma
- Erythema annulare centrifugum
- Granuloma annulare
- Lupus erythematosus
- Nummular eczema
- Parapsoriasis
- Pityriasis rosea (herald patch)
- Psoriasis

- Pyoderma
- Sarcoidosis
- Seborrheic dermatitis
- <u>Subacute cutaneous lupus erythematosus</u>
- Superficial pemphigus
- Syphilis
- Tinea versicolor

Treatment Options

- Topical imidazoles
- Terbinafine cream
- Butenafine cream
- Naftifine cream
- Ciclopirox
- <u>Terbinafine</u>
- Griseofulvin
- Itraconazole

Further reading:
- Ziemer M, Seyfarth F, Elsner P, Hipler UC (2007) Atypical manifestations of tinea corporis. Mycoses 50(Suppl 2):31–35

Tinea Cruris

Dermatophyte infection of the groin that is most commonly caused by *Trichophyton rubrum* and is characterized by pruritic, erythematous, annular scaly plaques that spare the scrotum

Differential Diagnosis

- Acanthosis nigricans
- Baboon syndrome
- <u>Candidiasis</u>

- <u>Contact dermatitis</u>
- Erythrasma
- Extramammary Paget's disease
- Hailey–Hailey disease
- <u>Intertrigo</u>
- Inverse pityriasis rosea
- Irritant dermatitis
- Langerhans cell histiocytosis
- Mycosis fungoides
- Pediculosis
- Pemphigus foliaceus
- <u>Psoriasis</u>
- Pyoderma
- <u>Seborrheic dermatitis</u>

Treatment Options

- Topical imidazoles
- Terbinafine cream
- Butenafine cream
- Naftifine cream
- Ciclopirox
- <u>Terbinafine</u>
- Griseofulvin
- Itraconazole

Further reading:
- Gupta AK, Chaudhry M, Elewski B (2003) Tinea corporis, tinea cruris, tinea nigra, and piedra. Dermatol Clin 21(3):395–400

Tinea Faciei

Dermatophyte infection of the face that is most commonly caused by *Trichophyton rubrum* and is characterized by annular, often unilateral scaly plaques (Fig. 6.118)

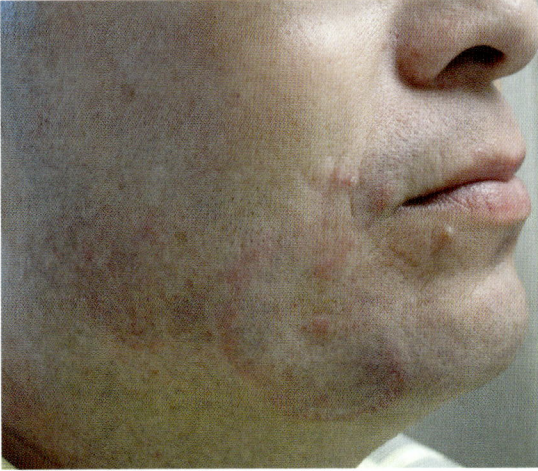

Fig. 6.118 Tinea faciei

Differential Diagnosis

- Actinic keratosis
- Atopic dermatitis
- Candidiasis
- Coccidioidomycosis
- Contact dermatitis
- Demodex folliculitis
- Granuloma annulare
- Impetigo
- Lupus erythematosus
- Lupus vulgaris
- Jessner's lymphocytic infiltrate
- Perioral dermatitis
- Pityriasis alba
- Polymorphous light eruption
- Psoriasis
- Pyoderma
- Rosacea

- Sarcoidosis
- <u>Seborrheic dermatitis</u>
- Syphilis

Treatment Options

- Topical imidazoles
- Terbinafine cream
- Butenafine cream
- Naftifine cream
- Ciclopirox
- <u>Terbinafine</u>
- Griseofulvin
- Itraconazole

Further reading:
- Lin RL, Szepietowski JC, Schwartz RA (2004) Tinea faciei, an often deceptive facial eruption. Int J Dermatol 43(6):437–440

Tinea Incognito

Refers to a dermatophytosis that has been modified by treatment with topical steroids and that mimics a variety of dermatoses

Differential Diagnosis

- Discoid lupus erythematosus
- Impetigo
- Lichen planus
- <u>Nummular eczema</u>
- <u>Psoriasis</u>
- Purpura
- Rosacea
- Seborrheic dermatitis

Treatment Options

- Topical imidazoles
- Terbinafine cream
- Butenafine cream
- Naftifine cream
- Ciclopirox
- Terbinafine
- Griseofulvin
- Itraconazole

Further reading:
- Romano C, Maritati E, Gianni C (2006) Tinea incognito in Italy: a 15-year survey. Mycoses 49(5):383–387

Tinea Manuum

Dermatophyte infection of the palm that is most commonly caused by *Trichophyton rubrum* and is characterized by erythema and scale which is predominantly localized to the palmar creases

Differential Diagnosis

- Atopic dermatitis
- Contact dermatitis
- Dyshidrotic eczema
- Keratolysis exfoliativa
- Palmoplantar pustulosis
- Psoriasis

Treatment Options

- Topical imidazoles
- Terbinafine cream

- Butenafine cream
- Naftifine cream
- Ciclopirox
- Terbinafine
- Griseofulvin
- Itraconazole

Further reading:
- Aste N, Pau M, Aste N (2005) Tinea manuum bullosa. Mycoses 48(1):80–81

Tinea Nigra

Superficial fungal infection that occurs most commonly in the tropics, is caused by the dematiaceous fungus *Hortaea werneckii*, and is characterized by an asymptomatic tan-to-black circular patch on the palm or sole

Differential Diagnosis

- Acral melanocytic nevi
- Addison's disease
- Chemical stain
- Fixed drug eruption
- Melanoma
- Pinta
- Postinflammatory hyperpigmentation
- *Scytalidium* infection
- Syphilis
- Talon noir
- Yaws

Treatment Options

- Topical imidazoles
- Terbinafine cream
- Butenafine cream

- Naftifine cream
- Ciclopirox
- Salicylic acid
- Topical retinoids
- Terbinafine
- Griseofulvin
- Itraconazole

Further reading:
- Gupta AK, Chaudhry M, Elewski B (2003) Tinea corporis, tinea cruris, tinea nigra, and piedra. Dermatol Clin 21(3):395–400

Tinea Pedis

Dermatophyte infection of the feet that is caused most commonly by *Trichophyton rubrum* and is characterized by erythema and scale with occasional bullae on the lateral aspects of the sole and/or interdigital area

Subtypes/Variants

- Interdigital
- Moccasin
- Ulcerative
- Vesiculobullous

Differential Diagnosis

- Acral lentiginous melanoma
- Atopic dermatitis
- Bacterial intertrigo
- Candidiasis
- Contact dermatitis
- Dyshidrotic eczema
- Erythrasma
- Erythema multiforme

- Friction blister
- <u>Gram-negative toe-web infection</u>
- Id reaction
- Juvenile plantar dermatosis
- Kaposi's sarcoma
- Localized bullous pemphigoid
- Mycosis fungoides palmaris et plantaris
- Pagetoid reticulosis
- <u>Psoriasis</u>
- Pyoderma
- Scabies
- Syphilis
- Weber–Cockayne syndrome

Treatment Options

- Topical imidazoles
- Terbinafine cream
- Butenafine cream
- Naftifine cream
- Ciclopirox
- <u>Terbinafine</u>
- Griseofulvin
- Itraconazole

Further reading:

- Ecemis T, Degerli K, Aktas E et al (2006) The necessity of culture for the diagnosis of tinea pedis. Am J Med Sci 331(2):88–90

Tinea Unguium

Type of onychomycosis representing a recalcitrant dermatophyte infection of the nails that is most commonly caused by *Trichophyton rubrum* and is characterized by nail thickening, discoloration, subungual debris, and onycholysis

Differential Diagnosis

- Bacterial paronychia
- Chronic mucocutaneous candidiasis
- Congenital malalignment of great toenails
- Contact dermatitis
- Darier's disease
- Lichen planus
- Melanoma
- Nail–patella syndrome
- Nondermatophyte onychomycosis
- Norwegian scabies
- Old age
- Onychogryposis
- Onycholysis
- Pachyonychia congenita
- Peripheral vascular disease
- Pincer nail deformity
- Pityriasis rubra pilaris
- *Pseudomonal* infection
- Psoriasis
- Traumatic nail dystrophy
- Twenty-nail dystrophy
- Yellow-nail syndrome

Associations

- AIDS
- Diabetes mellitus
- Elderly
- Peripheral vascular disease
- Smokers
- Tinea pedis
- Trauma

Treatment Options

- <u>Terbinafine</u>
- Griseofulvin
- Itraconazole
- Nail removal

Further reading:
- Scher RK, Tavakkol A, Sigurgeirsson B (2007) Onychomycosis: diagnosis and definition of cure. J Am Acad Dermatol 56(6):939–944

Tinea Versicolor (Pityriasis Versicolor, Eichstedt's Disease)

Superficial, recurrent fungal infection that is caused by *Malassezia globosa* and is characterized by asymptomatic, patchy scaly areas of hyperpigmentation or hypopigmentation on the upper chest, back, neck, and proximal extremities. An uncommon presentation of tinea versicolor is atrophic macules on the chest or upper back (pityriasis versicolor atrophicans) (Fig. 6.119)

Differential Diagnosis

- Anetoderma
- Bier spots
- Confluent and reticulated papillomatosis
- Epidermodysplasia verruciformis
- Erythema dyschromicum perstans
- Erythrasma
- Florid cutaneous papillomatosis
- Idiopathic eruptive macular pigmentation
- Lupus erythematosus
- Melasma
- Multiple tumors of the follicular infundibulum
- Mycosis fungoides
- Parapsoriasis

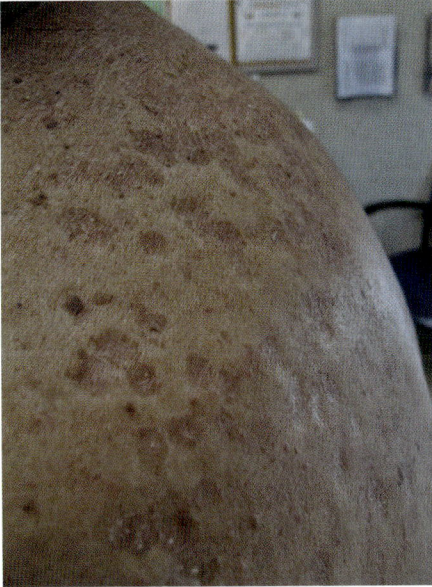

Fig. 6.119 Tinea versicolor atrophicans

- Pinta
- Pityriasis alba
- Pityriasis rosea
- Pityriasis rubra pilaris
- Progressive macular hypomelanosis
- Postinflammatory hyperpigmentation
- Postinflammatory hypopigmentation
- Seborrheic dermatitis
- Secondary syphilis (including syphilitic anetoderma)
- Tinea corporis
- Vitiligo

Treatment Options

- Topical ketoconazole
- Oral ketoconazole
- Selenium sulfide

Further reading:

- Crowson AN, Magro CM (2003) Atrophying tinea versicolor: a clinical and histological study of 12 patients. Int J Dermatol 42(12):928–932
- Gupta AK, Batra R, Bluhm R et al (2004) Skin diseases associated with *Malassezia* species. J Am Acad Dermatol 51(5):785–798

Toxic Shock Syndrome

Toxin-mediated syndrome associated with a focal *Staphylococcal* skin or visceral infection that is characterized by fever, hypotension, a diffuse morbilliform eruption, strawberry tongue, desquamation of the palms and soles, and variable internal organ manifestations (a more protracted variant that affects HIV-positive patients is called recalcitrant, erythematous, and desquamative (RED) disorder)

Differential Diagnosis

- Acute graft-vs-host disease
- Acute pyelonephritis
- Acute rheumatic fever
- Acute viral syndrome
- Capillary leak syndrome
- Drug reaction
- Gastroenteritis
- Hemolytic uremic syndrome
- Kawasaki disease
- Legionnaire disease
- Leptospirosis
- Lyme disease
- Meningococcemia
- Osteomyelitis
- Pelvic inflammatory disease
- Rocky Mountain spotted fever
- Scarlet fever

- Septic shock
- Staphylococcal scalded-skin syndrome
- Streptococcal toxic-shock-like syndrome
- Systemic lupus erythematosus
- Systemic mastocytosis
- Toxic epidermal necrolysis
- Typhus

Diagnostic Criteria

- Fever: temperature >39.6°C (or >102°F)
- Rash: diffuse macular erythroderma
- Desquamation: 1–2 weeks after the onset of illness (especially palms and soles)
- Hypotension: systolic blood pressure <90 mmHg for adults (less than fifth percentile for children)
- Involvement of three or more of the following organ systems:
  - Gastrointestinal
  - Muscular
  - Central nervous
  - Renal
  - Hepatic
  - Mucous membranes (erythema)
  - Hematologic (platelets <100,000/mm^3)
- Lack of evidence for other causes (if done):
- Negative blood, throat, cerebrospinal fluid cultures
- Negative serologic tests for Rocky Mountain spotted fever, leptospirosis, and measles

Associations

- Cellulitis
- Influenza
- Necrotizing fasciitis

- Postoperative wound infection
- Postpartum infection
- Sinusitis
- Thermal burns

Evaluation

- Blood cultures
- Cerebrospinal fluid cultures
- Chest radiograph
- Complete blood count
- Liver function test
- Renal function test
- Throat cultures
- Urinalysis

Treatment Options

- Supportive care
- Systemic antibiotics

Further reading:

- Herzer CM (2001) Toxic shock syndrome: broadening the differential diagnosis. J Am Board Fam Pract 14(2):131–136
- Nelson C (2004) Early recognition and treatment of staphylococcal and streptococcal toxic shock. J Pediatr Adolesc Gynecol 17(4):289–292

Traction Alopecia

Type of alopecia that is associated with styling, braiding, rolling, or tightening of the hair in such a way as to cause chronic mechanical forces that pull on multiple hair shafts and that is characterized by regional non-scarring (occasionally scarring) alopecia in the areas affected by the traction

Differential Diagnosis

- <u>Alopecia areata</u>
- Anagen effluvium
- Androgenetic alopecia
- Aplasia cutis congenita
- Frontal fibrosing alopecia
- <u>Central centrifugal cicatricial alopecia</u>
- Lupus erythematosus
- Occipital pressure alopecia
- Syphilis
- Telogen effluvium
- <u>Tinea capitis</u>
- Trichorrhexis nodosa
- Trichotillomania

Further reading:
- Hantash BM, Schwartz RA (2003) Traction alopecia in children. Cutis 71(1):18–20

Traction Folliculitis

Type of folliculitis that affects the scalp of patients with traction that is characterized by pustules only in the follicles affected by traction (Fig. 6.120)

Differential Diagnosis

- Bacterial folliculitis
- Occlusive folliculitis
- Tinea capitis

Evaluation

- Bacterial culture
- Fungal culture

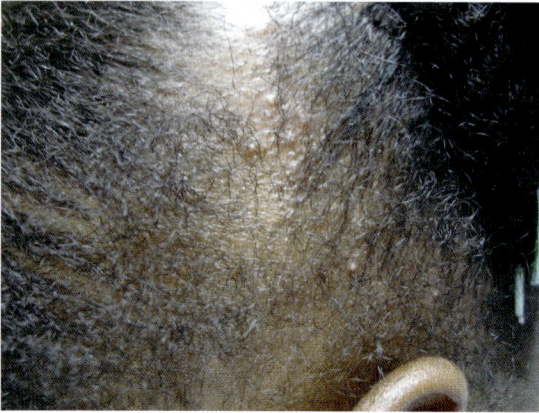

Fig. 6.120 Traction folliculitis

Treatment Options

- <u>Reduction of traction</u>
- Topical antibiotics
- Oral antibiotics

Further reading:

- Fox GN, Stausmire JM, Mehregan DR (2007) Traction folliculitis: an undereported entity. Cutis 79(1):26–30

Tragus, Accessory

Developmental anomaly representing a remnant of the first branchial arch that is characterized as a fleshy papule or papules located in the preauricular area

Differential Diagnosis

- <u>Acrochordon</u>
- Branchial cyst or sinus

- Bronchogenic cyst
- Epidermoid cyst
- Juvenile xanthogranuloma
- Melanocytic nevus
- <u>Neurofibroma</u>
- Preauricular cyst or sinus
- Rhabdomyomatous mesenchymal hamartoma
- Spitz nevus
- Thyroglossal duct cyst

Associations

- Goldenhar syndrome
- Townes–Brocks syndrome
- Treacher Collins–Franceschetti syndrome
- VACTERL association
- Wolf–Hirschhorn syndrome

Evaluation (Especially if Multiple)

- Hearing testing
- Renal/urinary tract ultrasound

Further reading:

- Jansen T, Romiti R, Altmeyer P (2000) Accessory tragus: report of two cases and review of the literature. Pediatr Dermatol 17(5):391–394

Transient Neonatal Pustular Melanosis

Benign dermatosis that affects predominantly African–American neonates, resolves within weeks to months, and is characterized by vesiculopustules that heal to hyperpigmented macules on the face, neck, and trunk but also the palms and soles

Differential Diagnosis

- Acropustulosis of infancy
- Candidiasis
- Eosinophilic pustular folliculitis
- <u>Erythema toxicum neonatorum</u>
- Impetigo
- Milia
- Miliaria
- Mongolian spots
- Neonatal acne
- Neonatal herpes simplex virus infection

Treatment Options

- Observation and reassurance

Further reading:
- Mengesha YM, Bennett ML (2002) Pustular skin disorders: diagnosis and treatment. Am J Clin Dermatol 3(6):389–400

Traumatic Tattoo

Accident-related tattoo that is caused by traumatic implantation of a pigmented foreign body into the skin and is characterized by solitary or multiple blue or black macules or papules with or without surrounding inflammation

Differential Diagnosis

- <u>Blue nevus</u>
- Drug-induced pigmentation
- Exogenous ochronosis

- Lentigo
- Melanocytic nevus
- <u>Melanoma</u>
- Talon noir

Further reading:
- Kang MJ, Kim MY, Kim YJ et al (2007) Traumatic tattoo associated with jet injector (Dermojet) use. J Dermatol 34(10):732–733

Trench Fever

Blood-borne bacterial infection that affects homeless persons, is caused by *Bartonella quintana* and transmitted by *Pediculus humanus* var. *corporis,* and is characterized by febrile episodes, bone pain, conjunctivitis, and a morbilliform eruption on the trunk

Differential Diagnosis

- Babesiosis
- Bacillary angiomatosis
- Cryptococcosis
- <u>Endocarditis</u>
- HIV infection
- Lyme disease
- Rat-bite fever
- Reactive arthritis with conjunctivitis and urethritis
- <u>Relapsing fever</u>
- Rocky Mountain spotted fever
- Q fever
- Schnitzler's syndrome
- Toxic shock syndrome
- Tuberculosis

Evaluation

- Bartonella ELISA and Western blot
- Blood cultures
- Echocardiography

Further reading:
- Brouqui P, Raoult D (2006) Arthropod-borne diseases in homeless. Ann N Y Acad Sci 1078:223–235

Trichilemmoma

Benign neoplasm derived from the outer root sheath that is characterized by a warty flesh-colored papule on the face

Differential Diagnosis

- Angiofibroma
- Basal cell carcinoma
- Clear cell acanthoma
- Eccrine acrospiroma
- Epidermal inclusion cyst
- Hidroacanthoma simplex
- Inverted follicular keratosis
- Neurilemmoma
- Poroma
- Seborrheic keratosis
- Trichoblastoma
- Trichoepithelioma
- Trichofolliculoma
- Wart
- Warty dyskeratoma

Associations

- Cowden's disease
- Nevus sebaceus

Further reading:
- Kurokawa I, Nishijima S, Kusumoto K et al (2003) Trichilemmoma: an immunohistochemical study of cytokeratins. Br J Dermatol 149(1):99–104

Trichinosis

Parasitic infestation with the nematode *Trichinella spiralis* that is acquired by ingesting larval cysts in uncooked pork and is characterized by muscle weakness and myalgias, fever, facial edema (especially of the eyelids), eosinophilia, urticaria, splinter hemorrhages, and palmar erythema

Differential Diagnosis

- Allergic reaction
- Angioedema
- Cysticercosis
- Dermatomyositis
- Eosinophilia–myalgia syndrome
- Hypereosinophilic syndrome
- Small vessel vasculitis
- Sparganosis
- Toxoplasmosis
- Visceral larva migrans

Evaluation

- Complete blood count
- Creatine kinase
- CT/MRI scan of brain or extremities

- Muscle biopsy
- Urinalysis

Further reading:
- Pozio E, Gomez Morales MA, Dupouy-Camet J (2003) Clinical aspects, diagnosis and treatment of trichinellosis. Expert Rev Anti Infect Ther 1(3):471–482

Trichodiscoma

Benign neoplasm of follicular derivation that is associated with Birt–Hogg–Dube syndrome (when multiple) and is characterized by small, often multiple flesh-colored papules on the head and neck, and often on the face

Differential Diagnosis

- Acrochordon
- Angiofibroma
- Basal cell carcinoma
- Fibrofolliculoma
- Fibrous papule
- Palisaded encapsulated neuroma
- Perifollicular fibroma
- Syringoma
- Trichilemmoma
- Trichoepithelioma
- Trichofolliculoma

Further reading:
- Collins GL, Somach S, Morgan MB (2006) CD-34-reactive trichodiscoma. J Cutan Pathol 33(10):709

Trichodysplasia Spinulosa

Facial skin eruption, possibly caused by polyoma virus, that affects patients on immunosuppressive therapy, especially transplant recipients, and that is characterized by erythematous follicular papules on the mid-face, chin, and glabella, as well as loss of eyebrows

Differential Diagnosis

- Acne vulgaris
- Drug-induced acne
- Follicular mucinosis
- Keratosis pilaris
- Keratosis pilaris atrophicans
- Lichen myxedematosus
- Sebaceous hyperplasia
- Trichostasis spinulosa

Treatment Options

- Valganciclovir
- Topical cidofovir
- Topical retinoids
- Systemic retinoids

Further reading:

- Schwieger-Briel A, Balma-Mena A, Ngan B, Dipchand A, Pope E (2010) Trichodysplasia spinulosa--a rare complication in immunosuppressed patients. Pediatr Dermatol 27(5):509–513

Trichoepithelioma

Benign neoplasm of follicular derivation that can be solitary or multiple (as a part of a hereditary syndrome) and is characterized by a small, flesh-colored dome-shaped papule on the face, especially around the nose (Fig. 6.121)

Differential Diagnosis

- Angiofibroma
- Basal cell carcinoma
- Basaloid follicular hamartoma syndrome

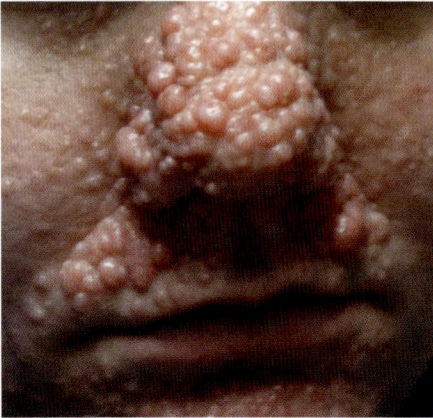

Fig. 6.121 Trichoepitheliomas

- Colloid milium
- Cylindroma
- Fibrofolliculoma
- Fibrous papule
- Microcystic adnexal carcinoma
- Milium
- Pilar cyst
- Steatocystoma
- Syringoma
- Trichilemmoma
- Trichoadenoma
- Trichoblastoma
- Trichodiscoma

Associations

- Brooke–Spiegler syndrome
- Myasthenia gravis
- Rasmussen syndrome
- Rombo syndrome
- Systemic lupus erythematosus

Further reading:

- Kim C, Kovich OI, Dosik J (2007) Brooke–Spiegler syndrome. Dermatol Online J 13(1):10

Trichofolliculoma

Benign hamartomatous tumor of the hair follicle characterized by a small, circumscribed papule with a central pore from which fine, white hairs are protruding

Differential Diagnosis

- Angiofibroma
- Basal cell carcinoma
- Colloid milium
- Cylindroma
- Dermoid cyst
- Dilated pore of Winer
- Fibrofolliculoma
- Folliculosebaceous cystic hamartoma
- Ingrown hair
- Microcystic adnexal carcinoma
- Midline nasal dermoid fistula
- Milium
- Molluscum contagiosum
- Perifollicular fibroma
- Pilar sheath acanthoma
- Pilar cyst
- Pili multigemini
- Syringoma
- Trichilemmoma
- Trichodiscoma
- Trichoepithelioma

- Trichostasis spinulosa
- Vellus hair cyst

Further reading:
- Kurokawa I, Kusumoto K, Sensaki H et al (2003) Trichofolliculoma: case report with immunohistochemical study of cytokeratins. Br J Dermatol 148(3):597–598

Trichomycosis Axillaris/Pubis

Superficial bacterial infection of the hair shafts of the axilla or pubic area that is caused by *Corynebacteria tenuis* and is characterized yellow granules that are firmly adherent to the hair shaft

Differential Diagnosis

- Antiperspirant residue
- Hair casts
- Pediculosis pubis
- Piedra

Associations

- Erythrasma

Treatment Options

- Removal of hair
- Topical clindamycin

Further reading:
- Lee PL, Lemos B, O'Brien SH et al (2007) Cutaneous diphtheroid infection and review of other cutaneous Gram-positive *Bacillus* infections. Cutis 79(5):371–377

Trichoptilosis (Split Ends)

Hair-shaft abnormality associated with distal trichorrhexis nodosa that is caused by excessive mechanical or chemical stress on the hair and is characterized by longitudinal splitting of the hair shaft from its most distal end in a proximal direction

Differential Diagnosis

- Pili bifurcati

Associations

- Monilethrix
- Netherton's syndrome
- Trauma
- Trichorrhexis nodosa
- Trichothiodystrophy

Further reading:
- Im M, Kye KC, Seo YJ et al (2006) Central trichoptilosis with onycholysis. Int J Dermatol 45(10):1187–1188

Trichorrhexis Invaginata

Inherited hair-shaft abnormality, associated with Netherton's syndrome and increased hair fragility, that is caused by invagination of the distal hair shaft into the proximal hair shaft and is characterized by sparse hair on the scalp

Differential Diagnosis

- Ectodermal dysplasia
- Monilethrix

- Trichorrhexis nodosa
- Trichoschisis

Evaluation

- Hair-shaft examination (highest yield from eyebrows)

Further reading:
- Sun JD, Linden KG (2006) Netherton syndrome: a case report and review of the literature. Int J Dermatol 45(6):693–697

Trichorrhexis Nodosa

Inherited or acquired disorder of hair fragility that is associated with a variety of metabolic and physical causes and is characterized by nodes along the hair shaft that represent portions that are frayed and prone to breakage

Subtypes/Variants

- Acquired distal
- Acquired localized
- Acquired proximal
- Congenital

Differential Diagnosis

- Anagen effluvium
- Hair casts
- Hypothyroidism
- Monilethrix
- Pediculosis
- Piedra
- Trichorrhexis invaginata

- Trichoschisis
- Trichotillomania

Associations

- Arginosuccinic aciduria
- Bazex–Dupre–Christol syndrome
- Chemical/physical hair treatments
- Citrullinemia
- Hypothyroidism
- Intractable infant diarrhea
- Menkes kinky-hair syndrome
- Netherton syndrome
- Neurodermatitis
- Trichoptilosis
- Trichothiodystrophy

Further reading:
- Burkhart CG, Burkhart CN (2007) Trichorrhexis nodosa revisited. Skinmed 6(2):57–58

Trichostasis Spinulosa

Follicular disorder caused by retention of telogen hairs within the follicle that is characterized by hyperkeratotic and hyperpigmented papules on the face (asymptomatic) or the trunk and extremities (pruritic)

Differential Diagnosis

- Comedonal acne
- Eruptive vellus hair cysts
- Favre–Racouchot disease
- Keratosis pilaris
- Keratotic spicules of myeloma
- Lichen spinulosus

- Nevus comedonicus
- Pili bifurcati
- Pili multigemini
- Pseudofolliculitis barbae
- Trichofolliculomas

Further reading:

- Strobos MA, Jonkman MF (2002) Trichostasis spinulosa: itchy follicular papules in young adults. Int J Dermatol 41(10):643–646

Trichothiodystrophy

Hereditary (AR) sulfur deficiency of the hair that is associated with several syndromes and is characterized by a tiger-tail appearance under polarized microscopy, brittle hair, pili torti, trichoschisis, and trichorrhexis nodosa

Differential Diagnosis

- Bloom syndrome
- Cockayne syndrome
- Kindler syndrome
- Menkes kinky-hair syndrome
- Netherton syndrome
- Nonbullous congenital ichthyosiform erythroderma
- Progeria
- Rothmund–Thomson syndrome
- Sjögren–Larsson syndrome
- Werner syndrome
- Xeroderma pigmentosum

Associations

- BIDS syndrome
- Cockayne syndrome

- Collodion membrane
- IBIDS syndrome (Tay syndrome)
- Marinesco–Sjögren syndrome
- PIBIDS syndrome
- Xeroderma pigmentosum

Further reading:
- Itin PH, Sarasin A, Pittelkow MR (2001) Trichothiodystrophy: update on the sulfur-deficient brittle hair syndromes. J Am Acad Dermatol 44(6):891–920

Trichotillomania

Neurotic disorder that affects people of all ages, is caused by compulsive plucking of hair shafts from the follicle, and is characterized by a patch of nonscarring alopecia in a geometric, often triangular pattern, that has growing hairs of variable length within the patch

Differential Diagnosis

- Alopecia areata
- Alopecia mucinosa
- Androgenetic alopecia
- Child abuse
- Lupus erythematosus
- Monilethrix
- Pili torti
- Pressure alopecia
- Syphilis
- Temporal triangular alopecia
- Tinea capitis
- Traction alopecia
- Traumatic alopecia

Diagnostic Criteria (DSM IV)

- Increasing sense of tension immediately before pulling out the hair or when attempting to resist the behavior
- Pleasure, gratification, or relief when pulling out the hair
- Recurrent pulling out of one's hair resulting in noticeable hair loss
- Disturbance is not better accounted for by another mental disorder and is not due to a general medical condition (e.g., a dermatological condition)
- Disturbance provokes clinically marked distress and/or impairment in occupational, social, or other areas of functioning

Treatment Options

- Psychotherapy
- SSRIs

Further reading:
- Hautmann G, Hercogova J, Lotti T (2002) Trichotillomania. J Am Acad Dermatol 46(6):807–821

Trigeminal Trophic Syndrome

Rare cause of ulceration that is associated with trigeminal nerve injury or pathology and that is characterized by a persistent, unilateral, painless ulcer near the nasal ala with associated numbness, paresthesias, and a history of picking or scratching the affected area

Differential Diagnosis

- Basal cell carcinoma
- Cocaine abuse
- Deep fungal infection
- Factitial ulcer
- Herpes simplex virus infection
- Infection

- Leishmaniasis
- Leprosy
- Malignancy
- Temporal arteritis
- Squamous cell carcinoma
- Syphilis
- Tuberculosis
- Wegener's granulomatosis
- Zoster

Associations

- Trigeminal nerve surgery
- Tumors of the trigeminal nerve
- Viral infection of the trigeminal nerve
- Zoster

Treatment Options

- Occlusive dressing
- Gabapentin
- Amitriptyline
- Carbamazepine
- Transcutaneous electric nerve stimulation

Further reading:
- Setyadi HG, Cohen PR, Schulze KE et al (2007) Trigeminal trophic syndrome. South Med J 100(1):43–48

Tropical (Phagedenic) Ulcer

Nonspecific term for any polymicrobial (including fusobacterium) infectious ulcer that affects malnourished children and adults in tropical areas and is characterized by a solitary, often trauma-related ulcer on the extremities

Differential Diagnosis

- Atypical mycobacterium
- Bacterial pyoderma
- Buruli ulcer
- Chromomycosis
- Cutaneous diphtheria
- Ecthyma
- Gummatous syphilis
- Leishmaniasis
- Pyoderma gangrenosum
- Squamous cell carcinoma
- Spider bite
- Venous stasis ulcer
- Yaws

Further reading:
- Robinson DC, Adriaans B, Hay RJ et al (1988) The clinical and epidemiologic features of tropical ulcer (tropical phagedenic ulcer). Int J Dermatol (1):49–53

Trypanosomiasis, African (African Sleeping Sickness)

Disease caused by the protozoa, *Trypanosoma brucei* (var. *rhodesiense* in east Africa or var. *gambiense* in west Africa), that is transmitted by the tsetse fly, *Glossina morsitans*, and is characterized by intermittent fever, generalized lymphadenopathy (especially posterior cervical; called Winterbottom's sign), angioedema, somnolence, and coma, with the east African form having a more rapid deterioration and worse prognosis

Differential Diagnosis

- Borreliosis
- Brucellosis
- Cryptococcal meningitis
- HIV disease

- <u>Malaria</u>
- Neurosyphilis
- Tuberculosis
- Typhoid fever
- Visceral leishmaniasis

Evaluation

- Complete blood count with peripheral blood smear
- Cerebrospinal fluid examination
- CT/MRI scan of the brain
- Sedimentation rate

Further reading:
- Maudlin I (2006) African trypanosomiasis. Ann Trop Med Parasitol 100(8):679–701

Trypanosomiasis, American (Chagas Disease)

Disease caused by the protozoan organism, *Trypanosoma cruzi*, that is transmitted by several species of reduviid bug, especially *Triatoma infestans*, and is characterized by an erythematous edematous bite called a chagoma (or Romana's sign when around the eye), fever, a morbilliform skin eruption, and in chronic forms, cardiomegaly, megaesophagus, and megacolon

Differential Diagnosis

- Angioedema
- Atypical mycobacterial infection
- Cutaneous tuberculosis
- Deep fungal infection
- Leishmaniasis
- Paracoccidioidomycosis
- <u>Periorbital cellulitis</u>

Further reading:
- Teixeira AR, Nitz N, Guimaro MC et al (2006) Chagas disease. Postgrad Med J 82(974):788–798

Tuberculosis, Cutaneous

Refers to the variable cutaneous presentation of infection with *Mycobacterium tuberculosis* that can be primarily cutaneous or disseminated to the skin from an underlying focus of infection

Subtypes/Variants

- Lupus vulgaris
- Miliary tuberculosis
- Scrofuloderma (tuberculosis cutis colliquativa)
- Tuberculosis cutis orificialis
- Tuberculosis verrucosa cutis (prosector's wart, Wilkes disease)
- Tuberculous cellulitis
- Tuberculous chancre (primary inoculation tuberculosis)
- Tuberculous gumma

Differential Diagnosis

Lupus Vulgaris
- Blastomycosis
- Colloid milium
- Discoid lupus erythematosus
- Granulomatous rosacea
- Leishmaniasis, lupoid type
- Leprosy
- Lichen simplex chronicus
- Sarcoidosis
- Squamous cell carcinoma
- Tertiary syphilis
- Wegener's granulomatosis

Miliary

- <u>Cryptococcosis</u>
- <u>Histoplasmosis</u>
- Papulonecrotic tuberculid
- Pityriasis lichenoides et varioliformis acuta
- Rickettsialpox
- Varicella
- Viral exanthem

Scrofuloderma

- Acne conglobata
- Actinomycosis
- Bacterial lymphadenitis
- Coccidioidomycosis
- <u>Hidradenitis suppurativa</u>
- Lymphoma
- <u>Osteomyelitis</u>
- Paracoccidioidomycosis
- Sarcoidosis
- Sporotrichosis
- Syphilitic gumma

Tuberculous Chancre, Primary Inoculation Type

- Cat-scratch fever
- Deep fungal infection
- Leishmaniasis
- *Mycobacterium marinum* infection
- Nocardiosis
- Pyoderma gangrenosum
- <u>Pyogenic ulcer</u>
- <u>Sporotrichosis</u>
- Syphilis
- Tularemia
- Yaws

Tuberculosis Verrucosa Cutis

- Blastomycosis
- Chromoblastomycosis
- Halogenoderma
- Hypertrophic lichen planus
- Majocchi granuloma
- *Mycobacterium marinum* infection
- Orf/milker's nodule
- Tertiary syphilis
- Verrucous carcinoma
- Warts

Evaluation

- Bacterial, mycobacterial, and fungal culture of lesional tissue material and blood
- Chest radiograph
- PCR of affected tissue
- Tuberculin skin test

Further reading:
- Bravo FG, Gotuzzo E (2007) Cutaneous tuberculosis. Clin Dermatol 25(2):173–180

Tuberous Sclerosis (Bourneville–Pringle Syndrome)

Inherited or sporadic genodermatosis caused by mutation of the genes encoding tuberin (TSC1) or hamartin (TSC2) that is characterized by hypopigmented macules, periungual fibromas, facial angiofibromas, shagreen patch, gingival fibromas, seizures, and mental retardation, among many other features

Differential Diagnosis

- Epidermal nevus syndrome
- Hunter and Hurler syndromes
- Hypomelanosis of Ito
- Multiple endocrine neoplasia, type IIb
- Neurofibromatosis
- Nevus depigmentosus
- Phylloid hypomelanosis
- Proteus syndrome

Diagnostic Criteria (Two Major or One Major+Two Minor)

- Major features
  - Facial angiofibromas or forehead plaque
  - Nontraumatic ungual or periungual fibromas
  - Hypomelanotic macules (three or more)
  - Shagreen patch
  - Multiple retinal nodular hamartomas
  - Cortical tubers
  - Subependymal nodules
  - Subependymal giant cell astrocytoma
  - Cardiac rhabdomyoma, single or multiple
  - Lymphangioleiomyomatosis
  - Renal angiomyolipoma
- Minor features
  - Multiple, randomly distributed pits in dental enamel
  - Hamartomatous rectal polyps
  - Bone cysts
  - Cerebral white matter radial migration lines
  - Gingival fibromas
  - Nonrenal hamartoma

- Retinal achromic patch
- Confetti skin lesions
- Multiple renal cysts

Evaluation

- CT/MRI scan of chest, brain
- Echocardiography
- Electrocardiography
- Electroencephalogram
- Genetic testing
- Neurodevelopmental testing
- Ophthalmologic exam
- Renal ultrasound

Further reading:

- Roach ES, Gomez MR, Northrup H (1998) Tuberous sclerosis complex consensus conference: revised clinical diagnostic criteria. J Child Neurol 13(12):624–628
- Schwartz RA, Fernandez G, Kotulska K et al (2007) Tuberous sclerosis complex: advances in diagnosis, genetics, and management. J Am Acad Dermatol 57(2):189–202

Tufted Angioma (Angioblastoma of Nakagawa)

Uncommon vascular tumor that can be complicated by Kasabach–Merritt syndrome, develops in the first decade of life, and is characterized by a red or purple vascular plaque most commonly located on the trunk

Differential Diagnosis

- Dabska tumor
- Hemangiopericytoma
- Infantile hemangioma
- Kaposi's sarcoma
- Kaposiform hemangioendothelioma

- Melanoma
- Venous malformation

Evaluation

- Complete blood count

Further reading:
- Kamath GH, Bhat RM, Kumar S (2005) Tufted angioma. Int J Dermatol 44(12):1045–1047

Tularemia

Blood-borne bacterial infection with *Francisella tularensis* that is acquired by contact with infected animals or via the bite of an infected tick, such as *Dermacentor andersoni* or *Amblyomma americanum*, and is characterized by fever and several different clinical presentations, the most common of which is the ulceroglandular form, in which there is a fever, an ulcerated cutaneous nodule, sporotrichoid lesions along the lymphatic drainage, and regional lymphadenopathy

Subtypes/Variants

- Glandular
- Oculoglandular
- Oropharyngeal
- Pneumonic
- Typhoidal
- Ulceroglandular

Differential Diagnosis

- Anthrax
- Atypical mycobacterial infection
- Blastomycosis

- Brucellosis
- <u>Cat-scratch disease</u>
- Coccidioidomycosis
- Diphtheria
- Ecthyma
- Endocarditis
- Foreign body granuloma
- Furuncle
- Glanders
- Leishmaniasis
- Lymphogranuloma venereum
- Majocchi's granuloma
- Malaria
- Melioidosis
- Mononucleosis
- <u>Nocardiosis</u>
- Orf/milker's nodule
- Paronychia
- *Pasteurella multocida* infection
- Plague
- Rat-bite fever
- Rocky Mountain spotted fever
- <u>Sporotrichosis</u>
- Syphilis
- Tuberculosis
- Typhoid fever

Evaluation

- Chest radiography
- Complete blood count
- ELISA and Western blot for tularemia antibodies

Further reading:
- Tarnvik A, Chu MC (2007) New approaches to diagnosis and therapy of tularemia. Ann N Y Acad Sci 1105:378–404

Tumor of the Follicular Infundibulum

Benign neoplasm of follicular derivation that arises in older patients and is characterized by a solitary, variably scaly, hypopigmented to flesh-colored papule, nodule, or plaque on the face

Differential Diagnosis

- <u>Basal cell carcinoma</u>
- Desmoplastic trichoepithelioma
- Eccrine syringofibroadenoma
- Microcystic adnexal carcinoma
- <u>Seborrheic keratosis</u>
- Trichilemmoma
- Trichodiscoma

Further reading:

- Cheng AC, Chang YL, Wu YY et al (2004) Multiple tumors of the follicular infundibulum. Dermatol Surg 30(9):1246–1248

Tungiasis

Type of infestation of the foot that is caused by the female *Tunga penetrans* flea, which burrows through the epidermis into the dermis, and is characterized by a pruritic or painful white papule with a central black dot

Differential Diagnosis

- Callus or clavus
- Creeping eruption
- Dracunculiasis
- Foreign body granuloma
- Insect-bite reaction
- <u>Myiasis</u>

- Squamous cell carcinoma
- Tick bite
- <u>Verruca plantaris</u>
- Verruga peruana

Further reading:

- Hager J, Jacobs A, Orengo IF, Rosen T (2008) Tungiasis in the United States: a travel souvenir. Dermatol Online J 14(12):3

Typhus, Epidemic

Louse-borne rickettsial disease that is caused by *Rickettsia prowazekii*, transmitted by *Pediculus humanus* var. *corporis,* and characterized by fever, headache, myalgias, and a centrifugally spreading, macular and petechial eruption that spares the palms and soles but that can become gangrenous

Differential Diagnosis

- Anthrax
- Dengue fever
- Ehrlichiosis
- Infectious mononucleosis
- Kawasaki disease
- Leptospirosis
- Malaria
- Meningococcemia
- <u>Relapsing fever</u>
- Rubella
- Rubeola
- Toxic shock syndrome
- Tularemia
- Typhoid fever
- <u>Viral exanthem</u>

Evaluation

- PCR
- Indirect immunofluorescence
- Rickettsia ELISA and Western blot

Further reading:

- Elston DM (2005) Rickettsial skin disease: uncommon presentations. Clin Dermatol 23(6):541–544

Typhus, Endemic

Flea-borne rickettsial disease that is caused by *Rickettsia typhi* or *Rickettsia felis*; is transmitted by the rat flea, *Xenopsylla cheopis*, or the cat flea, *Ctenocephalides felis*; and is characterized by fever, headache, and a centrifugally spreading, macular and petechial eruption that spares the palms and soles

Differential Diagnosis

- Anthrax
- Dengue fever
- Ehrlichiosis
- Infectious mononucleosis
- Kawasaki disease
- Leptospirosis
- Malaria
- Meningococcemia
- Relapsing fever
- Rubella
- Rubeola
- Toxic shock syndrome
- Tularemia
- Typhoid fever
- Viral exanthem

Evaluation

- PCR
- Indirect immunofluorescence
- Rickettsia ELISA and Western blot

Further reading:
- Elston DM (2005) Rickettsial skin disease: uncommon presentations. Clin Dermatol 23(6):541–544

Typhus, Scrub (Tsutsugamushi Fever)

Mite-borne rickettsial disease that is caused by *Orientia tsutsugamushi*, transmitted by the chigger (larval stage of the mite *Leptotrombidium akamushi*), and characterized by a tache noir at the site of the bite, fever, regional lymphadenopathy, and a centrifugally spreading macular and erythematous skin eruption

Differential Diagnosis

- Anthrax
- Dengue fever
- Ehrlichiosis
- Infectious mononucleosis
- Kawasaki disease
- Leptospirosis
- Malaria
- Meningococcemia
- Relapsing fever
- Rubella
- Rubeola
- Toxic shock syndrome
- Tularemia
- Typhoid fever

- <u>Typhus</u>
- Viral exanthem

Evaluation

- PCR
- Indirect immunofluorescence
- Rickettsia ELISA and Western blot

Further reading:
- Rajagopal R, Khati C, Vasdev V, Trehan A (2003) Scrub typhus: a case report. Indian J Dermatol Venereol Leprol 69(6):413–415

Ulerythema Ophryogenes (Keratosis Pilaris Atrophicans Faciei, Taenzer Disease)

Uncommon, idiopathic disorder of follicular keratinization and subtype of keratosis pilaris atrophicans that is characterized by erythematous, keratotic papules on the cheeks and lateral eyebrows that evolve to atrophic scars

Differential Diagnosis

- <u>Acne vulgaris</u>
- Atopic dermatitis
- Folliculitis
- <u>Keratosis pilaris</u>
- Keratosis pilaris rubra
- Keratosis pilaris spinulosa decalvans
- Lupus erythematosus
- Madarosis
- Pityriasis rubra pilaris
- Rosacea
- Seborrheic dermatitis
- Trichodysplasia spinulosa

Associations

- Cornelia de Lange syndrome
- Noonan syndrome
- Rubinstein–Taybi syndrome

Further reading:
- Callaway SR, Lesher JL Jr (2004) Keratosis pilaris atrophicans: case series and review. Pediatr Dermatol 21(1):14–17

Uncombable Hair Syndrome (Pili Trianguli et Canaliculi)

Inherited or sporadic hair-shaft disorder that becomes apparent in childhood, is possibly caused by premature keratinization of the inner root sheath, and is characterized by unruly, uncombable blond, shiny hair, which is shown to have a cross-sectional triangular shape and longitudinal grooves on microscopic examination

Differential Diagnosis

- Loose anagen hair syndrome
- Marie Unna syndrome
- Menkes kinky-hair disease
- Monilethrix
- Pili Torti
- Plica polonica (neuropathica)
- Progeria
- Woolly hair nevus

Associations

- Digital abnormalities
- Ectodermal dysplasia
- Enamel dysplasia
- Juvenile cataracts

- Loose anagen hair
- Wilson's disease

Further reading:
- Jarell AD, Hall MA, Sperling LC (2007) Uncombable hair syndrome. Pediatr Dermatol 24(4):436–438

Unilateral Laterothoracic Exanthem

Childhood exanthem possibly viral in etiology that is characterized first by an erythematous lesion with a surrounding halo in the axillary region that later spreads locally and becomes erythematous, eczematous, and coalescent, only to spontaneously resolve with desquamation

Differential Diagnosis

- Atopic dermatitis
- Contact dermatitis
- Dermatophytosis
- Drug eruption
- Gianotti–Crosti syndrome
- Inverse pityriasis rosea
- Miliaria
- Molluscum dermatitis
- Scabies
- Scarlet fever
- Tinea corporis

Treatment Options

- Observation and reassurance
- Topical corticosteroids

Further reading:
- McCuaig CC, Russo P, Powell J et al (1996) Unilateral laterothoracic exanthem. A clinicopathologic study of forty-eight patients. J Am Acad Dermatol 34(6):979–984

Urticaria

Acute or chronic disorder affecting children and adults that is caused by mast cell degranulation which is triggered by a variety of immunologic, physical, or idiopathic mechanisms and that is characterized by erythematous, pruritic, flat papules or plaques of dermal edema (wheals) without any epidermal change and with variable distribution and severity

Subtypes

- Acute ordinary (classic)
- Adrenergic (Fig. 6.122)
- Aquagenic
- Cholinergic (Grant syndrome)
- Chronic idiopathic
- Cold
- Contact
- Delayed pressure
- Dermatographism

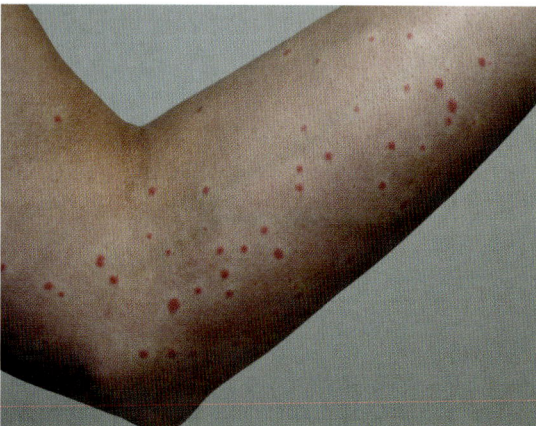

Fig. 6.122 Adrenergic urticaria

- Exercise induced
- Heat
- Solar

Differential Diagnosis

Classic

- Anhidrosis with pruritus
- Bullous pemphigoid
- Erythema marginatum
- Erythema multiforme
- Insect-bite reaction
- Mastocytosis
- Pruritic urticarial papules and plaques of pregnancy
- Rheumatoid neutrophilic dermatosis
- Serum-sickness-like reaction
- Still's disease
- Sweet's syndrome
- Urticarial vasculitis

Aquagenic

- Aquagenic pruritus
- Cholinergic urticaria (hot water)
- Cold urticaria (cold water)
- Dermatographism
- Heat urticaria

Cold

- Angioedema
- Aquagenic urticaria
- Cold panniculitis
- Cryoglobulinemia
- Perniosis

Persistent

- Urticarial bullous pemphigoid
- Urticarial erythema multiforme
- Urticarial vasculitis
- Urticarial dermatitis
- Urticaria pigmentosum

Associations

- Alcohol consumption
- Arthropod bites
- Autoimmune progesterone dermatitis
- Autoimmunity
- Candidiasis
- Chronic infection
- Cold
- Contact
- Dental infection
- Dermatographism
- Dermatophytosis
- Episodic angioedema with eosinophilia
- Exercise
- Foods
- Heat
- Hepatitis B vaccination
- Hypereosinophilic syndrome
- IPEX syndrome
- Medications
- Muckle–Wells syndrome
- Nicotine
- Parasitic infestation
- Pressure
- Upper respiratory infection
- Urinary tract infection

- Schnitzler syndrome
- Water

Cold

- Acute viral infection
- Atopy
- Cryoglobulins
- Familial cold autoinflammatory syndrome
- Monoclonal gammopathy
- HIV infection
- Syphilis

Foods

- Aspartame
- Caffeine
- Eggs
- Fish
- Fruits
- Ketchup
- Nuts
- Peanut oil
- Seafood
- Soybeans
- Spices
- Tea
- Tomatoes
- Vanilla
- Wheat

Associated Medications

- ACE inhibitors
- Aspirin
- Beta-lactam antibiotics

- NSAIDs
- Opiates
- Polymyxin B
- Radiocontrast media
- Tubocurarine

Evaluation

- Not recommended for duration <6 weeks
- See "Urticaria, Chronic Idiopathic"

Treatment Options

- <u>Antihistamines</u>
- Leukotriene inhibitors
- Systemic corticosteroids
- Doxepin

Further reading:
- Peroni A, Colato C, Schena D, Girolomoni G (2010) Urticarial lesions: if not urticaria, what else? The differential diagnosis of urticaria: part I. Cutaneous diseases. J Am Acad Dermatol 62(4):541–555; quiz 555–556

Urticaria, Chronic Idiopathic

Idiopathic, possibly immune-mediated type of urticaria with a variety of associated causes that is characterized by at least 6 weeks of recurrent, pruritic erythematous wheals on the trunk and extremities

Differential Diagnosis

- Allergic contact dermatitis
- Arthropod-bite reactions
- Atopic dermatitis

- <u>Early bullous pemphigoid</u>
- Erythema multiforme
- Hypereosinophilic syndrome
- Mastocytosis
- Rheumatoid neutrophilic dermatosis
- Scabies
- Schnitzler syndrome
- Serum-sickness-like reaction
- <u>Urticarial dermatitis</u>
- <u>Urticarial vasculitis</u>

Associations

- <u>Autoimmune thyroid disease</u>
- Dental infections
- Gastrointestinal candidiasis
- *Helicobacter pylori* infection
- Intestinal parasite
- Muckle–Wells syndrome
- Pernicious anemia
- Rheumatoid arthritis
- Schnitzler syndrome
- Systemic lupus erythematosus
- Stress
- Type I diabetes mellitus
- Vitiligo

Evaluation

- Antinuclear antibodies
- Complement levels
- Complete blood count
- Cryoproteins
- Dental radiography

- Sedimentation rate
- Viral hepatitis panel
- Epstein–Barr virus serology
- Pregnancy test
- Sinus radiography
- Stool examination for ova, cysts, and parasites
- Streptococcal serology
- Syphilis serology
- Thyroid function tests
- Thyroid microsomal and peroxidase antibodies
- Urinalysis

Treatment Options

- Antihistamines
- Leukotriene inhibitors
- Systemic corticosteroids
- Doxepin
- Nifedipine
- Thyroid hormone
- Cyclosporine
- Mycophenolate mofetil
- Intravenous immunoglobulin
- Plasmapheresis

Further reading:
- Zuberbier T, Maurer M (2007) Urticaria: current opinions about etiology, diagnosis and therapy. Acta Derm Venereol 87(3):196–205

Urticaria, Contact

Type of urticaria induced by physical contact with a variety of substances that is caused by either a type I hypersensitivity reaction (immunologic) or direct mast cell degranulation (nonimmunologic) and is characterized by rapid-onset, erythematous, edematous, pruritic plaques, with or without eczematous changes on the hands or other exposed areas

Differential Diagnosis

- Achenbach syndrome
- Airborne contact dermatitis
- Anaphylaxis
- Angioedema
- Aquagenic urticaria
- Cold urticaria
- Contact dermatitis
- Hand eczema
- Palmar hidradenitis
- Perniosis
- Pressure urticaria
- Protein contact dermatitis

Associations

Nonimmunologic

- Benzoic acid
- Cinnamic aldehyde
- Cobalt chloride
- DMSO
- Formaldehyde
- Histamine
- Sorbic acid
- Stinging nettles
- Spurges
- Turpentine

Immunologic

- Ammonium persulfate
- Animal dander

- Bacitracin
- Eggs
- Flour
- Grains
- Grasses
- Latex
- Nuts
- Plants
- Potatoes
- Spices
- Vegetables (especially celery)

Treatment Options

- Avoidance of triggering substance
- Antihistamines

Further reading:
- Bourrain JL (2006) Occupational contact urticaria. Clin Rev Allergy Immunol 30(1):39–46

Urticaria, Solar

Uncommon immune-mediated type of urticaria that is induced by ultraviolet or visible light and is characterized by pruritic, erythematous wheals on the exposed areas, shortly after sun exposure, with relative sparing of the face and hands

Differential Diagnosis

- Acute cutaneous lupus erythematosus
- Cholinergic urticaria
- Erythropoietic protoporphyria
- Exercise-induced urticaria

- <u>Heat urticaria</u>
- Photocontact dermatitis
- Photosensitive drug reaction
- <u>Polymorphous light eruption</u>
- Porphyria cutanea tarda

Treatment Options

- Sunscreen
- Antihistamines
- Hydroxychloroquine
- Intravenous immunoglobulins

Further reading:
- Beattie PE, Dawe RS, Ibbotson SH et al (2003) Characteristics and prognosis of idiopathic solar urticaria: a cohort of 87 cases. Arch Dermatol 139(9):1149–1154

Urticarial Dermatitis

Refers to the clinical manifestation of the dermal hypersensitivity reaction that is characterized by localized or widespread, pruritic, erythematous plaques with a combination of urticarial and eczematous features and excoriated papules

Differential Diagnosis

- Autoimmune progesterone dermatitis
- <u>Bullous pemphigoid</u>
- <u>Contact dermatitis</u>
- Drug reaction
- Hypereosinophilic syndrome
- Nummular eczema
- Prurigo
- Scabies

- <u>Urticaria</u>
- Urticarial vasculitis

Treatment Options

- Topical corticosteroids
- <u>Systemic corticosteroids</u>
- Antihistamines
- <u>Dapsone</u>
- Narrowband UVB

Further reading:

- Kossard S, Hamann I, Wilkinson B (2006) Defining urticarial dermatitis: a subset of dermal hypersensitivity reaction pattern. Arch Dermatol 142(1):29–34

Urticarial Vasculitis

Presentation of cutaneous small vessel (leukocytoclastic) vasculitis that resembles urticaria, except that it is more painful than pruritic, individual lesions last longer than 24 h, and it resolves with postinflammatory hyperpigmentation and bruising (Fig. 6.123)

Differential Diagnosis

- Acute hemorrhagic edema of childhood
- Allergic contact dermatitis
- Erythema multiforme
- Lyme disease
- <u>Ordinary urticaria</u>
- Pigmented purpuric dermatosis
- Schnitzler syndrome
- Serum-sickness-like drug reaction
- <u>Systemic lupus erythematosus</u>

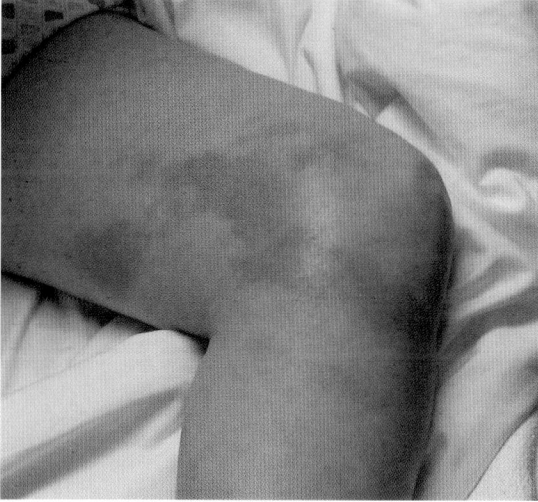

Fig. 6.123 Urticarial vasculitis (Courtesy of A. Record)

Associations

- Arthritis
- Chronic obstructive pulmonary disease
- Cocaine use
- EBV infection
- Fluoxetine
- HBV infection
- HCV infection
- Hypocomplementemia
- Idiopathic
- Inflammatory bowel disease
- Internal malignancy
- Interstitial lung disease
- Lyme disease
- Methotrexate (exacerbates)
- Mixed connective tissue disease
- Myeloma

- NSAIDs
- Pericarditis
- Polyarteritis nodosa
- Polycythemia vera
- Potassium iodide
- Pregnancy
- Schnitzler's syndrome
- Sjögren's syndrome
- Sun exposure
- Systemic lupus erythematosus
- Uveitis
- Viral infection
- Wegener's granulomatosis

Evaluation

- Anti-C1q antibodies
- Antinuclear antibodies (including SS-A and SS-B)
- Complement levels
- Direct immunofluorescence
- Renal function test
- Urinalysis
- Viral hepatitis panel

Treatment Options

- Antihistamines
- Dapsone
- Colchicine
- Hydroxychloroquine
- Azathioprine
- Mycophenolate
- Rituximab

Further reading:

- See Lee JS, Loh TH, Seow SC et al (2007) Prolonged urticaria with purpura: the spectrum of clinical and histopathologic features in a prospective series of 22 patients exhibiting the clinical features of urticarial vasculitis. J Am Acad Dermatol 56(6):994–100

Varicella (Chicken Pox)

Pruritic, childhood, centrifugally spreading exanthem that is caused by infection with the highly contagious varicella-zoster virus and is characterized by a widespread mucocutaneous eruption of lesions in various stages of evolution including erythematous macules, papules, vesicles, and crusts, some of which resemble a "dewdrop on a rose petal"

Differential Diagnosis

- Bullous pemphigoid
- Coxsackievirus infection
- Congenital syphilis
- Contact dermatitis
- Dermatitis herpetiformis
- Disseminated zoster
- Drug eruption
- Echovirus infection
- Erythema multiforme
- Herpes simplex virus infection
- Hydroa vacciniforme
- Insect bites
- Langerhans cell histiocytosis
- Monkeypox
- Papular urticaria
- Pityriasis lichenoides et varioliformis acuta
- Rickettsialpox
- Scabies

- Secondary syphilis
- Smallpox

Associations

- Lymphoma and leukemia (when hemorrhagic)
- Purpura fulminans
- Reye syndrome

Treatment Options

- <u>Observation and reassurance</u>
- Acyclovir

Further reading:
- McCrary ML, Severson J, Tyring SK (1999) Varicella zoster virus. J Am Acad Dermatol 41(1):1–14

Vasculitis, Cutaneous Small Vessel

Inflammation of the postcapillary venules of the skin with or without associated systemic vasculitis that is caused by depositing of immune complexes in the skin (predominantly in response to an acute infection or a medication), leading to inflammatory, palpable purpura typically located on dependent areas such as the legs or buttocks

Subtypes/Variants

- Bullous
- Erythema elevatum diutinum
- Erythema-multiforme-like lesions
- Livedo reticularis
- Necrotic/ulcerative lesions

- Palpable purpura
- Pustular
- Urticarial

Differential Diagnosis

- Amyloidosis
- Angiocentric T cell lymphoma
- Antiphospholipid antibody syndrome
- Arthropod bites
- Atrial myxoma
- Benign hypergammaglobulinemic purpura
- Buerger disease
- Cholesterol emboli
- Churg–Strauss syndrome
- Coagulopathy
- Cocaine-associated vasculopathy
- Disseminated candidiasis
- Drug eruption
- Eccrine syringosquamous metaplasia
- Erythema multiforme
- Gonococcemia
- Immune thrombocytopenic purpura
- Infective endocarditis
- Livedo reticularis
- Livedoid vasculopathy
- Meningococcemia
- Neutrophilic eccrine hidradenitis
- Perniosis
- Pigmented purpuric dermatosis
- Pityriasis lichenoides
- Polyarteritis nodosa
- Rocky Mountain spotted fever
- Scurvy

- Sneddon syndrome
- Sweet's syndrome
- Thrombotic thrombocytopenic purpura
- Urticaria
- Viral exanthem
- Wegener's granulomatosis

Associations

- Behçet's disease
- Chronic occult infections
- Cryoglobulinemia
- Cystic fibrosis
- Dermatomyositis
- Endocarditis
- Erythema elevatum diutinum
- Food and food additives
- Hairy-cell leukemia
- Hepatitis B and C
- Idiopathic
- Inflammatory bowel disease
- Internal malignancy
- Intestinal bypass
- Lymphomas
- Macroglobulinemia
- Medications
- Mycobacterial disease
- Myeloma
- Relapsing polychondritis
- Rheumatoid arthritis
- Sjögren's syndrome
- Systemic lupus erythematosus
- Streptococcal infection
- Systemic vasculitis syndromes

- <u>Upper respiratory infection</u>
- <u>Urinary tract infection</u>

Associated Medications

- Allopurinol
- Aspirin
- Barbiturates
- <u>Beta-lactam antibiotics</u>
- Cocaine
- Contrast dye
- Hydralazine (ANCA+)
- Minocycline (ANCA+)
- NSAIDs
- Phenothiazine
- Phenytoin
- Propylthiouracil (ANCA+)
- Quinidine
- Sulfonamides
- Thiazides

Evaluation

- Anticardiolipin antibodies
- Antineutrophilic cytoplasmic antibodies
- Antinuclear antibodies
- Blood cultures
- Chest radiograph
- Complement
- Complete blood count
- Creatine kinase and aldolase level
- Cryoglobulins
- Direct immunofluorescence

- Liver function test
- Lupus anticoagulant
- Nerve conduction studies
- Renal function test
- Sedimentation rate
- Serum protein electrophoresis
- Urinalysis
- Viral hepatitis panel

Treatment Options

- <u>Treat underlying cause</u>
- <u>Systemic corticosteroids</u>
- <u>Dapsone</u>
- <u>Colchicine</u>
- Azathioprine
- Mycophenolate mofetil
- Methotrexate
- Cyclophosphamide
- Intravenous immunoglobulin
- Rituximab
- Pentoxifylline

Further reading:

- Carlson JA, Chen KR (2006) Cutaneous vasculitis update: small vessel neutrophilic vasculitis syndromes. Am J Dermatopathol 28(6):486–506

Venous Lake

Venous ectasia associated with chronic sun exposure that affects older males and is characterized by a blue, compressible papule on the head and neck, especially the ear and lip

Differential Diagnosis

- Angiokeratoma
- Basal cell carcinoma
- Blue nevus
- Hemangioma
- Hidrocystoma
- Melanoma
- Mucocele
- Mucosal melanosis
- Traumatic tattoo

Further reading:

- Requena L, Sangueza OP (1997) Cutaneous vascular anomalies. Part I. Hamartomas, malformations, and dilation of preexisting vessels. J Am Acad Dermatol 37(4):523–549

Venous Malformation

Anatomic malformation that presents at birth or early childhood, arises through a variety of genetic mechanisms, can be solitary or multiple (in the setting of a variety of associated syndromes), and is characterized by a blue, compressible, occasionally painful (especially upon waking due to stasis overnight) nodule or mass most commonly located on the head and neck (but that can occur anywhere)

Differential Diagnosis

- Deep infantile hemangioma
- Extensive mongolian spots
- Glomuvenous malformation
- Kaposiform hemangioendothelioma
- Lymphangioma
- Nevus flammeus

- Nevus of Ota and Ito
- Spindle cell hemangioendothelioma
- Tufted angioma

Associations

- Bannayan–Riley–Ruvulcaba syndrome
- Blue rubber bleb nevus syndrome (Bean syndrome)
- Bockenheimer syndrome
- Cerebral cavernomas
- Familial cutaneous and mucosal venous malformation
- Gorham's syndrome
- Glomangiomas and familial glomangiomatosis
- Maffucci syndrome

Further reading:

- Garzon MC, Huang JT, Enjolras O et al (2007) Vascular malformations: part I. J Am Acad Dermatol 56(3):353–370

Verrucous Carcinoma

Low-grade type of squamous cell carcinoma that is associated with HPV types VI and XI and is characterized by an exophytic, markedly hyperkeratotic, verrucous nodule in the oral cavity (oral florid papillomatosis), on the hand or foot (epithelioma cuniculatum (Fig. 6.124)), the anogenital area (giant condyloma of Buschke–Lowenstein), or anywhere else (papillomatosis cutis carcinoides of Gottron)

Differential Diagnosis

- Actinomycosis
- Blastomycosis
- Eccrine porocarcinoma

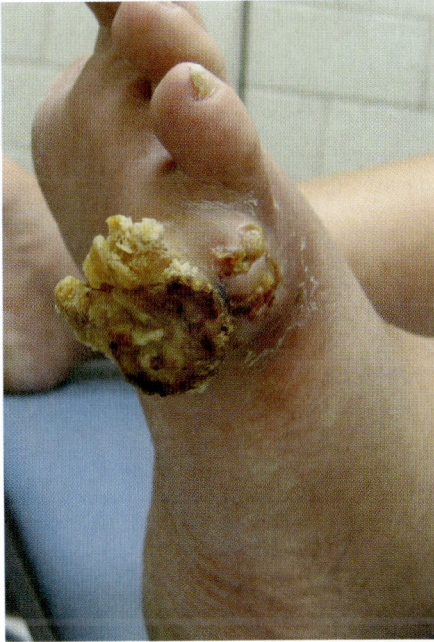

Fig. 6.124 Epithelioma cuniculatum

- Elephantiasis verrucosa
- Granular cell tumor
- Keratoacanthoma
- Leishmaniasis
- Leprosy
- Mycetoma
- <u>Squamous cell carcinoma</u>
- <u>Wart</u>
- Warty tuberculosis

Further reading:

- Lozzi GP, Peris K (2007) Carcinoma cuniculatum. Can Med Assoc J 177(3):249–251

Vibrio Vulnificus Infection

Blood-borne infection with the aquatic bacteria, *Vibrio vulnificus*, that results from consumption of contaminated raw shellfish or infection of a wound with contaminated water and is characterized by large hemorrhage, bullous lesions on the trunk and extremities, sepsis, and a high mortality

Differential Diagnosis

- *Aeromonas* infection
- Clostridial myonecrosis
- Necrotizing fasciitis
- Pseudomonal bacteremia
- Purpura fulminans

Associations

- Cirrhosis
- Diabetes
- Gastric surgery
- Glucocorticoid use
- Hemochromatosis

Further reading:
- Ralph A, Currie BJ (2007) *Vibrio vulnificus* and *V. parahaemolyticus* necrotizing fasciitis in fishermen visiting an estuarine tropical northern Australian location. J Infect 54(3):e111–e114

Vitiligo

Immune-mediated pigmentary disorder of uncertain cause that is characterized by depigmented macules and patches anywhere on the body, especially on the face (especially periorificially), hands, or genitalia, or in a generalized distribution

Subtypes/Variants

- Acrofacial
- Blue
- Focal
- Generalized (vulgaris)
- Inflammatory
- Lip tip
- Mixed
- Mucosal
- Ponctue
- Quadrichrome
- Trichrome (Fig. 6.125)
- Unilateral (segmental)
- Universal

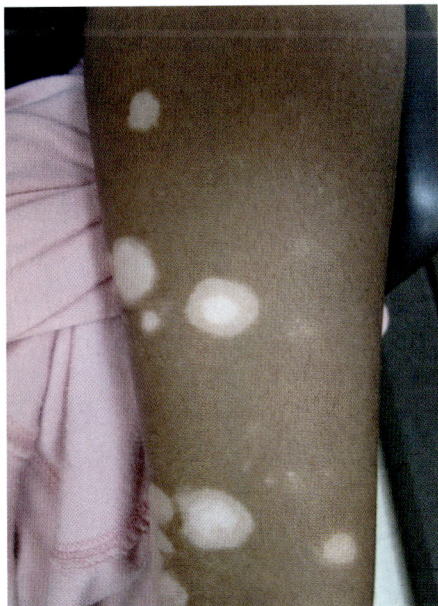

Fig. 6.125 Trichrome vitiligo

Differential Diagnosis

- Annular lichenoid dermatitis of youth
- <u>Chemical leukoderma</u>
- Discoid lupus erythematosus
- Halo nevus
- <u>Hypopigmented mycosis fungoides</u>
- Idiopathic guttate hypomelanosis
- Leprosy
- <u>Lichen sclerosus</u>
- Nevus anemicus
- Nevus depigmentosus
- Nevoid hypomelanosis
- Onchocerciasis
- Photodistributed vitiligo-like drug reaction in HIV patients
- Piebaldism
- Pinta
- <u>Postinflammatory depigmentation</u>
- Postinflammatory hypopigmentation
- Sarcoidosis
- Scleroderma-related leukoderma
- Tinea versicolor
- Topical steroid leukoderma
- Tuberous sclerosis
- Vogt–Koyanagi–Harada syndrome

Associations

- <u>Addison's disease</u>
- <u>Alopecia areata</u>
- Atrophic gastritis
- Candidiasis
- Chronic actinic dermatitis
- Dermatitis herpetiformis

- Diabetes mellitus
- Down syndrome
- <u>Halo nevus</u>
- Idiopathic T cell lymphopenia
- Interferon alpha
- Melanoma
- Pemphigus vulgaris
- <u>Pernicious anemia</u>
- Primary biliary cirrhosis
- Psoriasis
- Sarcoidosis
- Spondylarthritis
- <u>Thyroid disease</u>
- Twenty-nail dystrophy
- Uveitis

Evaluation

- Complete blood count
- Thyroid function test and antithyroid antibodies
- Fasting blood glucose

Treatment Options

- <u>Topical corticosteroids</u>
- <u>Tacrolimus ointment</u>
- <u>Narrowband UVB</u>
- Vitamin D analogues
- Excimer laser
- Skin grafts

Further reading:

- Sehgal VN, Srivastava G (2007) Vitiligo: compendium of clinico-epidemiological features. Indian J Dermatol Venereol Leprol 73(3):149–156

Vogt–Koyanagi–Harada Syndrome

Acquired, immune-mediated syndrome of unknown cause that affects young to middle-aged adults and is characterized by meningoencephalitis, followed by vitiligo, poliosis, uveitis, and hearing disturbance

Differential Diagnosis

- Alezzandrini syndrome
- Alopecia areata
- Piebaldism
- Vitiligo

Phases

- I: Prodromic or meningoencephalitic
- II: Uveitis
- III: Convalescent: poliosis and vitiligo
- IV: Recurrent uveitis

Diagnostic Criteria (Complete VKH: Criteria 1–5; Incomplete: 1–3+4 or 5; Probable: 1–3)

- 1. No history of penetrating ocular trauma or surgery preceding the initial onset of uveitis
- 2. No clinical or laboratory evidence suggestive of other ocular disease entities
- 3. Bilateral ocular involvement with evidence of a diffuse choroiditis, depending on the stage of the disease when the patient is examined
- 4. Meningismus, tinnitus, or cerebrospinal fluid pleocytosis
- 5. Alopecia, poliosis, or vitiligo

Associations

- Diabetes
- Hypothyroidism
- Interferon
- Melanoma
- Ulcerative colitis

Further reading:

- Read RW, Holland GN, Rao NA et al (2001) Revised diagnostic criteria for Vogt–Koyanagi–Harada disease: report of an international committee on nomenclature. Am J Ophthalmol 131:647–652

Vohwinkel Syndrome (Keratoderma Hereditaria Mutilans)

Inherited (AD) syndrome caused by mutation of the gene encoding either loricrin or connexin 26 that is characterized by diffuse palmoplantar keratoderma with the potential for pseudoainhum and starfish-shaped keratotic plaques on the dorsal hands and feet, elbows, and knees; ichthyosis (with loricrin mutation; Camisa's syndrome); and deafness (with connexin 26 mutation; classic Vohwinkel's syndrome)

Differential Diagnosis

- Congenital syphilis
- Hidrotic ectodermal dysplasia
- Leprosy
- Mal de Meleda
- Olmsted syndrome
- Palmoplantar keratoderma with deafness
- Progressive symmetric erythrokeratodermia
- Pseudoainhum
- Psoriasis
- Tertiary syphilis
- Yaws

Further reading:
- Ul Bari A (2006) Keratoderma hereditarium mutilans (Vohwinkel syndrome) in three siblings. Dermatol Online J 12(7):10

Waardenburg Syndrome

Inherited pigmentary disorder (AD) that is caused by failure of complete melanoblast migration as a result of several gene defects and is characterized by a white forelock; canities; dystopia canthorum (not type II); heterochromia iridis; spots of unpigmented skin on the face, trunk, and extremities; hearing loss (type II), limb defects (type III), and Hirschsprung's disease (type IV)

Differential Diagnosis

- Oculocutaneous albinism
- Hermansky–Pudlak syndrome
- Piebaldism
- Vitiligo
- Woolf syndrome
- Vogt–Koyanagi–Harada syndrome
- Ziprkowski–Margolis syndrome

Further reading:
- Karaman A, Aliagaoglu C (2006) Waardenburg syndrome type 1. Dermatol Online J 12(3):21

Warfarin Necrosis

Cutaneous necrosis that occurs within 5 days of initiating therapy with warfarin, is associated with underlying hypercoagulability that is exacerbated by warfarin-induced protein-C deficiency, and is characterized by purpuric, necrotic plaques in the areas of the body with abundant subcutaneous fat (Fig. 6.126)

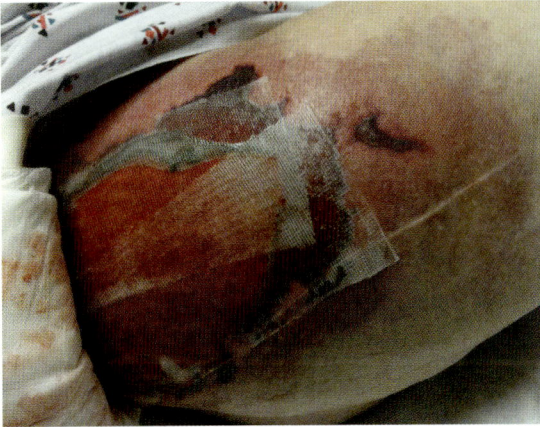

Fig. 6.126 Warfarin necrosis

Differential Diagnosis

- Anthrax
- Calciphylaxis
- Heparin necrosis
- Necrotizing fasciitis
- Pyoderma gangrenosum
- Spider-bite reaction
- Traumatic ulceration
- Vasculitis

Treatment Options

- Discontinuation of warfarin
- Vitamin K
- Heparin
- Activated protein C

Further reading:
- Jones A, Walling H (2007) Retiform purpura in plaques: a morphological approach to diagnosis. Clin Exp Dermatol 32(5):596–602

Wart (Verruca)

Benign growth that is caused by infection with various types of human papillomavirus and is characterized by a papule or nodule with a rough or verrucous surface

Subtypes/Variants

- Butcher's wart
- Common (verruca vulgaris)
- Cystic
- Filiform
- Flat (verruca plana)
- Focal epithelial hyperplasia
- Genital (condyloma acuminatum)
- Mosaic
- Myremecial
- Plantar (verruca plantaris)

Differential Diagnosis

Verruca Vulgaris
- Acne vulgaris
- Acquired digital fibrokeratoma
- Acrochordon
- Acrokeratosis verruciformis
- Actinic keratosis
- Amelanotic melanoma
- Angiokeratoma
- Arsenical keratosis
- Bowen's disease
- Callus/clavus
- Condyloma lata
- Cowden's disease keratoses
- Digital mucous cyst

- Eccrine syringofibroadenoma
- Keratoacanthoma
- Knuckle pads
- Lichen nitidus
- Lichen planus
- <u>Molluscum contagiosum</u>
- Mucinous syringometaplasia
- Periungual fibroma
- Poroma
- Prurigo nodularis
- Psoriasis
- <u>Seborrheic keratosis</u>
- Squamous cell carcinoma
- Syringocystadenoma papilliferum
- Trichilemmoma
- Tuberculosis verrucosa cutis
- Warty dyskeratoma

Plantar

- <u>Corn</u>
- Epidermal cyst
- Focal plantar keratoderma
- Melanoma
- Pitted keratolysis
- Poroma
- Punctate porokeratosis
- Syphilitic clavus
- Tungiasis
- <u>Verrucous carcinoma</u>

Associations

- Epidermodysplasia verruciformis
- Hyperimmunoglobulin M syndrome
- WHIM syndrome

Treatment Options

- <u>Cryotherapy</u>
- Salicylic acid
- Podophyllin
- Cantharidin
- Intralesional candida antigen
- <u>Electrodessication and curettage</u>
- 5FU cream
- Dibutyl squaric acid ester
- Oral zinc supplements
- Oral cimetidine
- Acitretin
- Duct tape
- Imiquimod
- Pulsed dye laser
- CO_2 laser
- Intralesional bleomycin

Further reading:

- Dalmau J, Abellaneda C, Puig S, Zaballos P, Malvehy J (2006) Acral melanoma simulating warts: dermoscopic clues to prevent missing a melanoma. Dermatol Surg 32(8):1072–1078

Warty Dyskeratoma

Benign epidermal neoplasm characterized by a hyperkeratotic papule with a central pore that is most commonly located on the face, or less commonly, on the oral mucosa or genital areas

Differential Diagnosis

- Acantholytic acanthoma
- Acantholytic actinic keratosis

- Acantholytic squamous cell carcinoma
- Basal cell carcinoma
- Darier's disease
- Epidermal nevus
- Familial dyskeratotic comedones
- Focal acantholytic dyskeratosis
- Grover's disease
- Hailey–Hailey disease
- Hypertrophic actinic keratosis
- Keratoacanthoma
- Pilar sheath acanthoma
- Seborrheic keratosis
- Solitary acantholytic keratosis
- Syringocystadenoma papilliferum
- Verruca

Further reading:

- Kaddu S, Dong H, Mayer G et al (2002) Warty dyskeratoma–"follicular dyskeratoma": analysis of clinicopathologic features of a distinctive follicular adnexal neoplasm. J Am Acad Dermatol 47(3):423–428

Weathering Nodule of the Ear

Small fibrous papule that arises on the ear of patients with a history of chronic sun exposure and is characterized by a white- or flesh-colored papule or multiple papules along the helical rim

Differential Diagnosis

- Amyloid
- Calcinosis cutis
- Chondrodermatitis nodularis helicis
- Colloid milium
- Elastotic nodule of the ear

- Gouty tophi
- Granuloma annulare
- Milia
- Rheumatoid nodules

Further reading:
- Kennedy C (2005) Weathering nodules are not the same as elastotic nodules. J Am Acad Dermatol 52:925–926

Wegener's Granulomatosis

Type of systemic necrotizing vasculitis that is associated with antineutrophil cytoplasmic antibodies (c-ANCA) and is characterized by granulomatous inflammation of the nasal passages (leading to chronic nasal discharge and sinusitis), lungs, and skin (ulcers, inflammatory purpura, and subcutaneous nodules)

Differential Diagnosis

- <u>Churg–Strauss syndrome</u>
- Cryoglobulinemia
- Henoch–Schonlein purpura
- Leishmaniasis
- Lymphomatoid granulomatosis
- Microscopic polyangiitis
- Natural killer cell lymphoma
- <u>Polyarteritis nodosa</u>
- Pyoderma gangrenosum
- Rhinoscleroma
- Sarcoidosis (lupus pernio)
- Sweet's syndrome
- Syphilis
- Temporal arteritis
- Yaws

Diagnostic Criteria (ACR; 2/4)

- Nasal or oral inflammation
- Chest X-ray showing nodules, infiltrates (fixed), or cavities
- Microscopic hematuria or red cell casts in urine
- Granulomatous inflammation on biopsy (within vessel wall or perivascular)

Evaluation

- Antineutrophilic cytoplasmic antibodies
- Chest radiograph
- Complement levels
- Complete blood count
- Renal function test
- Sedimentation rate
- Sinus radiograph or CT scan
- Urinalysis

Further reading:
- Fiorentino DF (2003) Cutaneous vasculitis. J Am Acad Dermatol 48(3):311–340

Werner Syndrome (Adult Progeria)

Inherited premature aging syndrome (AR) that is caused by a mutation of the RECQ2 DNA helicase repair gene and is characterized by onset in the second decade of poikilodermatous skin changes, leg ulcers, sclerodermatous face and hands, diabetes, tendency toward the development of various malignancies, including sarcomas, and death in middle age due to atherosclerosis or malignancy

Differential Diagnosis

- Acrogeria
- Diabetic cheiroarthropathy with stiff skin

- Hutchinson–Gilford progeria syndrome
- Rothmund–Thomson syndrome
- Scleroderma
- Systemic sclerosis

Diagnostic Criteria

Cardinal signs and symptoms (onset over 10 years old):
- Cataracts (bilateral)
- Characteristic dermatological pathology (tight skin, atrophic skin, pigmentary alterations, ulceration, hyperkeratosis, and regional subcutaneous atrophy) and characteristic facies ("bird" facies)
- Short stature
- Parental consanguinity (third cousin or greater) or affected sibling
- Premature graying and/or thinning of scalp hair

Further signs and symptoms:
- Diabetes mellitus
- Hypogonadism (secondary sexual underdevelopment, diminished fertility, testicular, or ovarian atrophy)
- Osteoporosis
- Osteosclerosis of distal phalanges of fingers and/or toes (X-ray diagnosis)
- Soft tissue calcification
- Evidence of premature atherosclerosis (e.g., history of myocardial infarction)
- Mesenchymal neoplasms, rare neoplasms, or multiple neoplasms
- Voice changes (high pitched, squeaky, or hoarse voice)
- Flat feet

Definite: All cardinal+two others
Probable: First three cardinal+two others
Possible: Either cataracts or dermatological alterations and any four others
Exclusion: Onset of signs and symptoms before adolescence (except stature)

Associations

- Cataracts
- Diabetes mellitus
- Internal malignancy
- Leg ulcers
- Osteoporosis

Further reading:

- Mohaghegh P, Hickson ID (2001) DNA helicase deficiencies associated with cancer predisposition and premature ageing disorders. Hum Molec Genet 10:741–746
- Oshima J, Martin G, and Hisama, F. Werner Syndrome. GeneReviews. Seattle (WA): University of Washington, Seattle; 1993–2002 Dec 02

White Sponge Nevus (of Cannon)

Autosomal-dominant familial disorder with onset early in life that is caused by a defect in the genes encoding keratin 4 or 13 and is characterized by a benign, white, keratotic, and thickened plaque on the buccal mucosa, often bilateral, with or without involvement of the surrounding areas of the oral cavity

Differential Diagnosis

- Cheek-bite keratosis
- Dyskeratosis congenita
- Hereditary benign intraepithelial dyskeratosis
- Leukoplakia
- Oral acanthosis nigricans
- Oral florid papillomatosis
- Pachyonychia congenita
- Smokeless-tobacco keratosis

Further reading:
- Martelli H Jr, Pereira S, Rocha T et al (2007) White sponge nevus: report of a three-generation family. Oral Surg Oral Med Oral Pathol Oral Radiol Endod 103(1):43–47

Wiskott–Aldrich Syndrome

X-linked recessive disorder that is caused by a defect in the WASP transcription factor which is important in lymphocyte and platelet function and is characterized by thrombocytopenic purpura and other bleeding problems, recurrent infections, eczema, and impaired cellular and humoral immunity

Differential Diagnosis

- Agammaglobulinemias
- Ataxia–telangiectasis
- Atopic dermatitis
- Chédiak–Higashi syndrome
- Chronic granulomatous disease
- DiGeorge syndrome
- Graft-vs-host disease
- Hermansky–Pudlak syndrome
- Hyper-IgE syndrome
- Langerhans cell histiocytosis
- Omenn syndrome
- Severe combined immunodeficiency
- Seborrheic dermatitis

Further reading:
- Notarangelo LD, Mori L (2005) Wiskott–Aldrich syndrome: another piece in the puzzle. Clin Exp Immunol 139(2):173–175

Woolly Hair Nevus

Sporadic congenital disorder of hair that is characterized by one or more discrete patches of curly, unruly hair that is different in color and consistency from surrounding normal hair

Differential Diagnosis

- Acquired progressive kinking of the hair
- <u>Carvajal syndrome woolly hair</u>
- Menkes kinky-hair syndrome
- <u>Naxos syndrome woolly hair</u>
- Plica polonica (neuropathica)
- Uncombable hair syndrome

Associations

- Epidermal nevi
- Incontinentia pigmenti
- Infantile diarrhea syndromes
- Precocious puberty

Further reading:

- Kumaran S, Dogra S, Handa S, Kanwar AJ (2004) Woolly-hair nevus. Pediatr Dermatol 21(5):609–610

Xanthoma

Dermatologic manifestation of hyperlipidemia that represents a focal, benign collection of lipid-laden histiocytes and is characterized by papular, nodular, or plaque-type lesions with variable size, morphologic features, and associated lipid abnormality

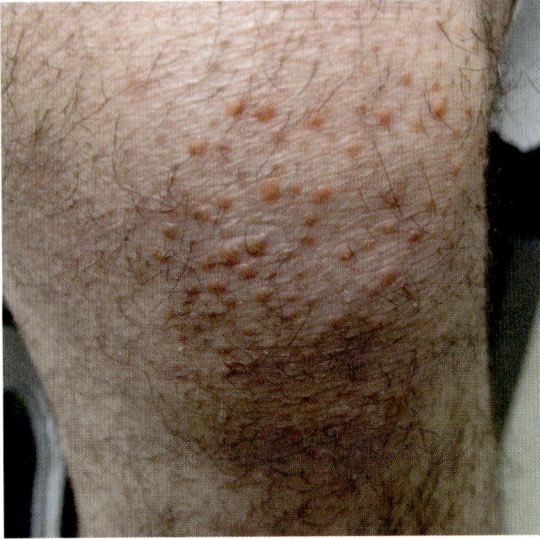

Fig. 6.127 Eruptive xanthomas

Subtypes

- Eruptive (Fig. 6.127)
- Intertriginous
- Papular
- Plane
- Tendinous
- Tuberous
- Verruciform
- Xanthelasma
- Xanthoma striatum palmare

Differential Diagnosis

Eruptive

- Cutaneous Rosai–Dorfman disease
- Erythema elevatum diutinum
- Eruptive histiocytomas

- Folliculitis
- Generalized eruptive histiocytoma
- <u>Granuloma annulare</u>
- Juvenile xanthogranuloma
- Molluscum contagiosum
- Multicentric reticulohistiocytosis
- <u>Papular sarcoidosis</u>
- Papular xanthoma
- Xanthoma disseminatum

Plane

- <u>Carotenoderma</u>
- Erythrasma
- Fox–Fordyce disease
- Lichenification
- Pseudoxanthoma elasticum
- Xanthelasma mastocytosis

Tendinous

- Erythema elevatum diutinum
- Ganglion cyst
- Giant cell tumor of the tendon sheath
- <u>Gouty tophi</u>
- Juvenile xanthogranuloma
- Lipoma
- <u>Rheumatoid nodule</u>
- Subcutaneous sarcoidosis

Tuberous

- <u>Erythema elevatum diutinum</u>
- Granuloma annulare
- <u>Gouty tophi</u>
- Histioid leprosy
- Juvenile xanthogranuloma

- Lymphoma
- Mastocytosis
- Neurofibromas
- <u>Rheumatoid nodule</u>
- Sarcoidosis

Verruciform

- Condyloma acuminatum
- Eccrine syringofibroadenoma
- Epidermal nevus
- Granular cell tumor
- Inflammatory linear verrucous epidermal nevus
- <u>Leukoplakia</u>
- Seborrheic keratosis
- Squamous cell carcinoma
- Verrucous carcinoma
- <u>Viral wart</u>
- Warty dyskeratoma

Xanthelasma

- Amyloidosis
- Lipoid proteinosis
- Milia
- <u>Necrobiotic xanthogranuloma</u>
- Nodular elastoidosis
- Sarcoidosis
- Sebaceous hyperplasia
- Syringoma
- Xanthoma disseminatum

Associations

Eruptive

- Alcohol abuse
- Diabetes mellitus

- Estrogen replacement
- High caloric intake
- <u>Hypothyroidism</u>
- <u>Obesity</u>
- Retinoid therapy
- <u>Type I hyperlipidemia (elevated chylomicrons)</u>
- Type IV hyperlipidemia (elevated VLDL)
- Type V hyperlipidemia (elevated chylomicrons and VLDLs)

Plane

- <u>Dysbetalipoproteinemia (palmar crease type)</u>
- Homozygous familial hypercholesterolemia (intertriginous type)
- Monoclonal gammopathy

Tendinous

- Cerebrotendinous xanthomatosis
- Dysbetalipoproteinemia
- <u>Familial hypercholesterolemia</u>
- Hepatic cholestasis
- Sitosterolemia

Tuberous

- Dysbetalipoproteinemia
- <u>Familial hypercholesterolemia</u>

Verruciform

- Bite keratosis
- Discoid lupus erythematosus
- Epidermolysis bullosa acquisita
- Graft-vs-host disease
- Lichen planus
- Pemphigus vulgaris

Evaluation

- Lipid panel
- Serum/urinary protein electrophoresis

Further reading:
- Sopena J, Gamo R, Iglesias L, Rodriguez-Peralto JL (2004) Disseminated verruciform xanthoma. Br J Dermatol 151(3):717–719

Xanthoma Disseminatum (Montgomery Syndrome)

Rare type of histiocytosis (non-Langerhans cell type) that arises primarily in adulthood and is characterized by diabetes insipidus and hundreds of yellow to brown keloid-like papules and nodules predominantly on the face and intertriginous areas, as well as in the oral cavity, airway, and bones

Differential Diagnosis

- Amyloidosis
- Eruptive xanthoma
- Generalized eruptive histiocytoma
- Juvenile xanthogranuloma
- Keloids
- Langerhans cell histiocytosis
- Lipoid proteinosis
- Multicentric reticulohistiocytosis
- Necrobiotic xanthogranulomas
- Papular xanthoma
- Pseudoxanthoma elasticum
- Pseudoxanthomatous mastocytosis
- Sarcoidosis

Further reading:
- Buyukcavci M, Selimoglu A, Yildirim U et al (2005) Xanthoma disseminatum with hepatic involvement in a child. Pediatr Dermatol 22(6):550–553

Xeroderma Pigmentosum (Kaposi's Dermatosis)

Group of autosomal-recessive disorders that have faulty DNA repair of UV-radiation-induced DNA damage, have a variety of gene defects in components of the nucleotide excision repair pathway, and are characterized by photosensitivity, skin cancers early in life, premature aging of the skin, chronic conjunctivitis, lentigines, freckling, poikiloderma, xerosis, progressive neurologic deterioration (not all patients), and early death

Differential Diagnosis

- Ataxia–telangiectasia
- Basal cell nevus syndrome
- Bloom syndrome
- Cockayne syndrome
- Congenital erythropoietic porphyria
- Erythropoietic protoporphyria
- Hartnup syndrome
- Hydroa vacciniforme
- Kindler syndrome
- LEOPARD syndrome
- Lupus erythematosus
- Polymorphous light eruption
- Rothmund–Thomson syndrome
- Trichothiodystrophy

Associations

- Cockayne syndrome
- Trichothiodystrophy
- Neurologic dysfunction (De Sanctis–Cacchione syndrome)

Further reading:
- Lichon V, Khachemoune A (2007) Xeroderma pigmentosum: beyond skin cancer. J Drugs Dermatol 6(3):281–288

X-Linked Dominant Chondrodysplasia
Punctata (Conradi–Hunermann–Happle Syndrome)

X-linked dominant disorder that is lethal in males, is caused by a defect in the emopamil-binding protein gene, and is characterized by collodion baby presentation, ichthyosiform erythroderma along the lines of Blaschko that is eventually replaced by follicular atrophoderma, stippling of the epiphyses on radiography, cataracts, and nail dystrophy

Differential Diagnosis

- CHILD syndrome
- Collodion baby
- Congenital ichthyosiform erythroderma
- Epidermal nevi syndrome
- Ichthyosis linearis circumflexa
- Incontinentia pigmenti
- Neutral lipid storage disease
- Other forms of chondrodysplasia punctata
- Sjögren–Larsson syndrome

Further reading:
- Trachea D, Read CP, Hull D et al (2007) A severely affected female infant with X-linked dominant chondrodysplasia punctata: a case report and a brief review of the literature. Pediatr Dev Pathol 10(2):142–148

X-Linked Reticulate Pigmentary Disorder
(Partington's Syndrome, Familial Cutaneous Amyloidosis)

X-linked pigmentary disorder of unknown cause that is characterized by brown pigmentation either along Blaschko's lines (in carrier females) or in a generalized distribution (in affected males), with males suffering from failure to thrive, colitis, and pneumonia and surviving adults demonstrating amyloid deposits in the skin

Differential Diagnosis

- Dyskeratosis congenita
- Dermatopathia pigmentosa reticularis
- Dowling–Degos disease
- Confluent and reticulated papillomatosis
- Incontinentia pigmenti
- <u>Linear and whorled nevoid hypermelanosis</u>
- Naegali–Franceschetti–Jadassohn syndrome
- Primary cutaneous amyloidosis
- Reticulate acropigmentation of Kitamura
- Rothmund–Thomson syndrome
- Weary–Kindler syndrome

Further reading:

- Anderson RC, Zinn AR, Kim J et al (2005) X-linked reticulate pigmentary disorder with systemic manifestations: report of a third family and literature review. Pediatr Dermatol 22(2):122–126

Yaws (Pian, Frambesia)

Nonvenereal tropical infection caused by *Treponema pertenue* and characterized by a cutaneous ulcer (primary, mother yaw), verrucous, raspberry-like nodules and plaques (secondary, daughter yaws), painful palmoplantar hyperkeratosis (crab yaws), and gummatous lesions of the skin and bone (tertiary yaws, gangosa, goundoa), especially the nasopharynx and palate

Differential Diagnosis

- Calluses
- Condyloma
- Eczema
- Endemic syphilis

- Idiopathic keratoderma
- Insect-bite reactions
- Leishmaniasis
- Leprosy
- Nutritional deficiency
- Osteomyelitis
- Paracoccidioidomycosis
- Psoriasis
- Rhinoscleroma
- Sarcoidosis
- Scabies
- Sickle cell disease
- Tuberculosis
- Tungiasis
- Venereal syphilis
- Vitamin deficiencies
- Warts

Evaluation

- Serologic tests for syphilis

Further reading:
- Lupi O, Madkan V, Tyring SK (2006) Tropical dermatology: bacterial tropical diseases. J Am Acad Dermatol 54(4):559–578

Yellow-Nail Syndrome (Samman Syndrome)

Acquired disorder of the nails that is associated with lymphedema, arises in adulthood, and is characterized by yellow color change of all nails, slowed growth of the nails, onycholysis, and nail thickening

Differential Diagnosis

- <u>Onychomycosis</u>
- Peripheral vascular disease
- Psoriasis
- Smoker's nails
- Twenty-nail dystrophy

Associations

- <u>Bronchiectasis</u>
- Chronic bronchitis
- <u>Lymphedema</u>
- Malignancy with lung involvement
- <u>Pleural effusions and empyema</u>
- Respiratory tract infection
- Sinusitis

Further reading:
- Hoque SR, Mansour S, Mortimer PS (2007) Yellow nail syndrome: not a genetic disorder? Eleven new cases and a review of the literature. Br J Dermatol 156(6):1230–1234

Zygomycosis

Term for mycotic infection due to several different types of ubiquitous, saprophytic fungi from the orders Mucorales and Entomophthorales that are characterized by an acute, rapidly spreading, angioinvasive infection, especially of the head and neck, including the orbit and sinuses (rhinocerebral type, which predominantly arises in ketoacidotic diabetes) with typical black pus and high mortality

Differential Diagnosis

- Anthrax
- <u>Aspergillosis</u>
- Ecthyma gangrenosum
- <u>Fusariosis</u>
- Nocardiosis
- Orbital cellulitis
- *Pseudallescheria boydii* infection

Further reading:

- Roden MM, Zaoutis TE, Buchanan WL et al (2005) Epidemiology and outcome of zygomycosis: a review of 929 reported cases. Clin Infect Dis 41(5):634–653

Aagenaes syndrome AR; hereditary cholestasis with eventual cirrhosis; hypoplastic lymphatics leading to lymphedema of the legs

Acanthamebiasis Amoebic infestation with the ubiquitous *Acanthamoeba* that affects AIDS patients and causes disseminated disease with nodular skin lesions, meningoencephalitis, and sinusitis

Acantholytic acanthoma Benign keratotic neoplasm that arises in older patients most commonly on the trunk; histopathologic examination reveals acantholysis

Acantholytic dyskeratosis of the vulva Benign pruritic papular eruption of the vulvar area with histologic features of transient acantholytic dermatosis

Acatalasemia (Takahara's disease) AR; catalase gene mutation; inability to detox bacterial hydrogen peroxide; painful oral ulcers; destruction of dental alveoli; loss of teeth

Acquired bilateral nevus of Ota-like macules (Hori's nevus) Acquired type of dermal melanocytosis that arises in middle-aged women of Asian descent and is characterized by darkly pigmented macules on the bilateral infraorbital cheeks (with absence of scleral or tympanic involvement)

Acquired brachial cutaneous dyschromatosis Acquired pigmentary disorder affecting the arm of middle-aged women that is characterized by hyperpigmented and hypopigmented macules on the dorsal aspect of the forearms

Acquired elastotic hemangioma Benign vascular neoplasm that arises in adulthood and is characterized by a slow-growing, angiomatous papule, nodular, or plaque on the sun-exposed areas

Acquired progressive lymphangioma Benign lymphatic proliferation that arises in children and young adults and is characterized by a localized, flat bruise-like plaque on the trunk or extremities

Acral ichthyosiform mucinosis Rare type of mucinosis associated with Sjögren's syndrome that appears on the lower legs and mimics pretibial myxedema

Acrogeria (Gottron syndrome) AR; atrophy and loss of subcutaneous fat on the extremities; short stature; no effect on longevity

Acute intermittent porphyria AD; porphobilinogen deaminase mutation; onset in puberty; acute episodes of abdominal pain, paresthesias, paralysis; SIADH; seizures; psychotic behavior; attacks precipitated by alcohol ingestion, infection, and starvation; no skin findings

Acute syndrome of apoptotic pan-epidermolysis (ASAP) Toxic epidermal necrolysis-like presentation of acute cutaneous lupus characterized by massive epidermal necrosis

ADULT syndrome AD; ectrodactyly, lacrimal duct obstruction, hypodontia, alopecia, and nail dystrophy

Aggressive digital papillary adenocarcinoma Aggressive type of eccrine carcinoma that arises on the distal, often volar, aspect of the fingers or toes

Alagille syndrome AD; jagged-1 gene mutation; hypoplastic intrahepatic bile ducts; xanthomas; photosensitivity; pruritus; typical facies; jaundice; numerous other anomalies

Albright's hereditary osteodystrophy AD; inactivating mutation of the G stimulatory protein; short metacarpals; osteoma cutis; hypocalcemia; pseudohypoparathyroidism

Alport's syndrome XLD; type-IV collagen mutation; deafness; kidney disease; genital leiomyomas; cataracts

Alstrom syndrome AR; ALMS1 gene mutation; retinitis pigmentosa; deafness; obesity; diabetes; acanthosis nigricans

Ambras syndrome Sporadic/AD; type of congenital hypertrichosis characterized by generalized hypertrichosis with diffuse, uniform involvement of the face; hairs are long and fine; dysmorphic facial features; dental abnormalities

Andogsky syndrome The association of anterior cataracts with adult atopic dermatitis

Angelman syndrome Sporadic; maternal partial deletion of chromosome 15; severe motor and intellectual retardation; ataxia; hypotonia; epilepsy; absence of speech; large mandible; open-mouthed expression; paroxysmal laughter

Angina bullosa hemorrhagica Asymptomatic, blood-filled blister of the oral cavity with uncertain etiology; most commonly involve the hard palate; heal without scarring

Angiocentric eosinophilic fibrosis Idiopathic, chronic fibrosing vasculitis of the upper respiratory mucosa that is probably a mucosal variant of granuloma faciale; affects middle-aged adults

Angiolipoleiomyoma Rare, benign mesenchymal tumor that can arise at any age and is characterized by a solitary subcutaneous nodule located most commonly on the acral areas, especially the ear

Anosacral amyloidosis Uncommon type of cutaneous amyloidosis that affects the perianal area and is characterized by a pruritic, lichenified plaque

APECED syndrome AR; AIRE gene mutation; autoimmune polyendocrinopathy; candidiasis; ectodermal defects; hypoparathyroidism; Addison's disease; chronic mucocutaneous candidiasis; alopecia

Apert syndrome AD; fibroblast growth factor receptor 2 (FGFR2) gene mutation; severe acne; craniosynostosis; syndactyly; mental retardation

Ascher syndrome Enlarged upper lip; blepharochalasis; thyroid goiter, and other endocrine abnormalities

Atrophia maculosa varioliformis cutis Idiopathic disorder of dermal connective tissue that affects young adults and is characterized by spontaneous varioliform and linear scars on the face

Autoimmune polyendocrine syndrome II (Schmidt syndrome) The association of Addison's disease with either autoimmune thyroid disease or type-I diabetes mellitus; arises in middle age; women more commonly affected

Babesiosis Tick-borne protozoan disease that is transmitted by Ixodes ticks, caused by *Babesia microti*, and characterized by intraerythrocytic infection, fever, chills, jaundice, and splenomegaly

Bandler syndrome Intestinal hemangiomatosis; mucocutaneous hyperpigmentation

Bannwarth's syndrome Neurologic manifestations of Lyme borreliosis; facial nerve neuropathy, often bilateral; meningoencephalitis

Barber–Say syndrome AD; macrostomia; hypertelorism; ectropion; atrophic skin; hypertrichosis; growth retardation

Bardet–Biedl syndrome AR; diabetes; obesity; mental retardation; digital anomalies; retinal disease; urogenital anomalies

Barraquer–Simons syndrome (acquired partial lipodystrophy) Sporadic or AD; childhood onset; associated with autoimmunity or preceding illness; C3 nephritic factor present; low complement; membranoproliferative glomerulonephritis; cephalothoracic lipoatrophy; sparing of lower extremities

Bart–Pumphrey syndrome AD; GJB2 gene mutation; knuckle pads; leukonychia; cochlear deafness; palmoplantar keratoderma

Beare–Stevenson cutis gyrata syndrome AD; FGFR2 gene mutation; cutis verticis gyrata; acanthosis nigricans; craniosynostosis; genital abnormalities; ear anomalies

Benign neonatal hemangiomatosis Sporadic; multiple cutaneous hemangiomas at birth or within the first month of life without any visceral involvement; spontaneously involute within the first few years of life

Berardinelli–Seip syndrome (congenital generalized lipodystrophy) AR; Seipin or AGPAT2 gene; onset at birth; loss of subcutaneous fat on the face, trunk and extremities with sparing of the palms, soles, and orbital fat; insulin resistance and diabetes; hypertriglyceridemia; liver failure

BIDS syndrome AR; ERCC2, ERCC4; brittle hair (trichothiodystrophy); intellectual impairment; decreased fertility; short stature

Bjornstad syndrome AR; BCS1L gene; pili torti; sensorineural deafness

Blaschkitis Inflammatory lichen striatus-like dermatosis that affects adults and occurs along Blaschko's lines

Bockenheimer syndrome (genuine diffuse phlebectasia) Venous ectasia of an extremity, with diffuse involvement of all levels of the venous circulation and with an upper extremity more commonly involved than a lower extremity

Book syndrome AD; premolar hypoplasia; palmoplantar hyperhidrosis; premature canities

Borst–Jadassohn phenomenon (intraepithelial epithelioma) Intraepidermal nesting that can be seen in a variety of benign or malignant epithelial neoplasms

Brachyonychia (Racket nails) Abnormality of nail development that is caused by early cessation of distal phalangeal growth and characterized by fingernails that are wider than they are long; seen in Rubenstein-Taybi syndrome; can be a benign finding

Branchio-oculo-facial syndrome AD; cleft lip; branchial sinus; lacrimal duct obstruction; scalp cysts; coloboma; premature canities; deafness

Branchio-oto-renal syndrome (Melnick–Fraser syndrome) AD; EYA1 gene mutation; deafness; branchial cleft cysts/sinuses; pre-auricular pits; renal anomalies

Brooke–Spiegler syndrome AD; CYLD gene; multiple trichoepitheliomas; cylindromas; spiradenomas

Brunsting–Perry cicatricial pemphigoid Type of cicatricial pemphigoid that is localized to the head and neck with minimal mucosal involvement

Bruton's agammaglobulinemia XLR; defect in tyrosine kinase needed for pre-B-cell to B-cell transition; decreased immunoglobulins, decreased B cells; frequent infections with encapsulated bacteria; eczema; autoimmune disease; enteroviral infections; dermatomyositis–encepha-itis syndrome

Bywater's lesions Nail-fold infarcts that occur in the setting of rheumatoid arthritis

Cantu syndrome AD; congenital hypertrichosis; palmoplantar hyperkeratosis; cutis laxa; osteochondrodysplasia; cardiomegaly

Carcinoma en curaisse Manifestation of cutaneous metastasis that resembles keloids, hypertrophic scars, or morphea, and that most commonly originates from breast carcinoma and is most commonly located on the chest wall

Carcinoma erysipelatoides Manifestation of cutaneous metastasis involving the dermal lymphatics that resembles erysipelas and most commonly originates from breast carcinoma

Carcinoma telangiectaticum Manifestation of cutaneous metastasis involving the dermal capillaries that presents with multiple grouped lymphangioma-like papulovesicles

Carvajal syndrome AR; desmoplakin gene mutation; striate and epidermolytic palmoplantar keratoderma; left ventricular dilated cardiomyopathy; woolly hair

Castleman's disease Acquired B-cell lymphoproliferative disorder associated with HHV-8 infection and IL-6 overproduction and characterized by lymphadenopathy in multiple sites, hepatosplenomegaly, fever, anemia, weight loss, and, uncommonly, paraneoplastic pemphigus

Catastrophic antiphospholipid antibody syndrome (CAPS, Asherson syndrome) Accelerated and life-threatening form of antiphospholipid antibody syndrome characterized by widespread thrombosis and multiorgan failure

Cellular angiofibroma of the vulva Rare type of angiofibroma that occurs on the vulva of middle-aged women and is characterized by a subcutaneous mass on the vulva that may be confused with Bartholin's gland cyst, lipoma, or leiomyoma

Cerebrotendinous xanthomatosis AR; sterol 27-hydroxylase gene mutation; lipid-storage disease; xanthomas; cerebellar ataxia beginning after puberty; spinal cord involvement; premature atherosclerosis; cataracts; deposits of cholesterol and cholestanol found in every tissue, including the Achilles tendons (tendinous xanthomas), brain, and lungs

CHANDS syndrome (Baughman syndrome) AR; curly hair, ankyloblepharon, nail dystrophy

Cheyletiella dermatitis An eruption caused by zoonotic, nonburrowing mites of the *Cheyletiella* genera that is characterized by pruritic, grouped, or widespread papules and is frequently transmitted via contact with dogs or cats

Chiclero ulcer Another name for New World cutaneous leishmaniasis caused by *Leishmania mexicana* that is characterized by a chronic ulcer that erodes the pinna of the ear

CHIME syndrome (Zunich neuroectodermal syndrome) AR; colobomas, congenital heart disease, ichthyosiform dermatosis, mental retardation, and ear anomalies/epilepsy

Chondrodysplasia punctata Refers to a developmental anomaly of the skeleton that is characterized by stippling of the epiphyses; also refers to a group of inherited disorders (AR, AR, XLR, or XLD) that, in addition to having chondrodysplasia punctata, have variable ichthyosis, mental retardation, cataracts, and shortened limbs (rhizomelia, AR type)

CINCA syndrome Chronic infantile neurologic, cutaneous, and articular syndrome; see NOMID

Clear cell papulosis Hypopigmented, macular to slightly papular eruption along the milk line, but especially in the pubic area; occurs in early childhood; lesions have intraepidermal clear cells that may be related to Paget's cells or Toker cells or may be of eccrine derivation

Coats' disease Exudative retinitis due to retinal telangiectasia that is associated with facial and conjunctival telangiectasias

Cobb syndrome (cutaneomeningospinal angiomatosis) Spinal cord angioma or arteriovenous malformation with port wine stain, angioma, angiokeratoma, angiolipoma, or lymphangioma in the associated dermatome

Cockayne–Touraine syndrome AD; type-VII collagen gene mutation; type of dominant dystrophic EB that differs from the Pasini type only by the absence of albopapuloid skin lesions

Coffin–Siris syndrome AR; absent nail on the fifth digits of the hands and feet; scalp hypotrichosis; body hypertrichosis; characteristic facies; developmental delay

Cogan syndrome Vestibuloauditory symptoms including sudden hearing loss; bilateral interstitial keratitis; headache; fever; arthralgias; associated with aortitis and systemic vasculitis

Cohen syndrome AR; COH1 gene; acanthosis nigricans; obesity; hypotonia; mental retardation; microcephaly; characteristic facial features; retinochoroidal dystrophy; myopia

Coma bullae Bullous skin lesions arising the comatose patient, especially in the setting of drug overdose (barbiturates); may arise from direct pressure and hypoxia or direct toxic effect of the drug; sweat gland necrosis

Condyloma lata Cutaneous manifestation of secondary syphilis that is characterized by highly infectious, moist, gray, flat papules and plaques on the anogenital areas

Congenital contractural arachnodactyly (Beals–Hecht syndrome) AD; fibrillin 2 gene mutation; arachnodactyly; contractures; crumpled ears; a highly arched palate; marfanoid body habitus

Congenital erosive and vesicular dermatosis Sporadic, erosive disorder and cause of infantile scarring that presents at birth with widespread erosions involving the trunk and extensor extremities; spares face; heals by 3 months of age; leaves reticulate scarring

Cook's syndrome AD; bilateral nail hypoplasia of the first, second, and third fingernails; absence of fourth and fifth fingernails; absence of all toe nails

Cornelia de Lange syndrome Sporadic; NIPBL gene; low-pitched cry; synophrys; mental retardation; facial and body hypertrichosis; characteristic facies; cutis marmorata; limb hypoplasia

Costello syndrome AR; HRAS gene mutation; acanthosis nigricans; periorificial papillomas; cutis laxa of the neck, palms, and soles; mental retardation; sociable, humorous behavior

Crandall's syndrome AR; pili torti; deafness; hypogonadism

Crigler–Najjar syndrome AR; UDP–glycuronosyltransferase gene; severe congenital jaundice and kernicterus; some with early death; unconjugated hyperbilirubinemia

Cross syndrome (Cross–McCusick–Breen syndrome) AR; silvery hair; generalized hypopigmentation; mental retardation; nystagmus, gingival fibromatosis; ataxia and spasticity

Crouzon's syndrome AD; FGFR3 mutation; acanthosis nigricans; craniosynostosis; exophthalmos

Crowe's sign Axillary freckling that is a diagnostic criteria for von Recklinghausen's disease

Cullen's sign Periumbilical purpura or hematoma that is associated with acute hemorrhagic pancreatitis and other causes of intraabdominal hemorrhage

Cutaeous pii migrans Rare condition in which a hair penetrates the stratum corneum, grows into the epidermis, and causes a painful creeping eruption

Cutis pleonasmus Refers to excess skin that results after rapid weight loss, as with bariatric surgery

Cyclic neutropenia Sporadic/AD; neutrophil elastase gene mutation; onset in childhood; 21-day cycle of neutrophil count changes; infections; fever; malaise; mucosal ulcers

De Barsy syndrome AR; congenital cutis laxa; corneal clouding, psychomotor retardation; hypotonia

Deck-chair sign Sparing of truncal skin folds that is associated with a variety of dermatoses, especially papuloerythroderma of Ofuji

Dermatopathia pigmentosa reticularis Pigmentary disorder characterized by diffuse reticulated hyperpigmentation, nonscarring alopecia, and nail dystrophy

Dermatopathic lymphadenitis Benign enlargement of the lymph nodes that occurs in the setting of erythroderma

Diabetic cheiroarthropathy/stiff skin Acquired scleroderma-like disorder associated with cutaneous induration of the distal aspects of the extremities; digital sclerosis and limited joint mobility (cheiroarthropathy); a characteristic feature is an inability to tightly oppose the middle aspects of palms (prayer sign)

Diffuse neonatal hemangiomatosis Multiple (can be hundreds) cutaneous and visceral (especially hepatic) hemangiomas; heart failure; hypothyroidism; hepatomegaly; early death

DiGeorge syndrome Sporadic/AD; TBX1 gene mutation; thymic aplasia with absence of T cells; candidiasis and other infections; absence of parathyroid glands with hypocalcemia; aortic arch anomalies; eczema; characteristic facies

Dirofilariasis Infestation with the filarial worm, *Dirofilaria repens/immitis*, which is acquired most commonly by arthropod bite, and characterized by a subcutaneous or subconjunctival nodule or creeping eruption

Disseminated intravascular coagulation Activation of the coagulation system due to a variety of causes (infection, trauma, etc.) that is characterized by purpura fulminans, simultaneous bleeding (due to consumption of coagulation factors) and clotting, and multiorgan failure

Distichiasis–lymphedema syndrome AD; FOXC2 gene mutation; bilateral lymphedema of the lower extremities with onset in the first or second decade of life; distichiasis (double row of eyelashes); occasionally, cardiac defects or spinal extradural cysts

Donahue syndrome AR; insulin receptor gene mutation; hyperinsuline-mia; mental retardation; hypertrichosis; acanthosis nigricans; large geni-talia; lipodystrophy

DOOR syndrome AR; deafness; onychoosteodystrophy; mental retar-dation; seizures; phalangeal abnormalities

Dowling–Meara type epidermolysis bullosa (EB herpetiformis) AD; keratin 5/14 gene mutation; skin fragility and herpetiform blistering with onset in the neonatal period; periorificial erosions; palmoplantar kerato-derma; dystrophic nails

Dubin–Johnson syndrome AR canalicular multispecific organic anion transporter (CMOAT) gene mutation; direct hyperbilirubinemia; jaun-dice by the second decade of life

Duncan's disease (X-linked lymphoproliferative disorder) XLR; SH2DIA gene mutation; inability to mount immune response against EBV; death due to EBV-induced lymphoma

Ectodermal dysplasia with absent dermatoglyphics (Basan syndrome) AD; hypohidrosis; absent dermatoglyphics; nail dystrophy

Ectodermal dysplasia with skin fragility syndrome (McGrath syn-drome) AR; plakophilin 1 gene mutation; skin fragility with extensive skin erosions; nail dystrophy; palmoplantar keratoderma; hypotrichosis; hypohidrosis

Eczematid-like purpura of Doucas and Kapetanakis (itchy purpura, disseminated pruriginous angiodermatitis) Type of pigmented purpu-ric dermatosis that shares features with Schamburg's disease but with more pruritus, tendency to begin on the lower legs and spread superiorly to the trunk, and tendency for relapse

EEC syndrome (Rudiger syndrome)   AD; p63 gene mutation; ectrodactyly ("lobster claw"); ectodermal dysplasia (sparse to absent hair; pegged teeth; nail dystrophy); cleft lip and/or palate; mental retardation; conductive hearing loss

Elejalde syndrome   AR; myosin Va gene mutation; severe mental retardation; hypotonia; silvery hair; generalized hypopigmentation

Ellis–Van Creveld syndrome   AR; EVC gene mutation; hypodontia; hyponychia; sparse hair; short limbs; chondrodysplasia; atrial septal defects; polydactyly; hypertelorism

Encephalocraniocutaneouslipomatosis(Haberlandsyndrome)   Sporadic; unilateral scalp fat hamartoma with overlying alopecia; ipsilateral intracranial lipomas; cerebral atrophy; porencephaly; mental retardation; seizures

Eosinophilic, polymorphic, and pruritic eruption associated with radiotherapy (EPPER)   Cutaneous eruption affecting cancer patients receiving radiotherapy that is characterized by a generalized, pruritic eruption with excoriations, erythematous papules and nodules, or wheals and bullae that is not confined to the treatment area

Epibulbar dermoids   Benign, congenital tumors containing choristomatous material and located on the conjunctiva

Erosio interdigitale blastomycetica   Candidal infection of the finger web spaces characterized by a white, macerated scaly plaque

Eruption of lymphocyte recovery   Cutaneous eruption that occurs after the recovery of peripheral lymphocytes following bone marrow ablation that is characterized by a macular or papular eruption that resembles acute graft-vs-host disease

Erysipelas melanomatosum   Cutaneous metastatic melanoma that presents as an erysipelas-like eruption

Erythrokeratodermia with ataxia (Giroux–Barbeau syndrome) AD; EKV-like erythrokeratodermia that resolves in early to middle adulthood; progressive ataxia with onset in middle age

Erythrokeratolysis hiemalis (Oudsthoorn disease) AD; winter-predominant eruption that affects South Africans; annular, scaly, erythematous plaques on the extremities and buttocks; recurrent erythema and peeling of the palms and soles

Espundia Refers to destructive changes of the nose and mouth that occur in mucocutaneous leishmaniasis

Esthiomene Elephantiasis of the genitals characterized by enlargement, thickening, and fibrosis most commonly referenced in the setting of chronic lymphogranuloma venereum or cutaneous tuberculosis

FACES syndrome The association of nevus spilus with facial features, anorexia, cachexia, and eye and skin anomalies

Familial cold autoinflammatory syndrome (familial cold urticaria) AD; cryopyrin gene mutation; hereditary periodic fever syndrome characterized by fever, arthralgias, and urticaria following cold exposure; onset in the first 6 months of life

Familial dysautonomia (Riley–Day syndrome) AR; IKBKAP gene mutation; autonomic dysfunction in a variety of organ systems; absent fungiform papillae of the tongue; decreased deep tendon reflexes; decreased response to pain or temperature; orthostatic hypotension; lack of tears with emotional crying

Fanconi anemia AR; FANA–FANN complementation group genes; pancytopenia; absent thumbs; hypoplastic radius; diffuse hyperpigmentation; horseshoe kidney; leukemia; café-au-lait macules; heart defects

Farber lipogranulomatosis AR; acid ceramidase gene mutation; visceral accumulation of ceramides; hoarseness; periarticular nodules and cutaneous infiltrates; painful joints; mental retardation; perianal telangiectasias; cherry-red macula

Fascioliasis Infestation with the liver fluke, *Fasciola hepatica*, which is acquired by ingesting uncooked aquatic vegetation and characterized by fever, right upper quadrant pain, intrahepatic cysts, and migratory skin lesions or cutaneous nodules

Felty's syndrome Rheumatoid arthritis; neutropenia; splenomegaly; leg ulcers

Ferguson–Smith syndrome AD; ESS1 gene mutation; multiple self-healing keratoacanthomas beginning early in life

Fibroblastic rheumatism Rare rheumatologic disease that mimicks multicentric reticulohistiocytosis and is characterized by rapidly progressive polyarthritis along with cutaneous nodules (with fibroblast proliferation) involving the hands and sclerodactyly

Fibrodysplasia ossificans progressiva Sporadic/AD; ACVR1 gene mutation; onset in childhood; endochondral type of primary osteoma cutis; characterized by hard subcutaneous nodules most commonly on posterior neck and back; monophalangic malformed great toes

Fibroma of the tendon sheath Benign myofibroblastic tumor that is characterized by a small, sometimes multinodular subcutaneous nodule on the hands or feet, often digital

Folliculitis spinulosa decalvans Subtype of keratosis pilaris atrophicans that is characterized by follicular papules on the scalp with pustule formation and scarring alopecia; onset in childhood with worsening at puberty

Forscheimer spots Enanthem of early rubella that is characterized by discrete rose-colored macules on the soft palate

Galli–Galli disease Acantholytic variant of Dowling–Degos disease that combines features of Dowling–Degos disease and transient acantholytic dermatosis (Grover's disease) and is characterized by reticulated hyper-pigmentation and pruritic keratotic and erythematous papules predominantly in the flexures but also on the trunk and extremities

Giant cell fibroblastoma Juvenile variant of dermatofibrosarcoma protuberans that presents as a painless, slow-growing soft tissue mass most commonly on the back or thigh

Generalized eruptive histiocytoma Benign type of non-Langerhans cell histiocytosis that is characterized by a widespread eruption of flesh-red-brown papules on the trunk and extremities; adult-onset and self-limited

Generalized eruptive keratoacanthomas (Gryzbowksi) Rare generalized eruption of hundreds of pruritic keratoacanthomas affecting cutaneous and mucosal surfaces with onset in adult life

Gilbert syndrome AR; UDP–glucuronosyltransferase gene mutation; unconjugated hyperbilirubinemia; mild jaundice; normal liver function tests

Gnasthostomiasis Infestation with a nematode, *Gnathostoma spinigerum*, that is endemic in southeast Asia and is characterized most commonly by migratory skin eruption or soft tissue swelling or nodule

Goldenhar syndrome Sporadic; accessory tragi; ear pits; deafness; eye, vertebral, and cardiac abnormalities; hemifacial microsomia; epibulbar dermoids

Goodpasture syndrome Autoimmune disease in which antibodies are generated against type IV collagen that is characterized by pulmonary hemorrhage and glomerulonephritis

Good syndrome Adult-onset immunodeficiency syndrome that coincides with the development of a thymoma; hypogammaglobulinemia and B-cell lymphopenia with or without T-cell lymphopenia are characteristic

Gopalan syndrome Peripheral neuropathy syndrome associated with malnutrition (deficiency of B vitamins) that is characterized by palmoplantar hyperhidrosis and burning pain in the soles of the feet

Gorham syndrome (vanishing bone syndrome) Breakdown of bone and subsequent fibrosis as a result of an overlying or adjacent vascular malformation

Gram-negative folliculitis Folliculitis caused most commonly by *Klebsiella*, *Enterobacter*, and *Serratia* that is a complication of long-term antibiotic treatment of acne, and is characterized by follicular erythematous papules and pustules that may be misdiagnosed as an exacerbation of acne

Grinspan syndrome The association of oral lichen planus with diabetes mellitus and hypertension; possibly drug induced

Haber syndrome AD; familial rosacea-like dermatosis; pitted scars; seborrheic keratoses

HAIR-AN syndrome The association of hyperandrogenism with insulin resistance and acanthosis nigricans

Haim–Munk syndrome AR; cathepsin C gene mutation; diffuse palmoplantar keratoderma; arachnodactyly; onychogryphosis; other features of Papillon–Lefèvre syndrome

Hallerman–Streiff syndrome (oculomandibulofacial syndrome) Sporadic; bird-like facies, natal teeth; microphthalmia; micrognathia; sutural alopecia and sparse hair; dyscephaly

Hallopeau–Siemens syndrome AR; type-VII collagen gene mutation; most severe form of recessive dystrophic epidermolysis bullosa; mitten deformity; generalized skin and mucosal blistering; squamous cell carcinoma

Harlequin color change   Peculiar, benign phenomenon that affects new-born infants that is characterized by well-demarcated hyperemia on one half of the body, including the face, with blanching of the contralateral side

Hay–Wells syndrome (AEC syndrome)   AD; p63 gene defect; anky-loblepharon; ectodermal dysplasia; cleft lip/palate; erosive scalp disease

Heck's disease (focal epithelial hyperplasia)   Oral infection with HPV types 13 and 32 that is characterized by multiple flesh-colored asymp-tomatic papules on the oral mucosa, especially the labial, buccal, and lin-gual mucosa

Heerfordt's syndrome   Association of acute sarcoidosis with fever, uveitis, and facial nerve palsy

Hennekam syndrome   AR; congenital lymphedema of limbs and geni-tals; intestinal lymphangiectasia; hypoproteinemia; lymphopenia; hypog-ammaglobulinemia; characteristic facies

Hepatoerythropoietic porphyria   AD; uroporphyrinogen decarboxy-lase gene mutation; homozygous, severe variant of porphyria cutanea tarda that presents in infancy

Hereditary benign telangiectasia   AD; multiple telangiectasias that arise in the first year of life in variable locations, with the sun-exposed areas the most common; tends to be more severe in women; lesions improve with increasing age

Hereditary coproporhyria   AD; coproporphyrinogen oxidase mutation; acute type of porphyria characterized by episodic abdominal pain, nausea/vomiting, constipation, photosensitivity, and neuropsychiatric symptoms

Hereditary painful callosities Autosomal-dominant, nummular type of keratoderma characterized by tender callosities over the pressure points of the palms and soles

Herpetic geometric glossitis Uncommon presentation of herpes simplex virus infection that affects the tongue of predominantly immunocompromised and that is characterized by painful linear fissures

Hibernoma Type of lipoma arising in adulthood that is derived from brown fat and is characterized by a subcutaneous mass on the interscapular back or neck

HID syndrome AD/AR; connexin 26 gene mutation; generalized ichthyosis hystrix with deafness

Homocystinuria Inherited metabolic disorder (AR) caused by deficiency of cystathionine synthase that is characterized by facial flushing, livedo reticularis, venous or arterial thrombosis, leg ulcers, marfanoid body habitus, ectopia lentis, osteoporosis, and variable neurologic disturbance and mental retardation

Huriez syndrome AD; TYS gene mutation; palmoplantar keratoderma in early childhood with progressive scleroatrophy; nail dystrophy; squamous cell carcinoma

Hyperimmunoglobulin D syndrome AR; mevalonate kinase gene mutation; high serum igd level on two occasions at least 1 month apart; periodic fever; cervical lymphadenopathy; abdominal pain; arthralgias; skin eruption of erythematous papules or purpura

Hyperimmunoglobulin M syndrome XLR; CD40 ligand gene mutation or NEMO gene mutation; high igm with other Ig's low; recurrent infections; numerous verruca vulgaris; ectodermal dysplasia (NEMO mutation only)

Ichthyosis hystrix-type epidermal nevus Type of epidermal nevus that is markedly hyperkeratotic with porcupine-like projections and bilateral distribution along Blaschko's lines

Ichthyosis hystrix, Curth–Macklin type AD; keratin 1 gene mutation; diffuse porcupine-like hyperkeratosis; palmoplantar keratoderma

Indeterminate cell histiocytosis Rare type of histiocytosis caused by an infiltrate of cells with both macrophage and Langerhans cell markers; affects all age groups; characterized by solitary or multiple red-brown papules or nodules on the face, trunk, or extremities

Inherited patterned lentiginosis AD; diffuse hyperpigmented macules on the face, lip, extremities, buttocks, palms, and soles without any internal manifestations

Jacquet's erosive diaper dermatitis Severe form of irritant diaper dermatitis characterized by erosions with elevated borders, giving them an umbilicated appearance

Jaffe–Campanacci syndrome The association of café-au-lait macules with nonossifying fibromas of the long bones and skeletal defects; may be a manifestation of neurofibromatosis

Johanson–Blizzard syndrome AR; aplasia cutis congenita of scalp; characteristic facies; imperforate anus; pancreatic insufficiency; failure to thrive; growth retardation; deafness

Johnson–Mcmillin syndrome AD; alopecia; hypogonadotropic hypogonadism; anosmia; conductive deafness; microtia; café-au-lait macules

Kallmann syndrome AD/XLR; KAL1,2 gene mutations; anosmia; cryptorchidism; hypothalamic hypogonadism; various anomalies

Kanzaki disease AR; alpha-galactosaminidase gene mutation; adult onset; angiokeratoma corporis diffusum; intellectual impairment

Kasabach–Merritt syndrome Syndrome associated with kaposiform hemangioendothelioma and tufted angioma that is characterized by consumption of platelets, bleeding tendency, purpura, and a high mortality

Keratotic spicules of myeloma Paraneoplastic phenomenon associated with myeloma that is characterized by filiform projections of hyperkeratotic, paraprotein-containing material arising from the follicles on the nose, scalp, or neck

Klinefelter syndrome Chromosomal disorder; XXY; hypogonadism; tall stature; psychiatric disturbance; leg ulcers; severe acne

Kobberling and Dunnigan syndromes (familial partial lipodystrophy) Two distinct types of familial partial lipodystrophy; Dunnigan type is autosomal dominant and associated with a lamin A/C gene mutation; inheritance and gene mutation in Kobberling type is unclear; both are associated with loss of subcutaneous fat on the extremities, with sparing of the face and variable involvement of the trunk

Koplik's spots Pathognomonic enanthem associated with measles that is characterized by erythematous macules or papules with a central white spot on the buccal and lingual mucosa

Kwashiorkor Acquired disorder caused by severe protein malnutrition; hypopigmentation; generalized edema; alternating light and dark bands in hair (flag sign); erosive and desquamating dermatitis with "pasted-on" scale (flaky paint sign)

Kyrle's disease Name for a type of perforating disorder that is associated with renal failure and diabetes mellitus and is characterized by multiple keratotic papules through which dermal material is perforating; term should be abandoned and replaced with acquired perforating dermatosis

Lawrence syndrome (acquired generalized lipodystrophy) Type of lipodystrophy that arises in childhood; may be associated with a preceding viral infection, panniculitis or autoimmune disease; characterized by loss of subcutaneous fat from the face, trunk, and extremities, including the palms and soles; acanthosis nigricans; liver disease; hyperinsulinemia and diabetes

Leiner's disease Cutaneous presentation of immunodeficiency characterized by generalized erythroderma; diarrhea, and failure to thrive; associated with Bruton's agammaglobulinemia, C3 and C5 deficiency, Hyper-ige syndrome, severe combined immunodeficiency, and Omenn's syndrome

Legius syndrome (NF1-like syndrome) Autosomal dominant disorder caused by mutation of the SPRED1 gene and characterized by cafe-au-lait macules, axillary freckling, lipomas, macrocephaly, and developmental delays, but no neurofibromas

Lelis syndrome Autosomal recessive disorder characterized by ectodermal dysplasia and acanthosis nigricans

Lennert's lymphoma (lymphoepithelioid cell lymphoma) Type of peripheral T-cell lymphoma characterized by epithelioid histiocytes that presents most commonly with cervical lymphadenopathy and uncommonly with nonspecific cutaneous features

Lesar–Trelat sign Controversial paraneoplastic phenomenon characterized by the eruption of hundreds of seborrheic keratoses on the trunk; association with pruritus and/or acanthosis nigricans should increase suspicious for underlying malignancy

Lesch–Nyhan syndrome XLR; HGPRT gene mutation; hyperuricemia and gout; mental retardation; self-mutilation behavior; choreathetosis

Lhermitte–Duclos disease CNS manifestations of Cowden's syndrome characterized by cerebellar gangliocytoma, ataxia, and seizures

Lichen aureus Type of pigmented purpuric dermatosis that occurs in younger patients; characterized by circumscribed collection of macules or flat papules with variable color, ranging from golden-yellow to bronze or brown

Limb–mammary syndrome AD; p63 gene mutation; hypoplasia of the mammary glands; lacrimal duct atresia; limb defects; hypohidrosis; nail dystrophy

Lipedematous scalp/alopecia Term for circumscribed or diffuse thickening of the subcutaneous layer of the scalp of adults that can manifest as localized or diffuse alopecia

Lipoatrophia semicircularis Localized lipoatrophy possibly caused by mechanical compression of the affected area that is characterized by semicircular depression, often bilateral, of the anteriolateral thigh

Lipoblastoma Localized or diffuse (lipoblastomatosis) soft tissue mass comprised of lipoblasts most often arising on the extremities shortly after birth

Lipodystrophia centrifugalis abdominalis infantalis Rare type of acquired localized lipodystrophy that affects Asians and is characterized by centrifugal loss of subcutaneous fat involving the abdomen and groin with peripheral panniculitis

Lipschutz ulcer Acute, nonvenereal vulvar ulceration predominantly affecting adolescent women as a manifestation of EBV infection

Loaiasis Type of filariasis caused by *Loa loa*; characterized by lymphedema, recurrent angioedema (Calabar swellings), urticaria, subconjunctival migratory lesions, and eosinophilia

Loeffler's syndrome Transient pulmonary eosinophilia and radiographic shadowing due to a variety of causes but often described in the setting of parasitic infestation or drug allergy

Lofgren's syndrome Syndrome associated with acute onset of sarcoidosis that is characterized by fever, arthritis, bilateral hilar lymphadenopathy, erythema nodosum, and uveitis

Lupus pernio Manifestation of cutaneous sarcoidosis that is characterized by an indolent, red-to-violaceous plaque on the nose, cheeks, lips, or ears with associated upper airway disease and bony cysts of the digits

Lupus vulgaris Type of cutaneous tuberculosis that most commonly results from hematogenous spread of the organism; occurs in patients with good immunity to the organism; characterized by apple-jelly-colored papules, nodules, or plaques on the face and ears

Lycopenemia Refers to yellow-orange discoloration of the skin that results from excessive consumption of dietary lycopene, usually from tomatoes

Lymphedema tarda AD; type of hereditary lymphedema of the legs with onset around age 35 years

Lymphoepithelioma-like carcinoma of the skin Uncommon primary cutaneous neoplasm that resembles lymphepitheliomatous tumors of the nasopharynx and that arises as a red or purple nodule on the face and scalp of middle-aged to elderly patients

Maculae cerulae Cutaneous manifestation of pediculosis pubis that is characterized by blue macules in the affected area representing louse-bite-induced purpura

MAGIC syndrome Mouth and genital ulcers with inflamed cartilage; combines features of Behçet's disease and relapsing polychondritis

Mal de meleda AR; SLURP1 gene mutation; diffuse transgrediens palmoplantar keratoderma; scrotal tongue; nail dystrophy; pseudoainhum; hyperkeratosis of the flexures; hyperhidrosis

Malignant peripheral nerve sheath tumor Malignant neural neoplasm of Schwann cell derivation and type of soft tissue sarcoma that arises most commonly in patients with neurofibromatosis, often in the setting of malignant degeneration of a plexiform neurofibroma

Marie–Unna hypotrichosis AD; MUHH gene mutation; hereditary hypotrichosis; milia

Marinesco–Sjögren syndrome AR; SIL1 gene mutation; sparse, brittle hair; trichoschisis; congenital cataracts; cerebellar ataxia; mental retardation

Mechanic's hands Cutaneous manifestation of the antisynthetase syndrome (Jo-1 antibodies; Raynaud's phenomenon; arthritis, and interstitial lung disease) characterized by hyperkeratosis and fissuring of the hands, particularly on the radial aspect

Meige lymphedema (lymphedema praecox) AD; hereditary lymphedema of the legs; onset around puberty

Melioidosis (Whitmore's disease) Rapidly fatal bacterial infection predominantly diagnosed in southeast Asia that is caused by *Burkholderia pseudomalle*; characterized by pulmonary and cutaneous abscesses and sepsis

Melorheostosis Radiographic finding in some patients with scleroderma, including localized forms, that is characterized by cortical or endosteal hyperostosis of the long bones, giving the bone the appearance of dripping candle wax

Metageria AR; premature aging syndrome; tall stature; poikiloderma; generalized lipoatrophy; diabetes; atherosclerosis

Meyerson's nevus (halo dermatitis) Eczematous eruption encircling a pre-existing melanocytic nevus

Microvenular hemangioma Benign, acquired vascular neoplasm that can be difficult to distinguish from Kaposi's sarcoma and is characterized by a small red-to-purple nodule on the forearm of a young to middle-aged adult

MIDAS syndrome XLD; microophthalmia; dermal aplasia (lesions of the upper half of the body); sclerocornea

Mikulicz syndrome Enlargement of salivary glands and lacrimal glands due to infiltration with granulomatous inflammation or lymphoma; associated with tuberculosis, sarcoidosis, lymphoma, and Sjögren's syndrome

Milroy disease AD; VEGFR3 gene mutation; congenital lymphedema of the extremities with onset at birth or early childhood

MORFAN syndrome Syndrome characterized by mental retardation, overgrowth, remarkable face, acanthosis nigricans

Morton's neuroma Term for localized neuropathic pain in the foot caused by chronic irritation of an intermetarsal nerve; typically involves the third metatarsal space

Moyamoya disease Disorder predominantly diagnosed in Japan that is characterized by progressive intracranial vascular stenosis of the circle of Willis; recurrent transient ischemic attacks and strokes; livedo reticularis

Muehrcke's lines Type of apparent leukonychia that results from chronic hypoalbuminemia that is characterized by paired white bands that are parallel to the lunula and do not grow out with the nail

Muckle–Wells syndrome AD; CIAS1 gene mutation (cryopyrin); urticaria; periodic fever; abdominal pain; polyarthralgias or arthritis; myalgias; sensorineural deafness; AA amyloidosis

Multiple endocrine neoplasia, type I (Wermer syndrome) AD; MEN gene mutation; tumors of the pituitary, pancreas; and parathyroid glands; lipomas; angiofibromas; collagenomas; café-au-lait macules

Multiple endocrine neoplasia, type IIA (Sipple syndrome) AD; RET gene mutation; tumors of the parathyroid, adrenal gland (pheochromocytoma), and thyroid (medullary thyroid carcinoma); macular amyloidosis/notalgia paresthetica

Myospherulosis, cutaneous (spherulocytosis) Subcutaneous disorder associated with degeneration of erythrocytes in spherule-like structures, often in the setting of petrolatum use on wound; characterized by pseudocystic nodules anywhere on the body

Naxos disease AR; plakoglobin gene mutation; diffuse palmoplantar keratoderma; woolly hair; arrhythmogenic right ventricular cardiomyopathy

Nelson's syndrome Complication of bilateral adrenalectomy for Cushing's syndrome that is characterized by rapid development of an ACTH and MSH secreting pituitary tumor; diffuse hyperpigmentation

NERDS syndrome The association of eosinophilia with articular nodules, rheumatism, dermatitis, and episodic swelling of the hands and feet

Neu–Laxova syndrome AR; severe intrauterine growth retardation; polyhydramnios; edema; ectodermal dysplasia and ichthyosis; severe CNS developmental defects

Neurofibromatosis, type II AD, schwannomin gene mutation (merlin); acoustic schwannomas; less cutaneous features than NF1; no Lisch nodules; can have cutaneous neurofibromas and schwannomas; less than 6 CALMS; posterior subcapsular lenticular opacities

Nevus mucinosis Type of connective tissue nevus containing mucin that can occur as a solitary finding or in combination with other features of Hunter's syndrome; characterized by flesh-colored papules on the trunk that are present at birth or erupt in early childhood

Nezelof syndrome Type of T-cell immunodeficiency due to absence of the thymus gland; associated with normal immunoglobulins

Nicolau syndrome (embolia cutis medicamentosa) Necrotic reaction occurring after intramuscular injection with penicillin, NSAIDs, or glucocorticosteroids; caused by compression or embolization leading to arterial compromise

Nicolau–Balus syndrome Eruptive micropapular syringomas, milia, and atrophoderma vermiculatum

Niemann–Pick disease AR; sphingomyelinase gene mutation; diffuse hyperpigmentation; xanthomas; hepatosplenomegaly; lymphadenopathy; cherry-red maculae; mental retardation; death in early childhood

Nijmegen breakage syndrome AR; NBS gene mutation; microcephaly; immunodeficiency; growth retardation; bird-like facies; no ataxia or telangiectasias

NISCH syndrome AR; claudin-1 gene mutation; neonatal ichthyosis; sclerosing cholangitis; hypotrichosis

Njolstad syndrome AR; congenital lymphedema of legs and face; pulmonary lymphangiectasia; hydrops fetalis

Noma (cancrum oris) Grotesque orofacial gangrene that results from progressive polymicrobial necrotizing gingivitis; predominantly affects malnourished children of sub-Saharan Africa

NOMID syndrome (neonatal onset multisystem inflammatory disease) Sporadic; CIAS1 (cryopyrin) gene mutation; migratory skin eruption; arthropathy with overgrowth of patella and distal femur; distinctive facies; chronic meningitis; progressive deafness and visual impairment

Noninvoluting congenital hemangioma Rare type of congenital hemangioma; GLUT-1 negative; fails to involute

Oasthouse syndrome (methionine malabsorption syndrome) AR; impaired absorption of methionine; urine smells like dried malt; canities; mental retardation; seizures

Oculocerebrocutaneous syndrome (Delleman syndrome) Sporadic; CNS cysts; congenital hydrocephalus; agenesis of the corpus callosum; aplasia cutis congenita; orbital cysts; microphthalmia

Oculodentodigital syndrome AD; connexin 43 gene mutation; microphthalmos; pitted teeth; syndactyly; sparse hair; neurologic disturbance

Oculoectodermal syndrome AD/AR; aplasia cutis congenita; epibulbar dermoids; cutaneous hyperpigmentation; giant cell granulomas

Odontotrichomelic syndrome AR; ectodermal dysplasia; malformed ears; four-limb hypoplasia; mental retardation; hypogonadism

Oliver–Macfarlane syndrome (congenital trichomegaly) Sporadic; chorioretinal degeneration; growth hormone deficiency; cerebellar dysfunction; long eyelashes and bushy eyebrows; sparse scalp hair

Ollier syndrome Sporadic; enchondromatosis; cartilaginous tumors (benign and malignant) in an asymmetric and random distribution; lacks the venous malformations seen with Maffucci's syndrome

Olmsted syndrome AD; diffuse mutilating palmoplantar keratoderma; pseudoainhum; periorificial hyperkeratosis

Omenn's syndrome AR; RAG1/2 gene mutation; Leiner's phenotype; severe combined immunodeficiency; lymphadenopathy; hepatosplenomegaly; failure to thrive

Oral–facial–digital syndrome XLD/AR; CXORF5 gene mutation (XLR); combination of oral anomalies (hyperplastic frenulum or dental abnormalities), facial anomalies, and syndactyly or polydactyly

Osteopathia straita Bony abnormality associated with Goltz syndrome; radiography reveals bilateral vertically oriented sclerotic striations extending from the metaphyses of the long bones to the diaphyses

Osteopoikilosis Asymptomatic bone abnormality associated with Buschke–Ollendorf syndrome; radiography reveals round or oval foci of increased density in the juxtaarticular areas

Otomycosis Superficial fungal infection of the external ear canal caused by a variety of fungi; causes include *Aspergillus* sp. and *Candida* sp.

Pallister–Killian syndrome Mosaic disorder; tetrasomy for chromosome 12p; hyperpigmentation and hypopigmentation along Blaschko's lines; mental retardation; seizures; characteristic facies

PAPA syndrome AD; PSTPIP1 gene mutation; destructive pyogenic arthritis; pyoderma gangrenosum; severe cystic acne

Papillon–Lefèvre syndrome AR; cathepsin C gene mutation; neutrophil dysfunction; diffuse palmoplantar keratoderma; periodontosis with premature loss of teeth; hyperkeratosis of the elbows and knees; dural calcification

Paragonimiasis Infestation with the trematode, *Paragonimus westermani*; occurs after ingesting raw shellfish; can affect any organ with invasion of the pulmonary system invasion most common; skin lesions are subcutaneous swellings or migratory lesions

Paraneoplastic acral vascular syndrome The association of Raynaud's phenomenon, gangrene, and acrocyanosis with an internal malignancy, most commonly adenocarcinoma; gangrene most common

Parry–Romberg syndrome Type of localized scleroderma (morphea profunda) that affects the face and is characterized by hemifacial atrophy involving the skin, fat, and bone

PELVIS syndrome The association of perineal hemangioma with external genitalia malformations, lipomyelomeningocele, vesicorenal abnormalities, imperforate anus, or skin tags

PFAPA syndrome Periodic fever syndrome occurring in early childhood; periodic fever; aphthous stomatitis; pharyngitis; adenitis

PHACES syndrome Posterior fossa malformation (Dandy–Walker malformation); segmental hemangioma of the face; arterial abnormality; cardiac abnormality (various); eye abnormality (various); sternal clefting or supraumbilical raphe; cleft palate

Phakomatosis pigmentokeratotica Type of epidermal nevus syndrome; nevus sebaceus along Blaschko's lines; nevus spilus; scoliosis; hemiatrophy; various ocular and CNS defects

Phylloid hypomelanosis Mosaic trisomy 13; hypopigmented macules resembling begonia leaves; agenesis of the corpus callosum; digital defects; deafness

PIBIDS AR; ERCC2, ERCC4; photosensitivity; ichthyosis; brittle hair; intellectual impairment; decreased fertility; short stature

Pigmented purpuric lichenoid dermatosis of Gougerot and Blum Type of benign pigmented purpura characterized by grouped lichenoid papules on the lower extremities, in addition to purpura

Pilar sheath acanthoma Benign follicular hamartoma most commonly occurring on the upper lip that is characterized by a pore-like papule or nodule, resembling a dilated pore or trichofolliculoma

Pili annulati AD; hair-shaft disorder; onset in early childhood; abnormally shiny hair with alternating light (representing air-filled cavities) and dark segments

Plasmacytosis, cutaneous Reactive polyclonal lymphoplasmacytic disorder characterized by infiltration of the skin with plasma cells and characterized by numerous erythematous to brown macules on the trunk or extremities

Plate-like osteoma cutis Type of primary osteoma cutis that occurs in newborns and young children; no associated calcium or phosphate abnormalities or preceding inflammation, trauma, or infection; characterized by a solitary, hard, dermal plaque most often located on the scalp

Plica polonica (neuropathica) Irreversible tangling and matting of the hair shafts of the scalp that is associated with malodor and crust; associated with pediculosis capitis and traction alopecia; occipital scalp involved most commonly

Plummer–Vinson syndrome Unknown cause; koilonychia; iron deficiency; esophageal web; dysphagia

Podoconiosis Nonfilarial endemic lymphatic filariasis; progressive bilateral fibrotic swelling of the lower extremities including the feet; affects predominantly the barefoot workers of Central and South America; caused by absorption of silica particles from the soil

Poikiloderma atrophicans vasculare Variant of cutaneous T-cell lymphoma characterized by plaques of hyperpigmentation, hypopigmentation, atrophy, and telangiectasia

Popliteal pterygium syndrome AD; IRF6 gene mutation; popliteal webs; lip pits; cleft lip/palate; cryptorchidism; nail dystrophy; digital anomalies

Prader–Willi syndrome Deletion of part of paternal chromosome 15; acanthosis nigricans; insatiable appetite; obesity; almond eyes; neonatal hypotonia; diffuse hypopigmentation; may also have oculocutaneous albinism type 2

Primary biliary cirrhosis (Hanot syndrome) Inflammatory disorder associated with destruction of the intrahepatic bile ducts that is associated with antimitochondrial antibodies, liver failure, pruritus, jaundice, and xanthomas

Proctalgia fugax Idiopathic anorectal pain disorder characterized by sudden-onset, intermittent, and recurrent episodes of rectal pain that lasts for at least 3 s

Progressive cribriform and zosteriform hyperpigmentation Localized hyperpigmentation similar to linear and whorled nevoid hypermelanosis but with onset typically in the second decade of life; no associated abnormalities

Progressive osseous heteroplasia AD; paternally inherited inactivating mutations of GNAS1 gene; primary intramembranous osteoma cutis that starts in infancy, is progressive, and can be associated with limited mobility later in life; lesions are asymptomatic papules, nodules, plaques on the trunk and extremities; can involve fascia and muscles

Prolidase deficiency AR; peptidase D gene mutation; leg ulcers; skin fragility; mental retardation; typical facies; lymphedema; purpura and telangiectasias

Pseudo-mycosis fungoides Lymphomatous condition often triggered by medications, especially carbamazepine and phenytoin, that is characterized by widespread patches and plaques with similar clinical and histological features to that of mycosis fungicides and that resolve after discounting the medication

Pustulosis acuta generalisata Refers to a generalized pustular eruption involving the trunk and extremities that arises following a group A streptococcal infection

Ramsay–Hunt syndrome Varicella–zoster virus reactivation syndrome with involvement of the facial and auditory nerves; zoster within the conchal bowl; deafness; facial nerve palsy

Rapidly involuting congenital hemangioma Rare congenital type of hemangioma; GLUT-1 negative; lack a proliferative phase; involute by 1–2 years

Rapp–Hodgkin syndrome AD; p63 gene mutation; anhidrotic ectodermal dysplasia; cleft lip/palate; ocular abnormality; hypospadias

Rasmussen syndrome Syndrome characterized by trichoepitheliomas, milia, and cylindroma

Reed syndrome (familial leiomyomatosis cutis and uteri) AD; fumurate hydratase gene mutation; cutaneous and uterine leiomyomas; papillary renal cell carcinoma

Refsum disease AR; phytanoyl-coa hydroxylase gene mutation; ichthyosis; ataxia; retinitis pigmentosa; peripheral neuropathy

Restrictive dermopathy AR; LMNA gene or ZMPSTE4 gene mutation; tight, thin translucent skin; flexion contractures; early death; fixed "O" face

Rhinoentomophthoromycosis Type of invasive zygomycosis of the rhinofacial region that is caused most commonly by *Conidiobolus coronatus*, a soil saprophyte, and is characterized by painless induration and swelling of the central face that begins via inhalation into, or traumatic inoculation of, the nasal passages

Richner–Hanhart syndrome (tyrosinemia, type II) AR; tyrosine aminotransferase gene mutation; focal, tender, palmoplantar keratoderma; herpetiform corneal erosions; photophobia; mental retardation

Riga–Fede disease (lingual traumatic ulceration, congenital autonomic dysfunction with universal pain loss) Chronic trauma-induced granulomatous and ulcerative disorder of the oral cavity, especially the tongue; affects infants at eruption of primary teeth; associated with autonomic dysfunction (Riley–Day syndrome)

Robert's syndrome AR; ESCO2 gene mutation; facial port wine stain; cleft lip/palate; hypotrichosis; limb defects

Rombo syndrome AD; basal cell carcinomas in childhood; atrophoderma vermiculatum; trichoepitheliomas; milia; vasodilation of the hands and feet with cyanosis

Ross' syndrome Acquired disorder of sympathetic degeneration presenting with generalized hypohidrosis, Adies' tonic pupil, and hyporeflexia

Rowell's syndrome Erythema multiforme-like lesions in a patient with discoid lupus erythematosus or systemic lupus erythematosus; positive La (SS-B) autoantibodies; positive rheumatoid factor

Rubenstein–Taybi syndrome AD; CREB binding protein gene mutation; broad thumbs; keloids; hypertrichosis; mental retardation; characteristic facies; cardiac and genitourinary anomalies; CNS tumors

Russell–Silver syndrome AD/AR; dwarfism; hemihypertrophy; clinodactyly; characteristic facies; ivory epiphyses

Sabra dermatitis Pruritic erythematous papular eruption that is caused by exposure to the fine needles of the prickly pear

SAHA syndrome The association of seborrhea, acne, hirsuitism, and alopecia that may reflect underlying hyperandrogenism in the setting of polycystic ovary disease or other endocrine disorder

SAPHO syndrome The association of synovitis, acne, palmoplantar pustulosis, hyperostosis, and osteitis

Schamberg's disease (progressive pigmentary dermatosis) Type of pigmented purpuric dermatosis predominantly affecting men that is characterized by yellow-brown patches on the legs with scattered cayenne-pepper-like macules

Schilder's disease (adrenoleukodystrophy) XLR; ABCD1 gene mutation; accumulation of very long chain fatty acids in the body; childhood and adult forms; adrenal insufficiency; diffuse hyperpigmentation; rapidly progressive cerebral demyelination

Schimmelpenning–Feuerstein–Mims syndrome Sporadic; type of epidermal nevus syndrome associated with extensive nevus sebaceus; seizures; coloboma; mental retardation; hypophospatemic rickets

Schopf–Schulz–Passarge syndrome AR; hypotrichosis; palmoplantar keratoderma; hidrocystomas; eccrine syringofibroadenoma; hypodontia

Scrofuloderma (tuberculosis cutis colliquativa) Type of cutaneous tuberculosis that predominantly affects children; results from direct extension of an underlying focus of infection to the skin; characterized by draining sinus tracts and scarring most often affecting the cervical lymph node basin

Seckel syndrome AR; ATR gene mutation; dwarfism; bird-headed facial appearance; mental retardation

Secretan syndrome (factitial edema) Self-inflicted or occupation-related hard edema of the dorsal hand

Setleis syndrome (facial ectodermal dysplasia, focal facial dermal dysplasia, Brauer lines) AD/AR; leonine facies; aplasia cutis congenita of the bilateral temples; redundant facial skin; frontal bossing

Shabbir syndrome (LOGIC syndrome, laryngoonychocutaneous syndrome) AR; laminin-alpha 3 (LAMA3) gene mutation; hoarseness; nail dystrophy; skin ulcers; hypodontia; conjunctival scarring; possibly related to junctional epidermolysis bullosa

SHORT syndrome AR; partial lipodystrophy; short stature; hyperextensibility of joints or hernia (inguinal) or both, ocular depression, Rieger anomaly (abnormal development of anterior segment of the eye), teething delay

Simpson–Golabi–Behmel syndrome XLR; glypican 3 gene mutation; supernumerary nipples; pre- and postnatal overgrowth; "bulldog" facies; congenital heart defects; numerous other defects

Sneddon syndrome Cerebrovascular accidents; livedo reticularis; vaso-occlusive disease of several different organ systems; antiphospholipid antibodies

Southern tick-associated rash illness (STARI) Lyme-disease-like illness occuring in the southern part of the United States that is transmitted by *Amblyomma americanum*, possibly caused by *Borrelia lonestari*, and characterized by an erythema migrans-like eruption with flu-like symptoms

Sparganosis Infestation with *Spirometra* tapeworm; subcutaneous swelling with variable muscle, ocular, urogenital, gastrointestinal, or CNS involvement

Stein–Leventhal disease Polycystic ovary disease; acanthosis nigricans; acne; irregular menstruation; obesity

Stewart–Bluefarb syndrome A type of pseudo-Kaposi's sarcoma (as opposed to acroangiodermatitis of Mali) that occurs in young, healthy adults with an underlying arteriovenous malformation of the lower extremity

Stewart–Treves syndrome Development of angiosarcoma in a chronically lymphedematous extremity; classically described in the post-mastectomy patient

Stickler syndrome AD; COL2A1 gene mutation; marfanoid body habitus; myopia; retinal detachments; cataracts; glaucoma; stiff or hyperflexible joints; cleft or high arched palate; micrognathia

Sturge–Weber syndrome Sporadic; port wine stain in the trigeminal nerve distribution, especially V1; leptomeningeal angiomatosis of the ipsilateral side; glaucoma; seizures; intracranial (tram-track) calcifications

Superior vena cava syndrome Edema, telangiectasia, and engorged veins on the chest, neck, and face as a result of blockage of the superior vena cava; typically occurs in the setting of intrathoracic malignancy

Sybert palmoplantar keratoderma (Greither's type) AD; diffuse type of palmoplantar keratoderma with erythema, peeling, and hyperkeratosis; transgrediens; hyperkeratosis over the elbows and knees

TAR syndrome AR; thrombocytopenia; absent radii; facial port wine stain; milk allergy; cardiac, cerebral, renal anomalies

Tay syndrome (IBIDS) AR; ERCC2, ERCC4; ichthyosis; brittle hair (trichothiodystrophy); intellectual impairment; decreased fertility; short stature

Thrombotic thrombocytopenic purpura (Moschcowitz disease) Acquired idiopathic disorder associated with deficiency of an enzyme which cleaves von Willebrand factor multimers; microangiopathic hemolytic anemia; thrombocytopenia and purpura; fever; renal failure; altered mental status or other CNS abnormality

Tietz syndrome AD; MITF gene mutation; diffuse hypopigmentation; congenital deafness

Townes–Brocks' syndrome AD; SALL1 gene mutation; imperforate anus; auricular pits, fistula, or skin tags; deafness; triphalangeal thumbs; other digital anomalies; urorenal anomalies

Toxic oil syndrome Scleroderma-like illness that is caused by consumption of denatured rapeseed oil

Treacher–Collins–Franceschetti syndrome (mandibulofacial dysostosis) Sporadic; TCOF1 gene mutation; accessory tragi; pre-auricular skin tags and pits; coloboma; facial bone hypoplasia; ear malformations; conductive hearing loss

Tricho-rhino-phalangeal syndrome AD; TRPS1 gene mutation; brittle, sparse hair; pear-shaped nose; cone-shaped epiphyses of the digits; short stature

Trimethylaminuria (fish-odor syndrome) AR; flavin-containing monooxygenase 3 gene mutation; impaired processing of trimethylamine; presents with self-declaration of a fishy body odor by the patient or family/friends of the patient

Tripe palms Refers to paraneoplastic phenomenon that occurs in the setting of gastric cancer or lung cancer; often accompanies malignant acanthosis nigricans; characterized by thickening of the palms with velvety or papillomatous textural changes

Tuberculosis, miliary Disseminated form that affects patients with an impaired immune response to *Mycobacterium tuberculosis*, especially children; characterized by multiple erythematous macules, papules, and nodules with or without ulceration

Tuberculous, primary inoculation (tuberculous chancre) Primary infection of the skin with accompanying lymphadenopathy in a patient previously unexposed to *Mycobacterium tuberculosis* and characterized by red papule that evolves to a nodule and then ulcer

Tuberculosis verrucosa cutis (prosector's wart) Results from exogenous infection of a patient with prior sensitization to *Mycobacterium tuberculosis*; characterized by a warty plaque affecting the hands or feet

Tumor necrosis factor receptor-associated periodic syndrome (TRAPS) AD; TNFRSF1A gene mutation; periodic fever; abdominal pain; myalgias; arthralgias; skin eruption during attacks; localized erythematous macules and papules or edematous, annular and serpiginous plaques; response to steroids, not colchicine

Turcot syndrome AD/AR; familial colorectal cancer with CNS tumors (glioma or medulloblastoma)

Unna–Thost palmoplantar keratoderma AD; keratin 1 mutation; diffuse nonepidermolytic palmoplantar keratoderma

Van der Woude syndrome AD; IRF-6 gene mutation; popliteal webbing; bilateral lower-lip pits; cleft lip or palate; limb defects

Variegate porphyria AD; protoporphyrinogen oxidase mutation; episodes of abdominal pain, neuropsychiatric symptoms, and blistering on the sun-exposed areas; combines features of porphyria cutanea tarda and acute intermittent porphyria; urinary copro greater than uro during attacks

VATER/VACTERL association Vertebral anomalies; anal atresia; cardiac defects; tracheo-esophageal fistula; radial anomalies; limb anomalies

Vilanova disease (subacute nodular migratory panniculitis, chronic erythema nodosum) Variant of erythema nodosum with significant clinical differences including unilateral lesions, peripheral migration of lesions, absence of pain, and less of an association with typical causative agents as in classic erythema nodosum

Von Hippel–Lindau syndrome AD; VHL gene mutation; adult onset; facial port wine stain; retinal, cerebellar, or spinal hemangioblastoma; pheochromocytoma; renal and pancreatic cysts; renal cell carcinoma

Vörner palmoplantar keratoderma AD; keratin 9 gene mutation; diffuse epidermolytic palmoplantar keratoderma

Waldenstrom's macroglobulinemia Type of lymphoplasmacytic lymphoma associated with an IgM monoclonal gammopathy; hepatosplenomegaly; lymphadenopathy; hyperviscosity; cryoglobulinemia; peripheral neuropathy; igm storage papules in skin; primary amyloidosis

Watson syndrome AD; NF1 gene mutation pulmonary stenosis; café-au-lait macules; mental retardation; short stature; neurofibromas

Weber–Cockayne syndrome (EBS, localized) AD; keratin 5/keratin 14 mutation; blisters localized to the hands and feet; induced by repeated trauma or friction

WHIM syndrome AD; CXCR4 gene mutation; warts; hypogammaglobulinemia; sinopulmonary infections; myelokathexis

Whipple's disease Infection with the Gram-positive bacteria, *Tropheryma whippelii*, that is characterized by diarrhea, malabsorption; vitamin deficiencies; diffuse patchy hyperpigmentation; arthritis; fever; weight loss

Wilson's disease (hepatolenticular degeneration) AR; ATP7B gene mutation; error in copper metabolism; neurodegenerative disease; cirrhosis; copper deposition in liver, brain; corneal Kayser–Fleischer rings; blue lunula

Winchester syndrome AR; matrix metalloproteinase 2 gene mutation; joint contractures; gingival hypertrophy; dwarfism, corneal opacities; mental retardation

Witkop's syndrome (tooth-and-nail syndrome) AD; MSX1 gene mutation; hypoplastic nails; hypodontia

Witten and Zak keratoacanthomas Familial keratoacanthoma syndrome characterized by both small, miliary, and eruptive (like Grzybowski type) as well as medium-sized (Ferguson–Smith type) keratoacanthomas

Wolf-Hirschhorn syndrome Chromosome 4p deletion; severe growth retardation and mental defect; microcephaly; "Greek helmet" facies; cleft lip or palate; coloboma; cardiac septal defects; aplasia cutis of the scalp; seizures

Wyburn-Mason syndrome (Bonnet–Dechaume–Blanc syndrome) Arteriovenous malformation of the brain and retina; ipsilateral port wine stain; seizures; mental retardation

Zellweger syndrome Rare syndrome caused by the decreased or absence of peroxisomes and that is characterized by faulty development of the CNS, hepatomegaly, characteristic facies, chondrodysplasia punctuate, and eye abnormalities

Ziprkowski–Margolis syndrome XLR; congenital deafness; piebaldism; light hair

Index